Pain: a Textbook for Therapists

Cover artwork by Matthew Nutt

For Churchill Livingstone:

Editorial Director, Health Professions: Mary Law
Project Development Manager: Mairi McCubbin
Project Manager: Jane Dingwall
Design Direction: Judith Wright

Pain: a Textbook for Therapists

Edited by

Jenny Strong BOccThy MOccThy PhD

Professor of Occupational Therapy, School of Health and Rehabilitation Sciences,
University of Queensland; Deputy President, Academic Board of the
University of Queensland, Brisbane, Queensland, Australia

Anita M. Unruh PhD RSW OT(c)RegNS

Associate Professor, School of Occupational Therapy, Dalhousie University, Halifax,
Nova Scotia, Canada

Anthony Wright BSc PhD GradCert Educ MPhtyST

Professor and Head of School of Physiotherapy, Curtin University of Technology, Perth, Australia;
Formerly Professor and Head, Division of Physical Therapy, School of Medical Rehabilitation,
University of Manitoba, Winnipeg, Manitoba, Canada

G. David Baxter TD BSc DPhil MCSP SRP

Professor, Head of School of Rehabilitation Sciences, Life and Health Sciences,
University of Ulster, Jordanstown, Northern Ireland, UK

Foreword by

Patrick D. Wall FRS DM FRCP

Professor Emeritus of Physiology, St Thomas' Hospital, London, UK

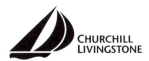

CHURCHILL
LIVINGSTONE

EDINBURGH LONDON NEW YORK PHILADELPHIA ST LOUIS SYDNEY TORONTO 2002

CHURCHILL LIVINGSTONE
An imprint of Elsevier Science Limited

First published 2002
Reprinted 2002

ISBN 0 443 05978 0

British Library Cataloguing in Publication Data
A catalogue record for this book is available from the British Library

Library of Congress Cataloging in Publication Data
A catalog record for this book is available from the Library of Congress

Note
Medical knowledge is constantly changing. As new information
becomes available, changes in treatment, procedures, equipment and
the use of drugs become necessary. The editors, contributors and the
publishers have taken care to ensure that the information given in this
text is accurate and up to date. However, readers are strongly advised
to confirm that the information, especially with regard to drug usage,
complies with the latest legislation and standards of practice.

The
publisher's
policy is to use
**paper manufactured
from sustainable forests**

Printed in China

Contents

Contributors

Shelley Allen BOcc Thy GradDipEd MOccThy
Lecturer, Occupational Therapy,
School of Health and Rehabilitation Sciences,
University of Queensland, Brisbane,
Queensland, Australia
14. Re-integration into work

Panos Barlas BSc(Hons) MCSP SRP Lic Ac PDD DPhil
Research Fellow – Clinical Trials, Primary Care
Sciences Research Centre, Keele University,
Keele, Staffordshire, UK
11. Electrophysical agents in pain management

G. David Baxter TD BSc DPhil MCSP SRP
Professor and Head of School of Rehabilitation
Sciences, Life and Health Sciences, University of
Ulster, Jordanstown, Newtonabbey,
Northern Ireland, UK
11. Electrophysical agents and pain management

Sally Bennett BOccThy(Hons)
Sessional Lecturer, Occupational Therapy,
School of Health and Rehabilitation Sciences,
University of Queensland, Brisbane,
Queensland, Australia
21. Cancer pain

Heather A. E. Benson BSc(Hons) PhD MPSNI
Western Australia Biomedical Research Institute and
School of Biomedical Sciences, Curtin University of
Technology, Perth, Western Australia,
Australia
16. Pharmacology of pain management

Mary P. Galea BAppSc(Phty) BA GradDip Physio(Neurol)
GradCert Clin Trials Management GradDip Neurosci PhD
Professor of Clinical Physiotherapy, School of
Physiotherapy, Faculty of Medicine, Dentistry and
Health Sciences, The University of Melbourne,
Victoria, Australia
2. Neuroanatomy of the nociceptive system

Libby Gibson BOccThy
Lecturer, Occupational Therapy, School of Health and
Rehabilitation Sciences, University of Queensland,
Brisbane, Queensland, Australia
14. Re-integration into work

Katherine Harman BSc (PT) MScPhD
Assistant Professor, School of Physiotherapy,
Dalhousie University, Halifax, Nova Scotia, Canada
 8. Generic principles of practice
12. Alternative and complementary therapies

Chris Henriksson MSc OT PhD
Lecturer, Department of Neuroscience and
Locomotion, Linköping University, Linköping,
Sweden
4. Psychological, environmental and behavioural
    dimensions of the pain experience

Julie Hides BPhty MPhtySt PhD
Clinical Supervisor, Mater Back Stability Clinic, Mater
Misercordiae Hospital, University of Queensland,
Brisbane, Queensland, Australia
13. Exercise and pain

Robert G. Large MBChB DPM PhD FFPsych (SA) FRANZCP
FFPMANZCA
Clinical Director and Psychiatrist, Auckland
Regional Pain Service, Auckland Hospital, Auckland,
New Zealand
22. Chronic pain and psychiatric problems

Frank New MB BS FRANZCP FFPMANZCA
Visiting Consultant to Royal Brisbane Hospital
Multidisciplinary Pain Centre; Clinical Senior
Lecturer, Department of Psychiatry,
University of Queensland, Brisbane, Queensland,
Australia
22. Chronic pain and psychiatric problems

James O'Callaghan MBBS FANZCA FFPMANZCA
Senior Visiting Specialist, Multidisciplinary
Pain Centre, Royal Brisbane Hospital, Brisbane,
Queensland, Australia
16. *Pharmacology of pain management*

Carolyn Richardson BPhty PhD
Associate Professor of Physiotherapy, School of
Health and Rehabilitation Sciences, University of
Queensland, St Lucia, Queensland, Australia
13. *Exercise and pain*

Patricia A. Roche MCSP BSc(Hons) MSc PSYCH PhD
Lecturer, Physiotherapy, School of Health and
Rehabilitation Sciences, University of Queensland,
Brisbane, Queensland, Australia
5. *Placebo analgesia – friend not foe*

Stephan A. Schug MD FANZCA FFPMANZCA
Associate Professor, Department of Anaesthesia,
University of Western Australia;
Director of Pain Medicine, Royal Perth Hospital,
Perth, Western Australia, Australia
19. *Pain in the acute care setting*

Tina Souvlis BPhty
Lecturer, Physiotherapy School of Health and
Rehabilitation Sciences, University of Queensland,
Brisbane, Queensland, Australia
17. *Musculoskeletal pain*

Jenny Strong BOccThy MOccThy PhD
Professor of Occupational Therapy, School of Health
and Rehabilitation Sciences, University of Queensland;
Deputy President, Academic Board of the University
of Queensland, Brisbane, Queensland,
Australia
1. *Introduction to pain*
7. *Pain assessment and measurement*
9. *Psychologically based pain management strategies*
14. *Re-integration into work*
15. *Lifestyle management*
20. *Chronic pain problems*
21. *Cancer pain*
22. *Chronic pain and psychiatric problems*

Jenny Sturgess BOccThy MOcoThy
PhD student, School of Health and Rehabilitation
Sciences, University of Queensland, Brisbane,
Queensland, Australia
7. *Pain assessment and measurement*

Anita M. Unruh PhD RSW OT(c) Reg NS
Associate Professor, School of Occupational Therapy,
Dalhousie University, Halifax, Nova Scotia, Canada
1. *Introduction to pain*
4. *Psychological, environmental and behavioural
   dimensions of the pain experience*
6. *Pain across the lifespan*
7. *Pain assessment and measurement*
8. *Generic principles of practice*
9. *Psychologically based management strategies*
12. *Alternative and complementary therapies*
22. *Chronic pain and psychiatric problems*

Bill Vicenzino BPhty MSc PhD Grad Dip Sports Phty
Senior Lecturer, Physiotherapy School of Health and
Rehabilitation Sciences, University of Queensland,
Brisbane, Queensland, Australia
7. *Pain assessment and measurement*
10. *Physical treatment*
17. *Musculoskeletal pain*

Deborah S. B. Watson MBBS (Lond)
Research Fellow, Division of Anaesthesiology, Faculty
of Medical and Health Sciences, University of
Auckland, Auckland, New Zealand
19. *Pain in the acute care setting*

Anthony Wright BSc(Hons) PhtyGradcert Edu MPhtyST PhD
Professor and Head, School of Physiotherapy, Curtin
University of Technology, Perth, Western Australia,
Australia.
Formerly, Professor and Head, Division of Physical
Therapy, School of Medical Rehabilitation, University
of Manitoba, Winnipeg, Manitoba, Canada
1. *Introduction to pain*
3. *Neurophysiology of pain and pain modulation*
10. *Physical treatments*
16. *Pharmacology of pain management*
17. *Musculoskeletal pain*
18. *Neuropathic pain*

Foreword

I am convinced that physiotherapy and occupational therapy are sleeping giants. This book is one of the welcome signs that the long sleep is over. For well over 2000 years classical physiotherapy was practised in every culture as a folk tradition. It was all there: heat, cold, massage, manipulation, acupuncture, reflexology, aromatherapy, etc. Since it was deeply embedded in every society and therefore attracted little intellectual attention, it was simply accepted as an empirical fact of life without the mechanisms being questioned. Occupational therapy is a newer profession: it emerged in response to the many veterans of the 20th century world wars who returned home traumatized, often disabled and in need of occupational rehabilitation. Still, a central tenet of occupational therapy, that humans have a need for meaningful occupation to cope and live with health problems, has been with us for centuries.

In the 18th century, a disaster hit the subsequent development of rehabilitative professions: it was the Age of Reason and the time when academic medicine was developing. This powerful and hugely successful movement was based on two essentials: diagnosis based on pathology and an obsessional search for cures based on rational therapy. Rehabilitation interventions lost out on both counts. The conditions treated often had a vague or non-existent pathology. Only the wildest who exhibited both charisma and the confidence of the charlatan claimed to effect permanent cure. The vast honest majority were proud of the ability to ameliorate the condition. Physiotherapists and occupational therapists were not the only professionals to be demoted by academic medicine. Palliative care, for example, had to wait for two centuries before regaining respectability, since it made no claim to cure. It climbed back to acceptance, once 'proper' doctors said, 'there is nothing more to be done'.

Physiotherapy and occupational therapy survived at the very bottom of the academic hierarchy. From the more-honest doctors, physiotherapists won a certain respect because it was clear that they were indeed helping some patients. For the less-honest doctors, physiotherapy represented a polite dumping ground for patients who had been labelled as unfit for appropriate rational medical or surgical therapy. Occupational therapy was considered useful to keep patients busy and diverted from their problems.

In the spirit of the times in the twentieth century, there was a partial move away from the traditional apprenticeship in which skills were taught by a senior physiotherapist who looked back with cosy pride to the traditional art. Bright younger physiotherapists and occupational therapists began to seek education to learn the rationale for what they were doing.

But what education? The answer seemed to be obvious: an abbreviated and dumbed-down version of what medical students were taught. This was a particularly unfortunate approach to the crucial subject of pain. Classical medicine had deliberately downgraded the study of symptoms, such as pain. Symptoms were regarded as no more than signposts that should not direct exploration of the only true road which led from diagnosis to cure. The phrase 'symptomatic medicine' became offensive, designating a low-grade practice that failed to face the deep professional problem of fundamental cure. This attitude condemned physiotherapists and occupational therapists to stick to the bottom of the academic ladder. It is symbolic that the physiotherapy and occupational therapy departments are often found in the windowless basement of most hospitals.

Medical school gave short shrift to an explanation of symptoms. Pain was inevitably caused by the pressure of damaged tissue which excited special nociceptor nerve fibres. These fibres fed a system in the central nervous system which was hard wired and modality dedicated, which triggered activity in a specific pain centre. This plan was completely accepted, and naturally directed the attention of the new academic physiotherapy entirely to the periphery. This resulted in a gaudy flowering of plausible but unlisted hypotheses to explain the aim and effect of the therapy. Since it was accepted that pain could be produced only by clearly pathological tissue and since physiotherapy was directed at that tissue, the hypotheses proposed tissue changes. Changes of arterial or venous or lymphatic flow, speeding the resolution of the inflammation by heating or cooling, release of trapped nerves by breaking adhesions or readjusting bones, relaxation of cramped muscles all make up the canon of courses in the intent and rationale of physiotherapy.

Four new areas of discovery have moved the emphasis from an entirely peripheral explanation for the source of pain and have opened up the field of debate to include the central nervous system. The first was the recognition of the crucial significance of referred pain. The site of the perceived pain and target therapy is not necessarily the site of causative pathology. For example, angina is undoubtedly caused by ischaemia in the heart and yet the arm may be the area of the troublesome disorders in spite of the fact that no pathology resides in the arm. The recognition of the phenomenon forced a conclusion that convergences occur within the central nervous system. Therapy may be directed successfully at both the primary and the secondary site.

Next, it was shown that widespread tenderness and muscle contraction associated with the peripheral damage can be caused by a rising secondary excitability in the spinal cord. This shows that the use of crippling pain may migrate from its original area in the periphery into central areas. This is one of the clear signs that the pain mechanism is not rigid, dedicated and hard wired, but plastic and changes with time.

The third change was the discovery that the pain producing messages reaching the brain are controlled descending symptoms originating in the brain. This opened the entire field to psychology, with the understanding that pain is not simply a mechanical response to the presence of tissue damage but is affected by the mood and the attitude of the one who suffers. The most obvious example is the role of attention, which must be directed to that area, if pain is to be felt. It also offers a rationale for the use of distraction and counter-stimulation, by cognitive therapies, which seize the opportunity to direct attention to some event other than pain. This advance shatters the old dualism in favour of an integrated whole, where mind and body or sensation and perception cannot be divided. This change had tremendous implication for occupational therapy in the area of pain: it provided a conceptual rationale for understanding how participating in activities that are meaningful to the patient might influence perception of pain and in turn decrease disability and improve function in daily life. For perhaps the first time, occupational therapy had a respected role in the management of pain particularly for the patient with chronic pain.

The last change comes from the new techniques of brain imaging, where we must now question the traditional separation of sensory and motor mechanisms. It becomes reasonable to propose that sensory events are analysed in terms of what might be the appropriate action. If this turns out to be reasonable, then therapies directed at active movement planning, posture and active participation in daily life may well influence perceived sensation. The chapter headings of this book show how the thinking of the editors and authors has expanded to incorporate this fundamentally new thinking about the origins of pain and the direction of new therapies.

Patrick D. Wall

Preface

Many people in our communities have ailments that cause pain. While some people receive appropriate interventions to help them alleviate and/or manage their pain, there are many people who suffer from pain. As Professor Ron Melzack has noted (1990), unrelieved pain kills. It is therefore encumbent upon health professionals to be knowledgeable about, and skilled in, the assessment and management of pain. Such is the case for physiotherapists and occupational therapists, whom we would contend are ideally placed to both help alleviate pain, and to help people to adjust to, and cope better with, ongoing pain. Yet, reports suggest that some suffering could be alleviated if professionals had better knowledge about pain. For example, Cousins (1991) found that postoperative pain was treated effectively in less than 30–50% of patients. Further, survey reports from a number of health professionals, including occupational therapists and physiotherapists, suggest that pain knowledge of newly graduating practitioners is less than adequate (Rochman 1998, Strong et al 2000, Unruh 1995).

The primary professional and research organisation concerned with the study and alleviation of pain, the International Association for the Study of Pain (IASP), has been actively involved in furthering an understanding about pain since its inception in 1975. One aspect of the IASP's activities has been the development of curricula to better equip health professionals to be good pain practitioners. In 1994, the IASP published the 'Outline Curriculum on Pain for Schools of Occupational Therapy and Physical Therapy'. Three of the editors of this book (Jenny Strong, Anita Unruh and David Baxter) were on the IASP Subcommittee that developed this curriculum (chaired by Anita Unruh), while the fourth editor (Anthony Wright) was a consultant to the Subcommittee's deliberations. Two other contributors to this book, Chris Henriksson and Pat Roche, also served on the Subcommittee or as a consultant to the Subcommittee.

Implementation of the OT/PT Pain Curriculum has been hampered by the lack of an integrated, comprehensive textbook to support our teaching and learning efforts. Hence, the idea for this book was born in 1996. Realising this idea has taken some time, with liaison and work across a number of countries – Australia, Canada, Ireland, Great Britain, New Zealand, and Sweden. The result is, we believe, a comprehensive textbook which will assist physiotherapists and occupational therapists (and other therapists) to become more informed about, and more sensitive and understanding towards, people with pain, and more effective and evidence-based in their approach to treating and managing people with pain.

This book has been designed to be used as a companion to the IASP pain curriculum developed for physiotherapists and occupational therapists. It provides a comprehensive discussion about the nature of the pain phenomenon including: its definition and epidemiology; the physiological, anatomical and psychological nature of pain; assessment and measurement of pain; management strategies for therapists; and common pain conditions. A lifestyle and lifespan perspective is used to discuss the pain phenomenon and its management. The text makes use of a number of learning strategies to help the student/reader, including chapter objectives, reflective exercises, case examples, and revision questions, along with comprehensive reference lists.

Finally, a word about the up-to-dateness of the information contained herein. Pain research is exploding with new discoveries and new understandings about pain, from many quarters. Basic science is unravelling many secrets about neurotransmitters and pain pathways. Applied research tells us much about people's anxieties and fears about pain, and the impact of these upon function. Therapists and students must keep up to date in their knowledge and their practice. This textbook is a starting point, from which each individual can develop a greater knowledge and understanding of pain. Therapists and students must never forget that pain is a uniquely subjective experience, which can have a profound impact on a person's dreams, responsibilities and capabilities in everyday life.

The publication of a textbook such as this has been an interesting one for us, the editors and authors. It has been a joy to work with experts across the globe. We thank all the contributors to this book for embracing the idea of a textbook for therapists, for providing expert content, and for cheerfully meeting deadlines. Also, thank you to our colleagues at Churchill Livingstone, Harcourt in Edinburgh, who eagerly agreed to publish such a text, and kept us focused and task oriented: to Mary Emmerson Law and Mairi McCubbin, thank you. Also, we thank our wonderful families, who endured so much time without us when we were engaged in 'finishing the book': Paul and Matthew, Pat and Mika, Heather, Tom and Sam, and Alice, Susan, Marian and Jennifer.

Finally, thank you, to those patients with pain who have taught us so much, to our students who have challenged us, and to our colleagues who have inspired our endeavours in this area.

Brisbane 2001	Jenny Strong
Halifax 2001	Anita M. Unruh
Winnipeg 2001	Anthony Wright
Jordanstown 2001	David Baxter

REFERENCES

Cousins M J 1991 Prevention of post-operative pain. In: Bond M R, Charlton J E, Woolf C J Proceedings of the VIth World Congress on Pain. Elsevier, Amsterdam

Melzack R 1990 The tragedy of needless pain. Scientific American 262: 19–25

Rochman D L 1998 Students' knowledge of pain: A survey of four schools. Occupational Therapy International 5: 140–154

Strong J, Tooth L, Unruh A 2000 Newly graduated occupational therapists and knowledge about pain. Canadian Journal of Occupational Therapy 66: 221–228

Unruh A M 1995 Teaching student occupational therapists about pain: A course evaluation. Canadian Journal of Occupational Therapy 62: 30–36

Understanding pain

SECTION CONTENTS

1

Introduction to pain

*Anita M. Unruh   Jenny Strong
Anthony Wright*

OVERVIEW

Pain is a common and growing problem in our societies. It is frequently associated with intentional and unintentional injuries, as well as illnesses and diseases that occur over a normal lifespan. Pain is a subjective symptom that cannot be objectively measured in the way that blood pressure or heart rate can be measured. How a person communicates about pain is influenced by factors such as age, gender, underlying disability, and social or cultural norms about acceptable pain behaviour. Pain is an intensely personal experience with major emotional and sensory components.

Many occupational therapists and physiotherapists work with people for whom pain has become a persistent and often disabling problem in everyday life. Persistent pain may have a major adverse affect on self-esteem, occupations of everyday life, relationships with others, physical function, emotional state, and on one's overall quality of life. In our professional experience, enabling individuals to regain control over pain and over their lives is a satisfying and fulfilling professional and personal challenge.

In this introductory chapter, we will provide the student with a brief orientation to this text, and then discuss the differences between acute and chronic pain. We will then review some epidemiological issues (discussed further in Chapter 6), and the multidimensional nature of pain. Lastly, we will outline and contrast the roles of occupational therapists and physiotherapists in their work with people who have pain, and provide an overview of service delivery, and the ethical and legal issues associated with practice in this area.

ORIENTATION TO THE TEXTBOOK

This textbook reflects an interprofessional collaboration between physiotherapists and occupational therapists. We believe that this type of collaboration provides an opportunity for students to consider the roles and contributions of each profession to the field of pain at their first exposure. Cooperation and collaboration strengthens each profession and enables us to offer the best possible care to clients and patients (see Box 1.1). This text is also an international effort involving experts from Canada, Australia, New Zealand, the UK and Sweden. We anticipate that the reader may appreciate the flavour of international examples. For this reason, we occasionally reject conformity to allow some international diversity. For example, at the end of each chapter, the reader will find Study questions/Questions for revision (northern hemisphere expression/southern hemisphere expression).

In 1993, the International Association for the Study of Pain (IASP) initiated an ad hoc committee to prepare a pain curriculum for students in occupational therapy or physiotherapy. Preparation of this curriculum involved an international committee of members or consultants from Canada, Australia, the USA, the UK, Sweden, New Zealand, Italy, India, Kenya, Columbia and Japan. The work of the committee and the consultants generated a curriculum that can be used by an entry-level professional programme in occupational therapy or physiotherapy (Ad Hoc Committee OT/PT Pain Curriculum 1994). This book is designed as a course text to be used in conjunction with the IASP occupational therapy/physiotherapy pain curriculum.

Many of the chapters in this text are relevant to both professions, but there are some chapters which are more specific to one profession. For example, chapters 10, 11 and 13 are most applicable to physiotherapists, while chapters 9, 14 and 15 are particularly relevant to occupational therapists.

Lastly, some chapters contain Reflective exercises. These exercises encourage the reader to think and reflect on her or his own pain experiences, experiences of family members or close friends, and experiences of clients or patients who have been encountered in fieldwork education, clinical placements or practice. Completion of the exercises will enable students to have a more personal understanding of some of the concepts and issues which are raised.

WHAT IS PAIN?

The IASP defined pain as, 'an unpleasant sensory and emotional experience associated with actual or potential tissue damage, or described in terms of such damage' (Merskey & Bogduk 1994 p 210). This definition highlights the duality of pain as a physiological and psychological experience. It is a physiological event within the body that is dependent on subjective recognition, that is, without psychological awareness, pain

---

Box 1.1 Key terms defined

Client vs patient – Occupational therapists and physiotherapists in different countries refer to people with whom they work as patients or clients. Preference is often embedded in philosophical positions and theoretical models about the nature of practice (Townsend 1998). For example, in Canada and in some other countries, occupational therapists prefer to use the term 'client' to reflect a more equal and collaborative therapeutic relationship, and to separate occupational therapy from medicine. 'Patient' is thought to connote a more passive approach to health that is inconsistent with a client-centred framework. In other countries, the term 'patient' is preferred. It is the most widely used term. Terms like 'client' or 'consumer' may also be equated with a commercial or business relationship that is inconsistent with problems of health. Although 'patient' is sometimes associated with passivity, it originates from the Latin word patiens, meaning to suffer (Stedman 1982). Many of the people who are seen by occupational therapists and physiotherapists seek out these services because they are suffering in some way. In this text, patient or client are used interchangeably depending on the authors of

the chapter, their preferences, and the contexts in which individuals with pain problems are seen (e.g. hospital or community).

Physical therapy vs physiotherapist – In the USA, 'physical therapy' is preferred to physiotherapy, but in most other countries 'physiotherapist' is used to designate this health professional whereas 'physical therapy' refers to interventions that have a primarily physical basis. In this text, we refer to this profession as physiotherapy.

Practioner vs therapist – In some countries, the term 'practioner' is preferred to 'therapist' (e.g. the USA). Practioner may be considered more in keeping with the other health professionals and may be seen as more professional. In this text we will use therapist and practitioner interchangeably. They refer to both occupational therapist and physiotherapist.

Pain terms – Throughout this text, we will be using definitions or concepts of pain as defined by the 1993–1994 International Association for the Study of Pain (IASP) taskforce on taxonomy (Merskey & Bogduk 1994).

cannot exist. It also highlights several other important aspects of the pain experience. Pain is usually considered as a warning signal of actual or perceived tissue damage. Nevertheless, pain can occur in the absence of tissue damage, even though the experience may be described as if the damage had occurred.

There are important distinctions between acute and chronic pain. Acute pain has an inherent biological function; it is a warning of actual or potential physiological harm (Melzack & Wall 1988). Acute pain usually stops long before healing is completed, a process that may take a few days or a few weeks (Loeser & Melzack 1999). In the past, chronic pain was defined as pain that persisted beyond the normal time of healing (Bonica 1953, Melzack & Wall 1988). Chronic pain was often considered as any pain that lasted more than 3–6 months. The IASP taskforce on taxonomy (Merskey & Bogduk 1994) maintained that this definition of chronic pain on the basis of a time interval and evidence of healing was inadequate. Physiological changes may contribute to the experience of many chronic pains (e.g. phantom limb pain), as well as recurrent episodic pains (e.g. migraines). Normal healing has not occurred for other chronic pains, such as pain associated with rheumatoid arthritis or metastatic carcinomas. Further, changes in the central nervous system due to injury may prolong and maintain pain long after the expected period of healing (Merskey 1988, Wall 1989). The nervous system may in fact be damaged by the original injury in such a way that it is unable to restore itself to normal functioning (Loeser & Melzack 1999). The IASP taskforce (Merskey & Bogduk 1994 p xii) proposed that chronic pain be considered as:

A persistent pain that is not amenable, as a rule, to treatments based upon specific remedies, or to the routine methods of pain control such as non-narcotic analgesics.

Loeser and Melzack (1999 p 1609) concluded:

It is not the duration of pain that distinguishes acute from chronic pain but, more importantly, the inability of the body to restore its physiological functions to normal homeostatic levels.

These distinctions between acute and chronic pain have important implications for pain assessment and intervention. Acute pain signals tissue damage, but chronic pain is markedly disassociated from tissue damage. It may be out of proportion to any initiating pathology or the degree of tissue damage. Chronic pain is associated with considerable suffering, with psychological, behavioural and environmental changes. In either case, pain must be recognized as a subjective experience. Pain exists when and where the client says it exists (McCaffery & Beebe 1989).

Epidemiology of pain

There is considerable variability in the rates reported for different types of pain from one setting to another. Some of this variability is due to the use of different indicators, different definitions for various pains, and the recall period used for the pain report.

Prevalence refers to all existing episodes of pain in a given period, whereas incidence rates refer only to new reports of pain in a given period (Mausner & Kramer 1985). Prevalence rates are easier to obtain and are more commonly reported in epidemiological studies. Prevalence may give an inflated estimate of pain, particularly when the reporting period is long, since some portion of the sample may be prone to have many more pain events. Definitions of some pains may be quite broad in epidemiological studies (e.g. headache and migraine). As more is known about a pain problem, definitions become more precise and narrow. Respondents may also be asked to report prevalence of pain over the past year, the past 6 months, the past month, or the previous 2 weeks. Such differences influence reported prevalence rates and their accuracy. In Chapter 6, we review prevalence of pain at different stages in the lifespan. It is worth noting at this point that back pain is the most common disabling pain associated with compensation and rehabilitation programme. Pain is also associated with a variety of diseases such as rheumatological diseases, multiple sclerosis, sickle cell disease, cancer, stroke, cardiovascular disease, spinal cord injury and bowel disorders. It may be a troubling complication following amputations. It may be due to physical or sexual abuse. It may also occur as a result of health procedures such as immunizations, venepunctures, bone marrow aspirations, lumbar punctures, dental procedures, surgery, debridement, splinting, manual examinations and so on.

The multidimensional experience of pain

Although the severity of pain or its intensity is often the first concern for the client and the health professional, there are many other dimensions of pain that are also important. The pain context must be considered to fully understand the pain experience of the client (see Reflective exercise 1.1). The physiology of the pain, the location and duration of the pain, the personality and the developmental history of the person, and the social/environmental context in which the pain occurs influence dimensions such as pain intensity, emotional upset due to pain, the sensory qualities of pain, the predictability and controllability of pain and other evaluative dimensions of pain.

The anatomy and the physiology of pain is complex and is discussed more fully in Chapters 2 and 3. Pain is often experienced at the site of tissue damage but the pain may radiate beyond this site and cause sensitization to noxious stimuli beyond this site. Sometimes, pain is felt in a different area than the site of tissue damage. Some pains, such as visceral pain, can be very difficult for the client to localize and may be diffuse in nature. The extent of the tissue damage is frequently not a reliable indicator of the severity of the pain that will be experienced. Apparently minor tissue damage can be associated with severe pain. Clients who have similar underlying tissue damage may report very different pain. Sometimes, what seems to be exactly the same pain, will seem more or less severe to the client than it did on a previous occasion. Some pains have characteristic sensory qualities that are useful to determine contributing causal factors. For example, headache is often described as a throbbing, stabbing pain; neuropathic pain may be described as burning whereas chest pain may feel heavy (Melzack & Katz 1994, Melzack & Torgerson 1971). Some pain experiences may have a greater affective component to the sensation. These variations in pain are only partially understood.

Emotional upset due to pain is influenced by many factors and is discussed in detail in Chapter 4. It is worth noting here that a hostile and doubting environment is likely to increase the anxiety, stress, and self-doubt of the person with pain, whereas a caring and supportive environment may decrease emotional upset and reinforce self-esteem and the positive coping behaviours that maintain function.

Other factors, such as the predictability and controllability of the pain, its duration, frequency of occurrence, fluctuations in severity, interference with mobility and everyday occupations, and the way in which the pain is appraised, may influence the severity of the pain experience (Unruh & Ritchie 1998, Unruh et al 1999). Belief that the pain is associated with a serious disease may increase anxiety and the perceived threat of the pain.

The social, cultural and physical context in which pain occurs is also an important influence on pain sensation and on behaviour in response to pain. For example, pain that occurs due to sports injuries, especially during competition, may be experienced very differently than pain due to disease or a health procedure or some unknown cause. Cultural or religious expectations about whether one should be stoic or expressive towards pain can have a powerful influence on pain response.

Extreme circumstances can have a dramatic effect on pain experience. For example, severely injured soldiers sometimes report very little if any pain from extensive wounds, or they may feel no pain until many hours later (Beecher 1959, Carlen et al 1978). Beecher reported that some of these men were not in a state of shock, and although they did not feel pain from injuries they did report pain due to venepunctures. Similarly, in a survey of people with injuries such as fractures, burns and major lacerations attending an emergency clinic, Melzack et al (1982) found that 38% of the patients did not feel pain due to their injuries. Such situational analgesia can occur at times of great crisis or when one is engaged in some intensely meaningful occupation. Melzack and Wall (1988) suggested that, at such times, areas of the brain that are essential for pain experience and response may be engaged on other matters and become inaccessible to receiving painful input, even if the person is aware of the injury.

THE ROLES OF OCCUPATIONAL THERAPY AND PHYSIOTHERAPY

Occupational therapists and physiotherapists often work collaboratively and often share similar principles of practice. The primary therapeutic objectives of occupational therapy and physiotherapy in the area of pain management are reduction of pain and associated disability, reduction or correction of impairments, promotion of optimal function in everyday living, enabling occupations that are meaningful to the client, and maintaining supportive family and social relationships. A range of cognitive–behavioural strategies, supportive/educational approaches and physical interventions for pain management may be implemented by occupational therapists and by physiotherapists to reduce pain and improve function and overall quality of life.

Therapists from both professions have a common commitment to person-centred care, the promotion of health and wellbeing, and the prevention of long-term disability and handicap resulting from pain. Client and family education about pain is an integral component of therapeutic programmes.

It is essential that occupational therapists and physiotherapists take a holistic and collaborative view of the needs of the person with pain. Therapists should be able to recognize the numerous misconceptions that prevail about pain and people with pain, and be able to challenge and refute the existence of such misconceptions.

Although there are similarities between occupational therapy and physiotherapy and many therapists work together through interprofessional teams, these two professions also differ considerably in their underlying theoretical foundations and in their overall approach to people in pain.

Theoretical perspectives of occupational therapy

Occupational therapists are concerned with those factors that contribute to the experience of productivity and meaning in the occupations that make up everyday life (Canadian Association of Occupational Therapists 1997). Although in common language 'occupation' is often thought of as paid work, occupational therapists consider occupation as a 'group of activities and tasks of everyday life, named, organized and given value and meaning by individuals and a culture' (Law et al 1997 p 34). In this sense, occupations refer to 'everything people do to occupy themselves, including looking after themselves (self-care), enjoying life (leisure), and contributing to the social and economic fabric of their communities (productivity)' (Law et al 1997 p 34). Many factors influence the capacity of an individual to engage in meaningful and productive occupations, including her or his physical, cognitive, and emotional health, and the physical, social, cultural, and economic factors of the individual's environment.

Occupational therapists are primarily concerned with the psychosocial and environmental factors that contribute to pain and the impact of pain on everyday life. Occupational therapists assess the impact of pain on occupational performance in the areas of self-care, paid and unpaid work, interests and leisure pursuits, customary habits and routines, and family relationships. Assessment will include evaluation of psychoso-

cial and environmental factors aggravating pain in the home and workplace. Occupational therapists work collaboratively with the person to develop an occupational therapy program to increase self-esteem, restore self-efficacy, and promote optimal occupational function despite pain. Intervention strategies may include assistive devices and adaptive equipment, purposeful and productive occupations/activities, and vocational rehabilitation or work hardening to improve endurance and work skills and re-establish roles, habits and routines of everyday life. Education about pain and supportive individual, family, or group counselling are utilized as needed.

Theoretical perspectives of physiotherapy

Physiotherapists apply a wide range of physical and behavioural treatments to reduce pain and prevent dysfunction. Physiotherapy assessment focuses initially on the evaluation of impairments related to the client's presenting condition, as well as undertaking a detailed appraisal of various aspects of the client's pain report, such as temporal pattern of pain and those activities that specifically aggravate or relieve pain. A major focus is on assessing and quantifying motor and sensory impairments. The assessment then extends to consider secondary biomechanical and or behavioural factors that contribute to pain, the pain–activity cycle and overall function. A physiotherapy treatment program is developed to provide pain relief, modify the effects of primary and secondary factors contributing to pain, reduce or reverse specific impairments, promote healing, and repair and minimize the influence of factors that may lead to recurrence of pain.

Physiotherapy intervention strategies may include education, exercise, manual therapy, movement facilitation techniques, and/or application of electrophysical agents based on thermal, mechanical, electrical or phototherapeutic modalities. Increasingly, physiotherapists adopt a cognitive–behavioural approach to the management of clients with chronic pain. Educational approaches focus on understanding pain, improving posture, body mechanics and gait, and on minimizing secondary contributing factors. Exercise is used by physiotherapists to activate specific muscle groups, re-educate motor control skills, increase muscle endurance, strengthen specific muscle groups and counteract the effects of generalized deconditioning. Movement is used to control and decrease pain and increase mobility.

Service delivery

Services for clients with pain provided by occupational therapists or physiotherapists can occur in a variety of settings. Clients for whom pain may be a primary or secondary problem can present themselves in any area or practice setting. However, it has become increasingly common to establish specialized pain services or clinics to deliver services for people with pain, especially chronic pain. The majority of such clinics provide specialized pain services for adults, but there are a growing number of pain clinics for children. Such pain services/clinics are typically multidisciplinary and offer a range of medical, psychological and rehabilitative assessments and interventions. In addition, there are many services provided outside of traditional medical facilities that are concerned with returning injured workers to the workplace. Many of these workers also struggle with problems of persistent pain, though the focus of intervention may be on return to work rather than pain relief per se. Increasingly, physiotherapists and occupational therapists act as primary care practitioners with an important role in providing pain management services for clients in the community.

ETHICAL AND LEGAL STANDARDS OF CARE

Unfortunately, pain research has demonstrated that clients are frequently given inadequate care for their pain. The subjectivity of pain can complicate pain assessment and intervention (see Reflective exercise 1.2). Health professionals make clinical judgements about the veracity of a client's *pain story*. These judgements are based on many factors such as professional experience, research familiarity and involvement in continuing education about pain, as well as personal beliefs about how people should respond to pain.

Reflective exercise 1.2

Subjective experiences like pain can be difficult for other people to understand. For this exercise, think about whether you, or a family member or a friend, have been in a situation in which you saw a health professional about a pain problem.

- Do you feel that the professional understood the experience and what was needed?
- What factors might have contributed to being believed or doubted?
- How did belief or doubt affect the type and quality of the care that was received?
- Did you receive the care you needed?

Occupational therapists and physiotherapists are also sometimes caught between perceived obligations to an employer and obligations to the client. Employers may expect the health professional to be particularly attentive to detect clients who may not have *real* pain or may be exaggerating pain complaints particularly for economic gain or to obtain medication for reasons other than pain relief. As a result, health professionals are often concerned about whether or not to believe the client's complaints about pain. On the other hand, clients expect to be believed when they complain about pain and to receive appropriate intervention.

Professional standards typically obligate an occupational therapist or physiotherapist to use a client- or patient-centred approach. Believing and accepting the client's perspective is crucial to such an approach. McCaffery and Beebe (1989 p 8) have suggested:

Pain is subjective and being fooled is simply a reality in dealing with something that can never be proved or disproved. This point must be acknowledged by all members of the health team. The risk of being fooled does not justify doubting the patient or withholding pain relief.

It is essential for health professionals to consider the following perspective in their approach to all clients who complain of pain and want assistance (McCaffery & Beebe 1989 p 8):

No matter which approach we use in responding to the patient's report of pain, we will eventually make a mistake. If we doubt some patients and withhold treatment, we may avoid being fooled by the minority who are addicts, abusers or malingerers, but we will eventually fail to help someone who does have pain. On the other hand, if we give everyone the benefit of the doubt and try to relieve pain in all who say they have it, we will be fooled by some who are addicts, abusers or malingerers, but we will never fail to help someone who does have pain. Either way we will make a mistake. Therefore we must address our professional responsibility and consider which mistake we can afford.

The dilemma that McCaffery and Beebe (1989) outline is very real and problematic. Therapists may find themselves alternating from one approach to the other because there are strengths and weaknesses to both positions. Being conscious of the potential pitfalls may be helpful.

Ethical obligations have personal and professional perspectives. Deciding how to approach clients with pain depends on values and ethical standards. National or regional occupational therapy and physiotherapy associations that govern professional standards will have a code of ethics that guide practice. Any practising occupational therapist or physiotherapist should be familiar with these ethical guidelines and consider them with respect to the concerns of their specific area of practice.

Clients do not typically sue health professionals for inadequate pain management. In 1993, in a keynote address at the IASP VIIth World Congress on Pain in Paris a Canadian ethicist, Dr Margaret Somerville, argued that leaving patients in pain, particularly at the end of life, should be considered an act of criminal negligence (Somerville 1993). Unfortunately, clients often approach healthcare situations trusting that health professionals know best about pain management. It is worth noting that when people are surveyed about pain, respondents who have had a recent experience with a person dying from cancer have less confidence that treatment of pain is adequate (Ashby & Wakefield 1993).

Legal actions for pain may occur under criminal or civil law (McGrath & Unruh 1993). Thus far, there have been very few criminal law suits for inadequate pain management. In November 1990 in the USA, US $15 million was awarded to a family of a man whose dying days were made intolerable by the decision of a nurse and her employer (nursing home) to withhold or reduce pain medication (Angarola & Donato 1991). Henry James had cancer of the prostate with metastases to the left femur and the lumbosacral spine. He was expected to live another 6 months. On admission to the nursing home a nurse assessed Mr James as addicted to morphine and implemented a plan to minimize the use of pain medication, substitute a mild tranquillizer, and delay or withhold the administration of an analgesic. A placebo was substituted for pain medication. The legal action in this case focused on the nursing staff and their employers, but legal action could conceivably involve any health professional who was involved in and agreed with the treatment plan for a given person.

Civil law involves settlements of disagreements between individuals, such as clients and health care providers (McGrath & Unruh 1993). These disputes often involve accepted standards of care, which may of course vary from country to country and profession to profession. We are not aware of any legal action in which an occupational therapist or a physiotherapist was a defendant in a criminal or civil action concerned with determining the adequacy of pain management. In this text, where contraindications to pain management strategies are indicated, they should be carefully noted and considered.

In addition to professional codes of ethics, occupational therapists and physiotherapists should also be cognisant of any position statements or standards for care that concern pain as might be published by the national professional association of their country, and their national pain society/association (all developed countries have such a body). Such documents provide evidence of standards of professional care that influence ethical and legal aspects of pain management. A number of professional associations have now produced position statements on the management of painful disorders. For example, the American Occupational Therapy Association (AOTA) has: 'Occupational Therapy guidelines for Chronic Pain' (AOTA 1999a) and 'Occupational Therapy Practice Guidelines for Adults with Low Back Pain' (AOTA 1999b), and the Australian Physiotherapy Association (APA) has produced a 'Neck Pain Position Statement' (APA 1999) and a 'Position Statement on the use of spinal manipulation/manual therapy and exercise for the treatment of Low Back Pain' (APA 1998).

Legal issues also affect health professionals and pain management practices in another way, through legislation that controls the prescription of opioids to manage pain. This legislation is typically concerned with preventing illegal drug use, but physicians' fear of legal action can create perceived and actual barriers to adequate pharmacological management for people with chronic pain (Clark & Sees 1993, Hill 1992, Hyman 1996, Johnson 1996, Mendelson & Mendelson 1991, Portenoy 1996, Shapiro 1996, Weissman 1993, Ziegler 1997). Even when pain is obviously due to an organic pathology such as cancer, fear of legal prosecution can hinder adequate pharmacological care for pain (Grossman 1993). The WHO Cancer Relief Program has provided important support for more accessible pharmacological control of pain (Takeda 1991). It is incumbent on therapists to be advocates for their clients in such situations. Inadequate pharmacological care reduces a client's capacity to have a meaningful and satisfying quality of life.

Lastly, end-of-life issues, euthanasia and physician-assisted suicide may concern therapists who work in palliative care. These questions often arise due to concerns about dying in great pain (Haugen 1997). Providing pain relief, even if it shortens life, is considered by many as ethical and humane, and in many countries it is legally permissible (Gostin 1997). Deliberately ending a person's life through euthanasia or physician-assisted suicide to end the person's suffering due to pain is also permitted in some countries and some jurisdictions, but not in others. When physicians are surveyed about euthanasia or physician-assisted suicide, alleviation of the person's pain is often the primary reason (Kuhse et al 1997, van Thiel et al 1997). Many ethicists and health professionals argue that requests for euthanasia or physician-assisted suicide reflect the current inadequate management of pain, even though it is currently possible to treat effectively most pain experienced at the end of life (Somerville 1993). They argue that much more aggressive research and attention should be given to adequate treatment of pain at the end of life, and that euthanasia or physician-assisted suicide are not appropriate moral alternatives. Although these issues may be the immediate responsibility of a physician or nurse, the person and family members, they concern all members on a health team and may require each member to have a position. Occupational therapists and physiotherapists who work in palliative care need to consider legal issues, professional ethics and their own personal values in this regard.

CONCLUSION

Pain is a complex and challenging problem for people who have it, and for the occupational therapists and physiotherapists who are involved in providing services. Pain is very common and affects people throughout life. Many occupational therapists and physiotherapists find that employment in the area of pain is a very challenging, satisfying and stimulating area of work. Often these two professions work closely together, since they are both concerned with restoring the individual to her or his normal level of function and occupational engagement. There are also important differences between these two professions which determine their specific responsibilities. Both occupational therapists and physiotherapists should be cognizant of the ethical and legal issues that concern pain management. Attention to professional codes of ethics and practice guidelines is important.

In the following chapters of this text, we will consider the many different components of the pain experience and the context in which it occurs, approaches and issues relevant to assessment and intervention, and some specific pain problems.

Study questions/questions for revision

1. What is the significance of defining pain as a sensory and an emotional experience?
2. What is the difference between acute and chronic pain?
3. Why is the difference between acute and chronic pain important to the client and to the therapist?
4. How should we provide care to a person who is dying and has severe pain?

REFERENCES

Ad Hoc Committee OT/PT Pain Curriculum 1994 Pain curriculum for students in occupational therapy or physical therapy. IASP Newsletter. International Association for the Study of Pain, Seattle

Angarola R T, Donato B J 1991 Inappropriate pain management results in high jury award. Journal of Pain and Symptom Management 6: 407

American Occupational Therapy Association 1999a Occupational therapy practice guidelines for chronic pain. American Occupational Therapy Association, Bethesda (www.aota.org)

American Occupational Therapy Association 1999b Occupational therapy practice guidelines for adults with low back pain. American Occupational Therapy Association, Bethesda (www.aota.org)

Ashby M, Wakefield M 1993 Attitudes to some aspects of death and dying, living wills and substituted health care decision-making in South Australia: public opinion survey for a parliamentary select committee. Palliative Medicine 7: 273–282

Australian Physiotherapists Association 1998 Position Statement on the use of spinal manipulation/manual therapy and exercise in the treatment of low back pain. Maher C, Latimer J, Refshauge K, on behalf of the Manipulative Physiotherapists Association of Australia.

Australian Physiotherapists Association 1999 Position statement on the efficacy of physiotherapy for the treatment of neck pain. Costello J, Jull G, on behalf of the Manipulative Physiotherapists Association of Australia.

Beecher H K 1959 Measurement of subjective responses. Oxford University Press, New York

Bonica J J 1953 The Management of Pain. Lea & Febiger, Philadelphia

Canadian Association of Occupational Therapists 1997 Enabling occupation. Canadian Association of Occupational Therapists, Ottawa, Ontario

Carlen P L, Wall P D, Nadvorna H, Steinbach T 1978 Phantom limbs and related phenomena in recent traumatic amputations. Neurology 28: 211–217

Clark H W, Sees K L 1993 Opioids, chronic pain and the law. Journal of Pain and Symptom Management 8: 297–305

Gostin L O 1997 Deciding life and death in the courtroom. From Quinlan to Cruzan, Glucksberg, and Vacco – a brief history and analysis of constitutional protection of the 'right to die'. Journal of the American Medical Association 278: 1523–1528

Grossman S A 1993 Undertreatment of cancer pain: barriers and remedies. Supportive Care in Cancer 1: 74–78

Haugen P S 1997 Pain relief. Legal aspects of pain relief for the dying. Minnesota Medicine 80: 15–18

Hill C S Jr 1992 The intractable pain treatment act of Texas. Texas Medicine 88(2): 70–72

Hyman C S 1996 Pain management and disciplinary action: how medical boards can remove barriers to effective treatments. Journal of Law, Medicine & Ethics 24: 338–343

Johnson S H 1996 Disciplinary actions and pain relief: analysis of the Pain Relief Act. Journal of Law, Medicine & Ethics 24: 319–327

Kuhse H, Singer P, Baume P, Clark M, Rickard M 1997 End-of- life decisions in Australian medical practice. Medical Journal of Australia 166: 191–196

Law M, Polatajko H, Baptiste S, Townsend E 1997 Core concepts of occupational therapy. In: Canadian Association of Occupational Therapists (ed) Enabling occupation. Canadian Association of Occupational Therapists, Ottawa, Ontario: 29–56

Loeser J D, Melzack R 1999 Pain: an overview. The Lancet 353 (May 8): 1607–1609

Mausner J S, Kramer S 1985 Epidemiology: an introductory text, 2nd edn. Saunders Company, Toronto

McCaffery M, Beebe A 1989 Pain: Clinical Manual for Nursing Practice. C V Mosby, St Louis

McGrath P J, Unruh A 1993 Social and legal issues. In: Anand K J S, McGrath P J (eds) Pain in the neonate. Elsevier, Amsterdam

Melzack R, Katz J 1994 Pain measurement in persons in pain. In: Wall P D, Melzack R (eds) Textbook of pain 3rd Edn. Churchill Livingstone, New York: 337–351

Melzack R, Torgerson W S 1971 On the language of pain. Anesthesiology 34: 50–59

Melzack R, Wall P D 1988 The challenge of pain. Penguin Books, London

Melzack R, Wall P D, Ty T C 1982 Acute pain in an emergency clinic: latency of onset and descriptor patterns. Pain 14: 33–43

Mendelson G, Mendelson D 1991 Legal aspects of the management of chronic pain. Medical Journal of Australia 155: 640–643

Merskey H 1988 Regional pain is rarely hysterical. Archives of Neurology 45: 915–918

Merskey H, Bogduk N 1994 Classification of chronic pain. Definitions of Chronic Pain Syndromes and Definition of Pain Terms, 2nd Edn. International Association for the Study of Pain, Seattle

Portenoy R K 1996 Opioid therapy for chronic nonmalignant pain: clinician's perspective. Journal of Law, Medicine & Ethics 24: 296–309

Shapiro R S 1996 Health care providers' liability exposure for inappropriate pain management. Journal of Law, Medicine & Ethics 24: 360–364

Somerville M 1993 Pain, suffering and ethics. Abstracts, VIIth World Congress on Pain in Paris. International Association for the Study of Pain, Seattle

Stedman T L 1982 Illustrated Medical Dictionary, 24th edn. Williams & Wilkins, Baltimore

Takeda F 1991 Changing attitudes towards narcotic use in cancer pain management in Japan. Postgraduate Medical Journal 67 (Suppl 2): S31–34

Townsend E 1998 Occupational therapy language: Matters of respect, accountability and leadership. Canadian Journal of Occupational Therapy 65: 45–50

van Thiel G J, van Delden J J, de Haan K, Huibers A K 1997 Retrospective study of doctors' 'end of life decisions' in caring for mentally handicapped people in institutions in The Netherlands. British Medical Journal 315(7100): 88–91

Unruh A M, Ritchie J A 1998 Development of the Pain Appraisal Inventory: psychometric properties. Pain Research and Management 3: 105–110

Unruh A M, Ritchie J A, Merskey H 1999 Does gender affect appraisal of pain and pain coping strategies? Clinical Journal of Pain 15: 31–40

Wall P D 1989 Introduction. In: Wall P D, Melzack R (eds) Textbook of Pain, 3rd edn. Churchill Livingstone, New York, pp 1–7

Weissman D E 1993 Doctors, opioids, and the law: the effect of controlled substances regulations on cancer pain. Seminars in Oncology 20(2 Suppl 1): 53–58

Ziegler D K 1997 Opioids in headache treatment. Is there a role? Neurologic Clinics 15: 199–207

2

Neuroanatomy of the nociceptive system

Mary P. Galea

OVERVIEW

This chapter is concerned specifically with the nervous system structures involved in nociception. The historical framework for studying pain has implied that there is a sensory channel for pain in the manner of sensory channels for other sensations (Willis & Coggeshall 1991). It will be clear from the following review that this is not strictly the case, and that pain is a complex multidimensional phenomenon, with pain signals being transmitted to many different regions of the nervous system. Melzack and Casey (1968) suggested that pain needs to be considered in three interacting dimensions: sensory–discriminative, cognitive–evaluative and motivational–affective. The sensory dimension refers to the capacity to analyse the intensity, location, quality and behaviour of pain. The cognitive–evaluative dimension is concerned with the phenomena of anticipation, attention, suggestion and the influence of previous experience and knowledge. Finally, the motivational–affective dimension is the emotional response (fear, anxiety) that controls responses to pain. A study of the anatomical connections of the nociceptive system provides a framework for understanding how all these dimensions of pain are registered and interact within the nervous system.

The physiological basis of nociception, particularly the mechanisms of signalling and modulating nociceptive stimuli will be covered more specifically in the next chapter. For the definitions and acronyms used in this chapter, refer to Box 2.1.

Learning objectives

At the end of this chapter, students will:

1. Appreciate the different types of peripheral nociceptors and their associated axons.

Box 2.1 Definitions and abbreviations

Key terms

Aδ fibre – small diameter myelinated afferent axon

C-fibre – unmyelinated afferent axon

Catecholamines – the neurotransmitters dopamine, adrenaline (epinephrine) and noradrenaline (norepinephrine)

Modulation – a term used to indicate the actions of neurotransmitters that do not directly evoke postsynaptic potentials in a neuron, but which modify its responses to other synaptic inputs

Neurotransmitter – a chemical that is released by a presynaptic element following stimulation and which activates postsynaptic receptors

Nociceptor – a receptor preferentially sensitive to noxious stimuli or to stimuli that would become noxious if prolonged

Polymodal nociceptor – a nociceptor that is responsive to a range of stimuli (mechanical, thermal, chemical)

Receptive field – the region of a sensory surface (e.g. skin) that, when stimulated, changes the membrane potential of a neuron

Sensitization – an increased responsiveness to stimuli

Acronyms

AMH receptor – A-fibre mechano-heat-sensitive receptor

CGRP – calcitonin gene-related peptide (neurotransmitter)

CL – central lateral nucleus of thalamus

CMH receptor – C-fibre mechano-heat-sensitive receptor

GABA – γ-aminobutyric acid (an inhibitory neurotransmitter)

HTM – high threshold mechanoreceptor

LTM neurons – low threshold mechanosensitive neurons that are only excited by low-threshold innocuous stimuli such as hair movement, touching or brushing the skin

MIA – mechanically insensitive afferent

NS neurons – nociceptive-specific neurons that are excited solely by nociceptors

PAD – primary afferent depolarization

PAG – periaqueductal grey

SI – primary somatosensory cortex

SII – secondary somatosensory cortex

SP – substance P (neurotransmitter)

VA – ventral anterior nucleus of thalamus

VIP – vasoactive intestinal peptide (neurotransmitter)

VL – ventral lateral nucleus of thalamus

VPL – ventral postero-lateral nucleus of thalamus

VPI – ventral posterior-inferior nucleus of thalamus

WDR neurons – wide dynamic range neurons responding to both nociceptive and mechanoreceptive input

WGA-HRP – wheatgerm agglutinin conjugated to horseradish peroxidase (an enzyme). This is taken up and transported by axons and is used to trace anatomical connections within the nervous system

---

2. Understand the organization of the dorsal horn and the termination patterns of afferent inputs.
3. Understand the pathways involved in transmitting nociceptive information within the nervous system.
4. Understand the areas of the nervous system involved in the perception, integration and response to nociception.

STRUCTURE AND FUNCTION OF PERIPHERAL NOCICEPTORS

A receptor is specialized nervous tissue sensitive to a particular change in the environment. A change in the environment provides the stimulus. Normally, a receptor responds preferentially only to one type of stimulus, called the 'adequate stimulus', not in the sense of magnitude, but rather its specificity to that receptor. Receptors convert the physical energy of the adequate stimulus into electrochemical energy that activates the associated neuron.

'Nociceptors' respond to tissue-damaging or potentially tissue-damaging stimuli (from Latin *nocere*, to injure). The skin is densely innervated by nociceptors, which are present in other body tissues, including bone, muscle, joint capsules, viscera and blood vessels, as well as the meninges and peripheral nerve sheaths. Nociceptors have not been found in articular cartilage, synovial membranes, lung parenchyma, visceral pleura, pericardium, brain or spinal cord tissue. The simplest type of sensory receptor has been called the 'free nerve ending', which terminates in a naked unmyelinated ending in cutaneous or other tissue. Historically, free nerve endings have been believed to subserve only pain, but this is not the case. Moreover, more recent studies of the ultrastructure of these receptors have indicated that their structure is more complex than this descriptive term implies. This will be considered further below.

The inference that specialized nociceptors existed was made on the basis of experiments on peripheral nerves in man, using graded electrical stimulation and differential nerve blocks (Adrian 1931, Bessou & Perl 1969, Burgess & Perl 1967). These experiments also indicated that pain was signalled by two sets of afferent fibres:

- Small-diameter thinly myelinated fibres (Aδ) with a conduction velocity of 5–30 metres/second. Activation of these fibres is associated with well-localized sensations of sharp, pricking pain.

- Small-diameter, unmyelinated C fibres that conduct slowly (0.5–2 metres/second). These fibres carry diffuse pain sensations that can be dull, poorly localized and persistent (Torebjörk & Ochoa 1980).

This terminology is used in relation to cutaneous and visceral axons (Erlanger & Gasser 1937). A different terminology applies in the case of muscle and joint nerves (Table 2.1).

Cutaneous nociceptors

Mechanical nociceptors (high threshold mechanoreceptors, HTM, Burgess & Perl 1967) respond to strong mechanical stimuli, but not to heat, irritant chemicals or extreme cold (in normal skin). These units respond with a slowly-adapting discharge to strong punctate pressure. In undamaged skin, they do not respond to heat or cold or to chemicals, and do not have any ongoing background firing. Their receptive fields are distinctive, consisting of a series of sensitive points that may be spread evenly over an area of several square centimetres in proximal areas. In distal areas, such as the glabrous skin of the hands and feet, or on the face, receptive fields are smaller and may comprise only a single point. These units have myelinated axons (Aδ) with a conducting speed of 5–25 metres/second, but with a few conducting more quickly in the Aα or Aβ range. This type of unit has

been found in hairy skin of several species (monkey, cat, rabbit and rat). Its terminals remain ensheathed by Schwann cell processes until they penetrate the epidermal basal lamina, suggesting that the term 'free nerve endings' for these nociceptive terminals is not appropriate (Kruger et al 1981). Mechanical nociceptors of this type are densely distributed over the skin (Table 2.2).

Mechanical nociceptors with C-axons have also been found, but there is little information about them. They lack the distinctive multipoint receptive fields of the large diameter units; instead their fields usually consist of a small zone of uniform sensitivity (Iggo 1960, Lynn 1984).

Polymodal nociceptors also respond to strong mechanical stimuli, and in addition, to noxious heat and to irritant chemicals, and sometimes to strong skin cooling. Bessou and Perl (1969) have shown that these are the predominant type of C-fibre nociceptor in mammalian skin, comprising about 90% of all afferent C-fibres. Since most systematic studies of nociceptors have involved the use of mechanical or heat stimuli, the terminology of AMH and CMH is now used to refer to A-fibre mechano-heat-sensitive nociceptors, and C-fibre mechano-heat-sensitive nociceptors respectively (Meyer et al 1994).

A-fibre mechano-heat receptors have been classified into two types. Type I AMHs have very high heat thresholds, usually 53°C or higher, are slowly adapting

Table 2.1 Classifications of mammalian nerve fibres used in the literature

Fibre type (Erlanger & Gasser 1937)	Function	Group (Lloyd 1943)	Function	Average fibre diameter (µm)	Average conduction velocity (m/s)
Aα	Primary muscle spindle afferents, motor fibres to motor neurons	I	Primary muscle spindle afferents	15	95
Aβ	Cutaneous touch and pressure afferents	II	Afferents from tendon organs, afferents from cutaneous mechanoreceptors	8	50
Aγ	Motor fibres to muscle spindles	–	–	6	20
Aδ	Cutaneous temperature and pain afferents	III	Afferents from deep pressure receptors in muscle	3	15
B	Sympathetic preganglionic fibres	– –	–	3	7
C	Cutaneous pain afferents (unmyelinated); sympathetic postganglionic fibres	IV	Unmyelinated nerve fibres	0.5	1

Table 2.2   Properties of nociceptors

Properties	Mechanical nociceptor (HTM)	Polymodal nociceptor
Axon size	$A\delta$	C
Stimulus	Pressure	Pressure
		Pinch
		Thermal
		Chemical (K^+ ions, histamine)
Neurotransmitter	L-glutamate	Substance P
		CGRP
Sensation	'First' (fast) pain	'Second' (slow) pain
	Well-localized	Diffuse
	Sharp	Dull
	Prickling	Aching
		Burning

(Treede et al 1991) and are prevalent in the glabrous skin of the primate hand (Campbell et al 1979). Type II AMHs have a substantially lower threshold and slower conduction velocity than Type I AMHs. They have been found in hairy skin and are thought to signal first pain sensation (Dubner et al 1977).

The chemosensitivity of C-polymodal nociceptors has not been studied to the same extent as their sensitivity to heat and pressure. They can be excited by potassium, histamine, serotonin, bradykinin, capsaicin, mustard oil, acetylcholine and dilute acids, by various means (topical application, intradermal injection, arterial injection), and all in doses that would be painful in man (see Willis & Coggeshall 1991 for review). Chemicals act on nociceptors by altering the conductance of ion channels in the cell membrane and causing depolarization (Rang et al 1991). This may result in sensitization of the nociceptors, such that they have an increased responsiveness to stimulation. Further information on peripheral sensitization will be presented in Chapter 3.

Cold nociceptors, transmitting along C-fibres, have been reported in the monkey (LaMotte & Thalhammer 1982) and in humans (Campero et al 1996). These respond strongly to prolonged cooling of the skin by ice and weakly to strong pressure, but are not responsive to heat. Cutaneous $A\delta$ nociceptors also respond to temperatures below 0°C and encode stimulus intensity (Simone & Kajander 1997). Cold pain is thought to be mediated by nociceptors located in cutaneous veins (Klement & Arndt 1992).

Mechanically insensitive afferents A good proportion of $A\delta$-fibre nociceptors and C-fibre nociceptors do not respond to or have very high thresholds for mechanical stimuli. This group is referred to as mechanically-insensitive afferents (MIAs). They have been reported in the knee joint (Schaible and Schmidt 1985), viscera (Häbler et al 1990) and cornea (Tanelian 1991). Some of the cutaneous MIAs may be chemospecific receptors, while others may respond to intense cold or heat stimuli (Meyer et al 1991). These receptors may become sensitized to mechanical stimuli after cutaneous injury or after joint inflammation.

Skeletal muscle nociceptors

The terminology of Lloyd (1943) is usually used in relation to muscle and joint nerves (Table 2.1). Group III afferent fibres are small diameter myelinated fibres; group IV fibres are unmyelinated. Numerous unencapsulated endings can be located in the connective tissue and in the wall of arterioles in skeletal muscle, and can be subdivided into mechanical and polymodal types (Stacey 1969). Effective stimuli are high intensity mechanical forces, as well as endogenous pain-producing substances such as bradykinin, serotonin and potassium ions. Hypoxia and impaired metabolism following trauma or unaccustomed exercise and increased levels of adrenaline may also activate nociceptors (Kieschke et al 1988, Mense 1993). Group III afferent fibres are responsive to mechanical stimulation of muscle, including stretch (Mense & Stahnke 1983), and many would be activated by exercise and therefore probably function as ergoreceptors. However, a significant proportion of these are nociceptive. Some group III afferents are responsive to the injection of chemicals such as hypertonic sodium chloride (Abrahams et al 1984). Few group IV afferents respond to muscle stretch or contraction, however some respond vigorously when muscle contractions occur during ischaemia (Mense & Meyer 1985), and many are readily activated by pain-producing chemicals (Mense & Meyer 1988) or thermal stimuli (Hertel et al 1976). Studies in humans have indicated that muscle nociceptors are sensitive to innocuous and noxious pressure in the projected area of pain induced by intraneural microstimulation (Simone et al 1994).

Joint nociceptors

Nociceptors in joints are located in the joint capsule and ligaments, bone, periosteum, articular fat pads and around blood vessels, but not in the joint cartilage. They have been studied predominantly in the knee joint. The terminals of group III and group IV sensory nerve endings comprise multiple axonal beads ensheathed by Schwann cell processes, except for some areas of exposed axon membrane containing structural specializations characteristic of receptive sites. The beads thus represent multiple receptive sites (Heppelmann et al 1990). Some of these receptors may be nociceptive.

Joint nociceptors can be classified as:

- High threshold units that discharge only in response to noxious pressure or extreme joint movement (Bessou & Laporte 1961)
- Units that respond to strong pressure but not to movement
- Units that do not respond to any mechanical stimulus in the normal joint (silent nociceptors) (Schaible & Schmidt 1988).

In the normal joint, only the first type are activated, but all joint afferents become sensitized if the joint becomes inflamed (see Chapter 3).

Visceral nociceptors

In somatic tissue such as skin and muscle there is a clear distinction between mechanoreceptive and nociceptive afferents. However, this is not the case in visceral tissue, for which pain may not be reported even in response to tissue-damaging stimuli. Nociceptors are located in visceral organs including the heart, gastrointestinal tract and reproductive organs and in the walls of blood vessels. Pain-producing stimuli in the viscera include inflammation, distension of hollow muscular-walled organs such as the gastrointestinal tract, the urinary tract and the gall bladder, ischaemia in organs such as the heart, and traction in the mesentery. Inflammation of visceral organs can induce central sensitization (see Chapter 3) of dorsal horn neurons and may lead to referred hyperalgesia. Visceral nociceptors are also sensitive to irritating chemicals. Afferent nociceptive fibres in viscera are found in association with both sympathetic and parasympathetic efferents (Meyer et al 1994)

ANATOMY OF REFERRED PAIN

The pain from stimulation of viscera is frequently localized to the surface of the body, a phenomenon termed 'referred pain'. This may be explained by the convergence of nociceptive input from deep and cutaneous tissues onto common somatosensory spinal neurons that also receive afferents from topographically separate body regions (the so-called projection–convergence theory, Ruch 1946). There are no separate ascending spinal pathways dedicated to the signalling of sensations from the viscera. These sensations are represented within the known somatosensory pathways. The level of the spinal cord to which visceral afferent fibres from the internal organs project depends on their embryonic innervation. Many viscera migrate well away from their embryonic origin during development, and therefore referred pain from the viscera may be perceived at locations remote from the actual site of the stimulus. For example, the heart is derived from endoderm in the neck and upper thorax, with the result that nociceptive afferents from the heart enter the spinal cord through the dorsal roots C3–T5 rather than lower down. Similarly, afferents from the gall bladder enter the spinal cord at T9 rather than at L1, its location later in life. The pain signals carried by these fibres may be referred to the areas of skin via Aδ fibres to the same segment of the spinal cord. Hence, a heart attack causing ischaemia of cardiac muscle can often present as pain in the left shoulder passing into the left arm (the cutaneous segments supplied by C3–T5). In the same way, an inflamed gall bladder can frequently cause pain at the tip of the right scapula, supplied by T9.

Pain may also be referred from tissues other than viscera, and frequently occurs in musculoskeletal conditions. This type of referred pain has been explained with reference to patterns of dermatomal, myotomal and sclerotomal territories. However, there is enormous individual variation in these territories, as well as variability in presenting symptoms (Grieve 1994).

DORSAL ROOT GANGLION CELLS

The somas of nociceptive afferents are located in the dorsal root ganglia (DRG) and the equivalent ganglia of cranial nerves V, VII, IX and X. DRG cells are pseudo-unipolar neurons conveying information from the periphery into the spinal cord. These cells can be grouped into two classes based on variations in soma size, diameter of axons, morphology of peripheral terminals and site of central terminations. The division into two size classes has a functional correlate in that, generally, large cells giving rise to large diameter axons relay low threshold mechanical and proprioceptive stimuli, and small cells relay nociceptive and thermal stimuli (Lawson 1992). Small DRG cells stain intensely and contain many organelles and peptides, including substance P (SP), somatostatin, calcitonin gene-related peptide (CGRP), vasoactive intestinal peptide (VIP) and galanin (Willis & Coggeshall 1991).

PRIMARY AFFERENTS

As primary afferent fibres in peripheral nerves travel towards the spinal cord, they group together to form spinal nerves, each spinal nerve supplying a discrete area of skin (dermatome), and overlapping to a greater or lesser degree the dermatomes of neighbouring spinal nerves. Each spinal nerve splits to form a ventral and dorsal root. The dorsal roots are purely sensory, but a considerable number of small diameter unmyelinated afferent fibres are located in the ventral root (ventral root afferents, Coggeshall et al 1974, Light & Metz 1978). The majority of these fibres appear to end blindly, with the rest either looping within the ventral roots or branching into the dorsal root (Willis & Coggeshall 1991). The function of the ventral root afferents is, as yet, unclear.

Sorting of primary afferent fibres occurs in the dorsal roots in primates (Snyder 1977). Large diameter afferents subserving mechanoreception enter the spinal cord in the medial division of the dorsal root, while small diameter fibres form a lateral bundle. The fibres enter the cord at the dorsal root entry zone. The bundle of small diameter fibres contains those involved in nociception, together with fibres involved in temperature and visceral sensation. They divide into short ascending and descending branches that run longitudinally in the dorsolateral fasciculus of Lissauer. Within several segments they leave the tract to synapse on neurons in the dorsal horn.

THE DORSAL HORN

The dorsal horn of the spinal cord is the first site for integration and processing of incoming sensory information. The dorsal horn has historically been divided into three broad regions: the marginal zone, the substantia gelatinosa and the nucleus proprius. Rexed (1952, 1954) divided the grey matter of the dorsal horn into six laminae based on cytoarchitectural criteria, the most dorsal being lamina I (Fig. 2.1). Further anatomical and physiological studies have since confirmed functional differences in dorsal horn neurons in different laminae, as well as different patterns of projections. In addition, cells, axons and terminals in the different laminae of the dorsal horn have a distinctive chemical profile which has been shown to change following a lesion (see Willis & Coggeshall 1991, for review).

Primary afferent fibres terminate in different laminae depending on their function (Fig. 2.2). Lamina I (the marginal zone) contains a high density of projection neurons that process nociceptive information. There are nociceptive-specific neurons that are excited solely by nociceptors, and wide dynamic range neurons (also in lamina V–VI), which respond to both nociceptive and mechanoreceptive input.

Lamina II is also called the substantia gelatinosa. The most prominent structures in lamina II are complex structures called glomeruli, through which a primary afferent terminal can make synaptic contact with several peripheral dendrites, axonal terminals and cell bodies (Kerr 1975). Glomeruli are key structures of the dorsal horn because they offer a morphological basis for both presynaptic and postsynaptic modulation of the primary afferent input. They comprise a central

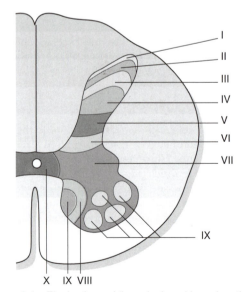

Figure 2.1 The laminae of the spinal cord based on the description of Rexed (1952, 1954). Laminae I–VI make up the dorsal horn.

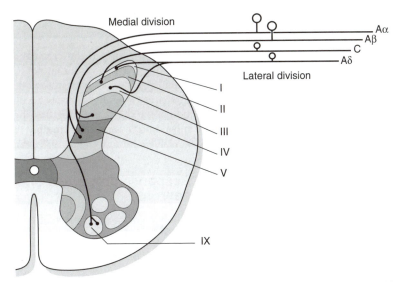

Figure 2.2 The terminations of afferent fibres in the dorsal horn vary by depth. Large fibres (Aα and Aβ) enter in the medial division and small fibres (Aδ and C) enter in the lateral division of the dorsal root.

primary afferent terminal that makes contact with a group of between four and eight surrounding dendrites and other peripheral axon terminals, and are set apart from the surrounding tissue by glial processes (Fig. 2.3). Using morphological criteria, the peripheral terminals appear to have the characteristics of inhibitory synapses and may contain the inhibitory neurotransmitters γ-aminobutyric acid (GABA) or enkephalin. The central terminals have the characteristics of excitatory terminals and may contain CGRP, glutamate, SP, cholecystokinin, or serotonin. The glomerulus therefore comprises a complicated arrangement of inhibitory synaptic terminals surrounding an excitatory primary afferent ending.

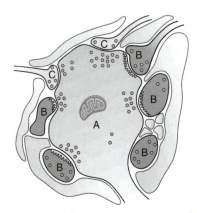

Figure 2.3 Diagram of a glomerulus based on the work of Kerr (1975). A = central terminal, B = dendrites, C = dendritic spines from lamina II neurons. Shaded areas represent glial processes.

The neuropil of lamina III resembles that of lamina II, but has slightly larger cells and myelinated axons. Laminae IV and V are characterized by neurons of various sizes. Lamina IV has prominent large cells, while lamina V is distinguished by longitudinally-oriented myelinated axons. Laminae III, IV and the upper part of lamina V comprise most of the nucleus proprius.

Lamina VI is present only in cervical and lumbosacral enlargements and is a transition zone between the primary afferent-dominated dorsal horn and the ventral horn, with descending input predominating.

A population of neurons responding to noxious mechanical and thermal stimuli has been reported in lamina X in the vicinity of the central canal of the spinal cord. In addition to these high threshold type cells, lamina X also contains neurons that are low threshold and have a wide dynamic range. Many of the cells have convergent input from visceral afferent fibres, and some of these respond only to visceral stimuli (Honda 1985, Honda & Perl 1985)

Terminations of afferent fibres in the dorsal horn

The incoming afferent fibres of all types establish a web of connections with dorsal horn neurons, exerting a changing pattern of excitatory and inhibitory inputs that determines the firing of dorsal horn projection neurons and of interneurons that mediate spinal reflex responses (Table 2.3). Normally there is a certain

Table 2.3 Terminations of afferent fibres in the dorsal horn

Afferents	Terminal zones in dorsal horn
Large diameter myelinated fibres	III, IV and V
Small diameter myelinated fibres (Aδ)	I and V
Unmyelinated fibres (C)	II, III
Visceral projections	II, IV–V and X

degree of segregation in the termination pattern for different afferent fibre classifications in the dorsal horn, however this may not be the case in pathological situations. Woolf et al (1992) showed that peripheral nerve injury triggers sprouting of myelinated afferents into lamina II, resulting in the possibility of functional contacts of low threshold mechanoreceptive afferents with cells that normally have only C-fibre input.

Large diameter myelinated fibres

Collaterals of the large Aβ fibres initially travel ventrally through the dorsal horn but reverse when they reach the deeper laminae, and break up to give rise to large flame-shaped arbours as they course dorsally. These terminations are dense in laminae III, IV and V. It has been shown that the distal parts of the arbours of hair-follicle afferents enter the innermost part of lamina II (Brown 1981).

Small diameter myelinated fibres

Collaterals of Aδ fibres terminate both superficially and deep within the dorsal horn. High threshold afferents terminate profusely with arborizations in lamina I. Low threshold hair afferents pass through lamina I to terminate in lamina V (Mense & Prabhakar 1986).

Unmyelinated fibres

Unmyelinated afferents terminate in the superficial dorsal horn. Lamina II is the site of termination of primary afferent fibres from the skin, with visceral afferents terminating in laminae I and II with some extension to lamina III (Gobel et al 1981, LaMotte 1977).

Visceral projections

Visceral afferent fibres terminate predominantly in lamina I, but have also been reported in laminae II, IV–V and X (Sugiura et al 1989).

Somatotopic organization of the dorsal horn

The dorsal horn in the cervical and lumbar enlargements appears to be somatotopically organized, with distal regions being represented medially and proximal areas laterally. There is a rostrocaudal representation of the digits, with the first digit being represented most rostrally and the fifth digit most caudally (Brown et al 1989, Florence et al 1988, Wilson et al 1986).

Response properties of dorsal horn neurons

Three major classes of dorsal horn neurons have been recognized (McMahon 1984):

1. Low threshold mechanosensitive (LTM), in which the cells are only excited by low threshold innocuous stimuli such as hair movement, touching or brushing the skin
2. Nociceptive-specific (NS), where only high threshold noxious or near-noxious levels of peripheral stimulation excite the cells
3. Wide dynamic range (WDR) or convergent cells, where the firing rate of the cells is increased by innocuous events, but further increased when stimulus intensity is raised to noxious levels.

This classification does not imply that each class of neurons is homogeneous. The properties of neurons in the dorsal horn depend to some extent on their location. A large proportion of lamina I neurons is NS (Christensen & Perl 1970), but WDR cells form the largest proportion of neurons in this lamina. The dendrites of lamina I cells remain within the lamina and these cells give rise to an ascending projection to the thalamus (Carstens & Trevino 1978). Lamina II cells are predominantly of the WDR type, while lamina III cells are predominantly LTM. Neither lamina II nor lamina III neurons give rise to ascending projections.

Wall (1967) demonstrated that lamina IV cells were predominantly of the LTM type and often received input from large diameter afferents only. Their receptive fields, located in distal regions of the body, tend to be smaller and have distinct edges. In lamina V, all three classes of cells are represented, but the WDR type more frequently. Many of these cells have long ascending axons that reach supraspinal levels, some of them directly reaching the thalamus. WDR cells are excited by C-fibres as well as by A-fibres, and this input reaches them either via lamina II cells or by synapses on their distant dendrites. Many lamina V cells have dendrites which reach lamina II.

SPINAL CORD TRANSMISSION PATHWAYS

Ascending tracts

Somatosensory signals are conveyed along two major ascending systems in the spinal cord, the anterolateral system, and the dorsal column–medial lemniscal system. The latter carries information about tactile sensation and limb proprioception. The anterolateral system relays information predominantly about pain and temperature, but also some tactile information. It comprises three pathways: the spinothalamic tract, the spinoreticular tract, and the spinomesencephalic tract (Fig. 2.4)

The spinothalamic tract (STT) originates from neurons along the length of the spinal cord with a particularly large concentration of STT cells in the uppermost cervical segments, including a large ipsilateral group of neurons in the ventral horn. Below this level, the majority of STT neurons are contralateral to their target. In the primate, STT neurons are located in three main regions, laminae I, V and VII–VIII, and comprise both nociceptive-specific and wide dynamic range neurons. Some STT neurons are also in laminae II, III and X (Apkarian & Hodge 1989a).

The axons cross the midline in the ventral white commissure at a level near the cell body and ascend to the thalamus in the lateral funiculus on the contralateral side. While most of the axons occupy the ventral lateral quadrant of the spinal white matter, some axons, particularly those originating from lamina I cells, ascend in the dorsal lateral quadrant (Apkarian & Hodge 1989b). The STT in the lateral funiculus has a somatotopic organization. Axons from the most caudal regions of the spinal cord occupy the most dorsolateral position, with axons from progressively more rostral levels joining the tract in more ventromedial positions (Applebaum et al 1975).

In the brain stem the STT passes dorsolateral to the inferior olivary nucleus in the medulla, then ascends dorsolateral to the medial lemniscus, through higher levels of the brain stem to the thalamus. The spinothalamic tract transmits nociceptive and thermal information, as well as touch sensations.

The spinoreticular tract (SRT) in the primate originates from neurons in laminae VII and VIII, as well as the lateral part of lamina V. Some neurons are in lamina X. The majority of neurons giving rise to the SRT are in the uppermost cervical segments, although

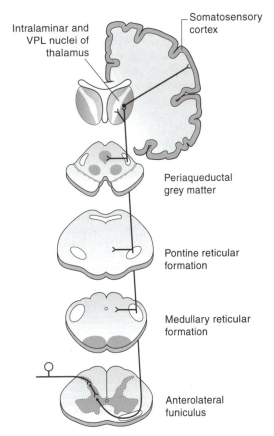

Figure 2.4 Organization of the anterolateral system. Primary axons terminate in the dorsal horn. Second-order axons cross the midline and ascend in the anterolateral funiculus in the spinal cord and the spinal lemniscus in the brainstem to terminate in the thalamus. Collaterals of these axons terminate in the reticular formation (spinoreticular axons) and in the periaqueductal grey matter (spinomesencephalic axons) (shaded). Thalamocortical axons then project to the somatosensory cortex.

cells from all levels of the spinal cord are involved (Kevetter et al 1982). There are two components: a projection to the lateral reticular nucleus (a precerebellar nucleus) and a projection to the pontine and medullary reticular formation, which give rise to descending pathways to the spinal cord.

Most of the projections from the cervical and lumbar enlargements cross the midline near the level of the cell bodies, however some axons originating from cervical segments remain uncrossed. They ascend in the ventral lateral column of the spinal cord with the STT and form a prominent bundle lateral to it in the brain stem.

The SRT has no obvious somatotopic organization, and terminates in the following nuclei of the reticular formation: nucleus medullae oblongatae centralis, lateral reticular nucleus, nucleus reticularis gigantocellularis, nucleus reticularis pontis caudalis and oralis, nucleus paragigantocellularis dorsalis and lateralis, and nucleus subcoeruleus (Mehler et al 1960).

The spinomesencephalic tract (SMT) is a collection of pathways from the spinal cord to several different midbrain nuclei. It originates primarily from neurons in laminae I, V, VII and X (Zhang et al 1990). The majority of axons cross the midline and ascend with the STT and SRT in the ventral lateral column. The SMT projects to the nucleus cuneiformis, the parabrachial nucleus, the intercollicular nucleus, the deep layers of the superior colliculus, the nucleus of Darkschewitsch, the anterior and posterior pretectal nuclei, the red nucleus, the Edinger–Westphal nucleus, the interstitial nucleus of Cajal and the periaqueductal grey (Yezierski 1988).

The SMT is roughly somatotopically organized, with the projection from the cervical enlargement terminating more rostrally than that from the lumbosacral region. The periaqueductal grey contains neurons that are part of a descending pathway that regulates pain transmission.

Other tracts in the dorsolateral funiculus and the dorsal columns also convey nociceptive information (Fig. 2.5).

The spinocervical tract (SCT) originates from laminae III and IV at all levels of the cord where neurons respond predominantly to tactile stimuli, but some are activated by noxious stimuli. The axons project ipsilaterally in the dorsolateral funiculus to the lateral cervical nucleus, located just ventrolateral to the dorsal horn in segments C1–C3. The lateral cervical nucleus is quite small in the primate (Mizuno et al 1967), and may be present in some humans, although it is possible that the nucleus may not be distinctly separate from the dorsal horn in some cases (Ha & Morin 1964, Kircher & Ha 1968, Truex et al 1965). Most of the neurons in the lateral cervical nucleus cross the midline in the ventral white commissure and ascend in the medial lemniscus to midbrain nuclei and to the thalamus.

The dorsal column–medial lemniscal system consists of branches of primary afferent fibres conveying tactile and proprioceptive information, as well as the axons of neurons in laminae IV–VI. However, recent reports indicate that there are unmyelinated primary afferent fibres that synapse in the dorsal column nuclei, presumably arising from nociceptors (Patterson et al 1990).

In addition, there is a visceral pain pathway ascending in the dorsal column (Al-Chaer et al 1998, Hirschberg et al 1996, Willis et al 1999). The medially located fasciculus gracilis contains a representation of

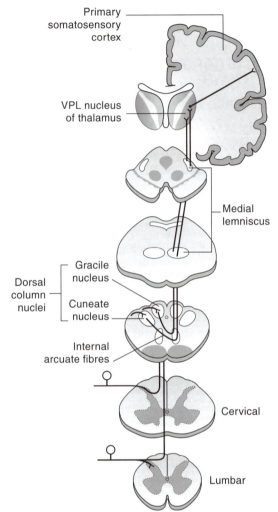

Figure 2.5 Organization of the dorsal column-medial lemniscal system. Large-diameter axons enter the spinal cord and ascend in the dorsal columns to the medulla, where they synapse in the dorsal column nuclei (nucleus gracilis and nucleus cuneatus). Second-order axons cross the midline and ascend in the medial lemniscus to terminate in the VPL nucleus of the thalamus. Thalamocortical axons then project to the somatosensory cortex.

the lower part of the trunk and lower extremity, whereas the fasciculus cuneatus lateral to it contains a representation of the upper part of the trunk and the upper extremity. This tract projects to the dorsal column nuclei in the medulla, from which axons ascend in the medial lemniscus to the thalamus. The sensory representation in the dorsal column nuclei is somatotopic with caudal parts of the body represented medially in the nucleus gracilis and the rostral regions laterally in the nucleus cuneatus. The trunk representation is in a region between the two nuclei. The distal extremities are represented dorsally and the proximal body ventrally (Johnson et al 1968).

TRIGEMINAL SYSTEM

Somatic sensation of the head and oral cavity is carried by four cranial nerves: the trigeminal nerve (innervates most of the head and oral cavity); the facial, glossopharyngeal and the vagus (innervate the skin of the external ear, pharynx, nasal cavity and middle ear). The meninges are innervated by the trigeminal and vagus nerves. The trigeminal nerve is the largest cranial nerve with four nuclei: the motor nucleus, the main sensory nucleus, the spinal nucleus and the mesencephalic nucleus. As is the case with sensory inputs to the rest of the body, tactile sensation is mediated by large diameter myelinated fibres, and pain and temperature sensations are mediated by small diameter myelinated and unmyelinated fibres.

The sensory nuclei of the trigeminal nerve consist of three different parts. From caudal to rostral these are the nucleus of the spinal tract, the main or principal sensory nucleus, and the mesencephalic sensory nucleus (Fig. 2.6). The fibres of the sensory root enter the pons and course dorsomedially towards the sensory nucleus. About half the fibres divide into ascending or descending branches as they enter the pons; the remainder ascend or descend without division. Many of the latter are very long and descend as the spinal tract of the trigeminal nerve to the caudal end of the medulla, where it fuses with the dorsolateral tract of Lissauer in the spinal cord. As the tract descends, collaterals are given off to a long nucleus lying immediately medial to it, the nucleus of the spinal tract, which is continuous with the substantia gelatinosa of the dorsal horn. The spinal nucleus extends caudally through the whole length of the medulla and into the spinal cord as far as the second cervical segment. In the medulla, the tract and its nucleus are situated just beneath the surface, with the upper part producing an elevation called the tuberculum cinereum.

Large diameter axons of the trigeminal nerve terminate in the main sensory nucleus. The majority of neurons in the main sensory nucleus give rise to axons that decussate in the pons and ascend dorsomedial to fibres from the dorsal column nuclei in the medial lemniscus. These ascending fibres (the trigeminal lemniscus) synapse in the medial division of the ventral posterior nucleus of the thalamus (VPM). From here, the axons of the thalamic neurons project to the primary somatosensory cortex. This is the principal pathway for tactile perception in the face and is analogous to the dorsal column–medial lemniscal system. The main sensory nucleus of the trigeminal nerve is functionally similar to the dorsal column nuclei.

Pain and temperature are conveyed by smaller diameter fibres terminating in the spinal part of the nucleus. The spinal trigeminal nucleus can be divided into three morphologically different parts: the nucleus caudalis, the nucleus interpolaris and the nucleus oralis. The nucleus caudalis mediates facial sensation. Like the dorsal horn, it plays an important role in pain and temperature senses, including dental pain, and a lesser role in tactile sensation. The nucleus interpolaris plays a role in mediating sensation from the teeth and the nucleus oralis is thought to be involved with discriminative touch sensation.

Structurally and functionally, the nucleus caudalis resembles the dorsal horn on the basis of a number of features: morphology and lamination, laminar distribution of afferent terminals and laminar distribution of projection neurons. The caudal nucleus is sometimes called the medullary dorsal horn (Fig. 2.7) because its laminar organization is similar to the spinal dorsal horn (Dubner & Bennett 1983, Martin 1996).

Lamina I is equivalent to the marginal zone of the dorsal horn, and the portion of the spinal tract overlying lamina I of the spinal nucleus is the rostral extension of Lissauer's tract. Lamina II is equivalent to the substantia gelatinosa, and laminae III and IV, termed the magnocellular nucleus in the trigeminal system, are equivalent to the nucleus proprius. Each of these structures is associated with neurons responding to various types of stimuli. Those in the deep regions respond to both nociceptive and innocuous stimuli (wide dynamic range neurons), while neurons responding specifically to nociceptive or thermal stimuli are located in the substantia gelatinosa. There is an 'onion skin' pattern of representation of parts of the face in the spinal trigeminal nucleus, where regions around the mouth and nose are represented rostrally in the nucleus, while those in more lateral regions of the face are represented more caudally (Brodal 1981).

The ascending pathway from the spinal nucleus (especially the caudal and interpolar regions) mediates facial and dental pain. The organization of this pathway is similar to that of the anterolateral system. This pathway is called the trigeminothalamic tract and

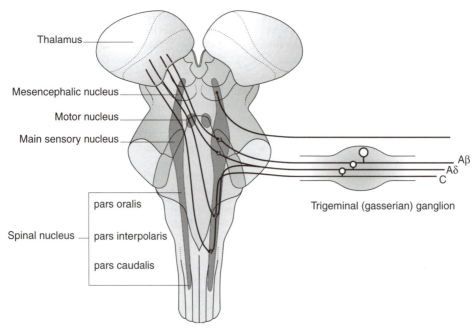

Figure 2.6 Nuclei of the trigeminal nerve and their afferent connections. The cell bodies of most of the primary sensory neurons are in the trigeminal (gasserian) ganglion, with the remainder in the mesencephalic nucleus. Small-diameter fibres subserving pain and temperature enter the spinal nucleus and synapse in the pars caudalis. Second-order axons cross the midline to form the trigeminothalamic tract.

is predominantly crossed, ascending with the axons of the spinothalamic tract to the thalamus.

SYMPATHETIC NERVOUS SYSTEM

The responses of an organism during pain and stress, which consist of autonomic, neuroendocrine and motor responses, are integral components of an adaptive biological system. They are important for the organism to function in a dynamic, challenging and possibly dangerous environment. The typical autonomic responses consist of an activation of various sympathetic pathways to skeletal muscle, skin, heart and viscera, thus leading to an increase of blood flow through skeletal muscle, increased cardiac output, piloerection, sweating and a reduction of bloodflow through skin and viscera (Jänig 1995). Under physiological conditions peripheral sympathetic pathways are distinct with respect to their target organs, and somatosensory pathways are functionally distinct with respect to the peripheral receptors and the corresponding sensations (Jänig 1992). However, following tissue damage this situation may radically change, such that the sympathetic and sensory channels are no longer separated (see below).

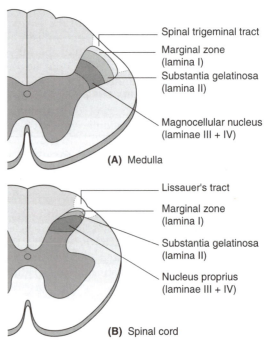

Figure 2.7 **A**. Section through the medulla illustrating the trigeminal dorsal horn. **B**. Corresponding areas of the spinal dorsal horn.

The hypothalamus

The hypothalamus has a major role in producing responses to emotional changes and needs, and is responsible for maintaining homeostasis. Through efferent pathways to autonomic ganglia in the brainstem and spinal cord, the hypothalamus controls sympathetic and parasympathetic functions. The hypothalamus receives inputs from the reticular formation in the brainstem and the amygdala, a collection of nuclei in the temporal lobe that are considered to be part of the limbic system.

The sympathetic pathways from the hypothalamus descend through the brainstem and spinal cord to synapse in the intermediolateral columns of the spinal cord between T1 and L2. In this area are the cell bodies of the preganglionic neurons. The preganglionic axons are myelinated and short (white rami), leaving the CNS via the ventral root and synapsing in the paravertebral sympathetic chain (ganglia). The sympathetic chain extends from the base of the skull to the coccyx (Fig. 2.8). The postganglionic axons are unmyelinated (grey rami) and rejoin the spinal nerves (Fig. 2.9), accompanying the peripheral nerves to innervate the body wall and blood vessels. Sympathetic axons innervating the face and brain arise from the inferior, middle and superior cervical ganglia and follow the carotid and vertebral arteries to their targets.

Clinical observations of changes in skin blood flow, and abnormal sudomotor activity affecting regions beyond the distribution of the injured part, have implicated sympathetic hyperactivity as a factor in neuropathic pain, which is commonly associated with peripheral nerve injury (see Chapter 18). Sympathetic fibre sprouting and hyperactivity might act partly through abnormal connections between sympathetic and sensory neurons.

Using an experimental peripheral nerve lesion model, McLachlan et al (1993) showed that noradrenergic axons in surrounding blood vessels sprout into dorsal root ganglia (on both injured and non-injured sides) and form basket-like structures around large diameter sensory neurons. Following peripheral nerve injury, both intact sensory neurons (Sato & Perl, 1991) and injured or regenerating axons (Wall & Gutnick 1974) develop an ectopic sensitivity to circulating adrenaline and noradrenaline released from postganglionic sympathetic nerve terminals, a process mediated by α-adrenoreceptors (Chen et al 1996) (see Chapter 18).

BRAIN AREAS INVOLVED IN PAIN PERCEPTION, INTEGRATION AND RESPONSE

Thalamus

The thalamus represents the final link in the transmission of impulses to the cerebral cortex, processing almost all sensory and motor information prior to its transfer to cortical areas. The thalamus consists of six groups of nuclei: lateral (ventral and dorsal), medial, anterior, intralaminar, midline and reticular (Fig. 2.10).

- The nuclei of the ventral tier of the lateral group are specific relay nuclei, each receiving specific sensory or motor input and projecting to specific regions of the cerebral cortex. Of this group of nuclei, the ventral posterolateral (VPL) and ventral posteromedial (VPM) nuclei are concerned with sensation from the body and the face respectively, while the ventral anterior (VA) and ventral lateral (VL) nuclei are concerned with motor function.
- The nuclei of the dorsal tier of the lateral group and the nuclei of the medial group (mediodorsal) are association nuclei, projecting to association cortex (prefrontal association cortex, limbic association cortex, parietal–temporal–occipital association cortex).
- The anterior nuclei are specific relay nuclei, with connections to the hypothalamus and the cingulate gyrus.
- The intralaminar, reticular and midline nuclei are non-specific nuclei, with widespread connections. The intralaminar nuclei receive inputs from the reticular formation in the brainstem.

Termination of spinothalamic afferents in the thalamus

Two subdivisions of the thalamic nuclei receive nociceptive input from spinal projection neurons.

The lateral nuclear group

Spinothalamic afferents from the contralateral side of the spinal cord terminate throughout VPL (Berkley 1980, Boivie 1979, Burton & Craig 1983, Mantyh 1983, Ralston & Ralston 1992). The terminals of spinothalamic axons overlap with those of the medial lemniscus in VPL of monkeys (Mehler et al 1960) and extend into the ventral posterior–inferior nucleus (VPI, Gingold et al 1991), rostrally into VL (Applebaum et al 1979, Berkley 1980, Boivie 1979, Burton & Craig 1983, Craig

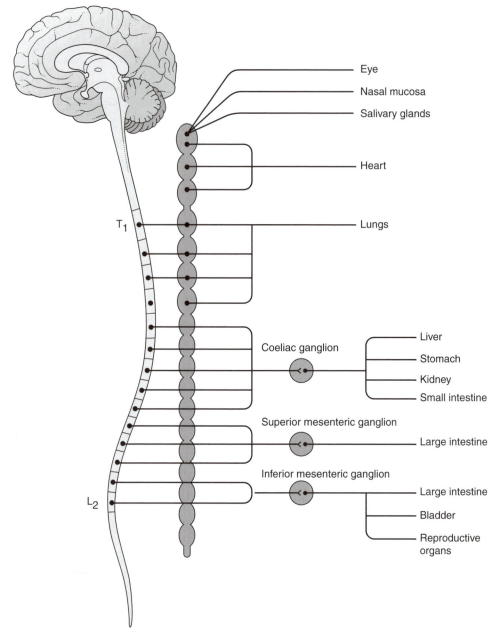

Figure 2.8 Plan of the sympathetic nervous system. Preganglionic neurons are red, postganglionic neurons are blue. The innervation of blood vessels, sweat glands and piloerector muscles is not shown.

& Burton 1981) and caudally into the posterior nuclei (Ralston & Ralston 1992). There is a somatotopic organization of spinothalamic terminals in VPL, which appear to be arranged in clusters across the nucleus (Boivie 1979, Mantyh 1983, Mehler et al 1960).

The receptive fields of thalamic neurons responsive to nociceptive stimuli are small and their discharge frequency can be related to the intensity and duration of the stimulus (Kenshalo et al 1980). These neurons mediate the sensory–discriminative aspects of pain. Neurons in VPI respond to innocuous mechanical stimuli (Kaas et al 1984), as well as to nociceptive stimuli (Casey & Morrow 1987). The spinothalamic inputs to the lateral thalamic nuclei, which have

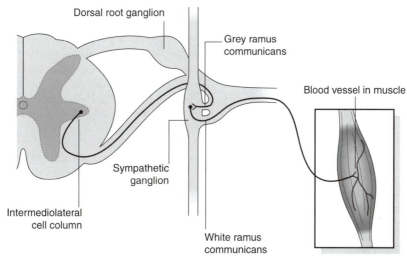

Figure 2.9   Relationship of sympathetic axons with peripheral nerves.

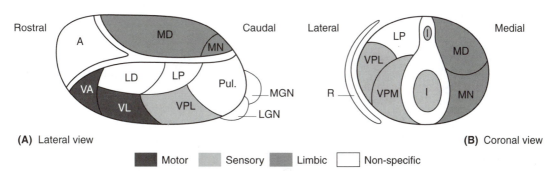

(A) Lateral view

(B) Coronal view

Motor | Sensory | Limbic | Non-specific

Figure 2.10   Nuclei of the thalamus in lateral (**A**) and coronal (**B**) views. Nuclei associated with limbic functions: A = anterior nucleus, MD = mediodorsal nucleus, LD = lateral dorsal nucleus. Nuclei associated with motor functions: VA = ventral anterior nucleus, VL = ventral lateral nucleus. Nuclei associated with sensory functions: VPL = ventral posterolateral nucleus, VPM = ventral posteromedial nucleus, LGN = lateral geniculate nucleus, MGN = medial geniculate nucleus. Nuclei associated with sensory integration: LP = lateral posterior, Pul = Pulvinar. Non-specific nuclei: MN = midline nuclei; IL = intralaminar nuclei.

direct projections to the primary somatosensory cortex (Gingold et al 1991), are known as the *neo-spinothalamic tract*. This structure appears to be most prominently developed in primates.

The medial nuclear group

The medial group of thalamic nuclei, particularly the central lateral nucleus (CL), the intralaminar complex and the mediodorsal nucleus, receives collaterals of the spinothalamic and trigeminothalamic tracts, as well as inputs from the medullary and pontine reticular formation (Apkarian & Hodge 1989c, Burton & Craig 1983, Craig & Burton 1981, Mantyh 1983), the cerebellum (Asanuma et al 1983), and globus pallidus (Nauta &

Mehler 1966). Neurons in CL are responsive to the intensity and duration of nociceptive stimuli, and have large, often bilateral receptive fields (Dong et al 1978).

Some spinothalamic tract axons project to both the intralaminar nuclei and VPL, and cells giving rise to these projections have small excitatory receptive fields, with surrounding larger inhibitory areas. Their discharge characteristics indicate that they could mediate discriminative aspects of noxious cutaneous stimulation, such as intensity, duration and localization.

The receptive fields of cells giving rise to projections to the intralaminar nuclei alone have large bilateral receptive fields (Giesler et al 1981). The diffuse projections of the intralaminar nuclei to many different areas of the cortex have been considered to be part of a non-specific arousal system, but it is also possible that their role is concerned with affective states induced by a painful stimulus. These nuclei are characterized by significant numbers of opiate receptors (see Jones 1985 for review). Because these medial projections to the thalamus appeared first in vertebrate evolution, they have been termed the *paleo*-spinothalamic tract.

Brainstem

Periaqueductal grey matter

The periaqueductal grey matter (PAG) surrounds the cerebral aqueduct of the midbrain. Anatomically, the PAG can be divided into medial, dorsal, dorsolateral and ventrolateral regions, each region forming longitudinal columns that have a high degree of functional specificity (Bandler & Keay 1996, Bandler & Shipley 1994, Bandler et al 1991, Henderson et al 1998). Through these longitudinal columns the PAG has reciprocal connections with all levels of the nervous system and plays an important role in integrating a large number of functions that are critical to survival, through its influence on the nociceptive, autonomic and motor systems (Bandler & Keay 1996, Bandler & Shipley 1994, Behbehani 1995, Bernard & Bandler 1998, Keay & Bandler 1993, Morgan et al 1998).

Functions controlled by PAG include pain facilitation, analgesia, fear and anxiety, vocalization, sexual behaviour, and cardiovascular control (Behbehani 1995, Bernard & Bandler 1998).

Pain modulation can be demonstrated from stimulation of various regions of the PAG. However, stimulation of the dorsolateral and ventrolateral subregions of the PAG produces different autonomic and motor responses (Lovick 1991, Morgan 1991), based on differing patterns of projections. In addition to the inputs from the spinal cord via the spinomesencephalic tract, the PAG also receives afferents from the parafascicular nucleus of the thalamus, the hypothalamus, the amygdala (Gray & Magnuson 1992), frontal and insular cortex (Hardy & Leichnetz 1981), the reticular formation, locus coeruleus (adrenergic projections) and other catecholaminergic nuclei in the brainstem (Herbert & Saper 1992).

The ascending projections from the dorsolateral PAG are to the central lateral and paraventricular thalamic nuclei and the anterior hypothalamic area (Cameron et al 1995a). The descending projections are to the locus coeruleus, the pericoerulear region and the nucleus paragigantocellularis (Cameron et al 1995b).

The ventrolateral PAG, on the other hand, projects rostrally to the parafascicular and centromedian thalamic nuclei, the lateral hypothalamic area (Cameron et al 1995a) and the orbital frontal cortex (Coffield et al 1992). The descending projections are to the pontine reticular formation and the nucleus raphe magnus (Basbaum & Fields 1984, Cameron et al 1995b).

Stimulation of the PAG or the nucleus raphe magnus inhibits spinothalamic tract cells (Fields & Basbaum 1994) (Fig. 2.11). This difference in anatomical connectivity between the dorsolateral and ventrolateral regions of the PAG may provide a basis for their distinct and opposite modulatory influences on pain, autonomic and motor functions (see Chapter 3).

Reticular formation

The reticular formation comprises a number of morphologically and biochemically different groups of neurons distributed throughout the medulla, pons and

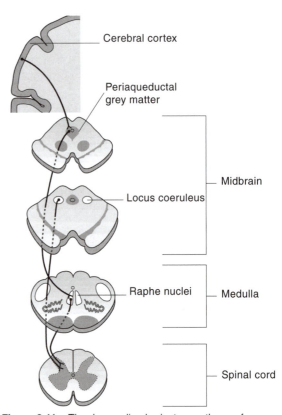

Figure 2.11 The descending brainstem pathways from periaqueductal grey matter, raphe nucleus and locus coeruleus involved in pain inhibition.

midbrain. There is a projection from the reticular formation to the intralaminar nuclei of the thalamus (Peschanski & Besson 1984), which are known to be involved in the processing of nociceptive information (Kenshalo et al 1980), as well as a projection to the spinal cord.

It is important to note that there are reciprocal connections between the reticular formation and the limbic system. As previously discussed, the nuclei of the reticular formation receive nociceptive inputs through the spinoreticular tract (Mehler et al 1960).

The reticular formation is involved in several different functions – activation of the brain for behavioural arousal, modulation of segmental stretch reflexes via the reticulospinal tracts, control of breathing and cardiac functions, and modulation of pain.

Two nuclei that are widely implicated in descending control of nociception are the nucleus raphe magnus and the dorsal raphe nucleus. The nucleus raphe magnus receives inputs from the PAG and the dorsal raphe nucleus and is believed to mediate some of the effects of PAG stimulation (Fig.2.12).

The raphe nuclei and adjacent nuclear groups contain serotonin (5HT) and project via the dorsolateral funiculus of the spinal cord to the superficial laminae of the dorsal horn, where the release of serotonin inhibits wide dynamic range neurons (Lipp 1991).

The dorsal raphe nucleus also has ascending projections to the thalamus and hypothalamus, the basal ganglia and the amygdala, and has been shown to modulate the activity induced by noxious stimulation of neurons in the thalamus (Wang & Nakai 1994).

The nucleus paragigantocellularis in the ventromedial medulla also receives input from the PAG and gives rise to a large projection to the locus coeruleus, as well as to the nucleus raphe magnus and the spinal cord (Stamford 1995).

Locus coeruleus

The locus coeruleus in the midbrain contains noradrenergic neurons and is also involved in the descending control of pain. It does this by inhibition of spinothalamic activity in the dorsal horn through binding of noradrenaline on the primary afferent neuron, which directly suppresses the release of substance P (Lipp 1991).

Limbic structures

Broca (1878) first described the 'limbic lobe' as consisting of the cingulate gyrus, the parahippocampal gyrus as well as the subcallosal gyrus and the hippocampal formation. Papez (1937) suggested that the limbic lobe formed a neural circuit providing the anatomical substrate for emotion.

It was MacLean (1955) who recommended the term 'limbic system', which refers to a much more extensive complex of structures including the limbic lobe, the temporal pole, the anterior portion of the insula, the posterior orbital surface of the frontal lobe and a number of subcortical structures, such as the thalamus, hypothalamus, septal nuclei and the amygdala (Fig. 2.12).

Evidence from lesion studies seems to indicate that the limbic structures may provide a neural basis for the aversive behaviours that comprise the motivational dimension of pain. Studies of transections of the brain at different levels in the 1920s demonstrated the importance of the hypothalamus for the expression of emotional behaviour, both with respect to the somatic component (control of facial and limb muscles) and the visceral component (control of glands and muscles by the autonomic nervous system).

Displays of intense emotional behaviour are accompanied by sympathetic responses, such as increased levels of adrenaline and noradrenaline, increased heart rate and piloerection, shunting of blood to the muscles and brain, and pupil dilation, in order to bring the animal to a high level of alertness and ready for any physical action.

The hypothalamus causes the release of hormonal endorphins (β-endorphins) from the pituitary gland; these bind to opiate receptors in the brain and spinal cord and are a potent source of pain inhibition.

Ablation of the amygdala and overlying cortex in the cat cause changes in affective behaviour, including reduced responsiveness to noxious stimuli (Schreiner & Kling 1953).

In humans, surgical section of the cingulum bundle, a tract connecting the frontal cortex with the hippocampus, was carried out to provide relief in cases of intractable pain, such as that from an inoperable carcinoma. Although still able to perceive the pain postoperatively, the patients seemed unconcerned about it. The aversive quality of the pain and the need to seek pain relief both appeared to be diminished.

Basal ganglia

Three large subcortical nuclei comprise the basal ganglia: caudate, putamen (together called the corpus striatum) and the globus pallidus (external and internal components). There are interconnections with the

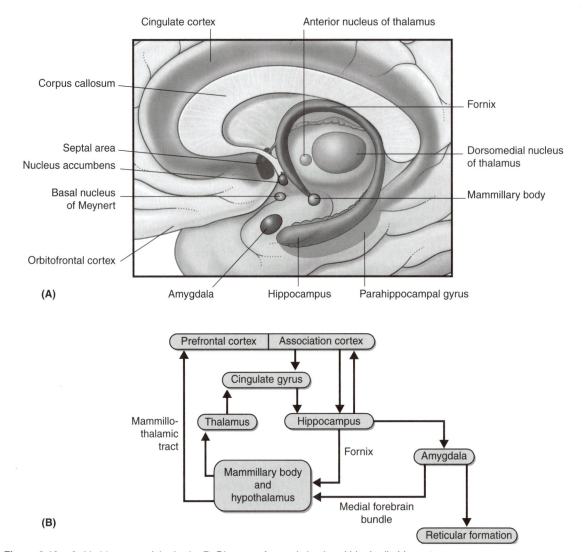

Figure 2.12 **A**. Limbic areas of the brain. **B**. Diagram of neural circuits within the limbic system.

subthalamic nucleus and the substantia nigra (comprising the pars reticulata and the pars compacta), which are also considered to be part of the basal ganglia (Fig. 2.13). The basal ganglia have a markedly heterogeneous structure structurally, neurochemically and functionally. Their role in movement control is evident from two common motor disorders affecting the basal ganglia, Parkinson's disease and Huntingdon's disease, both of which are caused by deficiencies in specific neurotransmitters.

The striatum receives afferent input from the entire cerebral cortex via the topographically organized corticostriate projection, as well as from other nuclei that comprise the basal ganglia, and projects to the ventral lateral, ventral posterior, mediodorsal and centromedian nuclei of the thalamus.

Through this circuit there are projections back to different regions of the cerebral cortex. There are at least four open-loop circuits between the cerebral cortex and basal ganglia: a motor loop concerned with regulation of movement, a cognitive loop concerned with aspects of memory, a limbic loop concerned with emotional aspects of movement and an oculomotor loop concerned with the control of saccadic eye movements (Côté & Crutcher 1991).

In the motor loop the putamen receives inputs from motor, somatosensory and parietal cortex, from the intralaminar nuclei of the thalamus, predominantly the centromedian nucleus and dopaminergic projections from the pars compacta of the substantia nigra. The putamen projects to the globus pallidus and substantia nigra and through these to the ventral anterior and ventral lateral nuclei of the thalamus, which in turn project to the prefrontal and premotor cortex.

The cognitive loop passes between the association areas of cortex, through the caudate, globus pallidus and ventral anterior nucleus of the thalamus which then projects to prefrontal cortex.

The limbic loop passes between the cingulate gyrus, lateral orbitofrontal cortex and amygdala through the nucleus accumbens (ventral striatum) and the ventral globus pallidus, returning via the mediodorsal nucleus of the thalamus to the premotor cortex and supplementary motor cortex. This loop is likely to be involved in giving motor expression to emotions, e.g. smiling, gesturing, adoption of aggressive posture, etc.

The striatum is not a homogeneous collection of cells but is organized in compartments: islands of cells called striosomes, and the surrounding regions called matrix (Goldman & Nauta 1977).

The majority of cortical projections to the striatum concerned with sensation and movement terminate in the matrix compartment. This compartment projects to the globus pallidus and the pars reticulata of the substantia nigra and inhibits the output from this

region to the cortex via the ventral anterior and mediodorsal nuclei of the thalamus. The result is a disinhibition of the target cells in the cortex.

The striosomes receive inputs from limbic regions, and project to the pars compacta of the substantia nigra where they inhibit dopaminergic cells which have a feedback loop onto matrix cells (Gerfen 1992).

In primates there is a third compartment (matrisomes), which receive complex combinations of inputs from ipsilateral and contralateral motor and somatosensory areas (Flaherty & Graybiel 1993). Cells projecting to the globus pallidus, through which the basal ganglia project to the thalamus, are characterized by various neurotransmitters and neuropeptides. Those projecting to the external segment express GABA, enkephalin and the D2 receptors for dopamine, while those projecting to the internal segment express GABA, substance P, dynorphin and the D1 receptors for dopamine (Graybiel 1991). These parallel systems, each with a unique combination of connections and neurotransmitters, provide the structural basis for modulating the responsiveness of the basal ganglia to cortical inputs (Gerfen 1992).

Electrophysiological, metabolic and bloodflow studies have demonstrated that neurons in the basal ganglia are responsive to noxious and non-noxious somatosensory information. Nociceptive neurons have been located in the substantia nigra, caudate, putamen and globus pallidus. There are neurons with large receptive fields that encode stimulus intensity, and another population of neurons responds selectively to noxious stimuli, but does not code stimulus intensity (Chudler et al 1993). Basal ganglia disease may be accompanied by changes in pain perception, and 10–29% of patients with Parkinson's disease complain of pain symptoms not associated with motor dysfunction (Sandyk et al 1988).

These observations, as well as the anatomical and neurochemical connections of the basal ganglia, have led to the suggestion that they have a role in the sensory–discriminative, affective and cognitive aspects of pain, as well as in the modulation of nociceptive information (Chudler & Dong 1995).

Cerebral cortex

The thalamocortical projections from the ventral posterolateral nucleus of the thalamus have as their target the primary somatosensory area of the cerebral cortex. This area (SI) of anthropoid primates is differentiable into three cytoarchitectonic subfields, areas 3, 1 and 2 of Brodmann. Each structurally distinctive cortical

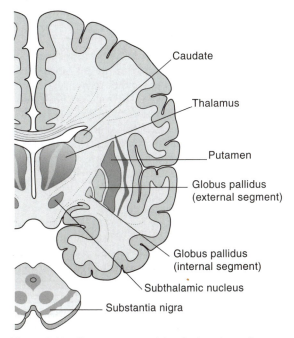

Caudate

Thalamus

Putamen

Globus pallidus (external segment)

Globus pallidus (internal segment)

Subthalamic nucleus

Substantia nigra

Figure 2.13   Structures comprising the basal ganglia (shaded).

field subserves a specific function, that is, there are functionally different neuron populations in each of these areas, with area 3a receiving proprioceptive inputs from muscle spindles, areas 3b and 1 receiving inputs from cutaneous receptors, and area 2 receiving input from deep pressure receptors (Kaas et al 1979). The contralateral body surface is represented sequentially in each of these cortical areas. The regions of the body surface with the greatest tactile acuity, the face and the hand, are maximally represented in the cortical projection to the postcentral gyrus (Fig. 2.14). These representational maps are dynamic and change as a result of experience (Buonomano & Merzenich 1998).

Fewer than 25% of ascending thalamocortical axons are capable of relaying nociceptive and thermal information to SI, and these project predominantly from the VPL, VPI and CL nuclei (Gingold et al 1991). Nociceptive information is most likely to be transmitted to areas 3b and 1, relayed from neurons located along the dorsal and ventral regions of the medial part of VPL. The VPI has connections with SI and SII (Cusick & Gould 1990), however it is not known whether nociceptive inputs to VPI are relayed only to SI or to both SI and SII. CL has diffuse cortical projections. Although stimulation of CL gives rise to motor responses (Schlag-Rey & Schlag 1984), spinothalamic projections to CL do not contact thalamocortical neurons projecting to primary motor cortex (Greenan & Strick 1986).

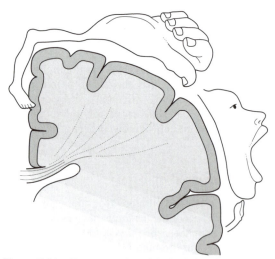

Figure 2.14 Representation of the body in primary somatosensory cortex.

Cortical representation of pain

In addition to the primary somatosensory cortex (Bushnell et al 1999), multiple cortical areas are activated by painful stimuli, including the secondary somatosensory cortex (SII), the anterior cingulate cortex (Talbot et al 1991), the insula, the prefrontal cortex (Treede et al 1999) and the supplementary motor area (Coghill et al 1994).

There is a distributed cortical system, involving parietal, cingulate and frontal regions, involved in the dynamic coding of pain intensity over time (Porro et al 1998). These cortical regions also give rise to corticospinal projection (Galea & Darian-Smith 1994) and are also activated during active movement (Colebatch et al 1991, Deiber et al 1991, Matelli et al 1993, Seitz & Roland 1992). Pain-related activation is more widely dispersed across both thalamic and cortical regions than that produced by innocuous vibratory stimuli, which is focused on SI. This distributed cerebral activation reflects the complex nature of pain, involving discriminative, affective, autonomic and motor components (Coghill et al 1994).

Parietal areas including SI are mainly involved in the sensory–discriminative aspects whereas frontal–limbic connections subserve the affective dimension of pain experience. For example, a recent study using positron emission tomography showed that hypnotic suggestion used to manipulate the unpleasantness of pain changed the regional cerebral bloodflow (rCBF) response in the anterior cingulate region but not in SI (Rainville et al 1997).

Little is known about the central mechanisms responsible for integrating incoming nociceptive information that results in a motor response (Chudler & Dong 1995). An ongoing barrage of nociceptive input, as in the chronic pain situation, may potentially affect motor output and control. The opposite might also occur whereby active movement (exercise) could potentially modulate nociception, presumably through corticospinal pathways (see Chapter 3).

Corticospinal projections

Corticospinal projections are the only direct link between the sensorimotor cortex and the spinal cord. The origin of corticospinal projections in the primate cortex is more extensive than is commonly recognized. They comprise parallel, somatotopically organized projections to each level of the spinal cord with unique, though overlapping, patterns of termination.

In addition to a dense projection from the motor cortex, corticospinal fibres arise from the premotor cortex, the postcentral cortex, especially the posterior parietal areas, the second somatosensory area and the caudal part of the insula. On the medial surface, there are extensive projections to the spinal cord from the supplementary motor area and the cortex within the cingulate sulcus (Dum & Strick 1991, Galea & Darian-Smith 1994) (Fig. 2.15).

Each of these cortical regions is distinguished not only by a characteristic cytoarchitecture, but also by a unique set of subcortical connections via the thalamus. The subcortical input to the precentral regions, including SMA and primary motor cortex, is mainly from the cerebellum and basal ganglia, whereas the input to the parietal corticospinal neuron populations is largely somatosensory (Darian-Smith et al 1990). The anterior cingulate cortex and insular cortex have connections with the limbic system (Baleydier & Maugiere 1980, Mesulam & Mufson 1982, Pandya et al 1981, Vogt & Pandya 1987), and may have particular relevance to

avoidance behaviour (Shima et al 1991). Furthermore, the regions giving rise to corticospinal projections have complex, often reciprocal cortico–cortical connections (Barbas & Pandya 1987, Cavada & Goldman-Rakic 1989, Preuss & Goldman-Rakic 1991). Both parietal and premotor cortical areas have converging inputs to the motor cortex (Leichnetz 1986, Matelli et al 1986, Muakkassa & Strick 1979, Petrides & Pandya 1984).

The direct cortical projections to the dorsal horn arise from postcentral cortical areas. However, there are corticospinal projections from other brain areas to other spinal cord laminae containing spinothalamic neurons. Areas 3b/1 and 2/5 have projections to laminae III–VI, with the greatest concentration medially (Cheema et al 1984, Coulter & Jones, 1977, Ralston & Ralston 1985). Cheema et al (1984) identified labelling in the superficial laminae of the dorsal horn (laminae I and II) after injections of WGA-HRP into the somatosensory cortex.

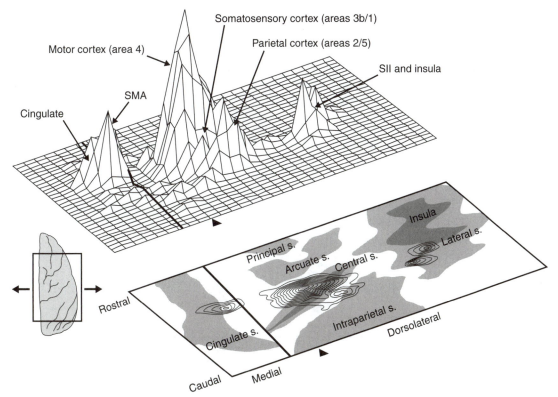

Figure 2.15 3-D map and the corresponding contour map of the contralateral corticospinal soma distribution, retrogradely labelled by a fluorescent dye injection in the cervical spinal cord. The contour map has been plotted onto the planar projection of the unfolded cortex. Sulci are indicated in light grey and are labelled in the middle map; area 3a and insular cortex are shown in a darker shade of grey. The heavy black line indicated by the arrowhead represents the sagittal midline, with the medial surface to the left. The maps show the variation in density of corticospinal projections terminating at mid-cervical levels. The most dense projection is from the primary motor cortex in the dorsal bank of the central sulcus, with smaller projections arising from the medial surface (SMA and rostral cingulate cortex), posterior parietal and insular cortex (including SII). Note the reduction of the corticospinal projection from areas 3a and 3b, compared with that from adjacent areas 4 and 2/5.

The precentral cortical areas have a very wide pattern of termination. Area 4, classical motor cortex, projects predominantly to the intermediate zone (laminae VII and VIII), but the terminals extend into the lateral and medial regions of the ventral horn (lamina IX), as well as extensively, though more sparsely, into the deeper laminae of the dorsal horn (laminae V and VI). The supplementary motor cortex has a similar pattern of termination mainly in the intermediate zone and among the motor neuron pools (Galea & Darian-Smith, 1997, Maier et al 1997).

The dorsal caudal cingulate area projects to the dorsolateral portion of the intermediate zone of the spinal cord (where spinothalamic neurons are located), while projections from the ventral caudal cingulate area terminate in the dorsomedial region (in the region of neurons projecting to the dorsal columns). However, there are sparse terminations in the dorsolateral region of the ventral horn and in the dorsal horn (laminae III and IV). These projections appear to be more dense in the rostral segments of the cervical spinal cord (Dum & Strick 1996) (Fig. 2.16).

Role of corticospinal projections

The corticospinal projections form a parallel, distributed system arising from areas with complex interconnections, and converging on different parts of the spinal circuitry. Their role in the modulation of activity in the dorsal horn, particularly in relation to pain, has not been investigated extensively.

It has been known for some time that stimulation of primary and secondary somatosensory areas can result in primary afferent depolarization (PAD) in fibres of the dorsal root (group Ib and II muscle afferents and cutaneous afferents, but not group Ia afferents) (Andersen et al 1964, Carpenter et al 1963). It appears that sensorimotor cortex stimulation depresses the response of superficial dorsal horn neurons to a subsequent stimulus from the Lissauer tract. This tract is therefore thought to mediate the PAD evoked from multiple neural pathways (Lidierth & Wall 1998).

Stimulation of sensorimotor cortex can also elicit both excitatory and inhibitory responses in dorsal horn neurons, particularly in laminae IV and V (Fetz 1968, Lundberg et al 1962, Wall 1967). These cells receive a wide convergence of cutaneous input, as well as afferent information from muscle and joints.

In a study in the monkey by Coulter et al (1974) stimulation of the pre- or postcentral gyrus produced either a depression of the activity of neurons in the dorsal horn, or an excitation followed by depression. Corticospinal projections from motor cortex may be excitatory to spinothalamic neurons, while those from postcentral cortex may inhibit them (Lidierth & Wall, 1998, Ralston & Ralston, 1985, Yezierski et al 1983). Corticospinal projections to the superficial laminae (arising predominantly from areas 3b/1) may directly modulate nociceptive-specific neurons (Cheema et al 1984).

Posterior parietal cortex has connections with the primary somatosensory cortex and other polymodal

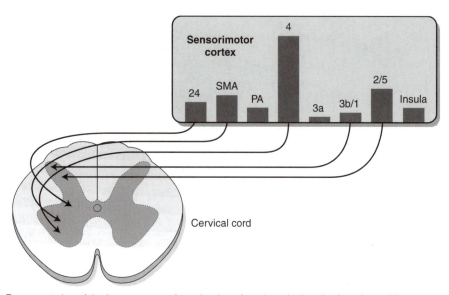

Figure 2.16 Representation of the known areas of termination of corticospinal projections from different cortical areas.

association areas, including the limbic system (Cavada & Goldman-Rakic 1989) and is part of a general attentional system. Activation of this region may reflect hypervigilance or superattentiveness to the sensory information accompanying chronic pain. The role of corticospinal projections from this region on dorsal horn neurons is unknown.

The role of the cingulate cortex is of particular interest, in that this region has been shown, using functional imaging studies, to be involved in the processing of painful stimuli (Hsieh et al 1995, Jones et al 1991, Treede et al 1999). The cingulate sulcus is a unique region of the limbic system, in that it appears to be involved in affect and regulating context-relevant motor behaviours (Devinsky et al 1995). It has been suggested that this region is critical for maintaining a working interaction between the limbic areas and motor areas of the cerebral cortex.

Stimulation in the cingulate area (area 24) may also be involved in autonomic responses, such as changes in respiration and cardiovascular function (Hoff et al 1963, Lofving 1961). Its role might be in linking emotional, motivational and memory-related information generated in limbic areas, directly to motor areas (Morecraft & van Hoesen 1998). A recent study by Koyama et al (1998) showed that the anterior cingulate cortex contained pain-anticipation-related neurons, and therefore has a role in the anticipation of pain that precedes avoidance behaviour.

Neurons in SII and the granular insula (Ig) are responsive to a wide range of somatosensory stimuli (Burton & Robinson 1981). The corticospinal projections from these areas terminate in the dorsal horn, but their specific role is unknown. The majority of neurons in SII respond to rapid, transient stimuli such as light touch.

'Complex zones' have been described, which become active during the performance of complex tasks (Burton & Robinson 1981). The posterior insula (Ig) receives converging information about all five sensory modalities. Its efferent connections include the limbic system through the cingulate gyrus and amygdala (Mesulam & Mufson 1982), as well as the spinal cord (Galea & Darian-Smith 1994). Therefore this area might have the function of providing the link between motivational and emotional states with relevant sensory information. Noxious heat has been found to activate a region of the anterior insula (Id), which has connections with SI, SII and the cingulate region (area 24) (Mufson & Mesulam 1982), as well as with the amygdala and perirhinal cortex (Friedman et al 1986). Although stimulation of the anterior insula produces predominantly visceral sensations, it also evokes unusual somatic sensations, movements and sometimes a sense of fear (Penfield & Rasmussen 1955).

The corticospinal neuron populations can produce indirect effects on the dorsal horn through collaterals to the dorsal column nuclei, where the effect is to diminish the postsynaptic responses of the dorsal column nuclei to somatic sensory nerve stimulation (Magni et al 1959).

In addition, there are collaterals to the PAG and the nucleus raphe magnus (Kuypers 1981), which have descending inhibitory connections with the spinal cord. Thus the cerebral cortex, through the corticospinal tract, may exert a modulatory effect on both motor and sensory functions, including pain.

CONCLUSION

This chapter has provided a review of the nervous system structures involved in nociception, and their connections. Nociceptors are involved in signalling painful stimuli. There are several kinds of cutaneous nociceptors that can be activated by one or more kinds of noxious stimuli: mechanical, thermal or chemical. Other nociceptors are found in muscle, joints and viscera.

Nociceptive and thermal signals are transmitted along unmyelinated (C) and small diameter myelinated ($A\delta$) axons that synapse in the dorsal horn. Second-order neurons arise from different regions of the dorsal horn, cross the midline in the ventral commissure and ascend to the brainstem and thalamus in the anterolateral column. They synapse in a number of brainstem nuclei (including the reticular formation and the periaqueductal grey) and in several thalamic nuclei (VPL, VPI, CL and the intralaminar nuclei). From the thalamus, nociceptive and thermal stimuli are relayed mainly to the primary somatosensory area (SI) of the cerebral cortex.

Multiple cortical areas are activated by painful stimuli, including the secondary somatosensory cortex (SII), the anterior cingulate cortex, the insula, the prefrontal cortex and the supplementary motor area. Pain signals may be modified through descending projections from the brainstem and cerebral cortex. The organization of these structures suggests that there is a distributed cortical system concerned with the perception of pain. This distributed cerebral activation reflects the complex nature of pain, involving discriminative, affective, autonomic and motor components. An understanding of this complexity can provide insights for the management of pain in the clinical setting.

Study questions/questions for revision

1. What classes of axons convey nociceptive and temperature information?
2. In which ways could nociceptive information be modulated at the level of the dorsal horn?
3. What spinal cord pathways convey nociceptive information to the brain? What are their targets?
4. Which regions of the brain subserve the sensory–discriminative and motivational–affective aspects of pain? How do their connections differ?
5. Name the descending projections to the dorsal horn? What is their role?

REFERENCES

Abrahams V C, Lynn B, Richmond F J R 1984 Organization and sensory properties of small myelinated fibres in the dorsal cervical rami of the cat. Journal of Physiology 347: 177–187

Adrian E D 1931 The messages in sensory nerve fibres and their interpretation. Proceedings of the Royal Society Series B 109: 1–18

Al-Chaer E D, Feng Y, Willis W D 1998 A role for the dorsal column in nociceptive visceral input into the thalamus of primates. Journal of Neurophysiology 79: 3143–3150

Andersen P, Eccles J C, Sears T A 1964 Cortically evoked depolarization of primary afferent fibers in the spinal cord. Journal of Neurophysiology 27: 63–77

Apkarian A V, Hodge C 1989a Primate spinothalamic pathways: I. A quantitative study of the cells of origin of the spinothalamic pathway. Journal of Comparative Neurology 288: 447–473

Apkarian A V, Hodge C 1989b Primate spinothalamic pathways: II. The cells of origin of the dorsolateral and ventral spinothalamic pathways. Journal of Comparative Neurology 288: 474–492

Apkarian A V, Hodge C 1989c Primate spinothalamic pathways: III. Thalamic terminations of the dorsolateral and ventral spinothalamic pathways. Journal of Comparative Neurology 288: 493–511

Applebaum A E, Beall J E, Foreman R D, Willis W D 1975 Organization and receptive fields of primate spinothalamic tract neurons. Journal of Neurophysiology 38: 572–586

Applebaum A E, Leonard R B, Kenshalo D R, Martin R F, Willis W D 1979 Nuclei in which functionally identified spinothalamic tract neurons terminate. Journal of Comparative Neurology 188: 575–586

Asanuma C, Thach W T, Jones E G 1983 Anatomical evidence for segregated focal groupings of efferent cells and their terminal ramifications in the cerebellothalamic pathway of the monkey. Brain Research Reviews 5: 267–297

Baleydier C, Maugiere F 1980 The duality of the cingulate gyrus in monkey: neuroanatomical study and functional hypothesis. Brain 103: 525–554

Bandler R, Keay K A 1996 Columnar organization in the midbrain periaqueductal gray and the integration of emotional expression. Progress in Brain Research 107: 285–300

Bandler R, Shipley M T 1994 Columnar organization in the midbrain periaqueductal gray: modules for emotional expression? Trends in Neurosciences 17: 379–389 [published erratum appears on 17: 445]

Bandler R, Carrive P, Zhang S P 1991 Integration of somatic and autonomic reactions within the midbrain periaqueductal gray: viscerotopic, somatotopic and functional organization. Progress in Brain Research 87: 269–305

Barbas H, Pandya D N 1987 Architecture and frontal cortical connections of the premotor cortex (area 6) in the rhesus monkey. Journal of Comparative Neurology 256: 211–228

Basbaum A I, Fields H L 1984 Endogenous pain control systems: brainstem spinal pathways and endorphin circuitry. Annual Review of Neuroscience 7: 309–338

Behbehani M M 1995 Functional characteristics of the midbrain periaqueductal gray. Progress in Neurobiology 46: 575–605

Berkley K 1980 Spatial relationships between the terminations of somatic sensory and motor pathways in the rostral brainstem of cats and monkeys. I. Ascending somatic sensory inputs to lateral diencephalon. Journal of Comparative Neurology 193: 283–317

Bernard J F, Bandler R 1998 Parallel circuits for emotional coping behaviour: new pieces in the puzzle. Journal of Comparative Neurology 401: 429–436

Bessou P, Laporte Y 1961 Étude des recepteurs musculaires innervés par les fibres afferentes du groupe III (fibres myelinisées fines), chez le chat. Archives Italiennes de Biologie 99: 293–321

Bessou P, Perl E R 1969 Response of cutaneous sensory units with unmyelinated fibres to noxious stimuli. Journal of Neurophysiology 32: 1025–1043

Boivie J 1979 An anatomical reinvestigation of the termination of the spinothalamic tract in the monkey. Journal of Comparative Neurology 186: 343–370

Broca P 1878 Anatomie comparée de circonvolutions cérébrales. Le grand lobe limbique et la scissure limbique dans le série des mammifères. Revue Anthropologique 1: 385–498

Brodal A 1981 Neurological Anatomy in Relation to Clinical Medicine. Oxford University Press, New York

Brown A G 1981 Organization in the Spinal Cord. Springer, Berlin

Brown P B, Brushart T M, Ritz L A 1989 Somatotopy of digital nerve projections to the dorsal horn in the monkey. Somatosensory and Motor Research 6: 309–317

Buonomano D V, Merzenich M M 1998 Cortical plasticity: from maps to synapses. Annual Review of Neuroscience 21: 149–186

Burgess P R, Perl E R 1967 Myelinated afferent fibres responding specifically to noxious stimulation of the skin. Journal of Physiology (London) 190: 541–562

Burton H, Craig A D 1983 Spinothalamic projections in cat, raccoon and monkey: a study based on anterograde transport of horseradish peroxidase. In: Macchi G, Rustioni A, Spreafico R (eds) Somatosensory Integration in the Thalamus. Elsevier, Amsterdam, pp 17–41

Burton H, Robinson C J 1981 Organization of the SII parietal cortex. Multiple somatic sensory representations within and near the second somatic sensory area of the cynomolgus monkeys. In: Woolsey C N (ed) Cortical Sensory Organization, Vol. 1. Multiple Sensory Areas. Humana Press, New Jersey, pp 67–119

Bushnell M C, Duncan G H, Hofbauer R K, Ha B, Chen J-I, Carrier B 1999 Pain perception: is there a role for primary somatosensory cortex? Proceedings of the National Academy of Sciences USA 96: 7705–7709

Cameron A A, Khan I A, Westlund K N, Cliffer K D Willis W D 1995a The efferent projections of the periaqueductal gray in the rat: a *Phaseolus vulgaris*-leucoagglutinin study. I. Ascending projections. Journal of Comparative Neurology 351: 568–584

Cameron A A, Khan I A, Westlund K N, Willis W D 1995b The efferent projections of the periaqueductal gray in the rat: a *Phaseolus vulgaris*-leucoagglutinin study. II. Descending projections. Journal of Comparative Neurology 351: 585–601

Campbell J N, Meyer R A, LaMotte R H 1979 Sensitization of myelinated nociceptive afferents that innervate monkey hand. Journal of Neurophysiology 42: 1669–1679

Campero M, Serra J, Ochoa J L 1996 C-polymodal nociceptors activated by noxious low temperature in human skin. Journal of Physiology 497: 565–572

Carpenter D, Lundberg A, Norrsell U 1963 Primary afferent depolarization evoked from the sensorimotor cortex. Acta Physiologica Scandinavica 59: 126–142

Carstens E, Trevino D L 1978 Laminar origins of spinothalamic projections in the cat as determined by the retrograde transport of horseradish peroxidase. Journal of Comparative Neurology 182: 161–165

Casey K L, Morrow T J 1987 Nociceptive neurons in the ventral posterior thalamus of the awake squirrel monkey: observations in identification, modulation and drug effects. In: Besson J-M, Guilbaud D, Peschanksi M (eds) Thalamus and Pain. Elsevier, Amsterdam, pp 211–226

Cavada C, Goldman-Rakic P S 1989 Posterior parietal cortex in rhesus monkey: II. Evidence for segregated corticocortical networks linking sensory and limbic areas with the frontal lobe. Journal of Comparative Neurology 287: 422–445

Cheema S S, Rustioni A, Whitsel B L 1984 Light and electron microscopic evidence for a direct corticospinal projection to superficial laminae of the dorsal horn in cats and monkeys. Journal of Comparative Neurology 225: 276–290

Chen Y, Michaelis M, Jänig W, Devor M 1996 Adrenoreceptor subtype mediating sympathetic-sensory coupling in injured sensory neurons. Journal of Neurophysiology 76: 3721–3730

Christensen B R, Perl E R 1970 Spinal neurons specifically excited by noxious or thermal stimuli. Journal of Neurophysiology 33: 293–307

Chudler E H, Dong W K 1995 The role of the basal ganglia in nociception and pain. Pain 60: 3–38

Chudler E H, Sugiyama K, Dong W K 1993 Nociceptive responses of neurons in the neostriatum and globus pallidus of the rat. Journal of Neurophysiology 69: 1890–1903

Coffield J A, Bowen K K, Miletic, V 1992 Retrograde tracing of projections between the nucleus submedius, the ventrolateral orbital cortex, and the midbrain in the rat. Journal of Comparative Neurology 321: 488–499

Coggeshall R E, Coulter J D, Willis W D 1974 Unmyelinated axons in the ventral roots of the cat lumbosacral enlargement. Journal of Comparative Neurology 153: 39–58

Coghill R C, Talbot J D, Evans A C, Meyer E, Gjedde A, Bushnell M C, Duncan G H 1994 Distributed processing of pain and vibration by the human brain. Journal of Neuroscience 14: 4095–4108

Colebatch J G, Deiber M-P, Passingham R E, Friston K J, Frackowiak R S J (1991) Regional cerebral blood flow during voluntary arm and hand movements in human subjects. Journal of Neurophysiology 65: 1392–1401

Côté L, Crutcher M D 1991 The basal ganglia. In: Kandel E R, Schwartz J H, Jessell T M (eds) Principles of Neural Science, 3rd edn. Elsevier, New York, pp 647–659

Coulter J D, Jones E G 1977 Differential distribution of corticospinal projections from individual cytoarchitectonic fields in the monkey. Brain Research 129: 335–340

Coulter J D, Maunz R A, Willis W D 1974 Effects of stimulation of sensorimotor cortex on primate spinothalamic neurons. Brain Research 65: 351–356

Craig A D, Burton H 1981 Spinal and medullary lamina I projection to nucleus submedius in medial thalamus: a possible pain center. Journal of Neurophysiology 45: 443–466

Cusick C G, Gould H J 1990 Connections between area 3b of the somatosensory cortex and subdivisions of the ventroposterior nuclear complex and the anterior pulvinar in squirrel monkeys. Journal of Comparative Neurology 292: 83–102

Darian-Smith C, Darian-Smith I, Cheema S S 1990 Thalamic projections to sensorimotor cortex in the macaque monkey: use of multiple retrograde tracers. Journal of Comparative Neurology 299: 17–46

Deiber M-P, Passingham R E, Colebatch J G, Friston K J, Nixon P D, Frackowiak R S J 1991 Cortical areas and the selection of movement: a study with positron emission tomography. Experimental Brain Research 84: 393–402

Devinsky O, Morrell M J, Vogt B A 1995 Contributions of anterior cingulate cortex to behaviour. Brain 118: 279–306

Dong W K, Ryu H, Wagman I H 1978 Nociceptive responses in medial thalamus and their relationship to spinothalamic pathways. Journal of Neurophysiology 41: 1592–1613

Dubner R, Bennett G J 1983 Spinal and trigeminal mechanisms of nociception. Annual Review of Neurosciences 6: 381–418

Dubner R, Price D D, Beitel R E, Wu J W 1977 Peripheral neural correlates of behaviour in monkey and human related to sensory-discriminative aspects of pain. In: Anderson D J, Mathews B (eds) Pain in the Trigeminal Region. Elsevier, Amsterdam, pp 57–66

Dum R P, Strick P L 1991 The origin of corticospinal projections from the premotor areas in the frontal lobe. Journal of Neuroscience 11: 667–689

Dum R P, Strick P L 1996 Spinal cord terminations of the medial wall motor areas in macaque monkeys. Journal of Neuroscience 16: 6513–6525

Erlanger J, Gasser H S 1937 Electrical Signs of Nervous Activity. University of Pennsylvania Press, Philadelphia

Fetz E E 1968 Pyramidal tract effects on interneurons in the cat lumbar dorsal horn. Journal of Neurophysiology 31: 69–80

Fields H L, Basbaum A I 1994 Central nervous system mechanisms of pain modulation. In: Wall P D, Melzack R (eds) Textbook of Pain. Churchill Livingstone, Edinburgh, pp 243–257

Flaherty A W, Graybiel A M 1993 Two input systems for body representations in the primate striatal matrix: experimental evidence in the squirrel monkey. Journal of Neuroscience 13: 1120–1137

Florence S L, Wall J T, Kaas J H 1988 The somatotopic pattern of afferent projections from the digits to the spinal cord and cuneate nucleus in macaque monkeys. Brain Research 452: 388–392

Friedman D P, Murray E A, O'Neill J B, Mishkin M 1996 Cortical connections of the somatosensory fields of the lateral sulcus of macaques: evidence of a corticolimbic pathway for touch. Journal of Comparative Neurology 252: 323–347

Galea M P, Darian-Smith I 1994 Multiple corticospinal neuron populations in the macaque monkey are specified by their unique cortical origins, spinal terminations and connections. Cerebral Cortex 4: 166–194

Galea M P, Darian-Smith I 1997 Corticospinal projection patterns following unilateral cervical spinal cord section in the newborn and juvenile macaque monkey. Journal of Comparative Neurology 381: 282–306

Gerfen C R 1992 The neostriatal mosaic: multiple levels of compartmental organization. Trends in Neurosciences 15: 133–139

Giesler G J, Spiel H R, Willis W D 1981 Organization of spinothalamic tract axons within the rat spinal cord. Journal of Comparative Neurology 195: 243–252

Gingold S I, Greenspan J D, Apkarian A V 1991 Anatomic evidence of nociceptive inputs to primary somatosensory cortex: relationship between spinothalamic terminals and thalamocortical cells in squirrel monkeys. Journal of Comparative Neurology 308: 467–490

Gobel S, Falls W M, Humphrey E 1981 Morphology and synaptic connections of ultrafine primary axons in lamina I of the spinal dorsal horn: candidates for the terminal axonal arbors of primary neurones in unmyelinated (C) axons. Journal of Neuroscience 1: 1163–1179

Goldman P S, Nauta W J H 1977 An intricately patterned prefronto-caudate projection in the rhesus monkey. Journal of Comparative Neurology 171: 369–385

Gray T S, Magnuson D J 1992 Peptide immunoreactive neurons in the amygdala and the bed nucleus of the stria terminalis project to the midbrain central gray in the rat. Peptides 13: 451–460

Graybiel A M 1991 Basal ganglia: input, neural activity, and relation to the cortex. Current Biology 1: 644–651

Greenan T J, Strick P L 1986 Do thalamic regions which project to rostral primate motor cortex receive spinothalamic input? Brain Research 362: 384–388

Grieve G P 1994 Referred pain and other clinical features. In: Boyling J D, Palastanga N (eds) Grieve's Modern Manual Therapy, 2nd edn. The Vertebral Column. Churchill Livingstone, Edinburgh

Ha H, Morin F 1964 Comparative anatomical observations of the cervical nucleus, *N. cervicalis lateralis*, of some primates. Anatomical Record 148: 374–375

Häbler H-J, Jänig W, Koltzenburg M 1990 Activation of unmyelinated fibres by mechanical stimuli and inflammation of the urinary bladder in the cat. Journal of Physiology (London) 425: 545–562

Hardy S G P, Leichnetz G R 1981 Cortical projections to the periaqueductal gray in the monkey: a retrograde and orthograde horseradish peroxidase study. Neuroscience Letters 22: 97–101

Henderson L A, Keay K A, Bandler R 1998 The ventrolateral periaqueductal gray projects to caudal brainstem depressor regions: a functional-anatomical and physiological study. Neuroscience 82: 201–221

Heppelmann B, Messlinger K, Neiss W F, Schmidt R F 1990 Ultrastructural three-dimensional reconstruction of group III and group IV sensory nerve endings ('free nerve endings') in the knee joint of the cat: evidence for multiple receptive sites. Journal of Comparative Neurology 292: 103–116

Herbert H, Saper C R 1992 Organization of medullary adrenergic and noradrenergic projections to the periaqueductal gray matter in the rat. Journal of Comparative Neurology 314: 34–52

Hertel H C, Howaldt B, Mense S 1976 Responses of group IV and group III muscle afferents to thermal stimuli. Brain Research 113: 201–205

Hirschberg R M, Al-Chaer E D, Lawand N B, Westlund K N, Willis W D 1996 Is there a pathway in the posterior funiculus that signals visceral pain? Pain 67: 291–305

Hoff E C, Kell J F, Carroll M N 1963 Effects of cortical stimulation and lesions on cardiovascular function. Physiological Reviews 43: 68–114

Honda C N 1985 Visceral and somatic afferent convergence onto neurons near the central canal in the sacral spinal cord of the cat. Journal of Neurophysiology 53: 1059–1078

Honda C N, Perl E R 1985 Functional and morphological features of neurons in the midline region of the caudal spinal cord in the cat. Brain Research 340: 285–295

Hsieh J-C, Belfrage M, Stone-Elander S, Hansson P, Ingvar M 1995 Central representation of chronic ongoing neuropathic pain studied by positron emission tomography. Pain 63: 225–236

Iggo A 1960 Cutaneous mechanoreceptors with C fibres. Journal of Physiology (London) 152: 337–353

Jänig W 1992 Pain and the sympathetic nervous system: pathophysiological mechanisms. In: Bannister R, Mathias C (eds) Autonomic Failure. Oxford University Press, Oxford, pp 231–251

Jänig W 1995 The sympathetic nervous system in pain. European Journal of Anaesthesiology 12 (Suppl. 10): 53–60

Johnson J I, Welker W I, Pubols B H 1968 Somatotopic organization of racoon dorsal column nuclei. Journal of Comparative Neurology 132: 1–44

Jones E G 1985 The Thalamus. Plenum Press, New York

Jones A K P, Brown W D, Friston K J, Qi L Y, Frackowiack R S J 1991 Cortical and subcortical localization of response to pain in man using positron emission tomography. Proceedings of the Royal Society, B 244: 39–44

Kaas J H, Nelson R J, Sur M, Lin C-S, Merzenich M M 1979 Multiple representations of the body within the primary somatosensory cortex of primates. Science 204: 521–523

Kaas J H, Nelson R J, Sur M, Dykes R W, Merzenich M M 1984 The somatotopic organization of the ventroposterior thalamus of the squirrel monkey, *Saimiri sciureus*. Journal of Comparative Neurology 226: 111–140

Keay K A, Bandler R 1993 Deep and superficial noxious stimulation increases Fos-like immunoreactivity in different regions of the midbrain periaqueductal gray of the rat. Neuroscience Letters 154: 23–26

Kenshalo D R, Giesler G J, Leonard R B, Willis W D 1980 Responses of neurons in primate ventral posterior lateral nucleus to noxious stimuli. Journal of Neurophysiology 43: 1594–1614

Kerr F W L 1975 Neuroanatomical substrates of nociception in the spinal cord. Pain 1: 325–356

Kevetter G A, Haber L H, Yezierski R P, Chung J M, Martin R F, Willis W D 1982 Cells of origin of the spinoreticular tract in the monkey. Journal of Comparative Neurology 207: 61–74

Kieschke J, Mense S, Prabhakar N R 1988 Influence of adrenaline and hypoxia on rat muscle receptors in vitro. In: Hamann W, Iggo A (eds) Progress in Brain Research. Elsevier, Amsterdam, pp 91–97

Kircher C, Ha H 1968 The nucleus cervicalis lateralis in primates including the human. Anatomical Record 160: 376

Klement W, Arndt J O 1992 The role of nociceptors of cutaneous veins in the mediation of cold pain in man. Journal of Physiology 449: 73–83

Koyama T, Tanaka Y Z, Mikami A 1998 Nociceptive neurons in macaque anterior cingulate activate during anticipation of pain. NeuroReport 9: 2663–2667

Kruger L, Perl E R, Sedivec M J 1981 Fine structure of myelinated mechanical nociceptor endings in cat hairy skin. Journal of Comparative Neurology 198: 137–154

Kuypers H G J M 1981 Anatomy of the descending pathways. In: Brooks V B, Brookhart J M, Mountcastle V B (eds) Handbook of Physiology Section 1: The Nervous System, Volume II, Motor Control, Part 1. American Physiological Society, Bethesda, pp 597–666

LaMotte C 1977 Distribution of the tract of Lissauer and dorsal horn root fibres in the primate spinal cord. Journal of Comparative Neurology 172: 529–562

LaMotte R H, Thalhammer J G 1982 Response properties of high-threshold cutaneous cold receptors in the primate. Brain Research 244: 279–287

Lawson S N 1992 Morphological and biochemical cell types of sensory neurons. In: Scott S A (ed) Sensory Neurons: Diversity, Development and Plasticity. Oxford University Press, Oxford, pp 27–59

Leichnetz G R 1986 Afferent and efferent connections of the dorsolateral precentral gyrus (area 4, hand/arm region) in the macaque monkey, with comparisons to area 8. Journal of Comparative Neurology 254: 260–292

Lidierth M, Wall P D 1998 Dorsal horn cells connected to the Lissauer tract and their relation to the dorsal root potential in the rat. Journal of Neurophysiology 80: 667–679

Light A R, Metz C B 1978 The morphology of the spinal cord efferent and afferent neurons contributing to the ventral roots of the cat. Journal of Comparative Neurology 179: 501–516

Lipp J 1991 Possible mechanisms of morphine analgesia. Clinical Neuropharmacology 14: 131–147

Lloyd D P C 1943. Neuron patterns controlling transmission of ipsilateral hindlimb reflexes in cat. Journal of Neurophysiology 6: 293–315

Lofving B 1961 Cardiovascular adjustments induced from the rostral cingulate gyrus. Acta Physiologica Scandinavica 53: 1–82

Lovick T A 1991 Interactions between descending pathways from the dorsal and ventrolateral periaqueductal gray matter in the rat. In: Depaulis A, Bandler R (eds) The Midbrain Periaqueductal Gray Matter. New York, Plenum Press, pp 101–120

Lundberg A, Norrsell U, Voorhoeve P 1962 Pyramidal effects on lumbosacral interneurons activated by somatic afferents. Acta Physiologica Scandinavica 56: 220–229

Lynn B 1984 The detection of injury and tissue damage. In: Wall P D, Melzack R (eds) Textbook of Pain. Churchill Livingstone, Edinburgh, pp 19–33

MacLean P D 1955 The limbic system ('visceral brain') and emotional behaviour. Archives of Neurology and Psychiatry 73: 130–134

Magni F, Melzack R, Moruzzi G, Smith C J 1959 Direct pyramidal influences on the dorsal column nuclei. Archives Italiennes de Biologie 97: 357–377

Maier M A, Davis J N, Armand J, Kirkwood P A, Philbin N, Ognjenovic N, Lemon R N 1997 Comparison of cortico-motoneuronal (CM) connections from macaque motor cortex and supplementary motor area. Society for Neuroscience Abstracts 23: 1274

Mantyh P W 1983 The spinothalamic tract in the primate: a reexamination using wheatgerm agglutinin conjugated to horseradish peroxidase. Neuroscience 9: 847–862

Martin J H 1996 Neuroanatomy Text and Atlas 2nd edn. Appleton & Lange, Stamford, Connecticut

Matelli M, Camarda R, Glickstein M, Rizzolatti G 1986 Afferent and efferent projections of the inferior area 6 in the macaque monkey. Journal of Comparative Neurology 251: 281–298

Matelli M, Rizzolatti G, Bettinardi V, Gilardi M C, Perani D, Rizzo G, Fazio F 1993 Activation of precentral and mesial motor areas during the execution of elementary proximal and distal arm movements: a PET study. NeuroReport 4: 1295–1298

McLachlan E M, Jänig W, Devor M, Michaelis M 1993 Peripheral nerve injury triggers noradrenergic sprouting within dorsal root ganglia. Nature 363: 543–546

McMahon S B 1984 Spinal mechanisms in somatic pain. In: Holden A V, Winlow W (eds) The Neurobiology of Pain. Manchester University Press, Manchester

Mehler W R, Feferman M E, Nauta W J H 1960 Ascending axon degeneration following anterolateral cordotomy. An experimental study in the monkey. Brain 83: 718–751

Melzack R, Casey K L 1968 Sensory, motivational, and central control determinants of pain. A new conceptual model. In: Kenshalo R (ed) The Skin Senses. Thomas, Springfield, Illinois, pp 423–443

Mense S 1993 Nociception from skeletal muscle in relation to clinical muscle pain. Pain 54: 241–289

Mense S, Meyer H 1985 Different types of slowly conducting afferent units in cat skeletal muscle and tendon. Journal of Physiology 363: 403–417

Mense S, Meyer H 1988 Bradykinin-induced modulation of the response behaviour of different types of feline group III and IV muscle receptors. Journal of Physiology 398: 49–63

Mense S, Prabhakar N R 1986 Spinal terminations of nociceptive afferent fibres from deep tissues in the cat. Neuroscience Letters 66: 169–174

Mense S, Stahnke M 1983 Responses in muscle afferent fibres of slow conduction velocity to contractions and ischaemia in the cat. Journal of Physiology 342: 383–397

Mesulam M-M, Mufson E J 1982 Insula in the Old World monkey: efferent cortical output and comments on function. Journal of Comparative Neurology 212: 38–52

Meyer R A, Davis K D, Cohen R H, Treede R-D, Campbell J N 1991 Mechanically insensitive afferents (MIAs) in cutaneous nerves of monkey. Brain Research 561: 252–261

Meyer R A, Campbell J N, Raja S N 1994 Peripheral neural mechanisms of nociception. In: Wall P D, Melzack R (eds) Textbook of Pain. Churchill Livingstone, Edinburgh, pp 13–44

Mizuno N, Nakano K, Imaizumi M, Okamoto M 1967 The lateral cervical nucleus of the Japanese monkey (Macaca fuscata). Journal of Comparative Neurology 129: 375–384

Morecraft R J, van Hoesen G W 1998 Convergence of limbic input to the cingulate motor cortex in the rhesus monkey. Brain Research Bulletin 45: 209–232

Morgan M M 1991 Differences in antinociception evoked from dorsal and ventral regions of the caudal periaqueductal gray matter. In: Depaulis A, Bandler R (eds) The Midbrain Periaqueductal Gray Matter. New York, Plenum Press, pp 139–150

Morgan M M, Whitney P K, Gold M S 1998 Immobility and flight associated with antinociception produced by activation of the ventral and lateral/dorsal regions of the rat periaqueductal gray. Brain Research 804: 159–166

Muakkassa K F, Strick P L 1979 Frontal lobe inputs to primate motor cortex: evidence for four somatotopically organized 'premotor' areas. Brain Research 177: 176–182

Mufson E J, Mesulam M-M 1982 Insula of the old world monkey. II Afferent cortical input and comments on the claustrum. Journal of Comparative Neurology 212: 23–37

Nauta W J H, Mehler W R 1966 Projections of the lentiform nucleus in the monkey. Brain Research 1: 3–42

Pandya D N, Van Hoesen G W, Mesulam M M 1981 Efferent connections of the cingulate gyrus in the rhesus monkey. Experimental Brain Research 42: 319–330

Papez J W 1937 A proposed mechanism of emotion. Archives of Neurology and Psychiatry 38: 725–743

Patterson J T, Coggeshall R E, Lee W T, Chung K 1990 Long ascending unmyelinated primary afferent axons in the rat dorsal column: immunohistochemical localizations. Neuroscience Letters 108: 6–10

Penfield W, Rasmussen T 1955 The Cerebral Cortex of Man. New York, Macmillan

Peschanski M, Besson J M 1984 A spino-reticulo-thalamic pathway in the rat: an anatomical study with reference to pain transmission. Neuroscience 12: 165–178

Petrides M, Pandya D N 1984 Projections to the frontal cortex from the posterior parietal region in the rhesus monkey. Journal of Comparative Neurology 228: 105–116

Porro C A, Cettolo V, Francescato M P, Baraldi P 1998 Temporal and intensity coding of pain in human cortex. Journal of Neurophysiology 80: 3312–3320

Preuss T M, Goldman-Rakic P S 1991 Ipsilateral cortical connections of granular frontal cortex in the strepsirrhine primate Galago, with comparative comments on anthropoid primates. Journal of Comparative Neurology 310: 507–549

Rainville P, Duncan G H, Price D D, Carrier B, Bushnell M C 1997 Pain affect encoded in human anterior cingulate but not somatosensory cortex. Science 277: 968–971

Ralston D D, Ralston H J 1985 The terminations of corticospinal tract axons in the macaque monkey. Journal of Comparative Neurology 242: 325–337

Ralston H J, Ralston D D 1992 The primate dorsal spinothalamic tract: evidence for a specific termination in the posterior nuclei (Po/SG) of the thalamus. Pain 48: 107–118

Rang H P, Bevan S, Dray A 1991 Chemical activation of nociceptive peripheral neurons. British Medical Bulletin 47: 534–548

Rexed B 1952 The cytoarchitectonic organization of the spinal cord in the cat. Journal of Comparative Neurology 96: 415–495

Rexed B 1954 A cytoarchitectonic atlas of the spinal cord in the cat. Journal of Comparative Neurology 100: 297–379

Ruch T C 1946 Visceral sensation and referred pain. In: Fulton J F (ed) Howell's Textbook of Physiology, 15th edn. Saunders, Philadelphia, pp 385–401

Sandyk R, Bamford C R, Iacono R 1988 Pain and sensory symptoms in Parkinson's disease. International Journal of Neuroscience 39: 15–25

Sato J, Perl E R 1991 Adrenergic excitation of cutaneous pain receptors induced by peripheral nerve injury. Science 251: 1608–1610

Schaible H G, Schmidt R F 1985 Effects of an experimental arthritis on the sensory properties of fine articular afferent units. Journal of Neurophysiology 54: 1109–1122

Schaible H G, Schmidt R F 1988 Time course of mechanosensitivity changes in articular afferents during a developing experimental arthritis. Journal of Neurophysiology 60: 2180–2195

Schlag-Rey M, Schlag J 1984 Visuomotor functions of central thalamus in monkey, I. Unit activity related to spontaneous eye movements. Journal of Neurophysiology 51: 1149–1174

Schreiner L, Kling A 1953 Behavioural changes following rhinencephalic injury in cat. Journal of Neurophysiology 15: 643–659

Seitz R J, Roland P E (1992) Learning of sequential and finger movements in man: a combined kinematic and positron emission tomography (PET) study. European Journal of Neurosciences 4: 154–165

Shima K, Aya K, Mushiake H, Inase M, Aizawa H, Tanji J 1991 Two movement-related foci in the primate cingulate cortex observed in signal-triggered and self-paced forelimb movements. Journal of Neurophysiology 65: 188–202

Simone D A, Kajander K C 1997 Responses of A-fiber nociceptors to noxious cold. Journal of Neurophysiology 77: 2049–2060

Simone D A, Marchettini P, Caputi G, Ochoa J L 1994 Identification of muscle afferents subserving sensation of deep pain in humans. Journal of Neurophysiology 72: 883–889

Snyder R 1977 The organization of the dorsal root entry zone in cats and monkeys. Journal of Comparative Neurology 174: 47–70

Stacey M J 1969 Free nerve endings in skeletal muscle of the cat. Journal of Anatomy 105: 231–254

Stamford J A 1995 Descending control of pain. British Journal of Anaesthesia 75: 217–227

Sugiura Y, Terui N, Hosoya Y 1989 Difference in distribution of central terminals between visceral and somatic unmyelinated (C) primary afferent fibers. Journal of Neurophysiology 62: 834–840

Talbot J D, Marrett S, Evans A C, Meyer E, Bushnell M C, Duncan G H 1991 Multiple representations of pain in human cerebral cortex. Science 251: 1355–1358

Tanelian D I 1991 Cholinergic activation of a population of corneal afferent nerves. Experimental Brain Research 86: 414–420

Torebjörk H E, Ochoa J L 1980 Specific sensations evoked by activity in single identified sensory units in man. Acta Physiologica Scandinavica 110: 445–447

Treede R-D, Meyer R A, Campbell J N 1991 Classification of primate A-fiber nociceptors according to their heat response properties. Pflügers Archives (Suppl. 1) 418: R42

Treede R-D, Kenshalo D R, Gracely R H, Jones A K P 1999 The cortical representation of pain. Pain 79: 105–111

Truex R C, Taylor M J, Smythe M Q, Gildenberg P L 1965 The lateral cervical nucleus of cat, dog and man. Journal of Comparative Neurology 139: 93–104

Vogt B A, Pandya D N 1987 Cingulate cortex of the rhesus monkey: II. Cortical afferents. Journal of Comparative Neurology 262: 271–289

Wall P D 1967 The laminar organization of dorsal horn and effects of descending impulses. Journal of Physiology 188: 403–423

Wall P D, Gutnick M 1974 Ongoing activity in peripheral nerves: the physiology and pharmacology of impulses originating from a neuroma. Experimental Neurology 43: 580–593

Wang Q-P, Nakai Y 1994 The dorsal raphe: an important nucleus in pain modulation. Brain Research Bulletin 34: 575–585

Willis W D, Coggeshall R E 1991 Sensory Mechanisms of the Spinal Cord, 2nd edn. Plenum Press, New York

Willis W D, Al-Chaer E D, Quast M J, Westlund K N 1999 A visceral pathway in the dorsal column of the spinal cord. Proceedings of the National Academy of Sciences USA 96: 7675–7679

Wilson P, Meyers D E, Snow P J 1986 The detailed somatotopic organization of the dorsal horn in the lumbosacral enlargement of the cat spinal cord. Journal of Neurophysiology 55: 604–617

Woolf C J, Shortland P, Coggeshall R E 1992 Peripheral nerve injury triggers central sprouting of myelinated afferents. Nature 355: 75–78

Yezierski R P 1988 Spinomesencephalic tract: projections from the lumbosacral spinal cord of the rat, cat and monkey. Journal of Comparative Neurology 267: 131–146

Yezierski R P, Gerhart K D, Schrock R J, Willis W D 1983 A further examination of effects of cortical stimulation on primate spinothalamic tract cells. Journal of Neurophysiology 49: 424–441

Zhang D, Carlton S M, Sorkin L S, Willis W D 1990 Collaterals of primate spinothalamic tract neurons to the periaqueductal gray. Journal of Comparative Neurology 296: 277–290

3

Neurophysiology of pain and pain modulation

Anthony Wright

OVERVIEW

In clinical practice, physiotherapists and occupational therapists often see the impact of pain on an individual. We see people rapidly transformed, from a situation in which they are experiencing no pain or minimal levels of pain, to a situation in which their pain experience is so severe and pervasive that it drives all of their behaviours. Pain can become the central focus of their existence.

Examples of patients who have sustained a whiplash injury, an acute back injury, a major fracture or a traumatic amputation or other acute trauma provide an indication of the impact of pain on previously pain-free individuals. The level of change that occurs in the behaviour of these individuals implies a very marked up-regulation of nociceptive system function, and consequent upon this, enormous neuroplasticity and change in many aspects of central nervous system function.

A large body of research has developed describing the ways in which nociceptive system function can be up-regulated, and pointing to the effects of up-regulation of the nociceptive system on somatomotor and somatosympathetic function. The nociceptive system is normally a very quiescent system requiring strong, intense, potentially damaging stimulation before it becomes activated. Yet, once an individual is experiencing pain, relatively innocuous stimuli activate the system and trigger pain perception. This altered perceptual state is encompassed by the phenomena of hyperalgesia, an exaggerated or increased response to a noxious stimulus, and allodynia, the production of pain by a stimulus that would not normally be painful (see Box 3.1). These phenomena and their neurophysiological basis will be discussed.

This chapter describes many of the processes that exist for up-regulation of the nociceptive system in response to tissue injury. The processes of peripheral and central sensitization are described. Potential interactions between the nociceptive, motor and autonomic systems are considered. The potential for psychosocial factors to influence neuroplasticity within the nociceptive system is also discussed. The functional importance of pain modulation systems will be considered in the context of mechanisms to down-regulate activity in the nociceptive system.

Learning objectives

Having studied this chapter students will:

1. Understand distinctions between primary and secondary hyperalgesia.
2. Understand the concepts of up-regulation and down-regulation of nociceptive system function.
3. Understand the processes of peripheral sensitization.
4. Understand the concept of 'inflammatory soup'.
5. Understand the concept of silent nociceptors or mechanically insensitive afferents.
6. Understand the processes of central sensitization.
7. Understand the interrelationship between the nociceptive system and the motor system.
8. Understand the interrelationship between the nociceptive system and the sympathetic nervous system.
9. Understand central integration of nociceptive inputs.
10. Understand the functional role of pain modulation systems.

Box 3.1   Key terms defined

Hyperalgesia – an increased response to a stimulus which is normally painful (Merskey & Bogduk 1994)

Allodynia – pain due to a stimulus which does not normally provoke pain (Merskey & Bogduk 1994)

Primary hyperalgesia – hyperalgesia present in the zone of tissue damage

Secondary hyperalgesia – hyperalgesia present in a region in which there is no evidence of tissue damage

Peripheral sensitization – altered transduction sensitivity of high threshold nociceptors

Central sensitization – increased excitability of pain-related central nervous system neurons

Up-regulation – mechanisms leading to increased sensitivity of the nociceptive system

Down-regulation – mechanisms leading to decreased sensitivity of the nociceptive system

---

Chapter 2 provided a detailed description of the neuro-anatomy of the nociceptive system and its intimate relationship with other major systems, such as the motor system and the sympathetic nervous system. While that description readily illustrates the distributed nature of the nociceptive system, it alone cannot provide an explanation of the plasticity of the system, and the degree to which it changes in response to an initial pain stimulus.

It is readily apparent that for the majority of people the nociceptive system is normally very quiescent, providing only a warning stimulus in response to extreme stimuli. Yet when pain becomes established it has a pervasive influence on all aspects of central nervous system function. It is now apparent that a number of mechanisms, at both the cellular and systems levels, contribute to this ability to dramatically alter the sensitivity of the nociceptive system.

This chapter will focus on mechanisms contributing to neuroplasticity in the nociceptive system, before considering the impact of altered nociceptive system activity on the function of the motor system and the sympathetic nervous system.

HYPERALGESIA

Since the 1930s, many researchers have investigated hyperalgesia (see Box 3.1) occurring as a result of peripheral injuries and visceral lesions. The hyperalgesic state is characterized by a decreased threshold for eliciting pain, increased pain with suprathreshold stimulation and spontaneous pain (Meyer et al 1985). The related phenomenon of allodynia also involves a reduced threshold for eliciting pain, although in this case there is also dissociation between the modality of the stimulus and the quality of pain produced (Merskey & Bogduk 1994). In most situations, the stimulus would be perceived as being non-painful. An example might be a situation in which a cold stimulus is perceived as a burning pain. The presence of allodynia implies some degree of neuroanatomical reorganization, as discussed in detail later in the chapter.

Primary and secondary hyperalgesia

It is widely recognized that noxious stimuli evoke two distinct forms of hyperalgesia that have been termed primary and secondary hyperalgesia (Hardy et al 1950). Noxious cutaneous stimulation initially produces a zone of primary hyperalgesia around the site of injury, after which a zone of secondary hyperalgesia gradually develops over a wide surrounding area. The zone of primary hyperalgesia is characterized by sensitivity to both thermal and mechanical stimuli, whereas the zone of secondary hyperalgesia is characterized by sensitivity to mechanical stimuli only (Raja et al 1984).

Microneurography studies

Utilizing capsaicin (the pungent ingredient in red pepper) as a nociceptive stimulus, Torebjörk and LaMotte conducted a series of studies to investigate the phenomena of primary and secondary hyperalgesia using microneurographic techniques (LaMotte et al 1992, Torebjörk et al 1992). Microneurography involves inserting fine electrodes into peripheral nerves to record from, or stimulate, individual nerve fascicles. Following intradermal injection of capsaicin, subjects developed mechanical and thermal hyperalgesia in an area surrounding the injection site (zone of primary hyperalgesia). Subsequently, a much wider area of mechanical hyperalgesia developed around the injection site (zone of secondary hyperalgesia). Distinct regions of mechanical hyperalgesia to pressure, punctate and brushing stimuli could be discerned (see Fig. 3.1) (Koltzenburg et al 1992).

Microneurographic recordings from unmyelinated

C-polymodal nociceptors, innervating the zone of primary hyperalgesia, indicated that these units were sensitized following the injection of capsaicin. Sensitization is characterized by increased impulse activity in response to a standardized stimulus and spontaneous impulse activity in the absence of stimulation. Recordings from unmyelinated C-polymodal nociceptors and myelinated A-fibres innervating the zone of secondary hyperalgesia showed that these units were not sensitized (La Motte et al 1992). However, intraneural electrical stimulation of myelinated afferents resulted in a report of pain and soreness (Torebjörk et al 1992). This response was more pronounced following stimulation with repetitive trains of stimuli leading to temporal summation. Since stimulation of myelinated afferents does not normally result in pain perception, it was proposed that the evoked soreness and associated mechanical hyperalgesia resulted from altered central processing of myelinated afferent inputs (Torebjörk et al 1992). It is suggested therefore that primary hyperalgesia is predominantly due to peripheral sensitization of nociceptors, whereas secondary hyperalgesia is dependent on the process of central sensitization in cells processing nociceptive information at the spinal-cord level.

Summary

Hyperalgesia is a psychophysical phenomenon, characterized by altered response thresholds for various forms of stimulation. It is clear that after injury there may be distinct differences between the mechanisms leading to hyperalgesia in injured and uninjured tissue. It is also apparent that the time course and extent of hyperalgesia is different for different forms of stimulation.

PERIPHERAL SENSITIZATION

There are now large bodies of research investigating both peripheral and central sensitization and it has become apparent that both processes are of great importance in up-regulation of the nociceptive system following injury.

Many early studies pointed to sensitization of peripheral nociceptors as a mechanism underlying the increased sensitivity to subsequent stimulation that takes place following tissue injury. Chapter 2 provides a detailed description of the ultrastructure of nociceptors and distinguishes specific groups of nociceptors. It is apparent that many peripheral nociceptors are polymodal, in the sense that they respond to chemical as well as mechanical and thermal nociceptive stimulation (Kumazawa 1996). It is also apparent that

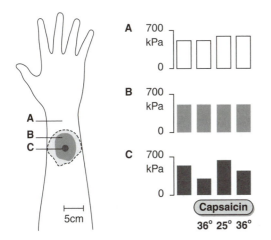

Figure 3.1 Spatial development of mechanical hyperalgesia 30 min after topical application of capsaicin to the volar skin of the forearm. The black area is the site of capsaicin application and the hatched and punctuated regions show the extent of mechanical hyperalgesia tested with cotton swabs or punctate stimuli. A, B and C indicate sites for testing pressure pain thresholds. Pressure pain thresholds only drop inside the skin area treated with capsaicin and this effect is temperature dependent. (Reprinted from Pain, 51, Koltzenburg et al, pp 201–219. © (1992) with permission from Elsevier Science.)

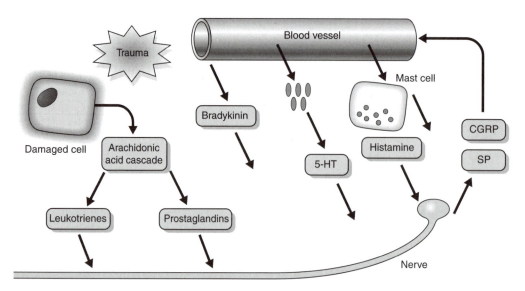

Figure 3.2 Chemical mediators contributing to peripheral sensitisation (CGRP = calcitonin gene-related peptide; SP = substance P; 5-HT = serotonin). (Reprinted from Maciewicz and Wittink, Physiology of pain, editors Wittink and Hoskins, Chronic Pain Management for Physical Therapists, Boston, MA, Butterworth-Heinemann, 1997 with permission.)

chemical mediators released into the tissues because of tissue injury promote sensitization of peripheral nociceptors. Some of the key mediators which have been identified include bradykinin, serotonin, histamine, potassium ions, adenosine triphosphate, protons, prostaglandins, nitric oxide, leukotrienes and cytokines (see Fig. 3.2) (Dray 1995).

The effects of these mediators involve binding to specific receptors, activation of ion channels for depolarization, activation of intracellular second messenger systems, release of a range of neuropeptides to promote neurogenic inflammation and alteration of neuronal properties by modifying gene transcription (Bevan 1996, Dray 1995). A number of receptors and second messenger systems may be activated following the release of different inflammatory mediators (Mizamura & Kumazawa 1996).

While polymodal receptors respond to a range of stimuli, it is apparent that different molecular receptors and second messenger systems are involved in excitation and sensitization for different stimulation modalities (Mizamura & Kumazawa 1996). It is therefore important to note that nociceptors may become differentially sensitized to thermal, mechanical and/or chemical stimuli. An individual nociceptor can potentially exhibit sensitization to thermal stimuli for example, while retaining normal sensitivity to mechanical or chemical stimuli.

'Inflammatory soup'

One of the most fundamental influences on nociceptor sensitivity is the pH of the surrounding tissue. High local proton concentrations are known to occur in many inflammatory states, and the consequent reduction in pH can contribute to sensitization of polymodal nociceptors (Handwerker & Reeh 1991, 1992, Reeh & Steen 1996). Altered pH of the local chemical environment of peripheral nociceptors is a particularly important factor in inducing mechanical sensitization and ischaemic pain (Dray 1995, Steen et al 1992). Combinations of inflammatory mediators, and the combination of chemical mediators with altered tissue pH, appear to be more effective in inducing sensitization than individual chemical mediators alone (Handwerker & Reeh 1991). Thus, in the natural situation, it appears to be a blend of chemical mediators, which Handwerker and Reeh have referred to as 'inflammatory soup', that produces sensitization of peripheral nociceptors (Handwerker & Reeh 1991).

Multiple forms of peripheral sensitization

Endogenous chemicals act on a variety of receptors, activate a number of different intracellular second messenger systems and influence different ion channels (Dray 1995, Mizamura & Kumazawa 1996), resulting in distinctions between thermal, mechanical and chemical sensitization in specific populations of noci-ceptors (Mizamura & Kumazawa 1996). For example, prostaglandins may induce sensitization to chemical mediators at much lower concentrations than those required to induce sensitization to heat stimuli (Mizamura & Kumazawa 1996). The vanilloid receptor, VR1 has been identified as a specific molecular mechanism for thermal hyperalgesia, as well as sensitization following capsaicin administration (Cesare et al 1999).

Peripheral sensitization can be produced through a number of different mechanisms. It can occur because of a direct influence of mediators, such as protons and serotonin, on membrane ion channels, particularly sodium channels, to increase membrane permeability and cellular excitability (Dray 1995). It is also apparent that many mediators act indirectly via G proteins, and a variety of second messengers, to induce changes in neuronal sensitivity. A range of chemical mediators play important roles in sensitization. The actions of these mediators normally fall into one of two categories; either direct activation of a nociceptive afferent, or sensitization so that subsequent stimulation leads to an enhanced response.

Direct influence on membrane ion channels

Increased proton concentration results in increased membrane permeability to cations, and sustained changes in mechanosensitivity and neuronal activation. The mechanism of action of protons appears to be very similar to that of exogenously applied capsaicin (Dray 1995). Adenosine triphosphate, bradykinin, serotonin and prostaglandins may act on receptors that produce changes in potassium ion permeability (Dray 1995).

G-protein-coupled intracellular cascades

It is also apparent that kinins such as bradykinin act on the B2 receptor causing phospholipase C activation, among other effects. This leads to the release of intracellular calcium and activation of ion channels to increase membrane permeability, particularly for sodium and calcium ions (Dray 1995). Increased intracellular calcium ion concentration also leads to the release of neuropeptides such as substance P, and stimulation of arachidonic acid production, leading to the production of prostaglandins and leukotrienes (Dray 1995).

Inhibition of hyperpolarization

Another mechanism by which peripheral sensitization can occur is inhibition of the hyperpolarization that occurs after impulse generation. This slow after-hyperpolarization limits the number of action potentials that can be generated following stimulation. Prostaglandins and bradykinin act to inhibit this phenomenon, allowing the neuron to fire repetitively (Dray 1995). This may also be one of the mechanisms activated by serotonin (Dray 1996).

Indirect mechanisms

Sensitization following the release of cytokines and leukotrienes appears to occur via indirect mechanisms, whereby these agents stimulate other cells to release sensitizing agents. For example, leukotriene B4 stimulates the release of 8R, 15SdiHETE from leukocytes, and this then acts to sensitize polymodal nociceptors (Levine et al 1993). Some of these agents may also act to induce receptors for other inflammatory mediators (Rang & Urban 1995).

In addition, Ca^{2+} and calmodulin can activate nitric oxide synthase to trigger the production of nitric oxide. Nitric oxide functions as a messenger between neurons and surrounding tissues. As it diffuses widely through the tissues, it can induce relaxation of vascular smooth muscle and may contribute to the spread of sensitization in the peripheral tissues (Anbar & Gratt 1997).

Action of trophic factors

There is increasing evidence for the role of nerve growth factor as a mediator of hyperalgesia (Anand 1995). Its actions include triggering mast cell degranulation, stimulating the release of neuropeptides and regulating other proteins such as proton-activated ion channels (Anand 1995, Dray 1995, 1996, Shu & Mendell 1999). The induced hyperalgesia may be reduced by the administration of anti-nerve growth factor antibodies (Woolf et al 1994). It has been suggested that nerve growth factor may be particularly important for thermal sensitization, and that it may condition the response of the VR1 receptor to capsaicin or thermal stimulation (Shu & Mendell 1999).

Mechanical hyperalgesia appears to be induced over a much longer time period (Shu & Mendell 1999). Blockade of nerve growth factor function by the administration of the nerve growth factor-specific tyrosine kinase receptor A, coupled to human immunoglobulin-γ (trkA-IgG), prevents the development of thermal and mechanical hyperalgesia following joint inflammation (McMahon et al 1995). The trkA-IgG fusion molecule has the effect of binding nerve growth factor and reducing the amount of free nerve growth factor present in the tissues.

Other neuroptrophic factors include brain-derived neurotrophic factor and glial cell line-derived neurotrophic factor. Although expressed by peripheral afferents, their primary effect appears to be related to modulation of central nervous system neurons. This will be discussed below.

Summary

The processes of peripheral sensitization are clearly one way in which nociceptive system activity can be up-regulated in response to tissue injury. It is apparent that the sensitization process is relatively complex, and that different forms of sensitization may develop depending on the nature of the injury or disease. Spontaneous discharge, reduced activation thresholds, inhibition of slow after-hyperpolarization and increased discharge rates in response to suprathreshold stimulation, contribute to increasing the nociceptive afferent input to the central nervous system.

OTHER MECHANISMS WHICH UP-REGULATE THE PERIPHERAL NOCICEPTIVE SYSTEM

Silent nociceptors

It is now well established that in many tissues there is a significant population of nociceptors that remain essentially inactive under normal conditions (see Fig. 3.3). These sleeping or silent nociceptors are activated because of tissue injury, with consequent release of chemical mediators and increased tissue hypoxia (Schmidt 1996). Schmidt estimates that they may represent approximately one-third of the total nociceptor population in joints (Schmidt 1996). They appear to be present in skin, joints, muscle and visceral tissue. At least 50% of visceral afferents may fall into this category (Mayer & Gebhart 1994). Once activated, these neurons exhibit marked sensitization, with increased spontaneous discharge rates, reduced thresholds for evoked discharge and increased discharge rates in response to stimulation.

Phenotype change

A further mechanism contributing to up-regulation of the nociceptive system has recently been described. Woolf and Costigan (1999) proposed that in the situation

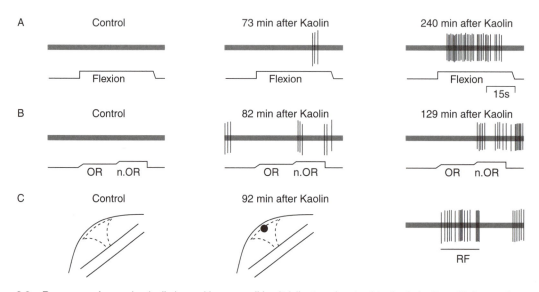

Figure 3.3 Response of a mechanically insensitive group IV unit (silent nociceptors) to the induction of inflammation (injection of kaolin and carrageenan) in the knee joint. **A:** Responses to flexion of the knee before and after inflammation. **B:** Responses to outward or external rotation of the knee before and after inflammation. **C:** Development of a receptive field after inflammation. (Reprinted from Pain, 55, Schaible and Grubb, pp 5–54. © (1993) with permission from Elsevier Science.)

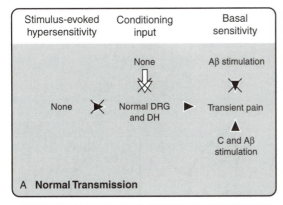

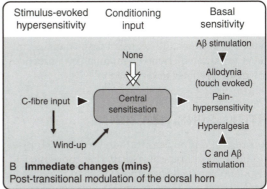

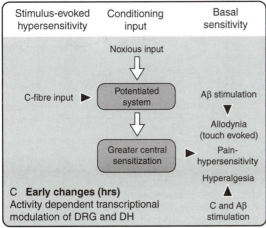

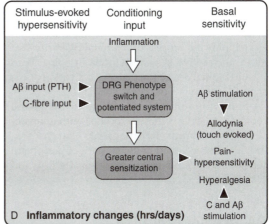

Figure 3.4 State-dependent sensory processing. **A:** The basal sensitivity of the system is normally such that only high-intensity stimuli produce pain. **B:** C fibre inputs produce immediate posttranslational changes in dorsal horn resulting in central sensitisation such that low-intensity stimuli result in pain. **C:** Conditioning C fibre inputs induce activity-dependent transcriptional changes in the DRG and dorsal horn, resulting in a potentiated system with augmented responsiveness to subsequent C fibre inputs. **D:** Inflammation results in both a potentiated system and phenotypic switches such that both C fibre and low-intensity Aβ fibre inputs can evoke central sensitization (from Woolf and Costigan, Transcriptional and posttranslational plasticity and the generation of inflammatory pain. Proceedings of the National Academy of Sciences of the USA 96: 7723–7730. © 1999, National Academy of Sciences, USA with kind permission).

where inflammation has been present for some time, transcriptional changes in gene expression might result in phenotype changes in some myelinated afferents, such that these fibres acquire the neurochemical properties of unmyelinated C fibres (See Fig. 3.4). Under these circumstances, myelinated afferents begin to express and release many of the neuropeptides that are important for inducing long-term changes in neuronal sensitivity. Importantly, this means that these fibres can contribute to nociception by inducing changes in central nervous system neurons (Woolf & Costigan, 1999). They may also contribute to the release of peptides and other chemical mediators responsible for peripheral sensitization. This conversion of myelinated afferents appears to be an additional

mechanism for up-regulation of peripheral nociceptive input.

Summary

Activation of nociceptors, sensitization of currently responsive nociceptors, recruitment of mechanically insensitive or silent nociceptors, and phenotype conversion of non-nociceptive afferents, represent four major mechanisms whereby tissue injury and inflammation can trigger both temporal and spatial summation of nociceptive afferent inputs to the central nervous system. Acting in concert, these mechanisms can contribute to substantial up-regulation of peripheral nociceptive system function. Ultimately, increased impulse activity in nociceptive neurons may be interpreted as pain at higher levels within the central nervous system. It is apparent, however, that there is not a constant link between the degree of tissue damage and the level of pain experienced; modulatory influences will be discussed later in this chapter.

CENTRAL SENSITIZATION

The process of central sensitization (Woolf 1994) is an important aspect of neuroplasticity that contributes to up-regulation of the nociceptive system in response to injury. This process may provide a link between the presence of pain, and sensorimotor and autonomic dysfunction in patients experiencing pain. Central sensitization describes the changes occurring at a cellular level to support the process of neuronal plasticity that occurs in nociceptive system neurons in spinal cord and in supraspinal centres, because of activation of the nociceptive system (Woolf 1994).

This process is initiated by activity in peripheral nociceptors, particularly those associated with unmyelinated afferent neurons, but it appears that the process can also be sustained in the absence of peripheral nociceptor input (Coderre & Melzack 1987, Woolf 1983).

NMDA receptor activation

Excitatory amino acid receptors, particularly those of the N-methyl-D-aspartate (NMDA) subtype have been strongly implicated in the generation of central sensitization (Dickenson 1995, Mao et al 1995, Woolf 1994). Release of excitatory amino acids such as glutamate, and concomitant release of excitatory neuropeptides, such as substance P and neurokinin A, from the presynaptic terminals of nociceptive afferents, initiates a cascade of changes in postsynaptic spinal cord neurons (Duggan et al 1988, 1990, Wilcox 1991). These include G-protein-mediated activation of phospholipase C, leading to the release of Ca^{2+} from intracellular compartments, as well as the production of diacyl glycerol, activating protein kinase C, which in turn modulates ion channel activity (see Fig. 3.5) (Mao et al 1995, Woolf 1994). These changes up-regulate NMDA receptors and enhance the neuron's responsiveness to subsequent excitatory amino acid release (Woolf 1994). One outcome of this up-regulation of NMDA receptors is an increased Ca^{2+} influx into the cell. Increased intracellular Ca^{2+} concentration reduces transmembrane potential, activates NMDA receptor ion channels and renders the cell more excitable.

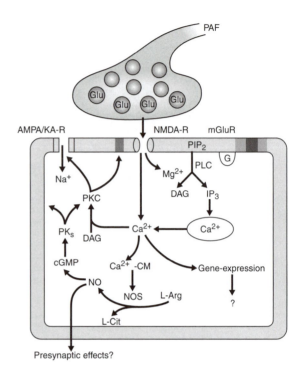

Figure 3.5 Release of glutamate from primary afferent fibres triggers many changes within spinal cord neurons. Activation of the NMDA receptor induces and influx of Ca^{2+} through Ca^{2+} channels, while activation of metabotrophic EAA receptors mobilizes Ca^{2+} from intracellular compartments. Increased intracellular Ca^{2+} concentration initiates a number intracellular cascades including PKC translocation/activation, NO production and regulation of gene expression. (PAF = primary afferent fibre; Glu = glutamate; AMPA/KA-R = α-amino-3-hydroxy-5-methylisoxazole-4-propanoic acid/kainic acid receptor; mGluR = metabotrophic glutamate receptor; G = guanosine triphosphate (GTP) binding protein; PLC = phospholipase C, Ca^{2+}-CM + calcium-calmodulin complex; NOS = nitric oxide synthase; L-Arg = L-arginine; L-Cit = L-citrulline; cGMP = cyclic guanosine monophosphate; PKs = protein kinases). (Reprinted from Pain, 62, Mao et al, pp 259–274. © (1995) with permission from Elsevier Science.)

Nitric oxide production

One other effect of increased intracellular Ca^{2+} concentration is to trigger the production of nitric oxide, which has important second messenger functions within the cell and is thought to be capable of diffusing out of the cell to bring about increased activation of the primary afferent neuron (Meller & Gebhart 1993).

Synthesis of nitric oxide is catalysed by the enzyme nitric oxide synthase, which is activated by binding of Ca^{2+}/calmodulin complexes (Gordh et al 1995). Nitric oxide, in turn, is thought to activate guanylate cyclase, triggering an intracellular cascade. The capacity of nitric oxide to diffuse may be an important factor in the spread of sensitization that appears to occur in spinal cord neurons.

Other glutamate receptors

While in recent years there has been a very strong emphasis on the role of the NMDA receptor in the central sensitization process, it has now become apparent that activation of NMDA receptors may not be critical to the development of all forms of central sensitization. It has been suggested that the NMDA receptor is particularly important in relation to thermal sensitization and that it plays a lesser role in mechanical sensitization (Meller et al 1996).

Co-activation of spinal α-amino-3-hydroxyl-5-methyl-isoxazoleproprionic acid (AMPA) and metabotrophic glutamate receptors induces an acute mechanical sensitization (Meller et al 1996). This is mediated through activation of phospholipase A_2 leading to the production of arachidonic acid. It appears to be the products of the cyclooxygenase pathway for metabolism of arachidonic acid that are of most importance in generating mechanical sensitization (Meller et al 1996). Activation of NMDA receptors, phospholipase C, protein kinase C and the production of nitric oxide do not appear to be important factors in the development of mechanical sensitization (Meller et al 1996).

Trophic factors

Brain-derived neurotrophic factor is released centrally from a sub-population of nociceptive neurons and has an important role in enhancing phosphorylation of NMDA receptors (Boucher et al 2000). It appears to be particularly important in facilitating the development of thermal hyperalgesia, since intrathecal administration of the fusion molecule tyrosine kinase receptor B–human immunoglobulin-γ (trkB–IgG), significantly reduces thermal hyperalgesia induced by carageenan inflammation (Boucher et al 2000, Thompson et al 1999). Current knowledge on the role of glial cell line-derived neurotrophic factor is limited, and while it appears likely that it may play a role in the development of sensitization, this has yet to be elucidated (Boucher et al 2000).

Neuroanatomical reorganization

Neuroanatomical reorganization within the central nervous system is another important factor that may contribute to up-regulation of the nociceptive system.

This mechanism appears to be particularly important when nerve injury has occurred. Under these circumstances, myelinated axons that normally terminate in laminae III and IV of the dorsal horn have been shown to sprout into lamina II of the dorsal horn, potentially developing synaptic connections with intrinsic neurons involved in the transmission of nociceptive afferent inputs (See Fig. 3.6) (Woolf et al 1992). It has been postulated that this may constitute a mechanism whereby normally innocuous afferent input could contribute to nociception (Woolf & Mannion 1999), and provide a neuroanatomical basis for the development of allodynia.

Summary

It is apparent that the process of central sensitization is a relatively complex one and that, in common with peripheral processes, the nature of molecular changes underlying central sensitization may vary, depending on the nature of the inducing stimulus. In both cases, it is increasingly clear that distinctions can be made between the processing of mechanical and thermal nociceptive information.

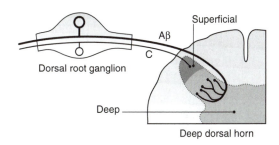

A   Normal terminations of primary afferents in the dorsal horn

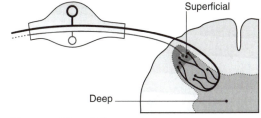

B   After nerve injury, C-fibre terminals atrophy and A-fibre terminals sprout into the dorsal horn

Figure 3.6   Sprouting of A fibre terminals into lamina II of the dorsal horn following peripheral nerve injury. (From Woolf & Mannion, Neuropathic pain: aetiology, symptoms, mechanisms and management. The Lancet, 353, 1959–64. © The Lancet Ltd., 1999.)

Central sensitization contributes to a number of aspects of neuroplasticity, including increased excitability of wide dynamic range cells (Woolf 1989), increased receptive field size (Cook et al 1987) and changes in somatic withdrawal reflexes (Woolf 1984). The development of tenderness (Tunks et al 1988), the spread of pain from a primary location (Simons & Travell 1983), increased guarding of an affected area and alterations in skin temperature (Diakow 1988) are among some of the clinical characteristics that may be manifestations of neuroplasticity due to central sensitization. The potential for neuroanatomical reorganization appears to exist in dorsal horn neurons. This may be an important factor contributing to the development of allodynia.

NOCICEPTIVE-SPECIFIC AND WIDE DYNAMIC RANGE CELLS

Chapter 2 described the existence of both wide dynamic range and nociceptive-specific neurons within the dorsal horn of the spinal cord.

Wide dynamic range cells are particularly prevalent in the deeper laminae of the dorsal horn. They receive input from both nociceptive and non-nociceptive afferent neurons and exhibit a graded response pattern related to the intensity of the afferent stimulus (see Fig. 3.7). If these neurons become sensitized and hyperresponsive, they may discharge at a high rate, following previously non-noxious stimulation (i.e. mild thermal or tactile stimulation) (Siddall & Cousins 1998). If the activity of wide dynamic range neuron exceeds a threshold, then the previously non-noxious stimulus will be perceived as painful. This may, in part, provide the neurophysiological basis for the phenomenon of secondary hyperalgesia, in which pain is perceived following stimulation of normal uninjured tissue.

As described in Chapter 2, nociceptive-specific cells are located predominantly in the superficial laminae of the dorsal horn, where they receive inputs from unmyelinated C-fibre afferents. Under normal conditions, their response characteristics include a lack of impulse generation in response to non-noxious stimu-

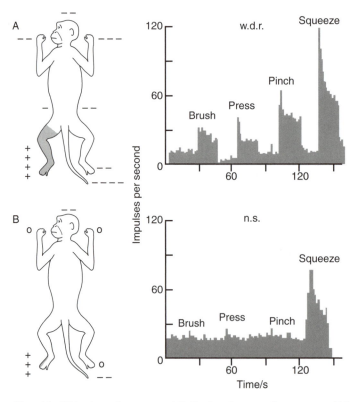

Figure 3.7 Response profiles of A: Wide-dynamic range and B: Nociceptive-specific neurons within the spinothalamic tract. The receptive fields of the cells are indicated on the figures to the left. Excitatory receptive fields are indicated by + signs and inhibitory receptive fields are indicated by – signs. (From Willis WD, Nociceptive pathways: anatomy and physiology of nociceptive ascending pathways, Phil Trans R Soc Lond B 308, 253–268, 1985, with permission.)

lation and a relatively sluggish response to intense noxious stimulation of their peripheral receptive fields (See Fig. 3.7). However, following stimulation of peripheral nociceptive afferents, and the development of central sensitization, the response characteristics of nociceptive- specific neurons change (Cook et al 1987). Subliminal inputs from myelinated afferent neurons are enhanced and the cells begin to exhibit response characteristics that are like those of wide dynamic range neurons.

Despite the fact that these cells can now be activated by non-noxious afferent inputs, it is likely that impulse activity generated by these neurons will contribute to pain perception at higher levels in the central nervous system. This may constitute another mechanism whereby normally non-nociceptive inputs, from injured or uninjured tissues, can contribute to pain perception.

Summary

The processes of central sensitization influence both wide dynamic range and nociceptive-specific cells in the dorsal horn of the spinal cord. Following tissue injury, the response characteristics of these cells change, such that normally non-nociceptive afferent inputs via myelinated afferents can generate impulse activity that is likely to trigger pain perception.

Thus, there are five major mechanisms by which tissue injury can up-regulate nociceptive system function, to contribute to nociception and pain perception.

Peripheral sensitization can reduce the response thresholds of peripheral nociceptors, increasing the likelihood that they will fire in response to peripheral stimulation. Peripheral sensitization can activate previously inactive or silent nociceptors, significantly increasing the population of nociceptors available to signal tissue injury.

Peripheral processes can also induce phenotype changes in myelinated afferent neurons so that they adopt the characteristics of nociceptors. Central sensitization can reduce the response thresholds of central neurons that process nociceptive inputs.

Finally, central sensitization can enhance the effects of previously non-nociceptive afferent inputs, such that afferent activity in large-diameter myelinated neurons can signal pain and tissue damage. This plasticity, and the ability to recruit additional nociceptors and normally non-nociceptive neurons to contribute to pain perception, constitute some of the main reasons why there can be such a substantial up-regulation of the nociceptive system following tissue injury.

SOMATOMOTOR DYSFUNCTION

The major consequences of molecular changes in spinal cord neurons are increased synaptic efficacy and increased neuronal excitability. Neuronal plasticity leading to increased synaptic efficacy and increased neuronal excitability in spinal cord neurons conveying nociceptive information is also likely to influence activity in other neuronal pools, with which the central nociceptive neurons make synaptic connections. This could account for changes in motor and autonomic nervous system function, which are clinical features of many pain states (Sterling et al 2001).

Enhanced withdrawal reflexes

It is clear that this hyperactive state of spinal cord neurons is associated with important changes in terms of sensorimotor function. Woolf (1984) has shown that the establishment of central sensitization is associated with facilitation of flexor withdrawal reflex responses. A prolonged increase in the response duration is maintained for several days, and in some cases may still be present weeks later, when tissue healing is presumed to have occurred (Woolf 1984).

Altered flexor withdrawal reflexes may be of clinical importance in tests such as the straight leg raise and the brachial plexus tension test. Increased muscle activity has been demonstrated in normal subjects when undergoing neural tissue provocation tests (Balster & Jull 1997). These studies support the proposal that muscle activity protects the nervous system from tensile forces. It has been suggested that this increase in muscle activity is due to activation of the flexor withdrawal reflex (Hall et al 1998, Wright et al 1994). Hall et al (1998) showed that the flexor withdrawal reflex is more easily elicited in chronic pain patients than in normal volunteers, during the straight leg raise test.

Vicious cycle model

In addition to increased muscle activation, attributable to the influence of pain and tissue damage on alpha motor neuron function, it has been suggested that pain may influence the excitability of gamma motor neurons contributing to the development of increased muscle tension or spasm.

The 'vicious cycle' model is often alluded to in the literature. As outlined by Johansson and Sojka (1991), the basic concept is that stimulation of nociceptive afferents from muscles excites dynamic and static fusimotor neurons, thus in turn enhancing the sensitivity of primary and secondary muscle spindle afferents (see Fig. 3.8).

Increased activity of primary muscle spindle afferents increases muscle stiffness; such increased muscle stiffness then leads to increased metabolite production and, following the vicious cycle formula, a further increase in muscle stiffness.

In addition, increased activity in the secondary spindle afferents projects back onto the gamma system, perpetuating enhanced muscle stiffness.

These effects are thought to be important in generating muscle spasm and pain (Johansson & Sojka 1991).

There are several studies demonstrating enhanced activity in primary and secondary spindle afferents following the application of chemical mediators such as potassium chloride, lactic acid, bradykinin and serotonin (Djupsjobacka et al 1995, Johansson et al

1993). In addition to altered responses following local muscle injection, these researchers have also demonstrated modulation of secondary muscle spindle afferents following injection of bradykinin into the contralateral muscle (Djupsjobacka et al 1995).

This model may provide some explanation of muscle spasm when it is a significant component of the clinical presentation. However, it provides very little explanation of situations in which we see muscle inhibition and wastage as a result of pain, and a number of studies have failed to show an increase in resting EMG activity, as might be postulated by this model.

Pain adaptation model

Lund and colleagues refute the 'vicious cycle' model, and suggest that pain reduces the ability to contract muscles, rather than making them hyperactive (Lund et al 1991).

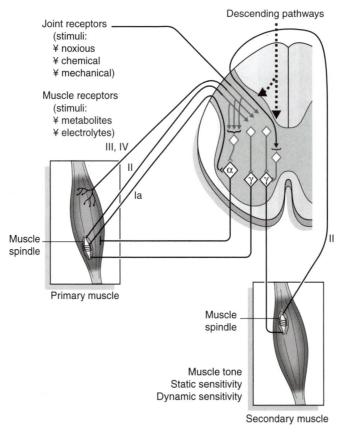

Figure 3.8 Pathophysiological model for mechanisms involved in the genesis and spread of muscular tension in occupational muscle pain and chronic musculoskeletal pain syndromes according to the vicious cycle hypothesis. (Reprinted from Medical Hypotheses, 35, Johansson H and Sojka P, Pathophysiological mechanisms involved in genesis and spread of muscular tension in occupational muscle pain and in chronic musculoskeletal pain syndromes: A hypothesis, 196–203. © 1991 by permission of the publisher Churchill Livingstone.)

Their model, termed the pain adaptation theory, is strongly linked to the phenomenon of central sensitization (see Fig. 3.9). They propose that the effect of noxious stimulation is to alter the activity of type II spinal cord interneurons, such that there is increased inhibition of agonist motor units and increased facilitation of antagonist motor units. This leads to an overall limitation of movement in any desired direction.

The proposed alterations in neural function would be manifest as a reduction in the ability to activate the agonist muscle, a time delay in activating the agonist muscle, and a reduction in the maximum force output from the agonist muscle.

Increased activity in antagonist muscles and a delay in producing reciprocal inhibition of these muscles might also be anticipated. Movement becomes slower, muscles appear to be weaker, and the overall range of movement accomplished may be reduced (Lund et al 1991).

Deficits of this type have been demonstrated in patients with low back pain, and in normal subjects following the injection of hypertonic saline into the lumbar paraspinal muscles (Arendt-Nielsen et al 1996) and the muscles of mastication (Svensson et al 1996). This model may represent a good explanation of the limitation of movement that occurs in the acute pain situation. It is apparent however, that motor dysfunction in chronic pain states may be a somewhat more complex phenomenon.

Emerging models

Recently, researchers have begun to investigate the influence of pain on patterns of neuromuscular activation and control. It has been suggested that the presence of pain leads to inhibition or delayed activation of muscles or muscle groups that perform key synergistic functions to limit unwanted motion (Sterling et al 2001). This produces alterations in the patterns of motor activity and recruitment during functional movement.

It has been suggested that this inhibition usually occurs in the deep muscles, local to the involved joint

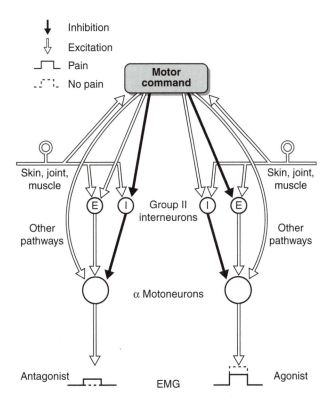

Figure 3.9 Hypothetical description of the pain adaptation model. The motor command facilitates an inhibitory pathway to agonist motoneurons and an excitatory pathway to antagonist motoneurons and disinhibition of the antagonist subgroups of interneurons. This results in reduced agonist motoneuron output and increased antagonist firing during movement. (From Lund et al, The pain adaptation model: a discussion of the relationship between chronic musculoskeletal pain and motor activity, Can J Physiol Pharmacol, 69, 683–694, 1991, with permission.)

that perform a synergistic function in order to control joint stability (Hides et al 1996, Hodges & Richardson 1996, Voight & Wieder 1991).

In both the lumbar and cervical spine, the dysfunctional muscles appear to be the deep muscles that attach directly to the vertebrae. These muscles span the vertebrae and perform important synergistic functions to stabilize articular segments, rather than being primarily responsible for movement production (Cholewicki et al 1997). It appears that while changes in the control of these muscles may be initiated in the presence of pain and tissue injury, they are often sustained beyond the acute pain phase, and may contribute to the chronicity of many musculoskeletal problems.

This model is discussed further in Chapters 13 and 20, as it relates to approaches to pain management using specific exercise programmes.

Summary

It is clear that pain can produce many changes in motor activity. Some of these changes can be explained by peripheral mechanisms in the muscles themselves and by mechanisms within the central nervous system. Certainly, pain has a potent effect on motor activity and control.

The dysfunction that occurs in the neuromuscular system, in the presence of pain, is complex. In addition to the more obvious changes, such as increased muscle activity in some muscle groups and inhibition of others, more subtle anomalous patterns of neuromuscular activation appear to occur.

Some elements of both the 'vicious cycle' and pain adaptation models may be important in acute and chronic pain states. However, neither of these models can fully explain the prolonged changes in motor function that are seen after tissue injury.

Loss of selective activation, and inhibition of certain muscles that perform key synergistic functions, leading to altered patterns of neuromuscular activation, and the ensuing loss of joint stability and control, are initiated with acute pain and tissue injury. However, these phenomena persist, and could be one reason for chronic symptoms.

SOMATOSYMPATHETIC DYSFUNCTION

Peripheral sensitization and central sensitization have also been implicated in changes in autonomic function that are a feature of many pain states. Several authors have recognized that a link may exist between the experience of pain and alterations of sympathetic function, and suggest that sympathetic outflow may influence or maintain afferent activity in nociceptive neurons (Campbell et al 1992, Devor 1995, Janig & Koltzenburg 1992, Perl 1999, Roberts 1986).

The potential role of the sympathetic nervous system (SNS) and postganglionic noradrenergic neurons in complex regional pain syndromes remains controversial (see Chapter 18 for a more detailed consideration of complex regional pain syndrome), and little consideration has been given to the role of such mechanisms in less severe musculoskeletal disorders. Nevertheless, alterations in sympathetic nervous system function have been noted, and abnormalities of somatosympathetic reflex responses have been demonstrated, in patients with musculoskeletal disorders (Mani et al 1989, Smith et al 1994, Thomas et al 1992).

Normal state

Under normal physiological conditions, there appears to be no communication between sympathetic postganglionic neurons and afferent neurons (Janig & Koltzenburg 1992). Afferent neurons are not sensitized or excited by activity in sympathetic efferents, or the release of noradrenaline (Shea & Perl 1985).

Under pathophysiological conditions however, increased alpha-adrenergic sensitivity in injured nociceptors has been demonstrated experimentally (Devor 1995, Janig et al 1996, Perl 1999, Sato & Perl 1991).

Pathological state

Several mechanisms may account for an interaction between sympathetic efferents and mechanoreceptor afferents in the case of peripheral nerve injury (Devor 1995, Janig et al 1996, Perl 1999, Sato & Kumazawa 1996). These include coupling between sympathetic fibres and afferent terminals in a neuroma, coupling between unlesioned postganglionic and afferent terminals following partial nerve lesion, and coupling due to collateral spreading in dorsal root ganglia following peripheral nerve lesion (Janig et al 1996, Perl 1999).

It is clear, however, that the process of peripheral sensitization is essential for the expression of noradrenergic sensitivity in the case of tissue injury or inflammation (Janig et al 1996, Sato & Kumazawa 1996). A form of indirect hyperalgesia, mediated by sympathetic postganglionic noradrenergic neurons, has been proposed and is referred to as sympathetic-dependent or maintained hyperalgesia (Levine et al 1992).

It appears that noradrenaline acts to stimulate prostaglandin release, which in turn induces nociceptor sensitization (Janig et al 1996, Sato & Kumazawa 1996). An important aspect of this model is that it does not require any increase in sympathetic nervous system efferent activity, but rather implies increased sensitivity of peripheral nociceptors to the normal release of noradrenaline.

Summary

It is apparent that activation and up-regulation of the nociceptive system induces changes in somatosympathetic function. However, further research is still required to bring about a comprehensive understanding of the linkages between these systems.

CENTRAL INTEGRATION OF NOCICEPTIVE INPUT

Pain and nociceptive inputs can exert a strong influence on motor function, autonomic function and emotional state. As well as interactions at spinal cord level, integration of nociception and other central nervous system functions must occur at higher centres.

It is also clear that pain perception can be strongly modulated by descending systems originating in various parts of the brain, and that the nociceptive system is normally in a state of tonic inhibition (Cervero & Laird 1996, Stamford 1995). This modulation can take the form of up-regulation of pain perception as well as down-regulation of pain perception, associated with analgesic effects (Cervero & Laird 1996).

It is now apparent that, as well as being influenced by pain, motor activity, autonomic functions and emotional state can in turn also influence pain perception (Dubner & Ren 1999). Consequently, the central nervous system is better viewed as an integrated cyclical system, rather than the simple cause and effect system enshrined in the distinction between afferent and efferent aspects of function.

Functional brain imaging

Functional brain imaging studies, investigating both experimentally-induced pain and clinical pain states, provide substantial evidence for the involvement of a number of key brain sites in pain perception. Some notable regions include the anterior cingulate cortex,

anterior insular cortex, primary somatosensory cortex, secondary somatosensory cortex, a number of regions in the thalamus, and (interestingly) areas such as the premotor cortex that are normally linked to motor function (Casey 1999).

There has been a good deal of controversy about the role of the primary somatosensory cortex in pain perception. Bushnell et al (1999) concluded that this area is involved in the sensory–discriminative aspect of pain perception, but that its involvement can be modulated by the attentional state of the person.

Functional imaging studies have provided abundant evidence of the distributed nature of the nociceptive system, and the potential for close association between areas of the nervous system responding to pain, and areas controlling autonomic and motor function and emotional state (Porro & Cavazzuti 1996). For example, it is clear that both the basal ganglia and the periaqueductal grey region receive nociceptive inputs as well as coordinating important aspects of movement and motor control (Chudler & Dong 1995, Lovick 1991).

Pain and emotional state

Those regions of the brain encompassing the limbic system and areas such as the periaqueductal grey region also provide a neuroanatomical substrate for interactions between nociception, emotional state and autonomic activity (Chapman 1996, Dubner & Ren 1999, Lovick 1991), indeed there is considerable overlap between the neuroanatomical and neurotransmitter systems modulating pain perception and those controlling emotional state (Chapman 1996).

Bandler and Shipley (1994) describe a model of columnar organization that projects from regions of the frontal cortex, the hypothalamus, thalamus and amygdala to the periaqueductal grey region of the midbrain. These neuroanatomical connections may provide the basis for the interaction between cognitive and emotional states, and pain perception, autonomic function and motor activity (Bandler & Shipley 1994).

Summary

Functional brain imaging studies increasingly provide a means of bridging the gap between psychological studies and basic neurophysiological studies, and allow us to gain some basic understanding of the way in which nociception is intimately integrated with many other aspects of central nervous system function. The work provides insights into the complex ways in which cognitive and emotional states can modulate pain perception. This is of considerable importance in understanding the influence of psychosocial factors on pain perception and pain report in the clinical situation.

MODULATION OF NOCICEPTIVE INPUT

The inherent capacity of the central nervous system to control the transmission of nociceptive afferent impulses, and thereby to limit the perception of pain, has been a focus of considerable scientific activity since the publication of Melzack and Wall's (1965) gate control theory. The resultant research has highlighted the importance of endogenous pain control systems and demonstrated that endogenous analgesia is a multifaceted phenomenon, involving a number of neuronal systems (Cannon & Liebeskind 1987, Lovick 1993, Morgan et al 1989).

It is widely recognized that the gate control theory emphasizes the importance of pain inhibition, but it is less widely recognized that the theory also allows for up-regulation of nociceptive input.

Research now clearly demonstrates an important role for the rostral ventromedial medulla in facilitating the development of central sensitization and hyperalgesia in inflammatory pain states (Urban & Gebhart 1999).

Both up-regulation and down-regulation of nociceptive system function due to the influence of systems projecting from the brain to the spinal cord will be discussed in this section.

Descending pain inhibition systems

The descending pain inhibitory systems have been extensively investigated, beginning with a seminal study by Reynolds (1969). This study highlighted the importance of the periaqueductal grey area in the control of nociception, and demonstrated that stimulation of discrete brain regions could produce profound analgesia. The analgesia induced by electrical brain stimulation in the periaqueductal grey region was sufficient to allow abdominal surgery to be carried out without apparent distress to the animals.

Following Reynolds' initial report, it rapidly became apparent that stimulation of a number of brain regions resulted in hypoalgesia in animals (Cannon & Liebeskind 1987, Jones 1992). Although the system involved in pain control is now known to be both extensive and relatively complex, the periaqueductal grey has retained its importance as a key control centre for endogenous analgesic mechanisms.

Distinct regions within the periaqueductal grey appear to be capable of eliciting at least two different forms of analgesia, which are distinguishable mainly in terms of their behavioural, physiological and pharmacological correlates (Cannon and Liebeskind 1987, Fanselow 1991, Lovick 1991, Morgan 1991).

The caudal periaqueductal grey can be divided into ventrolateral, lateral, dorsomedial and dorsolateral columns (see Fig. 3.10) (Bandler & Shipley 1994). Both the lateral and ventrolateral columns appear to be important for modulating pain perception, although they produce pain inhibition as part of two distinctly different behavioural responses (Bandler & Shipley 1994).

Ventrolateral column

Analgesia elicited from stimulation of the ventrolateral periaqueductal grey region is characterized by an association with immobility (Morgan 1991) or 'freezing' (Fanselow 1991), recuperative behaviour and sympathoinhibition (Lovick 1991). The analgesic effect is blocked by the administration of naloxone, particularly in the region of the dorsal raphe nucleus (Cannon et al 1982). It also exhibits tolerance with repeated stimulation (Morgan & Leibeskind 1987), and is consequently described as being an opioid form of analgesia. Ventrolateral periaqueductal grey analgesia appears to require a significant period of peripheral stimulation before it becomes apparent (Takeshige et al 1992).

Lateral column

In contrast, analgesia elicited from the lateral periaqueductal grey region is associated with fight/flight behaviour, aversive reactions (Besson et al 1991, Fanselow 1991, Morgan 1991) and sympathoexcitation (Lovick, 1991, Lovick & Li 1989).

Pharmacological studies indicate that lateral periaqueductal grey region analgesia is not blocked by the administration of naloxone (Cannon et al 1982) and does not exhibit tolerance (Morgan & Liebeskind 1987). It is consequently described as being a nonopioid form of analgesia. The onset of analgesia following stimulation of the lateral column is generally more rapid than ventrolateral column analgesia.

Noradrenergic and serotonergic systems

Fields and Basbaum (1989) highlighted the existence of two distinct projection systems, from the periaqueduc-

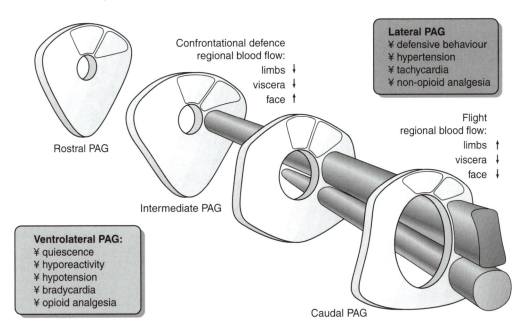

Figure 3.10 The lateral and ventrolateral columns within the periaqueductal grey region. Injection of excitatory amino acids within each of these columns elicits opposing response characteristics as indicated. (Reprinted from Trends in Neurosciences, 17, Bandler R and Shiplay MT, Columnar organization in the midbrain periaqueductal gray: modules for emotional expression? 379–389 (1994) with permission from Elsevier Science.)

tal grey and adjacent brain regions to spinal cord, that predominantly utilize two different neurotransmitters (see Fig. 3.11).

Projections from the lateral column via nucleus gigantocellularis, paragigantocellularis and paragigantocellularis lateralis utilize noradrenaline as a neurotransmitter, and are described as being noradrenergic. Significant projections from locus coeruleus also contribute to this system.

Projections from the ventrolateral column via nucleus raphe magnus, on the other hand, appear to use serotonin (5-hydroxytryptamine) as a neurotransmitter, and are described as being serotonergic. The dorsal raphe nucleus is also an important component of this system.

In a series of studies, Kuraishi and colleagues (Kuraishi 1990, Kuraishi et al 1983, 1991) demonstrated important differences between these control systems. For example, the noradrenergic system has a key role in mediating morphine analgesia in relation to mechanical nociceptive stimuli, whereas the serotonergic system is more important in relation to morphine analgesia directed against thermal nociceptive stimuli (Kuraishi et al 1983).

The descending noradrenergic system acts at spinal cord level to inhibit the release of substance P evoked by peripheral noxious mechanical stimulation, whereas the descending serotonergic system acts to inhibit the release of somatostatin, evoked by peripheral noxious thermal stimulation (Kuraishi 1990). Studies carried out by this group provide evidence of modality-specific control mechanisms for both mechanical and thermal nociception.

Descending pain facilitation systems

Studies investigating descending facilitation of pain and hyperalgesia have been a more recent development. It is now recognized that many of the same areas in the brainstem that are responsible for pain inhibition can also facilitate pain and hyperalgesia when stimulated appropriately (Urban & Gebhart 1999).

There appears to be a bi-directional response with low levels of stimulation (electrical or chemical) facilitating pain, while more intense stimulation produces pain inhibition. Fields et al (1983) characterized specific groups of cells in the rostral ventromedial medulla that may form the basis for this bi-directional control. They identified three distinct cell groups that show characteristically different responses during a thermal

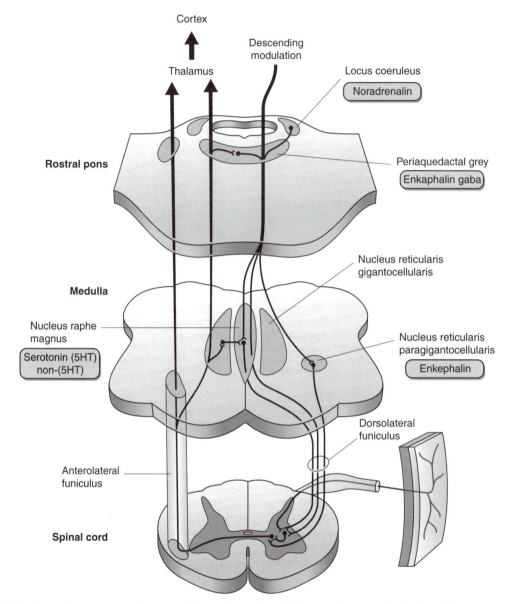

Figure 3.11 Ascending sensory pathways and descending pain modulatory pathways projecting through pons and medulla to spinal cord. Projections through nucleus raphe magnus use serotonin as a neurotransmitter whereas more lateral projections use noradrenaline as a neurotransmitter. (From Siddall and Cousins 1998.)

tail-flick test in the rat. The cells were described as off-cells which show continuous ongoing activity and pause just before the tail-flick response occurs, on-cells that are tonically inhibited but display a pronounced burst of activity just before the tail-flick response occurs, and neutral cells whose activity is not specifically related to the pain response (Fields et al 1983).

This group hypothesized that off-cells provide a tonic inhibition of nociceptive transmission cells in the spinal cord, that is disinhibited and then facilitated by on-cell activity when pain occurs. Subsequent research in a variety of inflammatory pain models has shown that blockade of rostral ventromedial medulla function effectively abolishes the development of hyperalgesia (Urban & Gebhart 1999).

Summary

The capacity for bi-directional control of pain perception mediated by a descending system from the brainstem suggests a number of interesting possibilities. Casey (1999) highlighted the relative importance of the human forebrain, compared to other animals. It is known that relevant anatomical connections exist from a number of forebrain regions to the periaqueductal grey region and the rostral ventromedial medulla (Bandler and Shipley 1994, Rizvi et al, 1991), suggesting that higher brain centres can influence these bulbospinal systems.

The capacity for forebrain regions to control spinal cord processing of nociceptive inputs, via descending bulbospinal tracts, provides a basis for bi-directional modulation of pain perception dependent on attentional, cognitive or emotional state, that may be of importance in some chronic pain states (Dubner & Ren 1999).

Impairments in these systems may be an important factor contributing to the development of chronic pain states such as fibromyalgia.

The influence of higher brain centres on nociceptive system function may also provide a basis for the influence of cognitive–behavioural approaches to pain management on pain perception; and this system is likely to provide the physiological basis for expression of placebo effects (see Chapter 5).

CONCLUSION

Recent advances in our knowledge of pain have provided a much greater insight into the many ways in which nociceptive system activity can be up-regulated in response to tissue injury. It is clear that both peripheral and central mechanisms are important, and that subtle variations in the mechanisms activated can result in different forms of altered sensitivity being induced.

Mechanisms exist to sensitize nociceptors, to recruit previously inactive nociceptors and to utilize afferent inputs via myelinated neurons to contribute to nociception. These mechanisms contribute to substantial spatial and temporal summation of nociceptive inputs. Central mechanisms appear to be particularly important in controlling the spread of sensitivity to uninjured tissues surrounding the region of tissue damage.

Rapidly developing areas of research are also improving our knowledge of the interrelationship between pain, motor and autonomic function, and emotional state.

We are beginning to move away from a largely peripheralist view of tissue injury, to a much more integrated understanding of the influence of pain and injury on the central nervous system, and the patient as a whole. This encompasses an emerging view of the nociceptive system as a highly distributed system that interacts many other neuronal systems.

We are beginning to understand the immense impact of pain and tissue injury on the central nervous system, and the plasticity induced by the presence of pain.

Ultimately this should lead to the development of a more comprehensive approach to the management of patients with pain.

Study questions/questions for revision

1. Describe the two different mechanisms that contribute to the development of primary hyperalgesia and secondary hyperalgesia.
2. List six chemicals that contribute to the development of peripheral sensitization.
3. What is meant by the term, 'inflammatory soup'?
4. What is meant by the term, 'silent nociceptor'?
5. Describe the mechanism by which the NMDA receptor becomes activated.
6. Compare and contrast wide dynamic range and nociceptive-specific cells.
7. Briefly describe the pain adaptation theory.
8. What is meant by the term, 'sympathetic-dependent hyperalgesia'?
9. Compare and contrast the ventrolateral and lateral columns of PAG.
10. What are the functions of off-cells and on-cells?

REFERENCES

Anand P 1995 Nerve growth factor regulates nociception in human health and disease. British Journal of Anaesthesia 75: 201–208

Anbar M, Gratt B M 1997 Role of nitric oxide in the physiopathology of pain. Journal of Pain Symptom Management 14: 225–54

Arendt-Nielsen L, Graven-Nielsen T, Svarrer H, Svensson P 1996 The influence of back pain on muscle activity and co- ordination during gait: a clinical and experimental study. Pain 64: 231–240

Balster S M, Jull G A 1997 Upper trapezius muscle activity during the brachial plexus tension test in asymptomatic subjects. Manual Therapy 2: 144–149

Bandler R, Shipley M T 1994 Columnar organization in the midbrain periaqueductal gray: modules for emotional expression? Trends in Neurosciences 17: 379–389

Besson J-M, Fardin V, Oliveras J-L 1991 Analgesia produced by stimulation of the periaqueductal gray matter: True antinociception versus stress effects. In: Depaulis A, Bandler R (eds) The Midbrain Periaqueductal Gray Matter. Plenum Press, New York, pp 121–138

Bevan S 1996 Signal transduction in nociceptive afferent neurons in inflammatory conditions. Progress in Brain Research 113: 201–213

Boucher T J, Kerr B J, Ramer M S, Thompson S W N, McMahon S B 2000 Neurotrophic factor effects on pain-signalling systems. In: Devor M, Rowbotham M C, Wiesenfeld-Hallin Z (eds) Proceedings of the 9th World Congress on Pain, Progress in Pain Research and Management, Vol. 16. IASP Press, Seattle, pp 175–189

Bushnell M C, Duncan G H, Hofbauer R K, Ha B, Chen J I, Carrier B 1999 Pain perception: is there a role for primary somatosensory cortex?, Proceedings of the National Academy of Sciences 96: 7705–7709

Campbell J N, Meyer R A, Davis K D, Raja S N 1992 Sympathetically maintained pain – a unifying hypothesis. In: Willis W D (ed) Hyperalgesia and Allodynia. Raven Press, New York, pp 141–149

Cannon J T, Prieto G J, Lee A, Liebeskind J C 1982 Evidence for opioid and non-opioid forms of stimulation-produced analgesia in the rat. Brain Research 243: 315–321

Cannon, J T, Liebeskind J C 1987 Analgesic effects of electrical brain stimulation and stress. In: Akil H and Lewis J W (Eds.), Neurotransmitters and Pain Control, Vol. 9, Karger, Basel, pp 283–294

Casey K L 1999 Forebrain mechanisms of nociception and pain: analysis through imaging. Proceedings of the National Academy of Sciences USA 96: 7668–7674

Cervero F, Laird J M A 1996 From acute to chronic pain: mechanisms and hypotheses. In: Carli G and Zimmerman M (eds) Progress in Brain Research, Vol. 110, Elsevier Science BV, Amsterdam, pp 3–15

Cesare P, Moriondo A, Vellani V, McNaughton P A 1999 Ion channels gated by heat. Proceedings of the National Academy of Sciences USA 96: 7658–7663

Chapman C R 1996 Limbic processes and the affective dimension of pain. Progress in Brain Research 110: 63–81

Cholewicki J, Panjabi M M, Khachatryan A 1997 Stabilizing function of trunk flexor-extensor muscles around a neutral spine posture. Spine 22: 2207–2212

Chudler E H, Dong W K 1995 The role of the basal ganglia in nociception and pain. Pain 64: 3–38

Coderre T J, Melzack R 1987 Cutaneous hyperalgesia: contributions of the peripheral and central nervous systems to the increase in pain sensitivity after injury. Brain Research 404: 95–106

Cook A J, Woolf C J, Wall P D, McMahon S B 1987 Dynamic receptive field plasticity in rat spinal cord dorsal horn following C primary afferent input. Nature 325: 151–153

Devor M 1995 Peripheral and central mechanisms of sympathetic related pain. The Pain Clinic 8: 5–14

Diakow P R P 1988 Thermographic imaging of myofascial trigger points. Journal of Manipulative and Physiological Therapeutics 11: 114–117

Dickenson A H 1995 Central acute pain mechanisms. Annals of Medicine 27: 223–227

Djupsjobacka M, Johansson H, Bergenheim M, Wenngren B I 1995 Influences on the gamma-muscle spindle system from muscle afferents stimulated by increased intramuscular concentrations of bradykinin and 5-HT. Neuroscience Research 22: 325–353

Dray A 1995 Inflammatory mediators of pain. British Journal of Anaesthesia 75: 125–131

Dray A 1996 Neurogenic mechanisms and neuropeptides in chronic pain. Progress in Brain Research 110: 85–94

Dubner R, Ren K 1999 Endogenous mechanisms of sensory modulation. Pain (Suppl 6): S45–53

Duggan A W, Hendry I A, Mortom C R, Hutchinson W D 1988 Cutaneous stimuli releasing immunoreactive substance P in the dorsal horn of the cat. Brain Research 451: 261–273

Duggan A W, Hope P J, Jarrot B, Schaible H-G, Fleetwood-Walker S M 1990 Release, spread, and persistence of immunoreactive neurokinin A in the dorsal horn of the cat following noxious cutaneous stimulation. Studies with antibody microprobes. Neuroscience 35: 195–202

Fanselow M S 1991 The midbrain periaqueductal gray as a coordinator of action in response to fear and anxiety. In: Depaulis A and Bandlier R (eds) The Midbrain Periaqueductal Gray Matter. Plenum Press, New York, pp 151–173

Fields H L, Basbaum A I 1989 Endogenous pain control mechanisms. In: Wall P D and Melzack R (eds): Textbook of pain, Churchill Livingstone, Edinburgh, pp 206–217

Fields H L, Bry J, Hentall I, Zorman G 1983 The activity of neurons in the rostral medulla of the rat during withdrawal from noxious heat. Journal of Neuroscience 3: 2545–2552

Gordh T, Karlsten R, Kristensen J 1995 Intervention with spinal NMDA, adenosine, and NO systems for pain modulation. Annals of Medicine 27: 229–234

Hall T, Zusman M, Elvey R 1998 Adverse mechanical tension in the nervous system? Analysis of straight leg raise. Manual Therapy 3: 140–146

Handwerker H O, Reeh P W 1991 Pain and inflammation. In: Bond M R, Charlton I E and Woolf C J (eds) Proceedings of the VIth World Congress on Pain, Pain Research and Clinical Management Elsevier, Amsterdam, pp 59–70

Handwerker H O, Reeh P W 1992 Nociceptors, chemosensitivity and sensitization by chemical agents. In: Willis W D (ed) Hyperalgesia and Allodynia, Raven Press Ltd, New York, pp 107–115

Hardy J D, Wolff H G, Goodell H 1950 Experimental evidence of the nature of cutaneous hyperalgesia. Journal of Clinical Investigation 29: 115–140

Hides J A, Richardson C A, Jull G A 1996 Multifidus muscle recovery is not automatic after resolution of acute, first-episode low back pain. Spine 21: 2763–2769

Hodges P W, Richardson C A 1996 Inefficient muscular stabilization of the lumbar spine associated with low back pain. A motor control evaluation of transversus abdominis. Spine 21: 2640–50

Janig W, Koltzenburg M 1992 Possible ways of sympathetic-afferent interactions. In: Janig W and Schmidt R F (eds) Pathological Mechanisms of Reflex Sympathetic Dystrophy. VCH, Weinheim, pp 213–243

Janig W, Levine J D, Michaelis M 1996 Interactions of sympathetic and primary afferent neurons following nerve injury and tissue trauma. Progress in Brain Research 113: 161–184

Johansson H, Sojka P 1991 Pathophysiological mechanisms involved in genesis and spread of muscular tension in occupational muscle pain and in chronic musculoskeletal pain syndromes: a hypothesis. Medical Hypotheses 35: 196–203

Johansson H, Djupsjobacka M, Sjolander P 1993 Influences of the gamma-muscle spindle system from muscle afferents stimulated by KCL and lactic acid. Neuroscience Research 16: 49–57

Jones S L 1992 Descending control of nociception. In: Light A R (ed) The Initial Processing of Pain and its Descending Control: spinal and trigeminal systems. Karger, Basel, pp 203–277

Koltzenburg M, Lundberg L E, Torebjörk H E 1992 Dynamic and static components of mechanical hyperalgesia in human hairy skin. Pain 51: 207–219

Kumazawa T 1996 The polymodal receptor: bio-warning and defense system. Progress in Brain Research 113: 3–18

Kuraishi Y 1990 Neuropeptide-mediated transmission of nociceptive information and its regulation. Novel mechanisms of analgesics. Yakugaku Zasshi 110: 711–726

Kuraishi Y, Harada Y, Aratani S, Satoh M, Takagi H 1983 Separate involvement of the spinal noradrenergic and serotonergic systems in morphine analgesia: the difference in mechanical and thermal algesic tests. Brain Research 273: 245–252

Kuraishi Y, Kawamura M, Yamaguchi T, Houtani T, Kawabata S, Futaki S, Fuji N, Satoh M 1991 Intrathecal injection of galanin and its antiserum effect nociceptive response of rat to mechanical but not thermal stimuli. Pain 44: 321–324

LaMotte R H, Lundberg L E, Torebjörk H E 1992 Pain, hyperalgesia and activity in nociceptive C units in humans after intradermal injection of capsaicin. Journal of Physiology (London) 448: 749–764

Levine J D, Yetunde O T, Heller P H 1992 Hyperalgesic pain: inflammatory and neuropathic. In: Willis W D (ed) Hyperalgesia and Allodynia, Raven Press Ltd, New York, pp 117–123

Levine J D, Fields H L, Basbaum A I 1993 Peptides and the primary afferent nociceptor. Journal of Neuroscience 13: 2273–2286

Lovick T A 1991 Interactions between descending pathways from the dorsal and ventrolateral periaqueductal gray matter in the rat. In: Depaulis A, Bandlier R (eds) The Midbrain Periaqueductal Gray Matter. Plenum Press, New York, pp 101–120

Lovick T A 1993 Integrated activity of cardiovascular and pain regulatory systems: role in adaptive behavioural responses. Progress in Neurobiology 40: 631–644

Lovick T A, Li P 1989 Integrated activity of neurons in the rostral ventrolateral medulla. Progress in Brain Research 81: 223–232

Lund J P, Donga R, Widmar C G, Stohler C S 1991 The pain adaptation model: a discussion of the relationship between chronic musculoskeletal pain and motor activity. Canadian Journal of Physiology and Pharmacology 69: 683–694

Maciewicz R, Wittink H 1997 Physiology of pain. In: Wittink H and Hoskins M T (eds) Chronic Pain Management for Physical Therapists, Butterworth-Heinemann, Boston, pp 27–42

Mani R, Cooper C, Kidd B L, Cole J D, Cawley M I D 1989 Use of laser doppler flowmetry and transcutaneous oxygen tension electrodes to assess local autonomic dysfunction in patients with frozen shoulder. Journal of the Royal Society of Medicine 82: 536–538

Mao J, Price D D, Mayer D J 1995 Mechanisms of hyperalgesia and morphine tolerance: a current view of their possible interactions. Pain 62: 259–274

Mayer E A, Gebhart G F 1994 Basic and clinical aspects of visceral hyperalgesia. Gastroenterology 107: 271–293

McMahon S B, Bennett D L, Priestley J V, Shelton D L 1995 The biological effects of endogenous nerve growth factor on adult sensory neurons revealed by a trkA-IgG fusion molecule. Nature Medicine 1: 774–780

Meller S T, Gebhart G F 1993 Nitric oxide (NO) and nociceptive processing in the spinal cord. Pain, 52: 127–136

Meller S T, Dykstra C, Gebhart G F 1996 Acute mechanical hyperalgesia in the rat can be produced by coactivation of spinal ionotrophic AMPA and metabotrophic glutamate receptors, activation of phospholipase A2 and generation of cyclooxygenase products. Progress in Brain Research 110: 177–192

Melzack R, Wall P D 1965 Pain mechanisms: a new theory. Science 150: 971–979

Merskey H, Bogduk N 1994 Classification of Chronic Pain: descriptions of chronic pain syndromes and definitions of pain terms. IASP Press, Seattle

Meyer R A, Campbell J N, Raja S N 1985 Peripheral neural mechanisms of cutaneous hyperalgesia. In: Fields H L (ed) Advances in Pain Research and Therapy, Vol. 9, Raven Press, New York, pp 53–71

Mizamura K, Kumazawa T 1996 Modification of nociceptor response by inflammatory mediators and second messengers implicated in their action – a study in canine testicular polymodal receptors. Progress in Brain Research 115–141

Morgan M M 1991 Differences in antinociception evoked from dorsal and ventral regions of the caudal periaqueductal gray matter. In: Depaulis A, Bandlier R (eds) The Midbrain Periaqueductal Gray Matter. Plenum Press, New York, pp 139–150

Morgan M M, Liebeskind J C 1987 Site specificity in the development of tolerance to stimulation-produced analgesia from the periaqueductal gray matter of the rat. Brain Research 425: 356–359

Morgan M M, Sohn J H, Liebeskind J C 1989 Stimulation of the periaqueductal gray matter inhibits nociception at the supraspinal as well as spinal level. Brain Research 502: 61–66

Porro C A, Cavazzuti M 1996 Functional imaging of the pain system in man and animals. Progress in Brain Research 110: 47–62

Perl E R 1999 Causalgia, pathological pain, and adrenergic receptors. Proceedings of the National Academy of Sciences USA 96: 7664–7667

Raja S N, Campbell J N, Meyer R A 1984 Evidence for different mechanisms of primary and secondary hyperalgesia following heat injury to the glabrous skin. Brain 107: 1179–1188

Rang H P, Urban L 1995 New molecules in analgesia. British Journal of Anaesthesia 75: 145–156

Reeh P W, Steen K H 1996 Tissue acidosis in nociception and pain. Progress in Brain Research 113: 143–151

Reynolds D V 1969 Surgery in the rat during electrical analgesia by focal brain stimulation. Science 164: 444–445

Rizvi T A, Ennis M, Behbehani M M, Shipley M T 1991 Connections between the central nucleus of the amygdala and the midbrain periaqueductal gray: topography and reciprocity. Journal of Comparative Neurology 303: 121–131

Roberts W J 1986 A hypothesis on the physiological basis of causalgia and related pains. Pain 24(3): 297–311

Sato J, Kumazawa T 1996 Sympathetic modulation of cutaneous polymodal receptors in chronically inflamed and diabetic rats. Progress in Brain Research 113: 153–159

Sato J, Perl E R 1991 Adrenergic excitation of cutaneous pain receptors induced by peripheral nerve injury. Science 251: 1608–1610

Schaible H-G, Grubb B D 1993 Afferent and spinal mechanisms of joint pain. Pain 55: 5–54

Schmidt R F 1996 The articular polymodal nociceptor in health and disease. Progress in Brain Research 113: 53–81

Shea V, Perl E R 1985 Failure of sympathetic stimulation to affect responsiveness of rabbit polymodal nociceptors. Journal of Neurophysiology 54: 513–519

Shu X Q, Mendell L M 1999 Neurotrophins and hyperalgesia. Proceedings of the National Academy of Sciences USA 96: 7693–7696

Siddall P J, Cousins M J 1998 Introduction to pain mechanisms: implications for neural blockade. In: Cousins, M J, Bridenbaugh P O (eds) Neural Blockade in Clinical Anesthesia and Management of Pain. Lippincott-Raven, Philadelphia

Simons D G, Travell J G 1983 Myofascial origins of low back pain. Postgraduate Medicine 73: 66–109

Smith R W, Papadopolous E, Mani R, Cawley M I D 1994 Abnormal microvascular responses in lateral humeral epicondylitis. British Journal of Rheumatology 33: 1166–1168

Stamford J A 1995 Descending control of pain. British Journal of Anaesthesia 75: 217–227

Steen K H, Reeh P W, Anton F, Handwerker H O 1992 Protons selectively induce lasting excitation and sensitisation to mechanical stimuli of nociceptors in rat skin, in vitro. Journal of Neuroscience 12: 86–95

Sterling M, Jull G, Wright A 2001 The effect of pain on motor activity and control. Journal of Pain *in press*

Svensson P, Arendt-Nielsen L, Houe L 1996 Sensory-motor interactions of human experimental jaw muscle pain: a quantitative analysis. Pain 64: 241–250

Takeshige C, Sato T, Mera T, Hisamitsu T, Fang J 1992 Descending pain inhibitory system involved in acupuncture analgesia. Brain Research Bulletin 29: 617–634

Thomas D, Siahamis G, Millicent M, Boyle C 1992 Computerized infrared thermography and isotopic bone scanning in tennis elbow. Annals of the Rheumatic Diseases 51: 103–107

Thompson S W, Bennett D L, Kerr B J, Bradbury E J, McMahon S B 1999 Brain-derived neurotrophic factor is an endogenous modulator of nociceptive responses in the spinal cord. Proceedings of the National Academy of Sciences USA 96: 7714–7718

Torebjörk E, Lundberg L, La Motte R 1992 Central changes in the processing of mechanoreceptive input in capsaicin-induced secondary hyperalgesia in humans. Journal of Physiology (London) 448: 765–780

Tunks E, Crook J, Norman G, Kalaher S 1988 Tender points in fibromyalgia. Pain 34: 11–19

Urban M O, Gebhart G F 1999 Supraspinal contributions to hyperalgesia. Proceedings of the National Academy of Sciences USA 96: 7687–7692

Voight M L, Wieder D L 1991 Comparative reflex response times of vastus medialis obliquus and vastus lateralis in normal subjects and subjects with extensor mechanism dysfunction. An electromyographic study. American Journal of Sports Medicine 19: 131–137

Wilcox G L 1991 Excitatory neurotransmitters and pain. In: Bond M, Woolf C J, Charlton J E (eds) Proceedings of the VIth World Congress on Pain, Pain Research and Clinical Management. Elsevier, Amsterdam, pp 97–117

Willis W D 1985 Nociceptive pathways: anatomy and physiology of nociceptive ascending pathways. Philosophical Transactions of the Royal Society of London B 308: 253–268

Woolf C J 1983 Evidence for a central component of post- injury pain hypersensitivity. Nature 306: 686–688

Woolf C J 1984 Long term alteration in the excitability of the flexion reflex produced by peripheral tissue injury in the chronic decerebrate rat. Pain 18: 325–343

Woolf C J 1989 Recent advances in the pathophysiology of acute pain. British Journal of Anaesthetics 63: 139–146

Woolf C J 1994 A new strategy for the treatment of inflammatory pain: Prevention or elimination of central sensitisation. Drugs 47: 1–9

Woolf C J, Costigan M 1999 Transcriptional and posttranslational plasticity and the generation of inflammatory pain. Proceedings of the National Academy of Sciences USA 96: 7723–7730

Woolf C J, Mannion R J 1999 Neuropathic pain: aetiology, symptoms, mechanisms, and management. Lancet 353: 1959–1964

Woolf C J, Shortland P, Coggeshall R E 1992 Peripheral nerve injury triggers central sprouting of myelinated afferents. Nature 355: 75–78

Woolf C J, Safieh-Garabedian B, Ma Q-P, Crilly P, Winter J 1994 Nerve growth factor contributes to the generation of inflammatory sensory hypersensitivity. Neuroscience 62: 327–331

Wright A, Thurnwald P, O'Callaghan J, Smith J, Vicenzino B 1994 Hyperalgesia in tennis elbow patients. Journal of Musculoskeletal Pain 2: 83–97.

4

Psychological, environmental and behavioural dimensions of the pain experience

Anita M. Unruh
Chris Henriksson

Here is perhaps the most difficult thought to accept about pain. We experience pain only and entirely as we interpret it. It seizes us as if with an unseen hand, sometimes stopping us in mid-sentence or mid-motion, but we too capture and reshape it. (Morris 1991 p 29)

OVERVIEW

It is often very tempting to separate an experience such as pain into biological and psychological components. But biology and psychology are interactive. They influence and change each other. All pain is dependent on a cortical recognition of a given stimulus as painful and this recognition of pain is shaped by many other factors such as the psychology of the person, the social context in which pain occurs, and the pain behaviours that are expected or discouraged. In Chapters 2 and 3, we reviewed the neuroanatomy and neurophysiological components of pain experience. In this chapter, we explore the psychological, environmental, and behavioural dimensions of pain experience (see Box 4.1 for terms used).

Learning objectives

At the end of this chapter, students will have an understanding of:

1. Psychological aspects of pain experience.
2. Environmental dimensions of pain and their relationship to psychological factors.
3. Behavioural expression of pain.
4. The impact of pain on occupational performance.

Box 4.1 Key terms defined

Noxious stimulus – A noxious stimulus is a stimulus that is perceived as aversive. The stimulus may or may not be initially painful but if the intensity increases, then the stimulus may become painful. In experimental pain, the noxious stimulus may be an electric shock, heat from a laser beam, pressure or immersion of the hand or forearm in cold water.

Catastrophizing – Catastrophizing is emotive thinking about pain that is concerned with ruminating, magnifying or exaggerating pain, and feeling helpless about pain (Sullivan et al 1995).

Occupational performance – Occupational performance is: 'the ability to choose, organize, and satisfactorily perform meaningful occupations that are culturally defined and age-appropriate for looking after oneself, enjoying life, and contributing to the social and economic fabric of a community'. Further, occupational performance results from: 'a dynamic relationship between persons, environment and occupation over a person's lifespan' (Canadian Association of Occupational Therapists 1997 p 181). The next two terms are two important research concepts. They are important to

clarify for the issues that we discuss in this chapter. In research and clinical practice, we are frequently concerned with whether psychological factors cause chronic pain or whether they are correlated with pain. The distinction is important for assessment and management of pain.

Correlation – Correlation is concerned with the extent to which two variables are related when they are measured at the same time (Hirsch & Riegelman 1992). A statistically significant correlation between two variables indicates that there may be a strong relationship between the two variables but it does not provide any evidence that the relationship is causal. Variable A may cause B but it may be that variable B causes A or there may be an unidentified variable that influences A and B.

Causality – Causality refers to the extent to which one can say that variable A causes a change in variable B. A causal relationship can be said to exist between these variables if all other alternative explanations have been considered and ruled out (Mausner & Kramer 1985).

INTERACTION OF PHYSIOLOGICAL, PSYCHOLOGICAL AND ENVIRONMENTAL COMPONENTS

In Chapter 1, we noted the IASP definition of pain as a sensory and emotional experience. The experience of pain is dependent on the person's perception or awareness of a noxious stimulus as pain. Many psychological and environmental factors may influence this perception of pain. Depending on these factors, a noxious stimulus of the same magnitude may feel more painful on one occasion than it will on another.

When there are strong competing cognitive stimuli, there may even be no perception of pain in the immediate situation. As noted in Chapter 1, soldiers on a battlefield may feel no pain due to their injuries but they may feel pain from an injection when being treated for these injuries. Observations such as this one contributed to the development of the gate control theory of pain (Melzack & Wall 1965).

Psychological and environmental factors can clearly have a powerful impact on the perception of an acute pain. Persistent and chronic pain in turn has a strong influence on psychological perceptions of the pain.

Practioners and researchers often feel a need to discern whether physiological, psychological, environmental or behavioural factors have a causal or contrib-

utory role in accounting for the occurrence of a given pain problem. In some cases, causal factors are readily apparent. If a person has a broken leg, physiological factors have an obvious causal role. However, psychological factors and environmental factors will have a contributory role influencing the perception of the pain. Physiological, psychological and environmental factors in turn determine the behavioural response to the pain.

When physiological factors are clearly visible, pain is more readily understood by practioners and clients. Unfortunately, many clients seen by occupational therapists and physiotherapists will have significant persistent pain for which physiological evidence as a primary causal explanation is absent or weak much to the frustration of practioners, clients, and family. Such pain is no less real for the client even though it is frequently doubted by practioners and family.

It is worth recognizing that our understanding of the physiology of pain, particularly persistent chronic pain, while increasing, is extremely limited. For many pains that were initially thought to be primarily caused by psychological problems (e.g. phantom limb pain, fibromyalgia), there is now growing evidence of underlying physiological factors. For example, recent research has identified biochemical abnormalities in serotonin metabolism and hormonal secretions in people with fibromyaligia (Bradley et al 1996).

However, even when there is some understanding of the causal physiological mechanisms, there is often no clear indication of a treatment that would cure the source of the pain.

For clients, the best option may continue to be a combination of interventions that are intended to control pain sensation, and to modify the psychological, environmental or behavioural factors that may contribute to the perception of the pain.

The reader will find it useful to complete Reflective exercise 4.1 in preparation for the remaining sections of this chapter.

PSYCHOLOGICAL COMPONENTS OF PAIN

Attitudes, beliefs, appraisals and coping strategies

Attitudes, beliefs, and appraisals about pain can have a strong influence on how pain is perceived and the way in which pain is managed by the person with pain (Unruh 1996, Unruh et al 1999). Acute pain is often perceived as a signal of tissue damage precipitating a search for the possible cause of the pain and its overall significance. Exposure to pain and learning enables the individual to make decisions about when pain signifies potential danger, or tissue damage, and what sources or degree of pain can be safely ignored.

Pain can persist and become chronic even though any underlying tissue pathology has healed. Often chronic pain exists without any evidence of a path-

ology requiring intervention. Nevertheless, a client may continue to appraise pain as a symptom of underlying tissue damage. This belief may hinder the person's recovery.

One important goal in pain management for clients with chronic pain is to shift appraisal of pain away from an acute pain model, focused on resolution of the underlying cause of the pain, to a coping model that incorporates management of pain with a problem-solving approach to regain a productive and functional daily life. Attitudes, beliefs, and appraisal of pain are also influenced by the person's age, gender culture, and family modelling about pain. Some of these factors are discussed in later sections of this chapter and in Chapter 6.

There are a variety of instruments that have been developed to measure attitudes, beliefs or appraisal of pain. These instruments include the 'Survey of Pain Attitudes' (Jensen & Karoly 1987, 1992, Jensen et al 1987), the 'Pain Beliefs and Perceptions Inventory' (Williams & Thorn 1989), the 'Chronic Pain Self-Efficacy Scale' (Anderson et al 1995), the 'Pain-Related Control Scale' (Flor et al 1993), the 'Pain and Impairment Relationship Scale' (Slater et al 1991), the 'Pain Appraisal Inventory' (Unruh & Ritchie 1998), the 'Meaning of Illness' (Browne et al 1988), the 'Arthritis Helplessness Index' (Smith & Wallston 1992) and the 'Pain Cognition List' (Vlaeyen et al 1990).

When people experience pain, they use a variety of behaviours to reduce the pain, to reduce its interference on daily life, and to limit the emotional distress caused by the pain. These behaviours are referred to as coping strategies. Attitudes, beliefs and appraisals of pain have an impact on the use of coping strategies. Appraisal that pain is a warning or a threat is associated with information-seeking, seeking social support, problem-solving, healthcare utilization, catastrophizing, decreased use of distraction strategies, and increased externalizing (e.g. getting angry at other people because of the pain) (Unruh 1996, Unruh et al 1999).

On the other hand, pain that is regarded as a challenge may be coped with by using distraction or positive self-statements (e.g. telling oneself that everything will be OK). Externalizing strategies can be problematic because they are likely to increase the interpersonal stress that a person experiences when in pain.

Catastrophizing is generally thought to be predictive of pain disability and poor coping (Bennett-Branson & Craig 1993, Turner & Clancy 1986). Recently, Sullivan et al (1995) found that catastrophizing was

---

Reflective exercise 4.1

For this exercise, identify a pain that you (or someone you know) have on a regular or episodic basis. Menstrual pain, headaches, abdominal pain and musculokeletal pains are common pains of this nature. If you have a chronic pain, you may want to consider it for this exercise. Ask yourself about the beliefs that you hold about this pain:

- Do you think the pain is likely associated with harm?
- How does the pain affect your overall mood and sense of well-being?
- What do you do to cope with the pain when it occurs?
- Do you think that there are any social or cultural norms that are associated with how you feel you should manage this pain?

more important in predicting disability than pain intensity, depression or anxiety. Catastrophizing reflects emotive thinking that is concerned with ruminating, magnifying or exaggerating pain, and feeling helpless about pain (Sullivan et al 1995).

There are a variety of instruments that can be used to measure coping strategies. The most frequently used instruments, all of which have good reliability and validity, include the 'Coping Strategies Questionnaire' (Rosenstiel & Keefe 1983), the 'Pain Coping Questionnaire' (Reid et al 1998), the 'Vanderbilt Pain Management Inventory' (Brown & Nicassio 1987), the 'Ways of Coping Checklist' (Folkman & Lazarus 1980) and the 'Pain Catastrophizing Scale' (Sullivan et al 1995).

Anxiety and fear

Anxiety is more likely to be associated with acute pain than with most chronic non-malignant pains. However, in the initial onset of a chronic non-malignant pain, an individual may be highly anxious because the pain is thought to be associated with underlying damage that will need assessment and intervention. If no evidence of substantive pathology can be found, then anxiety may be replaced by frustration, hostility and discouragement.

Anxiety about pain can be due to many factors. Exposure to repeated acute episodes of unrelieved pain increases anxiety about pain. The uncertainty of pain occurrence, especially if the pain is difficult to manage, may generate anxiety. Pain anxiety is also increased by painful medical or health procedures if these environments do not provide adequate relief from pain. If these procedures are carried out in an atmosphere of indifference about pain, then they also increase the client's anxiety about pain. For example, many adults have fears about dental pain or pain due to needles, in part due to negative childhood experiences with such pain exposure.

The disbelief of others about the legitimacy of the pain complaint also contributes to pain anxiety. Greg Lum who developed chronic pain following a motor vehicle accident wrote:

What I don't need (beside the physical pains) is to have to deal with someone else's 'attitude' or feel guilty and anxious about something I don't seem to be able to do anything about. (Lum 1997 p 68)

Chronic pain may be associated with fear about further pain, fear about re-injury, or fear about underlying disease progression. Often chronic pain is increased by activity, and if the pain is already severe, further pain will be feared and avoided. Clients often associate pain with tissue damage, and they may become fearful that persistent pain signifies more or continued tissue damage. If there is known a disease that is causing the pain, then the pain may be feared as an indicator of the progression of the disease. Fear of pain may be more disabling than the pain itself (Waddell et al 1993). This issue is discussed in more depth in Chapter 9.

Anxiety or fear of pain may produce crisis reactions to the pain that interfere with coping and may lead to pain disability beyond what may be expected by the severity of the pain (Cipher & Fernandez 1997). When anxiety or fear is present, careful assessment of possible physical, psychological and social factors is very important.

Suffering

Suffering is a difficult concept for many health professionals, but it is very evident that many clients with pain suffer greatly because of that pain. Chapman and Gavrin (1999) defined suffering as, 'the perception of serious threat or damage to the self, and it emerges when a discrepancy develops between what one expected of one's self and what one does or is' (Chapman & Gavrin p 2233).

Factors such as the severity of the pain and its unpredictability and uncontrollability add to suffering, but more importantly pain changes a person's sense of self in profound ways in much the same way as would any other chronic disease or difficulty. Much of what a person has envisioned for himself or herself may need to be modified and sometimes radically changed because of the persistence of pain. Chapman and Gavrin (1999) expressed this dilemma eloquently:

Now that I have unremitting pain, I can do less. As the task demands of everyday life increase, I can no longer match them. I am less than I once was and less than I should be . . . The disparity represents threat or damage to the integrity of the self, not only in the present but also in the future. This damage to the integrity of the self, which extends into the projected life trajectory, is the essence of suffering. (Chapman & Gavrin 1999 p 2236)

Chapman and Gavrin (1999) argued that understanding suffering and the way pain contributes to suffering is essential to deal with suffering adequately. They maintained that it is vital to prevent pain when at all possible and to relieve pain promptly when it occurs. Providing assessment and treatment in a caring environment, and enabling clients to reconstruct a meaningful and productive life are extremely important to reduce suffering.

Spirituality, meaning, hope and hopelessness

God is the God of pain as well as the God of enjoyment. To suffer is human – not divine, not personal and not deserved. We should never think of it as 'spiritual' to suffer, or exalt those who suffer. (Monihan 1996 p 32)

Little is currently known about the relationship between pain and spirituality, meaningfulness, hope or hopelessness. Nevertheless spiritual outlook, maintenance of a sense of meaningfulness, and feelings of hopefulness may be important to cope with and adapt to the presence of chronic pain in daily life. They may be particularly important to reduce the psychological suffering of chronic pain (Kahn 1986, Monihan 1996).

Most health professionals consider spirituality as separate and distinct from religion. In an extensive review of the literature on definitions of spirituality and religion, Gorsuch et al (1998) noted that spirituality is often thought to imply a more individualistic and experiential search for what is sacred in life, whereas religiousness refers to an organizational and institutional search for the sacred through a set of beliefs, practices and rituals. Other authors suggest that spirituality is a search for connectedness, meaning and purpose in life. Clearly there is also some overlap between religiosity and spirituality.

The presence of persistent pain that is difficult to manage can deeply shake a person's spirituality or religious faith. Overall perceptions of meaningfulness in life, particularly if pain limits the ability to engage in those occupations which are important to the spirituality of the person, may be seriously undermined. A person may lose his sense of self and connectedness with other people, particularly if the individual becomes isolated.

Intertwining of beliefs about pain with religious beliefs has been documented even in ancient civilizations (McGrath & Unruh 1987). Pain was often considered to result from the displeasure of God or gods. Although there are several texts related to pain, suffering and spirituality (e.g. Bakan 1968, Brena 1972, Lewis 1940), there is little research on the relationship between pain experience and spirituality. Unfortunately, we do not have a good understanding about the relationship between the experience of chronic pain, and spirituality or religious beliefs, particularly for religions other than Christianity.

Religious beliefs may increase feelings of guilt and unworthiness if the occurrence of chronic pain is perceived as punishment from a spiritual being. Sometimes the experience of pain is thought to have redemptive value. For example, some Christian writings suggest that the experience of pain and suffering draws the person closer to the suffering of Jesus Christ on the cross (Brena 1972, Lewis 1940). For some individuals, interpretation of pain in this way may be helpful in coping with pain, but for other people, such beliefs may perpetuate further feelings of failure and religious crisis.

Other writers suggest that prayer and seeking a closer relationship with God may enable more self-control over bodily processes, so that a person is less likely to experience chronic pain and suffering (Brena 1972).

Religious beliefs may influence the person's choice of pain-relief strategies. For example, if a person believes that suffering through pain brings one closer to God, then the person may be reluctant to take medication to relieve the pain. In fact, the Catholic church issued a directive in 1947 permitting Catholic parishioners to use pain-relieving methods, indicating that it was not an unChristian act to do so (McFadden 1947). Other documents from a variety of Christian publications suggest that while using pain-relieving methods, particularly medication, is permissible, rejecting medication and suffering through pain will enable deeper religious understanding. Interest in spirituality and pain experience is growing. Recently, Keefe et al (2001) reported that in a sample of people with rheumatoid arthritis, spiritual and religious coping had a positive impact on ability to control and decrease pain. Interest in spirituality raises questions about spiritual healing and pain (see Chapter 12). Recently, Abbott et al (2001) conducted a randomized, clinical trial of spiritual healing for chronic pain but were unable to demonstrate a significant positive effect.

Clients often appear to maintain an apparently unrealistic hope that the pain can be cured. They may have difficulty adjusting to life with chronic pain, or making lifestyle changes that may be needed to manage the pain, because a cure for the pain would eliminate the need for these changes.

Clients with unrealistic hope may also be more easily exploited by offers of magical cures for chronic pain. It is often very difficult for occupational therapists and physiotherapists to know how to respond to a client's expressions of hope or hopelessness. Some degree of hope that the pain may eventually dissipate, may become more manageable, or may be cured may be essential to maintain quality of life despite persistent pain.

Some clients experience considerable hopelessness. Apparent loss of control over the pain and its impact on daily life can produce deep feelings of helplessness. In these instances, clients may have little motivation to try new strategies. They may be particularly vulnerable to depression and suicidal thinking. They challenge therapists to find reasons for renewed optimism.

Crisis reactions and pain

There is some evidence that physical and/or sexual abuse in childhood is related to the development of chronic pain in adulthood, particularly chronic pelvic pain in women (Unruh 1996). In addition, posttraumatic stress disorder may be associated with recurrent pain (see Chapter 22). There is considerable speculation about the relationship between these traumatic experiences and pain, possibly suggesting the development of a pain-prone personality (see section on personality factors) (e.g. Roy 1998). However, there is no evidence that the explanation for a causal relationship is primarily due to psychological factors. It is possible that recurrent experience of traumatic and serious pain also alters underlying physiological mechanisms of pain, in conjunction with increased anxiety, fear and other psychological factors.

Stress and pain

The relationship between stress and pain is complex and more likely circular than linear. Chronic pain promotes an extended and destructive stress response that produces neuroendocrine dysregulation, fatigue, dysphoria, myalgia and impaired mental and physical performance (Chapman & Gavrin 1999).

Depression, fatigue, limitations in one's activities, and belief that the pain is uncontrollable lead to increased stress in daily life. Excessive stress in life may disrupt sleep, appetite and posture and may cause underlying muscle tension, all of which may contribute to ongoing chronic pain. Further, excessive stress affects psychological wellbeing and reduces the ability of the person to cope effectively with chronic pain.

Stress management strategies, particularly relaxation strategies and modification or resolution of psychological, social or physical factors that contribute to stress at home or work, may be very helpful to enable the person to cope better with chronic pain. They may also reduce acute exacerbations of chronic pain.

Depression, death-wish, suicidal risks

I think I have come to simply accept that the pain's here and it is unlikely to go away. I try to accept it as part of my being right now, because I really have only two choices: to endure it or die. Thus far, I've chosen to exist, but sometimes just barely. (Lum 1997 p 66)

Persistent, unrelieved pain can be a debilitating experience with substantial impact on self-esteem, occupations of daily life, and relationships with others including family, friends, and co-workers. For this reason, chronic pain is not infrequently associated with depression.

Depression may be more likely if the individual is exposed to the disbelief of others about the legitimacy of the pain. Sadly, many clients are made to feel that they themselves are to be blamed for the pain, particularly if medical investigations have failed to find any physiological cause for the pain or if the client does not have a positive response to offered treatments.

Many clients may also have been falsely and inappropriately accused of being addicted to pain medications, or using pain to obtain secondary social, psychological or financial benefits. Pain that is not adequately managed and is associated with depression increases the risk that a client will prefer to die. Some clients have said that they can adjust to unfortunate circumstance such as paraplegia or a terminal illness, but living or dying with severe pain is intolerable. Depression is discussed more fully in Chapter 22.

Suicidal risk increases with severe unrelieved pain, particularly if the person experiences isolation and abandonment (Somerville 1993). Therapists should consider suicidal risks of clients who have pain and clinical depression. A client who talks about losing the will to live or feels that family and friends would be better without him or her should always be taken seriously and provided with additional psychological support.

Grief

There is little known about grieving and chronic pain. However, some people with chronic pain may experience emotional reactions similar to those of people who are grieving a loss of some kind.

Many clients with chronic pain experience a variety of social, financial and productivity losses in their life. Grieving for such losses may be a prolonged process since chronic pain typically persists for a lengthy period of time. In addition, to manage chronic pain the client may need to make lifelong changes in habits and routines. Clients who are suffering may be grieving losses due to pain.

Personality factors

Much of the clinical and research interest in this area has been concerned with the identification of a pain-prone personality (Engel 1959). Engel argued that physical pain was essentially a metaphor for emotional distress or a defense against psychic conflict (Gamsa 1994a, Roy 1998). Engel's concept of a pain-prone personality generated considerable research and discussion to identify whether there were certain personality factors that caused a person to be at risk for developing migraines, abdominal pain or low back pain and so on.

Personality problems such as repressed hostility and aggression, rigid superego, guilt, resentment, defence against loss or threatened loss, early childhood deprivation or trauma, masked depression, neuroticism and other personality disorders have all been thought to have a causal relationship to the occurrence of chronic pain (Gamsa 1994a, 1994b). However, well-controlled studies in this area have generally failed to support the tenet that emotional conflict gives rise to bodily pain or that certain personality characteristics can be identified with the occurrence of chronic pain (Gamsa 1994a, 1994b, Gatchel 1996).

Psychological factors and causation of chronic non-malignant pain?

Severity of pain that is 'proportional' to the extent of tissue damage and is experienced at the site of the damage is easy to understand. But there are many pains that do not present in this way. As Turk and Flor (1999 p 19) wrote:

Pain in the absence of pathology, pathology in the absence of pain, individual differences in response to identical treatments, failure of neurosurgical procedures and potent analgesic agents to consistently eliminate pain, and the low association between impairment and disability fail to conform to a model of pain that presumes a direct transmission from the periphery to central nervous system structures.

The nature of the pain problems of clients who are seen by occupational therapists and physiotherapists often do not conform to a direct transmission model. As previously discussed, when researchers and practioners fail to find significant physiological evidence for the existence of chronic pain, psychological, environmental and behavioural factors are often relied upon to explain the existence of the pain.

Frequently research in this area uses a cross-sectional design in which pain and psychological distress are measured at the same time. These designs often find that there is a significant association between pain and psychological distress, but one cannot deduce that psychological distress causes pain or that pain causes psychological distress from these designs; either explanation would be plausible. In addition, a third factor may mediate the relationship between the two variables. In other words, cross-sectional studies may demonstrate associations but they do not provide evidence of causal mechanisms.

The relationship between psychological factors and pain is most convincing when there is close time-locking of psychological factors with pain (McGrath & Unruh 1987). For example, many people may experience abdominal pain before performing in public. Once the performance is complete, the pain dissipates. Such pain is very real and may be quite intense but its primary cause is psychological. It should be noted that even in these circumstance, physiological factors may also be influential. For example, if the person also made dietary changes coincidental with the occasion of the performance, then these dietary changes may be contributing to the experience of abdominal pain.

In an extensive review of the considerable body of research concerned with psychological factors, Gamsa (1994a, 1994b) found little convincing evidence that psychological factors have a causal role for the majority of chronic pain problems. The more convincing explanation for the significant correlational relationship between psychological factors and chronic pain is that pain causes substantial psychological distress and disability.

Teasell and Merskey (1997) argued, 'If physical and psychological causes cannot be established to the satisfaction of the clinician, the only proper thing to do is to recognize that the cause of the pain has not been established. Judgment has to be suspended if a diagnosis cannot be made' (Teasell & Merskey 1997 p 201). A biopsychosocial model of pain that avoids splitting pain experience into biological or psychological dichotomies is essential (Turk & Flor 1999).

Often health professionals and clients can identify psychological factors that have a negative impact on chronic pain, but most clients will feel misunderstood by suggestions that the pain is psychological or of their own creation. Enabling the client to understand that chronic pain often produces additional stress and dysphoria by wearing down personal psychological resources, that also eventually hinder effective coping and may exacerbate pain, is essential.

ENVIRONMENTAL COMPONENTS OF PAIN EXPERIENCE

Family influences

There is evidence that pain runs in families. In a prospective 2-week study of pain in families, Goodman et al (1997) found that when parents reported frequent pain, the children also reported frequent pain. Sternbach (1986) in a national survey found that adults who had parents with severe pain at some point in their lives were themselves likely to have back, muscle or joint pain. Genetics, a shared lifestyle related to activity and diet, and learning may all be influential factors.

Family members also influence each other with respect to communication about pain and behavioural response to pain. Parents socialize children about acceptable behaviour in response to pain and they may modify these expectations according to the age and gender of the child (Unruh & Campbell 1999). This modelling effect may be particularly influential for pains that are unfamiliar for the child.

Families also play a role in the degree of support, guilt or alienation that may be experienced by the person with pain. Persistent pain may necessitate some changes to the physical layout of a home to accommodate the person's needs. Family routines and activities may also be modified to some degree. In some situations, families will become overly solicitous and accommodating and may inadvertently hinder the client's adaptation to chronic pain in a more productive way.

At other times families may blame the client and disbelieve complaints of pain. Rejection of the client may also contribute to depression and reduced ability to function. While families play an important role in the person's experience of chronic pain, it is important to recognize that the influence of the family is also dependent on other factors such as the gender of the individual and the strength of their relationships (Flor et al 1989).

Most families are strongly motivated to help the family member to recover from pain. Family and friends also suffer by the painful living of someone they love. Observing severe pain in beloved family members may cause desperate actions within the family. In Canada, a father killed his severely disabled 10-year-old daughter because he could not bear her unrelenting pain and suffering and foresaw only more of the same for her future (Globe & Mail 1997).

Culture/ethnicity

Very little useful research has been conducted on the relationship between culture and pain experience (Bates et al 1993). The extent to which culture influences something like pain behaviour depends on many factors including the degree to which a cultural group has retained a distinct and separate identity.

Zborowski (1952) compared attitudes towards pain in three cultural groups from New York City by interviewing patients, doctors, nurses and other health professionals, as well as some healthy individuals from each of the cultural groups. The cultural groups were Italian-Americans, Jewish-Americans and Old-Americans.

Italians were preoccupied with the sensation of pain and complained a great deal while they were in pain with moaning and crying, but once the pain was treated they resumed their normal activities.

On the other hand, Jewish patients were also very emotional when in pain and tended to exaggerate pain symptoms. However, they worried more about the effect of the pain on their health and the overall welfare of their families than about the pain itself. At times, they had difficulty resuming their normal activities because of a preoccupation with the underlying cause of their pain.

The Old-American patients were more detached in their response to pain and they were more concerned with not bothering anyone. They also had more positive feelings about hospitalization.

This study was marred by the fact that the data collection was subjective and open to the biases and prejudices of the author and people interviewed.

First-generation immigrants may have different attributions for pain, coping strategies and pain behaviours than subsequent generations of their descendants (Bates et al 1993). Other characteristics of the cultural group such as traditional beliefs, locus of control and use of traditional health practices may also be important.

Bates et al (1993), who studied the influence of culture on pain among Hispanics, Polish, Irish, French-Canadian, Old-Americans and Italian individuals, found that ethnic group and locus of control significantly influenced reported pain intensity. People of Hispanic background reported external locus of control and higher pain intensity in this study.

Zborowski (1952) believed that attitudes towards pain are part of any culture's child-rearing practices. He found that both Jewish-American and Italian-American parents in his study were generally over-protective and overly concerned about their child's health and their children were frequently reminded to avoid fights, possible injuries and catching colds. Crying elicited considerable sympathy.

However, Old-American parents were less concerned and expected that the child would not run to the parent with a small problem. Children were taught to anticipate some pain while playing and they were expected not to show excessive distress. Once again we emphasize the subjective nature of the study which may reflect the author's biases more than the actual behaviour of the different cultural groups.

There are few studies which have been concerned with the influence of culture on pain expression in children. Abu-Saad (1984) conducted semi-structured interviews over a 6 month period with 24 children, aged 9–12 years, in each of three cultural groups: Arab-American, Latin-American and Asian-American. Although there was some variability among the three groups on causes of pain, descriptors of pain, colour of pain, and feelings about pain, the author provided no information about whether these differences reached statistical significance. The meaning of the variability of the children's responses on these items is also unclear.

Interestingly, children in all three groups chose medicine as their most common coping strategy, and girls in all three groups found being comforted as helpful. An important limitation of this study was its retrospective nature. Thus it is unknown how children of different cultures would respond during an actual painful experience.

It is important to note that observed cultural differences are more likely to concern the way in which pain is regarded, and the extent to which a person is permitted to express pain and under what conditions. These differences in pain behaviour are not evidence of differences in pain sensitivity, pain threshold or tolerance; they signify possible differences in the way people from different cultures may have learned to behave when they have pain.

In some cultures, painful experiences may be a test of the individual's strength in some way. For example, one of us (A. Unruh) was told by a Kenyan colleague that when a male was circumcised in his tribe, the child was expected to inhibit all expressions of pain as a test of his manliness. If the male child had high social status then his virility was tested further by adding salt to the wound. Similarly, women in some third world cultures appear to experience little pain during childbirth but in such cultures expression of pain by the woman may be socially prohibited.

Bernstein and Pachter (1993) noted that it is well accepted that culture is an important consideration with respect to the way a meaning of illness and pain is constructed and expressed through learned behaviour patterns and norms. Unfortunately, there is still no accepted model for understanding how one should think about cultural influences or how cultural considerations might be taken into account with clients.

Bernstein and Pachter (1993) advised that a culturally sensitive approach be utilized, avoiding reliance on stereotypes that may discount some pain experience or pain behaviour among some cultural groups as less important than it would be in others. They offered the following suggestions:

In the clinical setting, important cultural considerations may include beliefs about causes of illness and implications of pain, use of folk healers and remedies, acceptability and effectiveness of various pain management strategies (e.g. acupuncture, cognitive strategies) and expectations for normative styles of interaction with health care providers. Clinicians should become familiar with the beliefs and practices common to the cultural groups they serve, be willing to elicit information about these matters in a non-judgmental manner, and accommodate cultural practices in keeping with acceptable medical practice. (Bernstein & Pachter 1993 pp 119–120)

Secondary gain

Expectations about pain behaviour are transmitted through family and culture. In addition, co-workers, friends, strangers and health professionals convey expectations about how much sympathy or assistance might be acceptable on the basis of what is often a subjective perception about the credibility of the person's pain complaint.

A person with acute pain can expect to receive some degree of attention and temporary relief from responsibilities until the pain abates. If the pain persists and the individual continues to benefit to an excessive degree from having pain, then the person is said to be receiving secondary gain from the pain.

Secondary gain is not well-defined (Fishbain 1994). Fishbain noted that one of the problems with the concept of secondary gain is that it is often equated with disability and malingering. Often any possible benefit, such as compensation payments or attention from a family member or involvement in legal action, is taken as evidence of secondary gain and then used to cast doubt on the legitimacy of a pain complaint (Teasell & Merskey 1997). In addition, some behaviours such as not responding positively to treatment, or accepting some degree of disability, such as using pacing activities, are sometimes used as evidence of secondary gain.

Compensation is considered as the strongest form of secondary gain. However, Rohling et al (1995) in a meta-analysis of 32 studies comparing compensated patients with non-compensated patients found that compensation status accounted for only 6% of the pain experience. In other words, compensation has a very minor role in explaining anything about a client's pain.

Fishbain (1994) pointed out that chronic pain is often associated with many more secondary losses than secondary gains. People who are unable to work due to pain experience financial stress, boredom, anxiety, depression and significant loss in social status. Family and marital stresses are not uncommon.

Fishbain (1994), and Teasell and Merskey (1997) argue that, for clients/patients where secondary losses outweigh secondary gains, the utility of secondary gain as a causal factor in the persistence of pain or disability should be viewed skeptically.

Socioeconomic factors

Lower socioeconomic status is associated with increased frequency of musculoskeletal pains and low back pain, probably because of the more physically demanding and inflexible work of blue-collar workers (Teasell & Finestone 1999). People of lower socioeconomic status have an increased risk of disease and chronic health problems, and they also have an increased risk of becoming disabled when faced with these difficulties (Badley & Ibanez 1994). Teasell and Finestone (1999 p 91) commented:

The ideal solution to the dilemma of chronic pain and disability is to ensure that every worker has a postgraduate education, an adequate income (amount not defined) works in a highly supportive and flexible work environment where physically demanding work is avoidable and is able to pick and choose what tasks they are able to do and at what pace. More often, in the real world we must try to manage patients with limited skills and education levels who have jobs that require substantial physical effort and a workplace environment that is reluctant to make concessions.

Low socioeconomic status may also affect pain experience in another way. People living in poverty are likely to have more difficulty receiving appropriate pain management due to limitations in the accessibility of health care services, particularly when such services are provided through speciality pain clinics. Such clinics may be nonexistent in low-income or rural communities, and people may not have the resources to access or pay for these services.

Poverty may also influence the nature of the service people receive. For example, Grace (1995) found that the low socioeconomic status of women with chronic pelvic pain affected diagnosis, the communication between doctor and patient, information received and the appropriateness of treatment. Golletz et al (1995) reported that low-income mothers of school-aged children were less satisfied with the pain management that their children received for dental care than were mothers in higher income brackets.

Milgrom et al (1994) found that dentists in public clinics were less likely than dentists in private clinics to use local anaesthetics for paediatric dental restorations and extractions. Daneault and Labadie (1999), in a retrospective review of home care files of people with advanced HIV disease, reported that people living in extreme poverty were more likely to complain of uncontrolled pain in the last weeks of home visits.

For people who live in extreme poverty, such as those who are homeless, the problems are exacerbated even further. Ritchey et al (1991), who surveyed homeless men and women, reported high rates of headaches, abdominal pain, musculoskeletal pain, backache and dental pain. Many of these individuals had a history of previous physical and sexual abuse which might also contribute to current pain experiences. They also lived with high levels of stress, poor diet and minimal access to healthcare services.

Physical factors

The risk of pain is increased by many physical factors, particularly those concerned with the design of spaces for play, recreation, home and work, and the tools and equipment used in these spaces. Design issues are often focused on design aesthetics and efficiency. Ergonomic considerations tend to be applied when the design is intended for people who are already disabled in some way by disease, injury or pain.

Unfortunately, evaluation of the home or work environment to reduce risks of pain and disability typically occurs after the onset of chronic pain. Nevertheless, in some workplace settings efforts are made to address known physical contributors of workplace injury and pain. Guidelines for computer workstations are an important example.

Work factors

Poorly maintained equipment and sedentary and repetitive work increase the risk of injury. Tasks that require lifting of excessive weights, or that are difficult to do using proper lifting strategies, increase back strain. The type of work influences the risk for specific types of pain problems.

Light work which involves very frequent repetitive work with lightweight objects leads to progressive injury due to wear and tear on muscles and joints. These injuries may have a slow and insidious onset that may be difficult to locate to a specific point in time. Women are more likely to be employed in such work than men.

Men are often employed in heavy work that requires lifting and pulling of heavy weights. They are at risk for sudden, acute injury that is sometimes more compensable than injury due to light work that may be more insidious in onset.

Nurses, nursing assistants, home care workers, and caregivers at home who may be lifting and moving people are also engaged in heavy work that may result in chronic neck, shoulder and back pain.

Environmental factors, such as degree of work dissatisfaction, are thought to influence the occurrence of chronic low back pain, but this area remains controversial with conflicting data (Teasell & Merskey 1997). Bigos et al (1991, 1992) conducted a prospective study of industrial workers in the Boeing Company. Participants who reported that they hardly ever enjoyed their job tasks were 2.5 times more likely to report a back injury ($P = 0.0001$) than individuals who almost always enjoyed their work.

Several explanations are always possible to explain associations found in correlational studies. For example, in this study it is possible that workers with low work satisfaction were also more conscious of work-related pain. Dissatisfaction with work might cause workers to be less careful with job tasks; they may take more risks that lead to strain, injury and pain. Or these workers may be excessively attentive to minor and inconsequential pain to get out of work. Teasell and Merskey (1997) concluded that job dissatisfaction has yet to be shown to be causative of lower back pain.

The conflict between physiological and psychological explanations of pain are particularly problematic for individuals with workplace-related pain that may be compensatable. In recent years there have been stronger efforts to define such pain as activity intolerance, in other words, psychosocial pain that is treated primarily by use of an operant model (e.g. Fordyce 1995). Teasell and Merskey (1997 p 203) argued:

A wholesale denial of their (chronic pain syndromes') validity as clinical or biological entities and recent attempts to classify chronic pain disorders as solely psychosocial issues are misguided, particularly in the light of the evidence of organic causes for chronic pain conditions. Such an approach runs the risk of hurting those patients who can least afford it – individuals who perform jobs with heavier physical demands, are less well educated, lack transferable skills, are older and in a lower socioeconomic class. It seems more appropriate to take account of the needs of the individual patient and the social costs of denying compensation, and to focus more on issues of work structure, and worker education and retraining.

In a review of workplace interventions, Teasell and Finestone (1999) concluded that return to work interventions conducted close to the workplace, involvement of the workplace in return to work management,

supportive work and modified work strategies, a non-adversarial attitude and approach, and making the work environment more flexible for the worker, were all important qualities of successful programmes. Detailed discussion of work injuries, pain and rehabilitation is provided in Chapter 14.

BEHAVIOURAL COMPONENTS OF PAIN EXPERIENCE

The perception of a noxious stimulus such as pain often generates a behavioural response. For example, a person to whom a needle is being administered may wince, cry out, change his or her facial expression, or grab someone's hand, or the person may remain rigid and expressionless. Behavioural response to the injection depends on many factors such as the age and sex of the individual, the size of the needle, the volume and content of the needle, the amount of alcohol left on the skin after the swab, the reason for the injection, the skill of the health professional giving the needle, the quality of the interpersonal interaction, and the person's prior experience in receiving needles.

Behavioural response to pain is more visible for acute sharp pain, such as the experience of an injection. Often when pain is persistent, pain behaviours are dampened down. It is difficult to sustain continued behavioural distress. A person with prolonged severe pain may remain quite still because excessive movement may exacerbate pain. For this reason, behavioural measures of pain are not very useful for the evaluation of chronic pain. Often family members and health professionals are confused by the absence of behavioural expressions of pain even though the individual may complain of severe pain. Morris (1991 pp 67–68) wrote:

What surprised me most when I began my research at the pain clinic of a large university hospital was the apparently normal faces of the patients. I had steeled myself to expect agonized expressions and frightful cries ... It is not a pleasant trait, but we are sometimes suspicious of people who say they are in pain but who do not groan or writhe or pound the floor. Pain patients know what it means to face daily suspicion.

Although a person may exhibit little pain behaviour much of the time, sudden elevations in pain can produce sudden changes in pain behaviour. These changes in expressions of pain behaviour are also often misunderstood. How can someone look composed and not in pain at one moment and then appear in agony the next? It is possible to shift the mind away from pain by being attentive to more pleasant and engaging experiences, particularly if the pain is mild or moderate.

The possibility of shifting the mind away is the basis for many cognitive–behavioural interventions and occupational therapy strategies that are aimed at revitalizing meaningful and purposeful occupations of the client. A client who is engaged in something meaningful may say that the pain doesn't go away, it just 'moves over'. If the client stops concentrating, or comes to the end of the activity, or there is a sudden elevation in the pain, then the client may appear to be more visibly in pain.

Many clients who are seen in pain clinics will have difficulty with excessive pain behaviour, behaviour that increases risk of disability in self-care, leisure and productivity occupations. Such clients may also experience considerable loneliness and isolation from family, friends, and co-workers.

IMPACT OF PERSISTENT PAIN ON PERFORMANCE AND QUALITY OF LIFE

I simply want this to stop. I can't stand being out of control. I'm so tired of being in pain. I'm pained from being in pain. (Lum 1997 p 64)

As noted in Chapter 1, occupation refers to clusters of tasks and activities that give meaning to everyday life (Law et al 1997). Daily life consists of self-care occupations, leisure occupations, and productivity occupations. The quality of a person's engagement in occupations can be understood by considering the volition, habituation and performance aspects of human occupation, also referred to as the 'Model of Human Occupation' (Kielhofner 1985, 1995). This model of human occupation is utilized extensively in occupational therapy as an analysis of the interrelationship between the individual and the environment in relationship to occupations of daily life.

Another approach is the 'Canadian Model of Occupational Performance' (Law et al 1997). In this model, occupational performance is considered as the outcome of the interactional relationship between person, environment and occupation.

Volitional factors include awareness of oneself as an actor, and perception of control over ones' own behaviour. Interests and values influence choice of activities. Our values also affect our sense of obligation and conviction of what is important in life and how we experience and interpret life situations.

Habituation refers to the routines, habits and roles that organize daily activities into a time structure that gives regularity and identity. Performance is the integrated function of physical and mental factors that in a dynamic process forms the capacity for planned and goal-directed actions. Performance is made up of different skills and symbolic images learned through experiences.

People with chronic muscular pain usually experience limitations in performance of daily activities (Henriksson 1995a, Henriksson et al 1996). Tasks involving static or repetitive and eccentric movements such as carrying bags, climbing stairs, vacuum cleaning, peeling vegetables, stirring and holding tools are more difficult to perform. Also, certain movements and positions not normally thought of as tiring or difficult can be impossible to manage for clients in pain. Not only lifting and carrying small children but also dressing and undressing and feeding small children can be unmanageable. Holding a mug or a spoon when feeding involves static muscular work and is often reported as difficult.

Clients with chronic muscular pain need to learn to work in a dynamic fashion, avoiding static positions and repetitive tasks. Frequent pauses and relaxation techniques may be helpful and may decrease the level of pain during activity (Henriksson 1995b). The majority of clients with chronic muscular pain, regional or generalized, report that they need rest periods of half an hour or more in the afternoon, in order to be able to continue their scheduled activities in the late afternoon and evening (Henriksson et al 1996, Henriksson & Burckhardt 1996).

For many clients, pain will fluctuate from day to day or during the day, and on certain days may be more problematic than on others (Henriksson & Liedberg 2001). These variations in pain may be large. It is not unusual for clients to report that on 'a bad day' they may have problems getting out of bed and moving around, whereas, on 'a good day' the symptoms can be much less pronounced and most activities can be performed without problems.

Habits

Habits are the habitual ways in which we perform different tasks and activities of everyday occupations. Habits are the result of previous repetitions of a certain behaviour and they allow us to perform ordinary well-known tasks without having to concentrate on the performance or decide how the actions should be performed. Habits help us to organize our daily activities into stable patterns of behaviour and to regulate time.

When pain or injury occur, habits are often disrupted (Henriksson 1995a). Some movements cannot be performed in the usual way but have to be changed to lessen pain and fatigue-provoking procedures. Clients apply different strategies to cope with everyday life (Henriksson 1995b). All tasks take longer to perform and more attention has to be focused on the performance. This also means that simultaneous actions are more difficult to manage (Haglund & Henriksson 1995).

Roles

Roles give social identity and communicate obligations about how to behave in society and in social relationships. Roles contain expectations about the use of time and the performance of the various activities and tasks of occupations associated with these roles. Many roles can be affected by pain, but the two roles that receive the most attention in research and practice are worker and partner/spousal roles.

People with chronic pain often have serious limitations in their capacity to manage a work role. Often, heavy workload, repetitive work tasks and unsuitable work conditions are important factors that contribute to the development of the chronic pain condition. Return to the same work situation may not be possible. However, if work conditions can be adjusted and the demand of work is matched to the ability of the worker, many clients can continue to work and find satisfaction in their work (Henriksson & Liedberg 2001). The work role is for most clients an important part of their identity and serious consideration should be given to the client's ability to maintain a work role.

Control over the work situation is important and many clients can manage only if the work allows frequent changes of work positions and short rest periods when necessary. Often the work tasks or the work position may have to be changed or the work hours shortened. The work situation should be addressed as early as possible. Clients and their employees should be involved in examinations about adaptations, adjustments and preventive measures that would reduce the risk of re-injury, could compensate for limitations, and make work tasks easier to manage.

Chronic pain influences not only the client's life but also the life of other family members. Family activities such as going out, inviting guests for social occasions and leisure activities with children are all influenced. Sometimes traditions have to be changed and the family must find alternative ways to enjoy time together with relatives and friends. The role of the spouse is affected and consideration must be given to the adjustments that both partners must make to maintain a healthy relationship. By working together new ways of solving everyday challenges can be found.

Occupational performance

Occupational performance is the overall daily activity patterns organized into habits and roles. Occupational performance is disturbed by chronic pain because the previous structure has been disrupted. The previous time schedule must be adjusted to the client's limitations. People with chronic pain often need extra periods of brief rests during the day (Henriksson & Burckhardt 1996).

Many people find that regular light physical exercise distracts and decreases pain intensity and rebuilds stamina and endurance. Therefore, the occupational performance pattern must allow for extra periods of brief rest, relaxation or light physical activity.

Stress may increase the level of pain intensity and reduce occupational performance. Situations where stress is likely to occur should be avoided. Stress management training may also be helpful to improve the client's ability to identify personal stressors that affect pain and occupational performance, and to learn new ways to manage these stressors.

To be able to anticipate situations that may cause problems and to have alternative solutions may be one way to avoid stress or to cope with different situations.

Quality of life

Quality of life is usually rated as low by clients with chronic pain. However, individual clients may also report a high and sometimes increased quality of life. When the first critical period has passed and clients have adjusted their life situation to new limitations and feel more in control of their life, quality of life may increase.

Some clients revalue their life tasks and find new meaning and new arenas for developing social contacts and personal interests. Certain aspects of life may however be rated as low. Professional career, economic situations, physical activities and sexual satisfaction may represent areas of loss and limitations.

Linda Martinson, who is a poet and also lives with chronic pain, has expressed some of the feelings of happiness, grief, anger and sadness, that may be experienced by people with chronic pain (Martinson 1996). Her poetry about the ferociousness of pain eloquently illustrates the difficulty in maintaining quality of life:

Wading Through The Words

Throbbing.
Burning.
Pounding.
Shooting.
Stabbing.
Ceaseless.
These words are flat
Compared to the pain I feel.

There's an animal on my neck
and I can't shake it off.
The weight is heavy,
the teeth are sharp,
The claws dig in.
(Martinson 1996 p 1)

Leisure is a necessary part of a healthy lifestyle. Leisure time means time for relaxation, for physical exercise and mental stimulation. People with chronic pain have usually had to use their leisure time to compensate for everything that they have not been able to accomplish during the working hours. Weekends are used to catch up at work or at home. In the evening fatigue and pain is usually pronounced and any free time left is used for passive activities that do not give the necessary recreation and social contacts.

When the life situation for people with chronic pain is adjusted, active leisure occupations must be considered and clients given an opportunity and encouragement to develop healthy free-time occupations within their limitations and interest.

CONCLUSION

Psychological, environmental and behavioural factors have a very important and central role in the experience of pain. Together they shape the way that a person constructs a meaning of pain, and the way in which she or he will cope with the pain. They also influence the extent to which pain will interfere with the roles and responsibilities of daily life. They are also important issues to be considered in the assessment and management of pain.

Often in pain research and in clinical practice, we are tempted to separate physiological aspects of pain from these, often more complex, psychological, environmental and behavioural factors. But the separation is largely meaningless.

Psychological, environmental and behavioural factors are all interactive and all impact upon the physiological aspects of pain.

Study questions/questions for revision

1. To what extent does compensation affect pain experience?
2. What is the role of psychological factors in pain experience?
3. What happens to a person's behaviour as pain becomes more persistent and chronic?
4. Why might catastrophizing be associated with pain disability?
5. What effect does persistent pain have on occupational performance?

REFERENCES

Abbot N C, Harkness E F, Stevinson C, Marshall F P, Conn D A, Ernst E 2001 Spiritual healing as therapy for chronic pain: a randomized, clinical trial. Pain 91: 79–89

Abu-Saad H 1984 Cultural group indicators of pain in children. Children's Health Care 13: 11–14

Anderson K O, Dowds B N, Pelletz R E, Edwards W T, Peeters-Asdourian C 1995 Development and initial validation of a scale to measure self-efficacy beliefs in patients with chronic pain. Pain 63: 77–84

Badley E M, Ibanez D 1994 Socioeconomic risk factors and musculoskeletal disability. Journal of Rheumatology 21: 515–522

Bakan D 1968 Disease, Pain and Suffering: toward a psychology of suffering. University of Chicago Press, Chicago

Bates M S, Edwards W T, Anderson K O 1993 Ethnocultural influences on variation in chronic pain perception. Pain 52: 101–112

Bennett-Branson S M, Craig K D 1993 Postoperative pain in children: developmental and family influences on spontaneous coping strategies. Canadian Journal of Behavioural Science 25: 355–383

Bernstein B A, Pachter L M 1993 Cultural considerations in children's pain. In: Schechter N L, Berde C B, Yaster M (eds) Pain in Infants, Children and Adolescents. Williams & Wilkins, Baltimore, pp 113–122

Bigos S J, Battie M C, Spengler D M, Fisher L P, Fordyce W E, Hansson T H, Nachemson A L, Wortley M D 1991 A prospective study of work perceptions and psycho social factors affecting the report of back injury. Spine 1: 1–6

Bigos S J, Battie M C, Spengler D M, Fisher L D, Fordyce W E, Hansson T H, Nachemson A L, Zeh J 1992 A longitudinal prospective study of industrial back injury reporting. Clinical Orthopedics 279: 21–34

Bradley R A, Alberts K R, Alarcon G C, et al 1996 Abnormal brain regional cerebral blood flow (rCBF) and cerebrospinal fluid (CSF) levels of substance P (SP) in patients and non-patients with fibromyalgia (FM). Arthritis & Rheumatology 39: S212

Brena S 1972 Pain and Religion: a psychophysiological study. Charles C Thomas, Springfield

Brown G K, Nicassio P M 1987 The development of a questionnaire for the assessment of active and passive coping strategies in chronic pain patients. Pain 31: 53–65

Browne G, Byrne C, Roberts J, Streiner D, Fitch M, Corey P, Arpin K 1988 The Meaning of Illness Questionnaire: reliability and validity. Nursing Research 37: 368–373

Canadian Association of Occupational Therapists 1997 Enabling occupation: an occupational therapy perspective. Canadian Association of Occupational Therapists, Ottawa

Chapman C R, Gavrin J 1999 Suffering: the contributions of persistent pain. The Lancet 353: 2233–2237

Cipher D J, Fernandez E 1997 Expectancy variables predicting tolerance and avoidance of pain in chronic pain patients. Behaviour Research and Therapy 35: 437–444

Daneault S, Labadie J F 1999 Terminal HIV disease and extreme poverty: a review of 307 home care files. Journal of Palliative Care 15: 6–12

Engel G 1959 Psychogenic pain and pain-prone patient. American Journal of Medicine 26: 899–918

Fishbain D A 1994 Secondary gain. Definition, problems and its abuse in medical practice. American Pain Society Journal 3: 264–273

Flor H, Turk D, Rudy T E 1989 Relationship of pain impact and significant other reinforcement of pain behaviors: the mediating role of gender, marital status and marital satisfaction. Pain 38: 45–50

Flor H, Behle D J, Birbaumer N 1993 Assessment of pain-related cognitions in chronic pain patients. Behavior Research and Therapy 31: 63–73

Folkman S, Lazarus R S 1980 An analysis of coping in a middle-aged community sample. Journal of Health and Social Behavior 21: 219–239

Fordyce W E (ed) 1995 Back Pain in the Workplace. International Association for the Study of Pain, Seattle

Gamsa A 1994a The role of psychological factors in chronic pain. I. A half century of study. Pain 57: 5–15

Gamsa A 1994b The role of psychological factors in chronic pain. II. A critical appraisal. Pain 57: 17–29

Gatchel R J 1996 Psychological disorders and chronic pain – Cause-and-effect relationships. In: Gatchel R J, Turk D C (eds) Psychological Approaches to Pain Management: A practitioner's handbook. Guilford Press, London, pp 33–52

Globe & Mail February 7 1997 Euthanasia, mercy and Robert Latimer (see also www.newsworld.cbc.ca/archives/html/1997/10/29/latimer29c.html)

Golletz D, Milgrom P, Mancl L 1995 Dental care satisfaction: the reliability and validity of the DSQ in a low-income population. Journal of Public Health – Dentistry 55: 210–217

Goodman J E, McGrath P J, Forward S P 1997 Aggregation of pain complaints and pain-related disability and handicap in a community sample of families. In: Jensen T S, Turner J A, Wiesenfeld-Hallin Z (eds) Proceedings of the 8th World Congress on Pain, Progress in Pain Research and Management, Vol 8. IASP Press, Seattle

Gorsuch R L, Baumeister R F, de S Cameron N M 1998 Definitions of religion and spirituality. In: Larson D B, Swyers J P, McCullough M E (eds) Scientific Research on Spirituality and Health: A consensus report. National Institutes for Healthcare Research, Rockville

Grace V M 1995 Problems of communication, diagnosis, and treatment experienced by women using the New Zealand health services for chronic pain: a quantitative analysis. Health Care for Women International 16: 521–535

Haglund L, Henriksson C 1995 Activity – from action to activity. Scandinavian Journal of Caring Sciences 9: 227–234

Henriksson C 1995a Living with fibromyalgia: a study of consequences for daily activities. Linköping University Medical Dissertation No. 445, ISBN 91-7871-297-1

Henriksson C 1995b Living with continuous muscular pain – patient perspectives. Part I: Encounters and consequences. Scandinavian Journal of Caring Sciences 9: 77–86

Henriksson C, Burckhardt C 1996 Impact of fibromyalgia on everyday life – a study of women in the USA and Sweden. Disability and Rehabilitation 18: 241–248

Henriksson C, Liedberg G 2001 Factors of importance for work disability in women. Journal of Rheumatology, in press

Henriksson K G, Bäckman E, Henriksson C, de Laval J H 1996 Chronic regional muscular pain in women with precise manipulation work – a study of pain characteristics, muscle function, and impact on daily activities. Scandinavian Journal of Rheumatology 25: 213–223

Hirsch R P, Riegelman R K 1992 Statistical First Aid: interpretation of health research data. Blackwell Scientific Publications, Boston

Jensen M P, Karoly P 1987 Notes on the Survey of Pain Attitudes (SOPA): original (24-item) and revised (35-item) versions (unpublished manuscript). Arizona State University, Temple

Jensen M P, Karoly P 1992 Pain-specific beliefs, perceived symptom severity, and adjustment to chronic pain. Clinical Journal of Pain 8: 123–130

Jensen M P, Karoly P, Huger R 1987 The development and preliminary validation of an instrument to assess patients' attitudes towards pain. Journal of Psychosomatic Research 31: 393–400

Kahn D L 1986 The experience of suffering: conceptual clarification and theoretical definition. Journal of Advanced Nursing 11: 623–631

Keefe F J, Affleck G, Lefebvre J, Underwood L, Caldwell D S, Drew J, Egert J, Gibson J, Pargament K 2001 Living with rheumatoid arthritis: the role of daily spirituality and daily religions and daily coping. Journal of Pain 2: 101–110

Kielhofner G ed 1985 A Model of Human Occupation: theory and application. Williams & Wilkins, Baltimore

Kielhofner G 1995 A Model of Human Occupation: theory and application, 2nd edn. Williams & Wilkins, Baltimore

Law M, Polatajko H, Baptiste S, Townsend E 1997 Core concepts of occupational therapy. In: Canadian Association for Occupational Therapists (ed) Enabling Occupation: an occupational therapy perspective. Canadian Association of Occupational Therapists, Ottawa, pp 29–56

Lewis C S 1940 The Problem of Pain. G Bles, London

Lum G 1997 Prisoner of pain. In: Young-Mason J (ed) The Patient's Voice: experiences of illness. FA Davis, Philadelphia, pp 63–71

Martinson L 1996 Poetry of Pain. Poems of truth, acceptance and hope for those who suffer chronic pain. Simply Books, Lynnwood

Mausner J S, Kramer S 1985 Mausner & Bahn Epidemiology – an introductory text. WB Saunders, Philadelphia

McFadden C J 1947 Medical Ethics for Nurses. Davis, Philadelphia

McGrath P J, Unruh A M 1987 History of pain in childhood. In: McGrath P J, Unruh A M Pain in Children and Adolescents. Elsevier, Amersterdam, pp 1–46

Melzack R, Wall P D 1965 Pain and mechanisms: a new theory. Science 150: 971–979

Milgrom P, Weinstein P, Golletz D, Leroux B, Domoto P 1994 Pain management in school-aged children by private and public clinic practice dentists. Pediatric Dentistry 16: 294–300

Monihan R 1996 God of pain? Ability Network 5(1): 31–32

Morris D B 1991 The Culture of Pain. University of California Press, Berkeley

Reid G J, Gilbert C A, McGrath P J 1998 The Pain Coping Questionnaire: preliminary validation. Pain 76: 83–96

Ritchey F J, La-Gory M, Mullis J 1991 Gender differences in health risks and physical symptoms among the homeless. Journal of Health and Social Behavior 32: 33–48

Rohling M L, Binder L M, Langhinrichsen-Rohling J 1995 Money matters: a meta-analytic review of the association between financial compensation and the experience and treatment of chronic pain. Health Psychology 14: 537–547

Rosenstiel A K, Keefe F J 1983 The use of coping strategies in chronic low back pain patients: relationship to patient characteristics and current adjustment. Pain 17: 33–44

Roy R 1998 Childhood Abuse and Chronic Pain. A curious relationship? Toronto University Press. Toronto

Slater M A, Hall H F, Atkinson J H, Garfin S R 1991 Pain and impairment beliefs in chronic low back pain: validation of the Pain and Impairment Relationship Scale (PAIRS). Pain 44: 51–56

Smith C A, Wallston K A 1992 Adaptation in patients with chronic rheumatoid arthritis: application of a general model. Health Psychology 11(3): 151–162

Somerville M 1993 Pain, Suffering and Ethics. Abstracts of the World Congress on Pain, Paris: 1

Sternbach R A 1986 Survey of pain in the United States: the Nuprin Pain Report. Clinical Journal of Pain 2: 49–53

Sullivan M J L, Bishop S R, Pivik J 1995 The Pain Catastrophizing Scale: development and validation. Psychological Assessment 7: 524–532

Teasell R W, Finestone H M 1999 Socioeconomic factors and work disability: clues to managing chronic pain disorders. Pain Research & Management 4: 89–92

Teasell R W, Merskey H 1997 Chronic pain disability in the workplace. Pain Research and Management 2: 197–205

Turk D C, Flor H 1999 Chronic pain: a biobehavioral perspective. In: Gatchel R J, Turk D C (eds) Psychosocial Factors in Pain: critical perspectives. Guilford Press, New York

Turner J A, Clancy S 1986 Strategies for coping with chronic low back pain. Relationship to pain and disability. Pain 24: 355–362

Unruh A M 1996 Gender variations in clinical pain experience. Pain 65: 123–167

Unruh A M, Campbell M A 1999 Gender variation in children's pain experiences. In: McGrath P J, Finley G A (eds) Chronic and Recurrent Pain in Children and Adolescents. IASP Press, Seattle, pp 199–241

Unruh A M, Ritchie J A 1998 Development of the Pain Appraisal Inventory: psychometric properties. Pain Research & Management 3: 105–110

Unruh A M, McGrath P J, Cunningham S J, Humphreys P 1983 Children's drawings of their pain. Pain 17: 385–392

Unruh A M, Ritchie J A, Merskey H 1999 Does gender affect appraisal of pain and pain coping strategies? Clinical Journal of Pain 15: 31–40

Vlaeyen J W, Geurts S M, Kole-Snijders A M, Schuerman J A, Groenman N H, van-Eek H 1990 What do chronic pain patients think of their pain? Towards a pain cognition questionnaire. British Journal of Clinical Psychology 29: 383–394

Waddell G, Newton M, Henderson I, Somerville D, Main C J 1993 A Fear-Avoidance Beliefs Questionnaire (FABQ) and the role of fear-avoidance beliefs in chronic low back pain and disability. Pain 52: 157–168

Williams D A, Thorn B E 1989 An empirical assessment of pain beliefs. Pain 36: 351–358

Zborowski M 1952 Cultural components in responses to pain. Journal of Social Issues 8: 16–30

5

Placebo analgesia – friend not foe

Patricia A. Roche

OVERVIEW

Most people understand the word placebo as a term for mock medicine. Placebo effects are understood as any change in symptoms of illness that can be attributed to the giving of a placebo. Evidence-based practice requires that valid physical and occupational therapies must demonstrate beneficial therapeutic effect, above and beyond any effect derived from a placebo treatment. Health professionals prefer to attribute symptom relief to their therapies rather than to placebo effects. However, there is a large body of scientific evidence to show that placebo treatments can be just as effective as real treatments in reducing symptoms of pain and illness (Amanzio & Benedetti 1999, Marchand et al 1993, Ross & Olsen, 1982). It is therefore timely to re-examine the phenomenon of placebo and its scientific basis.

In this chapter, placebo (see Box 5.1) will be considered from both a historical and a current point of view. What is meant by placebo and placebo effects are considered next. Pain is the most common symptom known to respond to placebo. That is, the administration of

---

Box 5.1   Key terms defined

Placebo – A medicine having no therapeutic action, given to humour the patient or as a control during an experiment to test the efficacy of a genuine medicine (Hayward & Sparkes 1986).

Placebo effects – Change in symptoms or complaints which can be reliably attributed to the administration of a placebo (Shapiro & Morris 1978).

Nocebo effects – The production of negative effects, such as nausea, dizziness and increased pain, by suggestion (Max et al 1988).

Iatroplacebogenic – Sources of placebo response related to interpersonal–therapist–client interaction and environmental factors (French 1989).

---

some form of placebo therapy for pain frequently does result in analgesia. This chapter includes a tabular overview of selected research studies that demonstrate the nature of placebo effects in medical and physiotherapy studies on pain. Psychological and neurophysiological explanations of placebo effects in pain therapy are then discussed. The chapter concludes with the view that placebo analgesia has positive implications for pain research, and for practice in physiotherapy and occupational therapy.

Learning objectives

In this chapter, the student will:

1. Gain a historical perspective on placebo effects.
2. Review definitions of placebo and placebo effects.
3. Examine traditional attitudes toward placebo respondents.
4. Review placebo effects on physical, physiological and psychological symptoms of clinical and experimental pain.
5. Discriminate between placebo and nocebo effects.
6. Review psychological explanations for placebo analgesia.
7. Review neural pathways implicated in placebo analgesia.
8. Redefine placebo and consider the implications of placebo analgesia for therapeutic practice.

PLACEBO USE: YESTERDAY AND TODAY

A variety of organic and inorganic substances were prescribed in ancient times to treat symptoms of disease and illness. Crocodile dung, lizard's blood, putrid meat, gallstones from the intestines of animals, human perspiration and moss scraped from the skull of victims of violence, have all formed part of the pharmacopoeia of 'medicines' which have no known medical benefit but which improved symptoms of illness. Ancient Egyptians healed wounds with powdered mummy. European physicians in the sixteenth and seventeenth centuries prescribed worms, lozenge of dried viper, saliva of a fasting man and crab's eyes.

Despite these questionable, and presumably medically inactive treatments, patients were able to recover and the physicians who prescribed them continued to be held in high esteem (Shapiro 1959, Shapiro & Morris 1978). These early procedures and medicines are nowadays presumed to have had a psychological or placebo effect.

Today, a variety of medically unproven remedies remain an integral part of folk medicine. Little appears to have changed in the ability of people to accept that a substance or object they are informed is medicinal will heal, even though little or no evidence is produced. In 500 AD the 'Royal Touch' and the 'laying on of hands' by a royal or holy person were highly desired 'treatments' for a variety of ailments. It can be argued that these beliefs can still be seen today in the desire for personal contact with royalty, holiness or individuals with 'star' status. The present worldwide market in liquids, potions and inert objects, such as crystals and talismans, demonstrates the belief of new-age devotees in the curative, preventative or analgesic properties of scientifically unproven artefacts.

Interestingly, two differences exist in the belief-set of those who use allopathic (conventional) medicine and those who subscribe to alternative or complementary medicines (discussed in more detail in Chapter 12). The first difference is in the need to consult with qualified health practitioners. People who use conventional medicine have confidence in the ethical and knowledgeable health practice that comes with recognized professional registration.

Those who use alternative medicines may not have confidence in conventional healthcare, and may be less concerned about professional standards and regulations. They often consult practitioners who do not have recognized professional qualifications. They may accept the virtues of this or that potion from the word of non-accredited health advocates, such as the local health shop owner, and they may simply self-prescribe.

The second difference lies in the environmental surroundings in which healthcare is practised.

Conventional healthcare is most often practised within a specific and uniquely therapeutic environment; for example a physiotherapy or occupational therapy clinic, a physician's consulting room, a hospital ward or a surgical theatre. Each of these environments is filled with apparatus and the sounds, sights and smells which we have learned from personal experience (or even from televised hospital dramas), signal the practice of 'real' medicine or healthcare practice. The smell of disinfectant, the sound of instrument trolleys, the sight of a stethoscope or electrotherapy equipment, and importantly, medical uniforms, are all symbols of practice that is expected to be efficacious. Such stimuli are iatroplacebogenic, sources of placebo response related to interpersonal–therapist–client interaction and associated environmental factors (French 1989).

The conventional healthcare environment is replete with iatroplacebogenic stimuli, the alternative healthcare environment considerably less so. Placebos are nevertheless administered in both the conventional and alternative health settings, and in some cases, lead to effective symptom relief. Wall (1994) noted that these comparisons point to the single undeniable fact that no matter how we define placebo, it causes a response through a system of belief.

Definitions of placebo

The word placebo is derived from the Latin verb *'placere'*, which means to please (Shapiro & Morris 1978). The first registered use of the word placebo dates back to the works of Geoffrey Chaucer in the thirteenth century. Wall (1994) argued that placebo is derived from the Latin *'placebit'* meaning 'It will please'. He pointed out that placebo was in the first line of vespers for the dead in medieval times. The word fell into disrepute when priests and monks harassed the population for money to sing these vespers over their loved ones. From the sixteenth to eighteenth centuries it became a derisory term used to describe a servile flatterer, toady or parasite (Wall 1994).

In the eighteenth century, placebo entered western medical terminology. The 1785 edition of Motherby's New Medical Dictionary defined placebo as a 'commonplace method of medicine' (Routon 1983). By the beginning of the twentieth century, the word placebo was in common use. However, after the Second World War scientific interest in the placebo effect rose dramatically. The advent of scientific pharmacology and the increased number of therapeutically effective drugs led to the introduction of placebo-controlled trials in the 1950s (Richardson 1994). The definition of placebo was then narrowed to mean the administration of medically inert drugs or substances (Shapiro 1959).

Psychologists broadened the definition of placebo to be:

Any therapy or component of therapy that is deliberately used for it's non-specific psychological or psychophysiological effect, or that is used for its presumed effect, but is without specific activity for the condition being treated. (Shapiro & Morris 1978).

Subsequently, the most commonly accepted definition of the placebo effect has been, 'the psychological or psychophysical effects produced by placebos' (Plotkin 1985).

Nevertheless, there are still conceptual problems with these definitions. For example, Richardson (1994) noted that the terms 'specific' and 'non-specific' in the definition of placebo can be challenged because a reduction in pain from a placebo analgesic has no less a specific effect on pain than does analgesia from a drug such as morphine. Richardson also noted that the

pairing of placebo as, 'any therapy or any component of therapy . . . that is without specific activity' and 'placebo effects' suggested that the effect of a patient's arousal of hope from an injection of morphine should be labelled differently to the effect of their arousal of hope from an injection of placebo morphine. In summary, several researches have noted their dissatisfaction with the definition of placebo, although none have as yet entirely resolved the problem (Grunbaum 1981, Wilkins 1979).

Grunbaum (1981, 1985, 1986) suggested that the placebo phenomenon could be understood by differentiating between the 'characteristic' and 'incidental' ingredients of a given therapy. Characteristic ingredients are those ingredients that are remedial for a particular disorder. Incidental ingredients have no remedial effect. One author stated, 'for a therapy to be a non placebo, at least one of its characteristic ingredients should be remedial. Placebo effects are those which are produced by incidental ingredients, regardless of the presence of characteristic ingredients in the therapy' (Richardson 1994 p 16).

Under this model, there is a clearer acknowledgment that remedial effects from active (real) treatments are always combined with incidental effects. The emphasis of proof lies in demonstrating that the combined effect of incidental and characteristically remedial effects is significantly beyond that obtained from incidental effects alone.

Although at first glance this appears to be a restatement of the rationale behind the controlled clinical drug trial, it has the additional advantage of acknowledging the breadth of incidental effects contributing to the outcome of medical treatments.

Although there is some benefit in more clarity about the definition, not all researchers share this concern. For example, Wall (1994) saw difficulties in what he referred to as a general obsession with distinguishing mental from bodily sites of action to explain placebo effects. At this present stage, the safest statement is that debate continues over the specific language, concepts and definitions surrounding placebo.

ATTITUDES TOWARD PLACEBO

A predominantly negative attitude toward placebo and placebo effects has dominated medical circles in recent decades. Richardson (1994), citing Wall (1992), describes it thus:

Despite the existence of an extensive scientific literature attesting to the therapeutic potency of pharmacologically inert and theoretically ineffective treatments, the placebo effect continues to be widely regarded as at best a nuisance variable in therapy outcome research, and at worst an indication of medical charlatanism and quackery.

Wall (1992, 1994) discussed four related reasons for the discomfort provoked in medical circles by the topic of placebo and placebo effect. In summary, these are: the inference of quackery, the inferred challenge to the validity of 'real therapy', the inferred challenge to the reality of our own senses (that what does not seem real is real) and finally the unwelcome demonstration that the 'true' effect of therapy is complicated and made more expensive by the existence of this tiresome artefact.

It is important to recognize the detrimental consequences of these attitudes. Wall (1992, 1994) points to the myths surrounding placebo, and the effects that these myths have had on patient care. They can best be explained as mechanisms of professional self-defence. These myths include the following beliefs:

- Placebo differentiates between patients with organic and mental disease.
- Placebo affects mental and not organic symptoms of illness presentation.
- Placebo respondents have a special (by which is meant highly suggestible/neurotic or otherwise 'silly') mentality.
- A fixed fraction (33%) of patients respond to placebo.
- Placebo responses are short-lived.

The myths, separately and together, strongly imply that soma and psyche are separate, that 'real medical therapies' affect the soma, and consequently that patients whose symptoms are reduced by a placebo have a covert psychological component to their illness presentation. The implication that placebos have only a psychological benefit suggests that they would not be used in routine clinical practice (Blaschke et al 1985).

However, several surveys have found that use of placebos is far from rare (Goldberg et al 1979, Goodwin et al 1979, Gray & Flynn 1981). In a study of 300 nurses and physicians, 80% admitted to recent placebo administration, most commonly for pain relief (Gray & Flynn 1981). The most commonly cited reasons for giving a placebo included punishing 'difficult' or 'undeserving' patients, and proving that the patient's symptoms were imaginary (Goodwin et al 1979).

It should be evident that attitudes such as these lead directly to the label of psychosomatic illness; sadly, this label remains prevalent today. A label, or suggestion, of psychosomaticism in a patient's case notes holds a plethora of dangers for the patient. The practitioner who believes the patient to have a psychosomatic presentation may discredit the medical validity of the patient's complaint, verbally, or by withdrawal of the normal non-verbal body signals that signal compassion and interest. Since this is a confronting situation for practitioner and patient, the practitioner may refer the patient elsewhere. The new consultant, seeing the referring physician's suggestion of psychosomatic illness in the case notes is more likely to have a negative expectation of successful outcome in that patient and may also refer the patient on. Although infrequently discussed in allied health circles, physiotherapists and occupational therapists are not immune from a similar set of beliefs and responses concerning placebo responders.

Wall (1994) stated the case bluntly. Concerning the myth that placebo distinguishes between organic and mental disease he maintained, 'this is the most dangerous and cruel attitude which has been used by physicians and surgeons when they detect placebo responses'. It suggests to the physician that the pain is not real (i.e. organic). It suggests that diagnostic procedures to determine an organic cause of the pain are a waste of time.

Over 900 research papers containing the results of placebo-controlled trials were published in the literature prior to 1980 but none offered any scientifically sound explanation for the observed phenomena. Since then, we have fortunately entered an era of greater scientific interest and more rigorous research on placebo than has previously been the case.

In the following section, a brief selection of methodologically sound studies and their results are summarized, to illustrate that each of the standard myths about placebo has been demonstrated to be quite untrue.

EVIDENCE OF PLACEBO EFFECTS IN MEDICINE AND ELECTROTHERAPY

Table 5.1 reviews selected studies showing evidence of the existence and nature of placebo effects on pain. The studies were selected with a view to targeting the myths outlined above, and summarizing evidence regarding pain within the therapies of most direct interest to the reader. Nevertheless, considerable evidence of placebo effects exists in most fields of health care.

Table 5.1 emphasizes that placebo effects occur in physiological as well as in mental symptoms and across a range of health therapies. Perhaps the most dramatic of the experimental studies reviewed was the demonstration by Cobb et al (1959) of widespread

Table 5.1 Studies in medicine and physical therapy demonstrating placebo effects for pain

Authors/ Reference	Aims, conditions treatment	Methods	Findings	Conclusions and comment
Cobb et al 1959	To investigate the rationale for surgical relief of angina in the absence of proof from pathology. Real vs placebo surgery for angina pectoris	Double-blind trial Complete surgical ligation of mammary arteries vs sham surgery (skin incision and artery exposure) Neither the patients nor their physicians knew that sham surgery was conducted	The majority of each group showed improvement in the amount of pain, walking distance and consumption of drugs Electrocardiogram readings improved in some patients in both groups Each group maintained improvement over 6 months' observation	The first scientific evidence that: 1. The belief that surgery had been conducted was as effective as real surgery 2. Placebo surgery affected physical, functional and behavioural responses 3. Placebo surgery had long-lasting rather than brief effects 4. Placebo effects occur in people with real organic illness
Hashish et al 1988	To investigate the influence of ultrasound (US) on pain, jaw tightness and swelling following wisdom tooth extraction	Independent subjects design Comparison of outcome from different intensities of US including zero Double-blinded trial, neither patient or therapist knew when the treatment was or was not active	Significant reduction in pain, swelling and jaw tightness from non-emitting US, beyond that produced by active US The placebo effect was not due to the effect of the ultrasound-head massage of tissues The strongest effects occurred when the therapist and patient both believed that the US machine was on	A well designed experiment demonstrating the significant effect of placebo US on physiological swelling and tightness as well as acute pain Strengthens the evidence that placebo effects impact on physiological symptoms and do not impact on psychological components alone The results also indicate that the belief of the therapist is as important as the patient's (that the machine is on) in producing placebo effects
Roche et al 1984	Investigated the pain responses of healthy subjects to ischaemic pain when treated with TENS	Independent subjects design Induction of ischaemic pain with the sub-maximum effort tourniquet technique. Control, placebo (minimal intensity) and two active TENS conditions Subjects reported pain threshold and tolerance	Compared to controls, only the placebo group showed a significant increase in both pain threshold and pain tolerance Throughout the period of pain endurance, the placebo and active conditions showed the same pain intensity curve, which was lower than controls	Placebo effects occur in healthy individuals The effects can mimic the effects of real therapy in terms of duration and degree of analgesia
Langley et al 1984	TENS for patients with rheumatoid arthritis (RA) and chronic hand pain Patients had RA for 11 years on average	Double-blind trial Compared pain relief from high-frequency or acupuncture-like or placebo TENS while controlling for the factors of attention and suggestion of active therapy All patients viewed a TENS oscilloscope output	Significant decrease in resting grip pain in each group A non-significant decrease in joint tenderness in each group Placebo responses occurred in 54% of the placebo group	TENS and placebo TENS relieved two characteristic symptoms of inflammation Attention on the oscilloscope display may explain the similarity of results in each group Placebo effects occur in patients with chronic clinical disease and are not confined to 33% of a sample

Table 5.1 (continued)

Authors/Reference	Aims, conditions treatment	Methods	Findings	Conclusions and comment
Roche et al 1993	Explored the immediate and long-term effects of continuous or burst or placebo TENS in patients' spinal pain from malignant prostate cancer	Double-blind randomized study. Patient randomly assigned to one of three conditions. Patients taught to use daily diary records and home use of TENS. Patients self-recorded pain scores for 12 h after two daily home treatments, for 6–12 weeks	80% of 502 applications reduced pain intensity. Active TENS reduced pain by 44% compared with 12% in placebo responders, for up to 12 weeks. Placebo responders showed cumulative and/or complete pain relief for 12 weeks. Qualitative description with the McGill Pain Questionnaire showed that placebo reduced sensory and non-sensory word use when describing pain	The results suggest superior symptom relief from active TENS overall, but the placebo effect was powerful. In patients who did respond to placebo, some showed long-lasting benefit. Placebo effects can mimic properties of active interventions such as cumulative and time-curve effects. The placebo reductions of pain intensity and pain unpleasantness contradicted the myths that placebo affects do not occur in people with real organic disease, are short-lived and only influence the mental components of pain. Marchand et al (1993) showed similar results from TENS for chronic back pain
Moffet et al 1996	Investigated the effect of active and placebo short-wave diathermy (SWD) on pain and functional disability in ostearthritis of the hip and knee	Double-blind randomized study. Functional capacity was measured three times. Patients used diaries to record pain intensity and distress, mental health and perceived benefit, before and during treatment, and for a further 6 weeks	Scores of pain and disability did not differ between the groups before, during or after treatment. Placebo patients reported a marginal improvement in the benefit of treatment. Only the patients not on a waiting list for surgery showed some improvement	The results indicated no specific benefit from SWD but did show a trend toward the most beneficial effects from placebo therapy. The poorer results from patients on the surgical waiting list also suggested that these patients found SWD less credible compared to impending surgery and/or were concerned that a positive result would result in their removal from the surgical list. The patients' perception of the credibility of a treatment relative to the seriousness of their condition may affect treatment outcome
Roche and Tan (upublished)	Investigated the incidental effect of electrotherapy apparatus on pain in healthy volunteers	Independent subjects design. A randomized controlled study of pain threshold and pain tolerance in subjects with induced ischaemic pain and 'treatment' with placebo TENS or placebo Interferential (IF)	Compared with the no-treatment condition, placebo IF significantly increased pain threshold. Both placebo IF and TENS significantly increased pain tolerance. Pain intensity and unpleasantness were each lower in the placebo groups	The data confirmed the hypothesis that visual stimuli in the form of electrotherapy apparatus would be placebogenic. Analgesia was also confirmed in the sensory and non-sensory components of ischaemic pain. The importance of incidental effects on analgesia was confirmed

effects from sham surgery. These effects bridged physical, physiological and painful symptoms of angina; there is nothing subtle about the placebo effect.

The results of this study led to the abandonment of a popular but untenable and costly medical treatment for angina pectoris. Secondly, as outlined recently in a leading lay journal, the evidence of the power of placebo responses in core medical practice has become so overwhelming that placebo-controlled surgical trials have re-entered mainstream medical research (Thompson 1999).

As shown by several of the experiments outlined in Table 5.1, placebo administration for pain can have impressive outcomes. Placebo treatments not only reduce pain intensity and pain unpleasantness. They can be sufficiently long-lasting to be the envy of many a drug manufacturer or therapist concerned with alleviating pain with real therapy.

Visual cues can be potent in producing placebo analgesia. Langley et al (1984) (see Table 5.1) confirmed patients' expectation of medical treatment by having them attend to the visual evidence of treatment in the form of an oscilloscope output display. More than half of the patients in both the active and placebo groups responded with analgesia, thus making the results of active and placebo transcutaneous electrical stimulation (TENS) indistinguishable.

Roche & Tan (unpublished data) also demonstrated iatroplacebogenesis from a visual stimulus alone. Neither the TENS nor interferential machines they applied as treatment produced an active stimulus, although all visual stimuli emanating from the apparatus (e.g. flashing light in the TENS machine), were congruent with the idea that real therapy was being applied. The reported extension in pain threshold and tolerance (i.e. analgesia) could only be explained by the subject's sight of the apparently therapeutic apparatus. Amplifying belief in real treatment, by means of visually congruent stimuli enhances the placebo effect.

As indicated above, it is not difficult to give placebo applications of electrotherapy treatments. The apparatus is adjusted so that all normal visual displays of active treatment continue to function but the current to the output terminals is disconnected. Subjects can be informed that the trial investigates common forms of pain therapy but that, 'some applications may not be felt on the skin', and that, 'they may be included in a non-active therapy condition'. Even when no stimulus is felt and having been pre-warned that they may receive an inactive therapy, placebo analgesic effects occur. This should give physiotherapists food for thought, since electrotherapy treatments such as ultrasound and short-wave diathermy give little or no cuta-

neous sensation during their application. In addition, some machines such as ultrasound include a visual display of output.

Research has also dispelled other popular notions about placebo respondents. They do not differ in age, gender, personality or education from non-respondents (Evans 1985). Placebo effects cross a variety of disorders including diabetes, multiple sclerosis and Parkinsonism (White et al 1985). Several clinical and laboratory-based experiments in addition to Table 4.1 show placebo analgesia (Amanzio & Benedetti 1999, Marchand et al 1993). The phenomenon is common and potent.

Contrary to popular medical myth, placebo analgesia occurs, at least some of the time, in healthy people (Amanzio & Benedetti 1999, Voudouris et al 1990), who have normal personalities (Roche et al 1984, Stam & Spanos 1987), and in patients (Cobb et al 1959, Koes et al 1992) with painful malignant (Roche et al 1993, Houde et al 1966) or non-malignant disease (Langley et al 1984, Moffet et al 1996, Verdugo & Ochoa 1994), acute pain (Hashish et al 1988, Roche et al 1984, White et al 1985) and chronic pain (Fine et al 1994, Roche & Wright 1990, Roche et al 1993). The simple fact is that placebo responses occur in a variety of people and in a variety of painful conditions (Feine & Lund 1997).

Placebo analgesia can also be as powerful, and sometimes more powerful than pharmacological analgesia in relieving pain. Furthermore, individual responses vary from minimal to as much as 90% of the treatment's effect on pain (Fields 1981). The principal conclusion to be made is that the placebo effect is powerful and can be detected in any aspect of therapy (Wall 1994).

It is clear that placebo effects are a real and complex phenomena (Butler 1998), which tell us more about the interactive nature of the central nervous system (CNS) than we have previously known. Placebo effects must occur via the mechanisms of the central nervous system. To understand the mechanisms of placebo, we must examine the major theoretical propositions held to account for the placebo phenomenon and particularly the phenomenon of placebo analgesia. Psychological mechanisms, manifest via neural pathways in the central nervous system, are the principle explanations of placebo phenomena.

PSYCHOLOGICAL EXPLANATIONS OF THE PLACEBO EFFECT

Four psychological mechanisms are proposed to account for placebo effects. These are classical conditioning (Pavlov 1927, Wickramsekera 1985), expectancy (Evans 1985), anxiety and stress response (Wickramsekera 1985) and motivation (Jensen & Karoly 1991).

Conditioning

The earliest demonstration of classical conditioning was when dogs learned to associate the sound of a bell (conditioned stimulus) with the delivery of food (unconditioned stimulus). After only a few such stimulus–response pairings, the dogs salivated at the sound of the bell alone (Pavlov 1927).

Theorists now describe conditioning as, 'the learning of relations between events' (Montgomery & Kirsch 1997). The principal characteristics of such conditioning are:

1. Memory storage of the learned association
2. Reinforcement with repetition and, in time
3. Generalization of the response to a wider set of triggering stimuli (stimulus substitution)
4. Dormancy of the response with lack of reinforcement, but complete extinction is rare.

It is clear that classical conditioning is a first step in the establishment of learned associations, and paired associations undergo memory storage and reinforcement with repetition. Gifford (1998) notes that, 'physiological and environmental experiences are thus stored as memories during learning and can be recalled or remembered'. Items 3 and 4 above refer to responses elicited to stimuli, which are similar, or are only partially similar, to the original conditioned stimulus. There are hundreds of examples in our daily lives, which illustrate that recall of learned associations can induce physiological reactions and behaviour, for example, when we blush at the reminder of some embarrassing event.

I cannot resist giving a personal example of stimulus generalization and the absence of its extinction over time. In my youth I was fortunate to be raised with a species of South American monkey called the Humboldt's Woolly monkey – a delightful and gentle species which required considerable care and attention. Long after that period of my life, and long after the monkeys had died, I was absorbed in a book (in a physiotherapy common room), when the door of the room must have been blown slightly ajar in the breeze. The door hinges squeaked.

Without thought, but filled with apprehension, I was instantly out of the room and half way down the corridor to 'attend to the monkey' before I stopped and realised what I was doing, and why. The squeak of the door hinges had a tone, which was sufficiently

similar to the sound of a Woolly monkey's cry of distress to produce my instantaneous stress response and help behaviour. Such examples illustrate that conditioned responses may lie dormant for considerable periods of time but are not usually extinguished.

Montgomery and Kirsch (1997) summarize the stimulus substitution model of placebo effects in medicine (Turkaan 1989), as follows:

Active treatments are unconditioned stimuli (US) and the vehicles in which they are delivered (i.e. pills, capsules, syringes, etc) are conditioned stimuli (CS). The medical treatments which people experience during their lives constitute conditioning trials, during which the vehicles are paired with their active ingredients. These pairings endow the pills, capsules and injections with the capacity to evoke therapeutic effects as conditional responses. (Montgomery & Kirsch 1997).

Conditioned responses are assumed to occur automatically and to be outside the conscious thoughts going through our minds. Conditioned responses to drug administration have been shown in animals (Siegel 1985, Takeshige et al 1990). However, humans bring their thoughts, assumptions and expectations to the experience of pain and pain relief (Wall 1992). Two alternatives to conditioning models of placebo analgesia are expectancy and stress reduction.

Expectancy

The expectancy model of placebo analgesia involves the conceptualization that a given treatment will be effective or ineffective (Evans 1985). The phenomenon is facilitated through observational learning, self-learning and verbal instruction.

Conditioning and expectancy are closely related. Conditioning is likely to lead to positive or negative expectancies. Patients and persons in pain (including laboratory volunteers) are most likely to have expectations of positive outcomes from treatment, i.e. pain relief. 'Placebo' – to please – is therefore associated with (positive) pain relief.

Nocebo effects are the opposite of positive placebo effects. Nocebo effects are the production of negative effects such as nausea, dizziness and increased pain. These effects frequently occur in clinical trials in which subjects have been informed that adverse effects are likely to occur (Max et al 1988). Furthermore, the positive or negative direction of 'placebo' responses can be identified by simply asking subjects beforehand about what is expected (White et al 1985).

The results of Voudouris et al (1989, 1990) indicate that placebo analgesia is classically conditioned. Four groups of healthy subjects had ischaemic pain induced in their forearms and were given a series of electrical stimuli ranging from 0.1–2.0 mA to establish a baseline of pain expectation.

Prior to the next experimental session, positive or negative expectancies of pain relief were nurtured by means of a cream applied to the arm where pain would be felt. Groups 1 and 2 were told the cream was a 'safe, fast-acting and highly effective local pain killer'. Groups 3 and 4 were told the cream was neutral. In fact, the cream was always neutral. The groups were then conditioned in the direction they expected, i.e. the groups with 'analgesic cream' were given consecutive trials in which the severity of the pain stimulus was secretly reduced.

As expected the groups with the 'analgesic cream' reported significantly less pain compared with the others. Next, Voudouris and colleagues returned the pain stimuli to their original level. A strong carry-over effect was shown. The subjects who believed their cream was truly analgesic, continued to report less pain and seemed not to register the increased pain stimuli.

Montgomery and Kirsch (1997) challenged that conclusion. They believe that in addition to initial conditioning processes, placebo analgesia is mediated by information appraisal and experience, which result in the establishment of habitual directions of response or 'response expectancy'. They reasoned that if the conditioning model was responsible for placebo analgesia, it would not be affected by informing the subjects that their pain levels were being manipulated.

They proceeded to replicate the experimental method used by Voudouris et al (1990), with the single difference that they informed some of the participants (the informed group) that the stimulus was being lowered during the conditioning trials. Their results demonstrated significantly weaker placebo analgesia in the informed, compared to the uninformed group. By giving the subject information contrary to what he or she had expected they were able to prevent the conditioned process from occurring.

This group of researchers claim that their results gave stronger support to the response expectancy hypothesis of placebo analgesia than the conditioning hypothesis. It is most likely that both are true.

Conditioning is one step toward 'paired associations' leading to placebo analgesia, but it takes the establishment of expectations (a more sophisticated and cognate process) to activate the mechanisms of placebo analgesia.

Motivation

Motivation has received less attention in the literature on placebo, nevertheless, the motivational model is based on cognitive dissonance theory (Festinger 1957). Cognitive dissonance is the holding of two or more beliefs that are psychologically inconsistent. The state of tension created (dissonance) motivates the individual to reduce the inconsistency, by amplifying the belief(s) that he/she most wants to be true.

For example, if, after putting your entire savings into buying a wonderful new car, your neighbour proceeds to tell you that the latest motoring experts have found fault with the design and pronounced the model a flop, you will experience cognitive dissonance. Your likely reaction to this news, apart from wishing your neighbour would shut up, is to expound the attributes of the car, and, over the next few hours, to find several reasons to convince yourself that your purchase was a wise one, and that your neighbour is talking nonsense.

Richardson (1994) argued that when people seek medical care they do so in the belief that the care they receive will relieve symptoms, particularly if the physician says it will. The absence of relief is inconsistent with this belief and causes dissonance. A patient may endeavour to reduce this dissonance by changing his or her perception of the symptoms, in effect, becoming less sick.

Richardson (1994) also pointed out that, when a patient has made a strong personal commitment to treatment, and perhaps has had to make difficult choices between alternative treatments, dissonance and placebo effect will increase. He noted that nasty-tasting medicines and other unpleasant or difficult forms of treatment draw a similar response. Many of us recognize this phenomenon in the saying that, 'if it tastes bad, it must be good for you'. Most of us consider surgery as the most difficult form of treatment to have to undergo. Richardson (1994) suggests that the apparently enhanced effects of placebo surgery may also be due to high levels of cognitive dissonance, which would occur if the true nature of the surgery had been known.

Anxiety and stress reduction

Beecher (1960) and Wickramasekera (1985) proposed that reduction of anxiety and stress was the principle mechanism of placebo analgesia. Anxiety (regarding the cause and consequences of a pain) is the most common psychological symptom accompanying a new pain. Anxiety and pain each result in a general activation of sympathetic arousal and excessive motor behaviours (Gross & Collins 1981).

Pain-induced anxiety drives us to seek medical assistance and a diagnosis for the pain. It causes us to cancel our most urgent appointments and to obey our physician's or therapist's advice to rest the injured part and take medication so that pain can subside and healing can occur (Sternbach 1968). Pain-induced anxiety is therefore a principal mechanism of survival, by which we remove ourselves from the painful stimulus, seek appropriate medical advice and behave in a manner which is consistent with pain reduction, healing and the earliest possible resumption of normal activity (Wall 1979).

Nevertheless, significant stress results from pain and the accompanying anxiety. It seems entirely rational, therefore, to propose that placebo analgesia may be strongly linked to a desire to reduce anxiety. Nevertheless, the proposition that lowered anxiety has the direct effect of inducing placebo analgesia has not been well supported (White et al 1985); the relationship is likely to be more complex.

Although there is no solid evidence that reduced anxiety directly induces placebo analgesia, the concept is not without merit. Conditioning, expectation (of pain relief) and anxiety reduction are not mutually exclusive (Richardson 1994). Manipulations of cognitive dissonance, that are said to have a placebo effect (Totman 1989), could instead be affecting anxiety.

The study of specific psychological theories adds to our knowledge of the depth and complexity of mechanisms surrounding placebo analgesia. It is, however, accepted that several interrelated mechanisms account for the effect. No single model accounts fully for placebo phenomenon (Price 2000).

NEUROPHYSIOLOGICAL MECHANISMS

A unified and analytical system, modified by experience

Chapters 2 and 3 emphasized the current understanding of pain as a multidimensional and multilevel event that includes powerful descending control of any experience to do with pain. Gifford (1998) describes the pain system as constantly sampling the 'outside environment, it's own body and relevant past experience'. Wall (1996a) describes it as a 'unitary, integrated and constantly analysing system', which is 'modified by experience' (Wall 1996a).

These statements emphasize the unitary activation of systems subserving pain. It would therefore be nonsense to imagine that the experience of pain, medically-induced analgesia and placebo-induced analgesia are manifest by distinctly separate mechanisms. Instead, the systems involved in pain perception and in any form of pain relief, including the motor, sympathetic and neuroendocrine systems, work in complete unison. Therefore, the psychological elements, including conditioning and the cognitive components of learning, motivation, expectancy, attention and memory, are integrated and actively participating in any experience of pain and pain relief.

Prior to summarizing neurophysiological mechanisms believed to account for placebo analgesia, it is worth reminding the reader that a unitary explanation of pain and placebo analgesia was, until very recently, considered with disdain within medical science. It was not always the case. In the late eighteenth and early nineteenth century, the psychological aspects of pain and pain relief were frequently discussed (Gamsa 1994) and the authors did not separate the soma and psyche.

However, the establishment of the specificity (structure-oriented) model of pain in the latter part of the nineteenth century led to dualistic thinking, whereby pain was caused by either the soma or the psyche. The occurrence of placebo analgesia was relegated to a psychological response, distinct from a 'real' organic response to medical intervention. Emotions were relegated to a place of secondary importance. Organic causes were considered as the only medically legitimate explanations for pain, and organic treatments were the only legitimate reasons for pain relief. In brief, there was little understanding or acceptance that pain (and pain relief) is both a sensory and a psychological event, and that the central nervous system processes these components together.

Nowadays, we are in the more fortunate position of being able to utilize substantial scientific evidence, supporting unitary and multisystem explanations for pain, to suggest how psychological mechanisms, which appear to be primarily responsible for the occurrence of placebo effects, can be translated into actual reductions in pain.

The physiological component of the placebo effect

Table 5.1 outlined physiological changes in addition to pain relief induced by placebo electrotherapies. Physiological changes induced by placebo treatment, although of varying magnitude, can be shown in other physical therapy techniques, for example in manual therapy. Peterson et al (1993) evaluated sympathetic outflow to the upper limb in normal subjects following active cervical 5/6 posteroanterior joint mobilization (experimental group), manual contact at the neck without cervical mobilization (placebo group) and a no contact group (control). The results showed a

50–60% increase in skin conductance in the actively treated group, compared with a 15% increase in the placebo group and a negligible increase in the control group. The placebo response in this study, although weak, nevertheless underlines that placebo effects include demonstrable changes in physiological functions.

Brain pathways and placebo analgesia

As discussed in Chapters 2 and 3, nociception from the periphery is controlled at spinal cord segments and via ascending and descending pathways to the midbrain. There is also some research exploring the neural links between the midbrain and the cortex. It seems increasingly likely that some areas of brain activity are common to analgesia and placebo analgesia.

The midbrain and placebo analgesia

The periaqueductal grey region is an important region in the midbrain that controls analgesia and other functions that are important for preservation of life. Electrical or chemical stimulation of the ventrolateral periaquedutal grey causes profound analgesia (Reynolds 1969). Evidence suggests that analgesia via acupuncture (Takeshige et al 1990) and manipulative therapy (Vicenzino et al 1998) is mediated via descending pathways, directly or indirectly linking the periaqueductal grey and brainstem with the dorsal horn of the spinal cord.

Analgesia is considered to be opioid based if it can be reversed by the opioid antagonist naloxone, if it exhibits tolerance, and if it shows cross-tolerance with morphine analgesia. Analgesia that does not exhibit this phenomenon is said to be non-opioid (see Chapter 3). The results of several studies conducted in the 1980s and early 1990s indicated that placebo analgesia could be reversed by naloxone and was therefore opioid-based, but the results were inconclusive. Recent studies show intriguing evidence that placebo analgesia is mediated by the endogenous opioid system, but only when expectation is involved (Amanzio & Benedetti 1999).

The cortex and placebo analgesia

The clear involvement of expectancy, motivation and affect in placebo analgesia supports Wall (1996b), who argued against limiting the location of supraspinal mechanisms of analgesia to the midbrain. Studies employing a variety of brain imaging techniques have indicated wider regions of changed activity in the cortex and subcortical structures during a pain stimulus than had previously been known (Wall 1996b). There is now sufficient evidence to suggest that the prefrontal cortex and other areas of the brain that are involved in memory, arousal, expectation, conditioning, perception and motivation, may have either direct or indirect input to the periaqueductal grey region and other brain centres capable of altering pain experience (Bandler & Shipley 1994, Treede et al 1999). The relevance of these projections to our discussion of placebo analgesia is that they highlight the neuroanatomical pathways whereby psychological responses consequent to learning, motivation and cognitive appraisals, may access the periaqueductal grey region and brainstem areas related to analgesia (See Chapters 2 and 3).

The prefrontal cortex also has extensive anatomical connections with the occipital, parietal and temporal lobes. Therefore it has access to sensory experiences and to information from past experiences that also influence pain perception. The prefrontal cortex has been associated with emotional arousal, motivation, conditioning, conceptualization and cognitions and it has reciprocal connections with other brain structures involved in pain perception (Fuster 1989). Cortical and subcortical regions, including the thalamus, hypothalamus and amygdala of the limbic system, play important roles in the emotional responses to situations, including pain and relief from pain (Fuster 1989, Treede et al 1999).

It may be that placebo responses associated with conditioning and expectancy also activate the limbic system and trigger the same analgesic centres that can be accessed from the periphery via acupuncture, electrotherapy and manipulative therapy. Certainly, the evidence points to widespread links between neural, psychological and physical systems subserving pain and analgesia. We can be certain that the current evidence in relation to placebo supports the known plasticity of the central nervous system in altering individual experiences of pain (Wall 1994, 1996a, 1996b). Placebo analgesia is but a component of that plasticity and involves the individual's conditioning, expectancy, stress, anxiety and motivation to be rid of pain.

PLACEBO ANALGESIA: WHAT IS IT?

In previous sections of this chapter, we examined the component parts of the placebo phenomenon but have not yet made a clear statement about the whole entity. An analogy would be to have listed the component parts of a car; the chassis, the engine, the wheels, the seating and the petrol needed to activate these, without stating that it is a vehicle of transport.

The evidence presented in previous sections points to placebo analgesia as one example of the central nervous system's bias toward inhibiting pain. Chapter 3 showed that the central nervous system is naturally biased toward inhibiting nociception by means of tonic inhibitory systems. It takes powerful nociceptive inputs to switch the 'off' system off and switch pain transmission on. When nociception is processed, the endogenous systems that deal with it are, by nature, primarily inhibitory. The neurophysiological systems and psychological processes involved in placebo analgesia link directly or indirectly with this inhibitory system.

It makes intuitive sense, therefore, to suggest that placebo analgesia is just one more face of this naturally occurring inhibitory system. Perhaps its most interesting aspect is that the inhibitory effect is triggered by a belief state or learned expectancy. Butler (1998) notes that, 'a deep-rooted and universal belief exists in the willingness of physicians and health therapists to help (relieve pain)'. In addition, the clinical setting contains iatroplacebogenic stimuli, which reinforce an individual's belief in a positive outcome from therapy. Finally, there is nothing more important to our daily survival and comfort than the avoidance and inhibition of pain. Indeed, it would be impossible for our species to survive and progress if it were otherwise. Imagine, for a moment, what would happen if the central nervous system was biased toward accentuating rather than inhibiting pain. Our daily lives would be an immense struggle. Happiness and the motivation to work and study would be virtually impossible under those circumstances.

The significance of placebo analgesia lies in the demonstration that analgesic responses are controlled to some degree by cognitions, particularly beliefs and expectations. Real biophysical changes occur due to the individual's cognate response. Pain relief from a placebo is therefore a vital demonstration of every individual's inner capacity for cognately triggered pain control. It is a potentially valuable source of pain control, which physiotherapists and occupational therapists should understand and utilize in the most appropriate manner, in their care of the patient and treatment of pain.

IMPLICATIONS FOR PHYSIOTHERAPISTS AND OCCUPATIONAL THERAPISTS

Research implications

The notion of placebo analgesia as an illustration of the body's principal evolved system of analgesia raises many interesting issues for therapists. Placebo analgesia demonstrates the combined workings of the psychological and neurophysiological actions of the central nervous system, in bringing about a switch from pain into non-pain. Physiotherapists and occupational therapists combine psychological and physiological techniques to do the same thing. A major goal of our treatment is to influence our patient's cognitive–behavioural outcomes toward less pain and improved function, i.e. to help the patient learn or re-learn well-behaviours (to exercise, to return to work and social activities).

Our primary tools of pain management are physical and educational. Our methods of pain therapy are non-invasive. In contrast to pharmaceutical or surgical therapies for pain they have limited risk of producing unwanted side-effects. Placebo analgesia is also a non-invasive form of pain therapy. It works via the individual's own psychological and neurophysiological mechanisms. We are still a long way from a complete understanding of the mechanisms of placebo analgesia. Nevertheless, it would seem that considerable similarities exist between the mechanisms of action of placebo analgesia and those which account for some of the outcomes of physical therapies. In conclusion, placebo analgesia is an important research topic for the physiotherapist and occupational therapist interested in exploring the body's own mechanisms of pain therapy.

Practice implications

There are a number of important practice implications for therapists that are based on our preceding discussion on the nature of placebo analgesia. The first is the thorny issue of whether placebo therapy (in terms of its conventional meaning as an inert/false medicine deliberately applied to fool the patient) should be deliberately employed in the non-experimental clinical setting. I support Wall's (1994) view that to do so would be unethical and, 'a lie'. Patients expecting treatment are entitled to receive treatments which are believed, via clinical or experimental evidence, to be truly medicinal, i.e. to have a characteristically remedial effect for the disorder under treatment. If however, we believe that placebo analgesia, as demonstrated by experimentation, illustrates the effect of learned expectations, then our focus should be on maximizing such learned effects in a positive direction. This provides one rationale for our current endeavours to provide evidence-based practice. The more we can prove that our treatments are reliably effective, the more we will meet the patient's expectations of effective treatment. Conversely, there is every reason to avoid viewing placebo in a negative light, we can instead view it as a gateway toward a better understanding of the role of cognitions in the therapeutic outcome for pain. Since learned expectancy is the basis to the psychophysiological phenomenon of placebo analgesia, we can now consider how best to harness and apply such expectancies toward the best outcome from clinical practice.

Early success boosts successful outcomes

The medical setting alone and the individual's trust in their carer's commitment can engender expectations of symptom relief. The literature also shows that consistent reductions in pain from a placebo can be quickly and reliably conditioned (or primed) in subjects who first experience, and then expect, reduced pain (Amanzio & Benedetti 1999, Montgomery & Kirsch 1997, Voudouris 1990). Learned expectancy is easily generalized to associated stimuli. The conclusion is that a positive mental set or expectancy about the outcome of a specific, or similar, therapeutic interventions, is common in individuals seeking medical care. Early success in pain therapy is likely to further prime expectancy in a positive direction, and consequently to contribute to future success with subsequent treatments.

Once good pain relief has been established, the expectation of continuing success is likely to influence the central nervous system towards pain inhibition in subsequent treatments. To date, we cannot be sure what contribution such a priming effect makes towards successful pain therapy. Nevertheless, the evidence clearly indicates that it is there. Furthermore, and as demonstrated in the studies shown in Table 5.1, the effect can be long-lasting, sometimes extending over several months. The implication for therapists is that in order to best utilize the effect of learned expectancy in therapy, treatments for pain must give efficient analgesia as quickly as possible, and certainly within the first few sessions of treatment.

Early failure primes the system for failed outcomes

Just as early success primes the system for continued success, early failure can have the opposite effect.

Learning in this case may be even more powerful because of the considerable physical, psychological and social distress associated with persistent pain. There is also no reason to believe that negative learning has a shorter duration. Indeed the problem of negative priming is that it can have long-term consequences and may become generalized. A patient who experiences early failure may find it difficult to be hopeful about the therapeutic benefit of other treatment strategies.

Failure of pain therapy contributes to the development of chronic pain

The implications of failed early treatment are serious. Lack of pain relief lessens the individual's trust in their therapist's capacity to help and may induce anxiety and fear. Patients with pain, which is unresponsive to treatment, often worry that the pain is due to undiagnosed and more serious pathology. If failure continues, learned helplessness (Abramson & Seligman 1978, see Chapter 4) may occur.

Learned helplessness (the sense of having no personal control over pain) heightens the individual's level of pain. For example, in 120 out-patients under regular medical review for rheumatoid arthritis, learned helplessness contributed at least as much to the patient's pain levels as did the clinical severity of the disease (Roche 1995, 1998). Helplessness and increased depression reduce motivation to exercise and maintain fitness, despite pain. Unrelieved pain, combined with increasing psychological distress and deterioration in physical health therefore contributes to the development of overall disability in many patients with chronic pain.

The implications are that in addition to relying on physiotherapy or occupational therapy techniques for reducing pain and improving function, therapists should actively prime expectancy mechanisms in a positive direction.

Using the learned expectancies to best effect

From the discussion so far it will be evident that we should be reasonably confident that those strategies that we use in pain management are reliably effective. Using evidence-based practice, as discussed in Chapter 8, can help ensure that we are knowledgeable of the extent to which any particular strategy is likely to be effective for individual patients. The information (that the treatment he/she will receive is known from research to have good effect) should be imparted to patients as one method of priming positive expectations. In addition, therapists can make better use of pain education, and strategies that reduce anxiety and stress, such as relaxation, imagery and distraction. Each and all of these strategies improve the patient's sense of personal control over pain. They are particularly important for patients with chronic pain, in whom negative priming due to poor pain relief has already occurred. For example, simple explanations about the cyclical nature of pain and psychological distress assist patients with cancer, and their families, to better understand and cope with pain (de Wit et al 1997).

Therapists can also examine their own attitudes and behaviours towards patients as a means of positive priming. The therapist's understanding of pain as a physical and psychological (e.g. often worrying and depressing) event can convey a positive message to patients if it is accompanied by a comment that is credible and does not imply any psychosomatic source to the patients pain. Brief and simple statements such as, 'research has shown us the links between the brain and the spinal cord which help us understand why pain is so distressful' or, 'research has shown us why feelings of depression make pain worse, can indicate to the patient that there is scientific justification for the stressful emotions which pain can induce. Such statements also signal the therapist's understanding of the mind–body link. They can be of immense value. Chronic pain patients, particularly those for whom a diagnosis for the pain is unclear, are acutely conscious of the negative psychological effects of pain on their lives and emotions. They are however, often fearful of being labelled as having a psychosomatic cause for their pain.

Therapists who maintain a positive and respectful perspective, which acknowledges the mind–body link, reinforce the patient's perception of the therapist's ability and commitment to help. There are several studies that indicate that positive priming arises from interpersonal factors (Dinnerstein & Holm 1970, Evans 1985) such as a warm personality and interest in the patient (Shapiro 1960). Careful use of body language, considerate listening and questioning, good eye-contact and goal-setting that is meaningful to the patient, signal that he/she is entering a collaborative therapeutic relationship. Interaction in this way heightens the patient's sense of participation and control. It also ensures that the therapist has an opportunity, when appropriate, to have a better understanding of issues that may worry the patient and impact on his or her ability to comply with therapeutic instructions (Butler 1998).

The therapist who shows appropriate concern and interest, and engages the patient in goal-setting, creates an environment in which the patient may share adverse beliefs or apprehensions about their therapeutic capacity and work with the therapist to improve outcome. Cognitive re-training and encouragement of appropriate positive self-statements such as, 'I can complete this task if I take it more slowly', 'I am having a setback, but it will improve' 'I know I can do these exercises with my therapist's guidance' are important to re-setting a positive expectation, particularly amongst those with chronic pain.

Finally, a word about the physical environment of the therapeutic interaction. Some treatment settings, for example hydrotherapy, can be expected to have positive psychological as well as physical benefits, due to the calming and relaxing effects of warm water and buoyancy. Even on land, it makes sense to appeal to the analgesic system with an environment which signals comfort and caring. Environments that are bright, comfortable and engaging are likely to have a positive therapeutic influence.

CONCLUSION

Placebo analgesia is a demonstration of the body's natural tendency to reduce pain. Historical myths have denigrated placebo effects as a purely psychological response. However, a growing body of evidence indicates that placebo analgesia is one expression of endogenous analgesia, and that it is activated by psychological mechanisms of learning and expectancy. Principle explanations for placebo analgesia were discussed. Numerous clinical and experimental demonstrations of placebo analgesia demonstrate our capacity for a positive mind-set to be learned, expected and established.

The neural links exist in the central nervous system to action changes in physical symptoms due to expectancy. Pain, among other symptoms of illness, can be reduced or increased by the individual's expectancy. A positive expectancy contributes to positive results from pain therapies. The effects of positive expectancy can be long-lasting and may generalize to the outcome of other treatment modalities.

Failed treatment is also likely to have a long-lasting but negative effect, which may contribute to the development of chronic pain and general disability due to pain. In this chapter, several reasons were given for the physiotherapist and occupational therapist to view the placebo response as an ally in pain management.

Study questions/questions for revision

1. List five factors in physiotherapy or occupational therapy practice that could be considered iatroplacebogenic.
2. List five characteristics of the nature of placebo analgesia as demonstrated by clinical or experimental research.
3. List four psychological explanations for placebo analgesia. Which has the greatest validity according to current experimental evidence, and why?
4. Which structures of the brain are associated with placebo analgesia?
5. How could failed therapy for pain contribute to chronic pain disability?
6. List three ways to enhance positive expectancy and three ways to induce negative expectancy of treatment outcome in your approach to the patient in pain.

REFERENCES

Abramson L Y, Seligman M E P 1978 Learned helplessness in humans; critique and reformulation. Journal of Abnormal Psychology 87: 49–74

Amanzio M, Benedetti F 1999 Neuropharmacological dissection of placebo analgesia: expectation-activated opioid systems versus conditioning-activated specific subsystems. The Journal of Neuroscience 19: 484–494

Bandler R, Shipley M T 1994 Columnar organisation in the midbrain periaqueductal gray: modules for emotional expression? Trends in Neuroscience 17: 379–389

Beecher H K 1960 Increased stress and effectiveness of placebos and active drugs. Science 132: 91–92

Blaschke T F, Nies N S, Mamelok R D 1985 Principles of therapeutics. In: Gilman A, Goodman L S, Rall T W, Murad F (eds) The Pharmacological Basis of Therapeutics, 7th edn. New York, MacMillan, New York, pp 49–65

Butler D 1998 Integrating pain awareness into physiotherapy – wise, action for the future. In: Gifford L (ed) Topical Issues in Pain 1, Whiplash: science and management. Fear-avoidance beliefs and behaviour, Physiotherapy Pain Association Yearbook. CNS Press, Falmouth, pp 1–27

Cobb L A, Thomas G I, Dillard D M, Merendino K A, Bruce R A 1959 An evaluation of internal mammary artery ligation by a double-blind technique. New England Journal of Medicine 260: 1115–1118

Dinnerstein A J, Holm J 1970 Modification of placebo effects by means of drugs: effects of aspirin and placebos on self-rated moods. Journal of Abnormal Psychology 75: 308–314

de Wit R, van Dam F, Zanbelt L, van Buuren A, van der Heijden K, Leenhouts G, Loonstra S A 1997 Pain Education Program for chronic cancer pain patients: follow-up results from a randomised controlled trial. Pain 73: 55–69

Evans F J 1985 Expectancy, therapeutic instructions and the placebo response. In: White L, Tursky B and Schwartz G E (eds) Placebo-theory, research and mechanisms Guildford Press, New York, pp 215–218

Feine J S, Lund J P 1997 An assessment of the efficacy of physical therapy and physical modalities for the control of chronic musculoskeletal pain. Pain 71: 5–23

Festinger L 1957 A theory of cognitive dissonance. Stanford University Press, Stanford, California

Fields H L 1981 Biology of placebo analgesia. American Journal of Medicine 70: 745–746

Fine P G, Roberts W J, Gillette R G, Child T R 1994 Slowly developing placebo responses confound tests of intravenous phentolamine to determine mechanisms underlying idiopathic chronic low back pain. Pain 56: 235–242

French S 1989 Pain: some psychological and sociological aspects. Physiotherapy 75: 255–260

Fuster J M 1989 The Prefrontal Cortex: Anatomy, Physiology and Neuropsychology of the Frontal Lobe, 2nd edn. Raven Press, New York

Gamsa A 1994 The role of psychological factors in chronic pain. 1. A half century of study. Pain 57: 5–15

Gifford L 1998 The mature organism model. In: Gifford L (ed) Topical Issues in Pain 1: Whiplash: science and management. Fear-avoidance beliefs and behaviour, Physiotherapy Pain Association Yearbook. CNS Press, Falmouth, pp 45–65

Goldberg R J, Leigh H, Quinlan D. 1979 The current status of placebo in hospital practice. General Hospital Psychiatry 1: 196–201

Goodwin J S, Goodwin J M, Vogel J M 1979 Knowledge and use of placebo by house officers and nurses. Annals of Internal Medicine 91: 106–110

Gray G, Flynn P 1981 Survey of placebo use in a general hospital. General Hospital Psychiatry 3: 199–203

Gross R T, Collins F L 1981 On the relationship between anxiety and pain: a methodological confounding. Clinical Psychology Review 1: 375–386

Grunbaum A 1981 The placebo concept. Behaviour Research and Therapy 19: 157–167

Grunbaum A 1985 Explication and implications of the placebo concept. In: White L, Tursky B, Schwartz G E (eds) Placebo: Theory, Research and Mechanisms. Guildford Press, New York, pp 37–58

Grunbaum A 1986 The placebo concept in medicine and psychiatry. Psychological Medicine 16: 19–38

Hashish I, Feinman C, Harvey W 1988 Reduction of postoperative pain and swelling by ultrasound: a placebo effect. Pain 83: 303–313

Houde R W, Beaver W T, Wallenstein S L, Rogers A 1966 A comparison of the analgesic effects of pentazine and morphine in patients with cancer. Clinical Pharmacology and Therapeutics 7: 740–751

Hayward A L, Sparkes J J 1986 The Concise English Dictionary, Omega Books, London, p 867

Jensen J P, Karoly P 1991 Motivation and expectancy factors in symptom perception: a laboratory study of the placebo effect. Psychometric Medicine 53: 144–152

Langley G B, Sheppeard H, Johnson M, Wigley R D 1984 The analgesic effects of transcutaneous electrical nerve stimulation and placebo in chronic pain patients. Rheumatology International 2: 1–5

Marchand S, Charest J, Jinuxe Li, Chenard Jean-Rene, Lavignolle B, Laurencelle L 1993 Is TENS purely a placebo effect? A controlled study on chronic low back pain. Pain 54: 99–106

Max M B, Schafer S C, Culnane M, Dubner R, Gracely R H 1988 Association of pain relief with drug side-effects in postherpetic neuralgia: a single dose study of clonidine, codeine, ibuprofen and placebo. Clinical Pharmacology Therapy 43: 363–371

Moffet J A, Richardson P H, Frost H, Osborn A 1996 A placebo controlled double blind trial to evaluate the effectiveness of pulsed short wave diathermy for osteoarthritic hip and knee pain. Pain 67: 121–127

Montgomery G H, Kirsch I 1997 Classical conditioning and the placebo effect. Pain 72: 107–113

Pavlov I 1927 Conditioned Reflexes, England, Oxford University Press

Peterson N, Vicenzino B, Wright A 1993 The effects of cervical mobilisation technique on sympathetic outflow to the upper limb in normal subjects. Physiotherapy Theory and Practice 9: 149–156

Price D D 2000 Factors that determine the magnitude and presence of placebo analgesia. In: M Devor M, Rowbotham M C, Wiesenfeld-Hallin Z (eds) Proceedings of the 9th World Congress on Pain, Progress in Pain Research and Management, Vol 16. IASP Press, Seattle, pp 1085–1095

Plotkin W B 1985 A psychological approach to placebo: the role of faith in therapy and treatment. In: White L, Tursky B, Schwartz G E (eds) Placebo: Theory, Research and Mechanisms. New York: Guildford Press, New York, pp 237–254

Reynolds D V 1969 Surgery in the rat during electrical analgesia by focal brain stimulation. Science 164: 444–445

Richardson P H 1994 Placebo effects in pain management. Pain Reviews 1: 15–32

Roche P A, Gijsbers K, Belch J J F, Forbes C D 1984 Modification of induced ischaemic pain by transcutaneous electrical nerve stimulation. Pain 20: 45–52

Roche P A, Wright A 1990 An investigation into the value of TENS for arthritis pain. Physiotherapy Theory and Practice 6: 25–33

Roche P A, Heim H, Oei T, Ganendran A, Summers S 1993 Transcutaneous electrical nerve stimulation (TENS) for pain from metastatic carcinoma of the prostate: an interim report. Abstract 1126, 7th World Congress on Pain, Paris, France. IASP Publications, Seattle, p 421

Roche P A 1995 Anxiety, depression and the sense of helplessness: their relationship to pain from rheumatoid arthritis. In: Shacklock M O (ed) Moving in on Pain. Butterworth-Heinemann Australia, pp 90–97

Roche P A 1998 The course and prediction of pain in rheumatoid arthritis: a six year study, PhD study. University of Queensland, Australia

Routon J 1983 The placebo response. In: Brena S F, Chapman S L (eds) Management of Patients with Chronic Pain. Spectrum Publications Inc, Jamaica, pp 205–211

Ross M, Olsen J M 1982 Placebo effects in medical research and practice. In: Eiser J R (ed) Social Psychology and Behavioural Medicine. Wiley, Chichester, pp 441–458

Shapiro A K 1959 The placebo effect in the history of medical treatment: implications for psychotherapy. American Journal of Psychiatry 116: 298–304

Shapiro A K, Morris L A 1978 The placebo effect in medical and psychological therapies. In: Bergin A E, Garfield S (eds) Handbook of Psychotherapy and Behavioural Change, 2nd Edn. John Wiley, New York, pp 369–410

Shapiro A K 1960 A contribution to a history of the placebo effect. Behavioural Science 5: 109

Siegel S 1985 Drug-anticipatory responses in animals. In: White L, Tursky B, Schwartz G E (eds) Placebo: Theory, Research and Mechanisms. Guildford Press, New York, pp 288–305

Stam H J, Spanos N P 1987 Hypnotic analgesia, placebo analgesia and ischaemic pain: the effects of contextual variables. Journal of Abnormal Psychology 96: 313–320

Sternbach R 1968 Pain: a Psychophysiological Analysis. Academic Press, New York

Takeshige C, Tanaka M, Sato T, Hishida F 1990 Mechanisms of individual variation in effectiveness of acupuncture analgesia based on animal experiments. European Journal of Pain 11: 109–113

Thompson D 1999 Real knife, fake surgery. Time Magazine February 22: 52

Totman R 1989 Cognitive dissonance in the placebo treatment of insomnia – a pilot experiment. British Journal of Medical Psychology 49: 393–400

Turkaan J S 1989 Classical conditioning: the new hegemony. Behavioural Brain Science 12: 121–179

Treede RD, Kenshalo, D R., Gracely RH, Jones AKP 1999 The cortical representation of pain. Pain 79: 105–111

Verdugo R J, Ochoa J L 1994 Placebo response in chronic, causalgiform, 'neuropathic' pain patients: study and review. Pain Review 1: 33–46

Vicenzino B, Collins D, Benson H, Wright A 1998 An investigation of the interrelationship between manipulative therapy-induced hypalgesia and sympatho-excitation. Journal of Manipulative and Physiological Therapies 21: 448–453

Voudouris N J, Peck G L, Coleman G 1989 Conditioned response models of placebo phenomena: further support. Pain 38: 109–116

Voudouris N J, Peck G L, Coleman G 1990 The role of conditioning and verbal expectancy in the placebo response. Pain 43: 121–128

Wall, P D (1979) On the relation pain to injury. Pain 6: 253–264

Wall P D 1992 The placebo effect: an unpopular topic. Pain 51: 1–3

Wall PD 1994 The placebo and placebo response. In: Wall PD and Melzack RC (eds) The Textbook of Pain, pp 1297–1307. Churchill Livingstone, Edinburgh

Wall P D 1996a Comments after 30 years of the Gate Control Theory. Pain Forum 5: 12–22

Wall P D 1996 b Imaging of pain in humans. Abstracts, 7th International Symposium, October 2–6, The Pain Clinic, Istanbul, p 126

White L, Tursky B, Schwartz G E (eds) 1985 Placebo: Theory, Research and Mechanisms. Guildford Press, New York, pp 37–58

Wickramsekera I 1985 A conditioned response model of the placebo effect: predictions from the model. In: White L, Tursky B and Schwartz G E (eds) Placebo: Theory, Research and Mechanisms. Guildford Press, New York, pp 255–287

Wilkins W 1979 Getting specific about non-specifics. Cognitive Therapy Research 3: 319–329

6

Pain across the lifespan

Anita M. Unruh

OVERVIEW

Unless a person is born with a congenital insensitivity to pain, a rare and serious problem, pain affects us across our lifespan from the moment of birth. In this chapter we will examine the prevalence of pain for infants, children, adolescents, adults and the elderly. The experience of pain is also influenced by a person's sex or gender (see Box 6.1), her or his race, and the presence of special needs or disease. We will consider some of the specific concerns related to these aspects. Readers are invited to reflect about how age, sex, race, and special needs might be viewed in relationship to pain in their own particular settings.

In each section, we will consider the implications of age, sex, race and special needs on the assessment, measurement and management of pain. In Chapter 7, we will discuss the three primary components of pain assessment.

Box 6.1 Key terms defined

Sex – Sex refers to the biological, hormonal, anatomical and other physiological differences between women and men that may affect brain chemistry and body metabolism (Phillips 1995).

Gender – Gender denotes a broader, more complex, psychological, sociological and political framework which shapes attitudes, perceptions or beliefs that tell people how to think, feel and act as women or men in a particular society, on the basis of their sex (Phillips 1995).

Special needs – Specific characteristics of an individual that affect her or his health and wellbeing and usually require healthcare intervention. The special need may be minor or major, and is often associated with some degree of disability, handicap or challenge. In this chapter, special needs refer specifically to severe cognitive and communication impairments.

Learning objectives

On completing the chapter, readers will have an understanding of:

1. The prevalence of pain across the lifespan and its unique features at different life stages.
2. The distinction between sex and gender and their influence on pain experience.
3. The influence of age, sex, gender, race and special needs on the adequacy of pain management.
4. The implications of age, sex, gender, race, and special needs for occupational therapy and physiotherapy.

PAIN IN INFANCY AND CHILDHOOD

If a new skin in old people be tender, what is it you think in a new born Babe? Doth a small thing pain you so much on a finger, how painful is it then to a child, which is tormented all the body over, which hath but a tender new grown flesh? If such a perfect Child is tormented so soon, what shall we think of a Child, which stayed not in the wombe its full time? Surely it is twice worse with him (Wurtz, 1656, quoted in Ruhräh, 1925 p 205–205).

Children are not strangers to pain. Virtually all infants will have a heel-prick within the first few days of life to collect the few drops of blood required for PKU and adrenal screening. Many male infants will be circumcised in the first week of life. In their first 2 years, most children will also be given a series of immunizations against a variety of serious diseases. As children develop their gross motor skills, they also experience the many bumps and falls of childhood.

Observational studies of incidents of everyday pain among preschoolers and young school-aged children on a daycare playground yield mean rates between 0.34 and 0.41 incidents per hour per child (Fearon et al 1996, von Baeyer et al 1998).

Prevalence of pain in childhood

In addition to the many minor pains associated with the bumps and falls of childhood, many of the common recurrent pains of adulthood occur also among children, though they are less common. Headache and migraine are reported by about 3–7% of school-age children but increase after puberty, particularly for girls (Unruh & Campbell 1999). Ten to fifteen percent of children have recurrent abdominal pain. Four percent of school-children have limb pains and 15% report growing pains (Goodenough 1998, Naish & Apley 1950). Growing pains are characterized by deep aching sensations in the muscles of the lower limbs late in the day or at night.

Some children will experience pain resulting from serious injuries. Injury prevention programmes to identify and eliminate hazards at home, playgrounds, daycare centres and schools fill an important role in protecting infants and children from such occurrences (McGrath & Unruh 1987). Sadly, some children will experience pain due to physical or sexual abuse, or torture and experiences associated with conflict and revolution.

Fortunately, children are less likely than adults to develop serious acute or chronic health problems that are commonly associated with pain. However, some children have cancer, AIDS, neurodegenerative disorders or rapidly progressive forms of cystic fibrosis (Berde & Collins 1999). Children with cancer often experience pain from the growth of tumours, and from procedures used to diagnose and treat cancer. In addition, long-term survivors of childhood cancer may have chronic pain, such as causalgia, phantom limb pain, postherpetic neuralgia, and central pain following spinal-cord tumour resection, even though the cancer appears to be cured (Berde & Collins 1999). Neurological degeneration associated with AIDS may be painful and many of the diagnostic and treatment procedures are also invasive and painful (Hirschfeld et al 1996). Headache and chest pain are common in children with cystic fibrosis, particularly if the disease is rapidly progressive, and in the last 6 months of life (Berde & Collins 1999). All of these pains are complicated by the associated fear and anxiety of life-threatening disease and require sensitivity and skillful management.

The most common childhood disease that is accompanied by pain is juvenile chronic arthritis (JCA). Approximately 25% of children with JCA have moderate to severe pain due to the disease (Schanberg et al 1997). Other children may experience pain due to contractures or physical deformities associated with an underlying problem such as muscular dystrophy, cerebral palsy or scoliosis.

Often the disease or injury is itself painful, but the procedures to treat it may also inflict pain. Lumbar punctures, bone-marrow aspirations, injections and so on can be painful experiences if not adequately managed. Many occupational therapists and physiotherapists, who have worked with children suffering from burns, are conscious of the severe pain children may experience during debridement, splinting and range-of-motion exercises. Some pain is also associated with healing. For example, children often feel considerable discomfort from the itching that occurs with recovery from burns.

Special issues concerning pain in infants and children

Unfortunately, numerous surveys have demonstrated that infants and children are frequently given inadequate treatment for their pain (Beyer et al 1983, Eland & Anderson 1977). For example, children are often given considerably less pain medication than adults for post-surgical pain. Until the late 1980s it was not uncommon for infants to receive only muscle relaxants and nitrous oxide (light anaesthesia) for surgical procedures (Anand & McGrath 1993). Anaesthesia was considered risky for newborns and there was considerable doubt that infants were capable of feeling pain.

Infants and children are unable to complain about the quality of their care, and parents often assume that all that can be done is being done. If parents do not challenge the quality of care, then care can be slow to change (McGrath & Unruh 1993). Responsibility for managing children's pain can also be unclear. Whose responsibility is it to relieve the pain of a child with burns during range-of-motion activities? Further, applying an adult model of pain to children is inadequate in understanding children's pain. There are unique features about infants and children, due to their developmental immaturity, that alter the way children might experience and communicate their pain. These differences between adults, infants and children are a challenge to ensuring the adequacy of pain management for this age-group.

Challenges to providing adequate pain management

One of the first challenges to paediatric pain management is the question, 'Are infants capable of feeling pain?'. Most parents would readily answer such a question in the affirmative, but the question is quite complex and has concerned clinicians and researchers for centuries (Unruh 1992). How can we determine whether an infant feels pain and not some other sensation, such as hunger? Is it possible that pain sensitivity might be more or less acute at this point in life than at later stages? What stimuli would be likely to cause pain in an infant? Is the pain sensitivity of an infant changed by disease or disability? Knowledge about neonatal pain sensitivity influences how minor procedures such as heel-pricks and immunizations, and more invasive procedures such as circumcision, heel lance or surgery, are performed with infants. It also raises issues about handling and stimulation for seriously ill neonates and premature infants.

Thus far, the evidence is clear that while the central and peripheral nervous system is immature in early life, the basic connections in nociceptive and pain pathways are formed before birth (Fitzgerald 1993). There are also important postnatal changes that affect pain sensitivity and perception. The infant does not appear to have the segmental control mechanisms within the spinal cord or the descending controls from the cortex that are present in an adult (Fitzgerald 1993). What this means is that the infant will have very little, if any, ability to dampen down a pain stimulus using cortical mechanisms. The implication is that infants may be extremely sensitive to all stimuli and may have heightened pain sensitivity and arousal.

It has been argued that, although infants may have the physiological capacity to receive and transmit noxious stimuli to the brain, this stimulus may not be perceived as 'pain' (see Cunningham 1993). Unfortunately, we can only determine whether the infant actually feels pain indirectly, that is, by behavioural changes such as crying, avoidance behaviour, body movements, facial grimaces, or by physiological changes, such as the mounting of a stress response when the infant is exposed to a painful procedure. However, behavioural or physiological changes could be the result of other factors besides pain. If an infant is crying when given a heel lance, it could be argued that the infant was frightened rather than in pain.

Evidence of a physiological stress response following a procedure might be suggestive of pain but it could also be argued that it is the result of blood-loss. Nevertheless, the growing body of research in this area demonstrates that although infants are unable to provide a self-report of pain, they do demonstrate behavioural and physiological changes in response to procedures that in adults would be regarded as painful. Although we may not know whether the infant recognizes what she or he feels as pain, it would be more humane to assume that the infant is feeling pain and to treat the infant accordingly.

Another important question about infants' and children's pain experiences is whether early pain events have consequences on later pain experiences. There are at least two ways in which pain in early infancy might be influential. The first is through memory and learning. Although it is obvious that at some point in our life we remember and learn from negative painful experiences, it is not clear when such learning begins to occur. It is a part of NICU folklore that infants who are subjected to numerous invasive procedures soon develop the tendency to 'go off' when their incubator is approached by anyone (McGrath & Unruh 1993). These babies demonstrate anticipatory anxiety behaviour.

Recently, it has been argued that infants are also capable of developing a physiological memory of pain (e.g. Taddio 1999). In a series of studies, Taddio and colleagues found that male infants who were circumcised had higher pain scores at their routine 4 and 6 month immunization than male infants who were not circumcised (Taddio et al 1995, 1997). In addition, infants who were given EMLA, a local anaesthetic, had lower pain scores at immunizations than infants who were circumcised with a placebo. Taddio (1999) argued that circumcision may produce long-lasting changes in infant pain behaviour because of changes to the infant's central nervous system processing of painful stimuli. This argument was based on two points. The infants demonstrated these changes months after the circumcision when the surgical site was already healed, and the site of the immunization differed from the location of the circumcision.

Unfortunately, the belief that infants and children do not remember pain or, if they do remember it, then the memory is not long-lasting, has contributed to the inadequate management of children's pain (Cunningham 1993). Aversive pain experiences in childhood can have lasting negative effects even in adulthood, as can be demonstrated by adult fear of needles and dental anxiety.

Psychological factors are frequently thought to be more important in children's than in adult's experience of pain. Children are often vulnerable to beliefs that they are exaggerating their pain or that their pain has primarily a psychological origin (McGrath & Unruh 1987). There is no evidence to support such attitudes. As was discussed in Chapter 4, psychological attributions for pain are more convincing when they are time-locked with the onset and the cessation of pain. For example, if a child complains of abdominal pain before going school, does not complain of pain when allowed to stay home and complains of pain next morning before going to school, then it may be important to enquire about events at school. The abdominal pain may be very real for the child but the causation of the pain may be due to school difficulties. It is important to note, though, that there can be more than one cause for pain. If there are dietary changes in the family and the child is having school problems, then abdominal pain may be due to both factors.

Children are more readily distracted from pain than adults. Distraction is one of the strategies that children will often use on their own initiative to manage pain and other difficulties (Brown et al 1986). For this reason, a child in pain who is playing may appear to have little pain. Children also make good use of their imagination to understand and cope with pain. For example, when children draw pictures of pain, it is not uncommon for them to draw personification drawings, in which the pain appears as something alive that can inflict pain (Unruh et al 1983). However, this does not mean that children have less pain.

In the past 15 years, a rapidly growing body of research concerned with pain in infants and children has drawn considerable attention to these special issues about pain in infants and children, and the inadequacy of paediatric pain management (McGrath 1990, McGrath & Unruh 1987, Ross & Ross 1988, Schechter et al 1993), and practice has begun to change. Advances have been made in paediatric pain measurement and intervention. Papers about various aspects of pain in infants and children are now common in leading pain journals and at national and international meetings.

Guidelines for assessment and measurement of pain in children

Assessment and measurement of pain in infants and children is complicated by the developmental status of the child. Self-report measures which are considered the gold standard in pain measurement are not possible to apply to an infant or very young child (McGrath & Unruh 1999). Children with early verbal skills are able to communicate pain experience but the very young child will still have a relatively limited cognitive understanding about pain and limited language with which to express it. Words such as 'boo-boos' or 'hurt' may be better understood by the child than the word 'pain'. At this stage, it is extremely important to question the child directly about pain and to use language that is developmentally appropriate to the child. It is also important not to underestimate the child's understanding about pain, because of the diversity with which children learn and mature. The following comments are an illustration of a preschooler's explanation of another child's pain:

I know what is like a pain, hurt is like a pain. Maybe he cut himself. He should go to the doctor. Maybe he is sad. (Matthew, 3 years, 5 months old)

Matthew's comments indicate that pain is unpleasant, that it may be related to an injury and that it may cause one to feel upset. He suggests a possible way of dealing with the pain. His understanding of pain is quite sophisticated at $3\frac{1}{2}$ years.

Pain measures for young children reflect the developmental pain language of the young child. The Poker Chip Tool (Hester 1979) based on 'pieces of hurt' has been used successfully with children aged 4–8 years. Several faces scales have also been developed based on changing facial expressions. The Oucher Scale (Beyer 1984) uses photographs of children's faces and can be used with children aged 3–12 years. Variants of the Oucher have been developed for African-American and Hispanic children (Beyer & Knott 1998), and a First Nations version is also in development. Other faces scales use representational drawings. The Bieri Faces Scale (Bieri et al 1990) uses drawings based on children's own drawings of pain faces. It can be used successfully with children aged 6–8 years.

Visual analogue scales (VAS) consisting of a 10-cm vertical or horizontal line with 'no pain' at one anchor and 'pain as bad as it could be' at the other anchor can be used for children over 5 years. However, the VAS does require a child to translate pain intensity into an analogue format and to understand proportionality (McGrath & Unruh 1999). Numerical scales (i.e. 0–5, 0–10, 0–100) use numbers to represent increasing pain. These scales are particularly easy to use in a clinical setting, depending on the child's grasp of number concepts, because they don't require any extra materials and are easy to enter on a child's chart.

Pain thermometers superimpose numerical ratings on a VAS that is shaped like a thermometer with anchors of 'no hurt' and 'most hurt possible'. This measure of pain intensity has been successfully used with children with pain due to burns (Szyfelbein et al 1985).

Behavioural measures of pain can also be used and they are particularly useful for infants and pre-verbal children (McGrath & Unruh 1987). Behaviours such as facial expression, vocalization and body movement are typically associated with pain, but there is always the challenge of distinguishing them from other distress such as anxiety, hunger or thirst (McGrath & Unruh 1999). For short, sharp pain the Children's Hospital of Eastern Ontario Pain Scale (McGrath et al 1985) and the Toddler-Preschool Postoperative Pain Scale (Tarbell et al 1992) can be used. For longer-lasting pain in children aged 2–6 years, the 15-item scale developed by Gauvain-Piquard et al (1987) may be useful. Two more recently developed measures, the Premature Infant Pain Profile (Stevens et al 1996) and the COMFORT Scale (Ambuel et al 1992) combine behaviour and physiological items. Both scales have excellent psychometric properties.

There are a variety of pain measures that can be used with infants and children. The major impediment to their use is the failure to assess and measure pain routinely with children who are at risk for pain (McGrath & Unruh 1999).

Guidelines for management of pain in children

It is very helpful to begin by examining the child's understanding of his or her pain, and to clarify the child's understanding of pain, if needed. Children develop a concept of pain that is initially concrete and based primarily on the sensory aspects of pain, that is, the soreness and where the soreness might be, and the general location of the pain (Gaffney 1993). Young children have limited understanding about pain, particularly causal factors. For this reason, pain may be appraised by young children as highly threatening, until experience and learning enable the child to discriminate more accurately between truly harmful pain (such as a burn) and minor pain (such as bumps in a playground) (Unruh & Ritchie 1998).

School-aged children develop a more complex view of pain and its affective qualities. The older child has the capacity for introspection and abstraction about pain and is able to perceive that pain has sensory and affective dimensions, and psychosocial as well as physical consequences (Gaffney 1993). Social factors, particularly the influence of parents, play an important role in how the child learns to think about pain and cope with it. For example, hostility and ridicule about pain add to fear and anxiety about pain.

It is very useful to talk to the child about pain and to use the child's understanding and his imagination to plan interventions or strategies. Children are sometimes not given sufficient information about pain in language that they can understand. In addition, because they are in an unfamiliar situation in which they often feel powerless, they will have heightened anxiety about the therapeutic situation, particularly if it may involve pain. To illustrate, the author was referred a 12-year-old child with spastic diplegia who was considered severely depressed because he typically cried during range-of-motion exercises and was accompanied to the clinic by his divorced parents. However, the child had no evidence of depression, and upon direct questioning, conveyed that he had no understanding of the purpose of range-of-motion exercises. He was afraid of injury to his limbs, and indeed range-of-motion examination was terminated only when he cried. When given an explanation about the purpose of the examination, and assured that his verbal statements about range-of-motion endpoints would be believed, he no longer cried during examination.

Explanations about interventions and possible pain should be geared to a child's level of understanding, using language with which the child is familiar.

Children should never be lied to or tricked into a painful experience. Deceiving children will hinder development of any therapeutic relationship and will likely increase children's anxiety about future activities that may also be painful. Children should have reasonable control over therapeutic examinations, exercises and activities, to maximize their motivation and decrease the possibility that fear, anxiety or hostility will increase a child's experiences of pain.

Most children prefer to have a parent present during therapy, particularly if there is some possibility of pain from the child's perspective (Ross & Ross 1988). Health professionals often prefer to have parents absent, as children may appear to be more disruptive if a parent is present (Brown & Ritchie 1990). A parent can be instructed about how she or he can be most helpful to the child during the therapeutic intervention. For example, the parent can be taught to give relaxation instructions or engage the child in a distracting activity while the therapist is fashioning a splint (von Baeyer 1997).

Indulgent and excessive attention to pain by parents or other caregivers may reduce active coping behaviour and may promote disability. Family members may need assistance with knowing how to provide appropriate support and encouragement for the child.

Many of the strategies used to manage pain and reduce disability in adulthood can be used with children, but the intervention typically requires adaptation to a more child-centred format (Unruh & McGrath 2000). Information should be broken into smaller, developmentally-appropriate pieces, with more opportunities for practice. Cautela and Groden (1978) wrote a detailed manual for teaching children to relax.

McGrath et al (1990a) developed a patient manual which includes a relaxation tape and a corresponding professional manual (McGrath et al 1990b). This programme has been shown to be effective in the treatment of migraine headache but can also be modified for use with children with other pain problems (McGrath et al 1992). The patient and professional manuals by McGrath et al (1990a, 1990b) discuss the use of cognitive methods (distraction, imagery, thought-stopping and transformation) to manage pain in children. Images for visualization should incorporate images that are meaningful to the child. Play and art may enable the child to talk about thoughts and worries about pain, as well as underlying disease or pain. In some case, pain drawings may help the child to understand pain and may provide images that can be used in cognitive–behavioural interventions (Unruh et al 1983).

Hypnosis can also be used by children to manage pain (Kuttner 1988). Young children (below age 8 or 9 years) may not be able to initiate hypnosis on their own and would require coaching by a trained parent. Texts by Hilgard and Le Baron (1984) and Olness and Gardner (1988) provide detailed and helpful information about the use of hypnosis for children. Patrick Wall and Ron Melzack have produced four editions of the 'Textbook of Pain', a leading publication in this field. The 1994 and 1999 editions have had a series of chapters concerned with pain in infants, children and adolescents. In addition, there are a number of other resources which may be helpful to the occupational therapist or physiotherapist concerned about pain in this age-group (see Table 6.1).

PAIN IN ADOLESCENCE

Prevalence of pain in adolescence

As children enter the late school years and early adolescence, their risk for pain increases, particularly for girls, with the onset of puberty (see section on sex, gender and pain). The prevalence of headache, migraine, abdominal pain and musculoskeletal pains all increase. Several studies identify increased prevalence rates of back pain through the adolescent years with rates of 1–6% in the school-age years (Taimela et al 1997) but reaching 50% and higher by late adolescence (Balagué et al 1988, Leboeuf-Yde & Kyvik 1998, Newcomer & Sinaki 1996, Taimela et al 1997). These rather high rates are troubling, since back pain in adulthood is linked with high disability rates (Teasell & Merskey 1997).

Several researchers have found increased risk of back pain to be linked with sports and other physical activities, particularly those associated with musculotendinous or ligamentous strains caused by excessive loading (Burton et al 1996, Kujala et al 1996, 1997, Leboeuf-Yde & Kyvik 1998, Newcomer & Sinaki 1996). The impact of competitive sports, sport injuries and pain at this stage of life on later life experiences with pain is also unknown.

Some chronic pains that occur in adults are also reported in early adolescence. Complex regional pain syndrome type I (CRPS-I, also known as reflex sympathetic dystrophy) and fibromyalgia occur in this age-group. Buskila et al (1993) reported that 6.2% of a sample of healthy schoolchildren, aged 9–15 years, had fibromyalgia. Berde (1998) reported that many children and adolescents with CRPS-I are dancers, gymnasts or competitive athletes. Some children and adolescents experience pain associated with sickle cell

Table 6.1 Resources about pain in infants, children and adolescents

Resource	Title	Description
Recent Books		
Anand & McGrath 1993, neonatal 1999	Pain in Neonates	Edited book concerning basic science relevant to neonatal pain, assessment, intervention, social, legal and ethical issues
Finley & McGrath 1998	Measurement of Pain in Infants and Children.	Edited book based on keynote papers presented at the first International Pediatric Pain Forum
McGrath & Finley 1999	Chronic and Recurrent Pain in Children and Adolescents	Edited book based on keynote papers presented at second International Pediatric Pain Forum
Series		
McGrath & Finley (editors)	Pediatric Pain Letter	Series of abstracts and commentaries on issues of clinical concern. Contact Patrick..McGrath@dal.ca
Videos		
Kuttner 1999	No Fears, No Tears – 13 years later children coping with pain	For review see Pask 1999, Pediatric Pain Letter, 3, p. 22–23. Contact Dr. Leora Kuttner, fax 604-294-9986, Email: leora-kuttner@sfu.ca
Internet/Web Resources		
Electronic list	pediatric-pain	The owner is Allen Finley. To subscribe send an email message to mailserv@ac.dal.ca In the message write sub pediatric-pain
http://is.dal.ca/~painsrc	Pediatric Pain Sourcebook of Protocols, Policies and Pamphlets	Up-to-date database of pain assessments, measurements and management strategies
Conferences		
Special Interest Group on Pain in Childhood, IASP	International Symposium on Paediatric Pain	Conference is concerned with all issues relevant to pain in childhood
McGrath & Finley	Biennial International Forum on Paediatric Pain	Each meeting is focused on a specific topic, contact Kate Finlayson of Conventional Wisdom, Fax: 1-902-423-5232; Email: katefin@chebucto.ns.ca

disease. Shapiro et al (1995), in a prospective diary study of seven girls and 11 boys aged 8–17 years, found that pain was reported on 30% of days. In addition to these pains, many adolescent girls experience menstrual pain with the onset of menstruation. Menstruation also increases the probability of the occurrence of headache, migraine, back pain and abdominal pain due to constipation.

Special issues concerning pain in adolescents

Much less is known about pain in adolescents and its unique features than the pain experience of infants and children. Although it is evident that the risk of serious pain begins to increase in this age-group, there is little evidence of attention to this problem. For example, the reasons for back pain in this population are not well understood and should receive much more attention, since early intervention may reduce some of the burden of back pain in adulthood.

Adolescents are also in transition between relying on parents to direct their healthcare and assuming responsibility for their own healthcare. It is possible that, as adolescents assume responsibility for their healthcare, at least initially their use of pain management strategies would be modeled on the practices of their parents. There is insufficient research at present to help us understand how parents manage their children's various pain experiences, with the exception of medication use. However, there is evidence that parents do not provide adequate medication for their children's pain, even for post-surgical pain when the parent believes the child is in pain, and when the parent has been given specific instructions and information about pain management (Chambers et al 1997, Finley et al 1996). There are several reasons for parents' reluctance to use medication, including fear of addiction (see Chapter 7) and concern that using pain medication will teach a child to rely on medication to solve problems and may thereby increase the risk of drug abuse.

Unfortunately, as a result, adolescents may have an inadequate understanding of how to use pain medication when they become responsible for managing their own health problems. The best illustration of this problem is menstrual pain. Many adolescent girls experience substantial menstrual pain but they do not seek out medical or parental advice about pain relief, and they do not appear to use medication in a way that will provide sufficient pain relief. Severe menstrual pain is associated with increased disability, that is, with more severe pain girls are more likely to restrict their school, home, work and social activities (Campbell & McGrath 1997). Klein and Litt (1981) found that only 14.5% of adolescents seek medical assistance for menstrual pain including only 29% of adolescents with severe dysmenorrhoea. Only 30% of these adolescent girls even told their mothers about their menstrual pain. Teperi and Rimpela (1989) found that 31% of girls with severe pain did not use any medication for pain relief. When used appropriately, non-steroidal anti-inflammatory drugs (NSAIDs) such as ibuprofen and naproxen sodium relieve 60–100% of dysmenorrhoea (Chan et al 1979, Henzl et al 1980, Jay et al 1986, Morrison et al 1980). Use of these medications for menstrual pain is associated with improvements in daily activities (Henzl et al 1980, Morrison et al 1980). However, in a recent survey of over-the-counter (OTC) medication use, while the majority of the adolescents, particularly those with greater symptom severity and disability, reported using OTC medications to manage their menstrual discomfort, the majority also used medication less often than recommended on the package label (Campbell & McGrath 1997). Only 17% of these adolescents had used a prescription medication to manage menstrual discomfort.

Healthcare utilization practices for some pain problems in adolescence may be influenced, in part, by embarrassment about some aspects of the pain. Adolescent girls may perceive that menstrual pain is too commonplace and too embarrassing to ask for advice, and adolescent boys may feel that being stoic about pain is a necessary part of the masculine image (Unruh & Campbell 1999). Nevertheless, menstrual pain, or other pain during the monthly cycle, often benefits from intervention and may be associated with other more problematic issues that need medical attention, such as endometriosis.

Guidelines for assessment and intervention

Assessment strategies and pain measures that are used with adults can be successfully used with adolescents. There is some research evidence that males change the way that they talk about their pain according to the sex of the questioner and also that males are influenced by perceived male role expectations that they should be stoic in response to pain (Unruh & Campbell 1999, Unruh et al 1999). It's not known whether these perceptions influence adolescent male clients in a clinical setting, but therapists may want to consider this possibility in assessing pain.

Intervention approaches that are used for adults can also be used for adolescents. However, whereas children benefit from and often need the support and assistance of their parents, adolescents may want more independence. The adolescent's needs should be assessed individually to determine what is most helpful and desirable. Similarly to children, the primary productivity occupation for the adolescent will be school-related and intervention should be directed to reducing handicap in this area. Some adolescents may also be employed and may need attention to workplace factors that put her or him at risk for pain or aggravate pain. Lastly, the increased prevalence of back pain through the adolescent years is of serious concern. Back education and preventive programmes organized through schools may be very helpful.

PAIN IN ADULTHOOD
Prevalence of pain in adults

As people enter the adult years, the prevalence of pain increases. Approximately 30–45% of adults have one or more headaches per month. Fifty percent of adults report muscle or joint pain in the previous year. Eighty percent of women have moderate to unbearable pain with menstruation (Unruh 1996a). Thirty percent of adults have at least one episode of back pain in the previous year; 70% will have back pain at least once in a lifetime. Many people who experience troublesome and worrying pain never seek out specialized services for pain. They may see a family physician or a disease specialist but manage to live with pain with minimal disruption. Other people will have much greater difficulty coping with pain. The most common pain problem of clients seen by an occupational therapist or physiotherapist will be back pain.

Special issues concerning pain in adulthood

There are many possible explanations for the increase in pain during the adult years. An important explanation is the wear and tear on the body through problems of workplace design, the ways in which people complete work, and the stresses associated with the pace of work and the milieu associated with work. For many occupational therapists and physiotherapists these issues have opened up new areas of employment through injury-prevention programmes, ergonomic consultation, stress management, in addition to the more traditional workers' compensation programmes.

Although the majority of pain research and the majority of pain clinics are concerned with pain management in adulthood, it is not at all clear that pain at this stage of life is adequately managed even when there is clear evidence of a physiological source of the pain. For example, numerous studies have reported that adult clients routinely receive less analgesia following surgery than they actually need (Choinière et al 1990, Cohen 1980, Donovan et al 1987, Oates et al 1994, Salmon & Manyande 1996).

There are many factors which may contribute to inadequate management of pain in adulthood. Concerns about addiction influence prescription of medications for pain, particularly if the pain is likely to be persistent over a long period of time. Often medication in hospitals is also prescribed on a PRN basis which means that a client will receive medication on request. This arrangement results in a complex interpersonal negotiation between a patient and nurse about whether the pain is sufficiently serious enough to warrant giving the medication. Nurses may underestimate the patient's pain, and they may have negative views about patients who complain about pain (Salmon & Manyande 1996).

The preceding problem concerns clients with acute pain due to surgery, but there is also evidence that many adults with other chronic pains are not given adequate care for pain. In a large national study, Cleeland et al (1994) found that adults with metastatic cancer also received inadequate medication for pain. Clients who have chronic pain with inadequate evidence of organic pathology are particularly vulnerable to inadequate care for pain, often complicated by the denial of chronic pain by health professionals (Teasell 1997, Teasell & Merskey 1997, Thompson 1997).

So far, we have discussed the adequacy of pain management adults receive via medication. Unfortunately, there is little information about the access adults have to other services, such as occupational therapy and physiotherapy, to manage their pain. Often, but not always, access to these services are controlled through medical referrals. Governmental and private insurance programmes may also restrict the amount of time that is available to a client for these services. The client's use of private community services may depend on his or her awareness of the role of these services in providing pain management and assistance with managing occupations of daily life and the client's financial resources.

Guidelines for assessment and management of pain in adulthood

Many of the issues concerning the physiology of pain, the psychological, emotional and behavioural components of pain, and their bearing on assessment and intervention, reflect an adult model of pain experience, and are addressed in other chapters of this text. A comprehensive assessment that considers all of these factors is important in ensuring that the adult client receives the best possible service.

Pain management in adulthood is often provided through multidisciplinary pain clinics. An advantage of such a service is the team approach and the provision of multiple strategies to manage pain and reduce disability. However, several issues are extremely important to ensure maximum benefit. There is some compelling research to suggest that early intervention for pain is much more likely to have a beneficial impact on pain. Breaking the pain cycle early may be extremely important to interrupt the physiological sequelae of pain and the psychological consequences that are often associated with chronic pain.

PAIN IN THE ELDERLY

Prevalence of pain in the elderly

The elderly are often considered to be those individuals aged 65 years and older, although in geriatric medicine the age of 75 years may be considered more appropriate (Ferrell 1996). In research, 65 years is often used as the demarcation of age-groups for purposes of analysis. Ageing is not a uniform process around the world (Ferrell 1996). Differences in healthcare, diet, activity levels, environmental conditions, risks and rates of diseases and many other factors affect pain experience in the elderly. In particular, the incidence of many diseases associated with pain, such as heart disease, diabetes, nephritis, cancer, arthritis and orthopaedic impairments increase with age.

The prevalence of some types of pains do decrease in these later years. For example, headache, migraine, abdominal pain and low back pain decrease with age. However, the prevalence of musculoskeletal pain increases (Ferrell & Ferell 1996). Much of this musculoskeletal pain may be associated with arthritic diseases. Approximately 80% of people over the age of 65 years have arthritis (Davis 1988). Almost all types of cancer are more prevalent in old age and 80% of people with cancer still have substantial pain (Foley 1994).

Special issues concerning pain in the elderly

Ferrell (1996) noted that problems such as depression, decreased socialization, sleep disturbance and impaired ambulation and increased use of healthcare services are also associated with pain in the elderly. Some problems, such as deconditioning, gait disturbances, falls, slow rehabilitation, cognitive dysfunction, malnutrition and inappropriate use of multiple medications, may be made worse by pain that is poorly managed (Ferrell 1991). At this stage of life, problems that may exacerbate pain and increase disability, such as poverty and adequate access to healthcare, and other problems related to racism and sexism, also become problematic.

Unfortunately, there is some evidence that the elderly are also inadequately treated for pain. Cleeland et al (1994) who surveyed pain treatment for people with metastatic cancer found that respondents over 70 years-of-age were the least likely to receive adequate analgesia for pain. Elderly people with chronic pain also appear to have reduced access to multidisciplinary rehabilitation clinics. In an American study of 96 such facilities, no facility had an explicit exclusion of older people but 6.3% did exclude people with no chance of return to work (Kee et al 1996). In addition, respondents were given a series of paired case scenarios in which the individuals in the pairs differed primarily by age. Respondents were asked about the probability that the person would be admitted to the program. People who were older were significantly less likely to be admitted. In addition, the majority of rehabilitation clinics offer only out-patient services. Older people are more likely to be treated as in-patients rather than out-patients either because there is better insurance coverage for in-patient services (e.g. the USA), or the practical organization of travel and accomodation to attend out-patient services may be more difficult for the older person (Kee et al 1996).

Ensuring that elderly people receive appropriate attention for pain is hindered by stereotypes that elderly people feel less pain (Ferrell 1996). These stereotypes are fostered in part by the reluctance elderly people sometimes demonstrate about complaining about pain. Elderly people may sometimes under-report pain because they expect pain with ageing and disease, or they are afraid that the pain means progression of disease (Ferrell 1996, Nishikawa & Ferrell 1993). Past experience with poor pain management may also cause elderly people to feel that there is no point in mentioning pain because nothing will help.

Elderly people may not have pain in association with some illnesses that do present with significant pain in younger adults. For example, an elderly person may have painless myocardial infarction or painless intra-abdominal catastrophes (Ferrell 1996). There are substantial physiological changes at this stage of life but there is no reliable evidence about how these changes affect pain perception. In a review of pain perception and the elderly, Harkins (1996) concluded that there were no age-related changes in pain threshold or tolerance.

One of the difficulties in achieving adequate control of pain in this age-group is also inadequate use of analgesics by the elderly. Pahor et al (1999) found that even with severe osteoarthritic pain, 41% of older disabled women were using less than 20% of the maximum analgesic dose. Again, inadequate use of analgesics may be related to fears about addiction and concerns that if medication is taken before pain is severe, then the medication may be ineffective if pain worsens.

Lastly, Ferrell and Ferrell (1996) argue that in many countries, even with economic variation and differences in the structure of healthcare systems, there are two important issues that place the elderly at greater risk for inadequate treatment of pain. One problem is the increased difficulty for elderly people to seek healthcare given other financial problems associated with aging. The other problem is the lack of family support for many elderly people, or a family advocate who is able to help in seeking pain relief. As a result of these difficulties, elderly people have much more limited access to health professionals who are able to provide pain management services.

Guidelines for assessment and intervention for pain in the elderly

It is extremely important to take enough time to complete a thorough assessment of pain with an older person. The therapist needs to be attentive to potential problems such as fatigue, language difficulties, hearing problems or cognitive limitations, that may require modification in assessment of the person's pain. Family members may also provide assistance in understanding the nature of the elderly person's pain and the extent to which it is interfering with her or his daily occupations, activity and quality of life.

A cognitive–behavioural perspective can be used with an older client to examine the way that pain can affect activities, bodily responses and thoughts and feelings. Ensuring that the client understands the purpose in relationship to the pain, of any occupational therapy or physiotherapy strategies is important. Strategies such as relaxation training, pacing, distraction and cognitive restructuring can also be used with this population, but these strategies may require some modification (Keefe et al 1996).

Older clients may be more likely to fall asleep using relaxation and they may worry about falling if they relax too much (Keefe et al 1996). Modification of relaxation training by keeping the eyes open, and ensuring that relaxation is used in a safe environment will be helpful. If pain is due to arthritic disease then relaxation strategies that do not require tension of muscles may be preferable. Brief relaxation strategies are also helpful because they are less likely to induce sleep and can be used throughout the day (Keefe et al 1996).

Involvement of families may be particularly important to help the client make changes in the home environment or modify habits and routines that reduce pain and improve coping.

Some studies have found that strategies such as biofeedback are not helpful to manage pain in the elderly. However, Kee et al (1996) in their review of this literature argued that methodological problems do not justify these conclusions. Indeed, designs with treatment protocols that are adapted specifically for the elderly client have found that biofeedback is effective to reduce pain due to headache in the older person (Arena et al 1991, Kabela et al 1989. Middaugh et al 1991, 1992). Making an effort to talk more slowly, simplifying instructions, avoiding jargon, checking that the client has understood, brief summaries and repetition in subsequent sessions and allowing for extra time, were all important adaptations to the intervention programmes (Kee et al 1996).

Use of medication for pain is more complex because of age-related changes in pharmacokinetics and pharmodynamics in older people, and these interactions in turn may be complicated by underlying disease and the use of other therapies (Popp & Portenoy 1996). Medications for pain also have increased risk of side-effects for elderly clients (Levy et al 1980). The risk of adverse reactions for people older than 60 years is 2–3 times higher than for people younger than 30 years (Popp & Portenoy 1996). Elderly individuals may have multiple health problems which increase the risk of drug interactions. Poor compliance with medications is also increased with elderly clients, usually due to a lack of understanding, financial constraints, or in an effort to simplify a complex medication regimen (Popp & Portenoy 1996). Occupational therapists and physiotherapists who work with elderly people in the area of pain should be attentive to possible problems in the client's use of medications, such as waiting to take medication until pain is severe, combining medications without medical or pharmacist guidance, addiction fears, and possible adverse drug reactions. These problems should be referred to the client's physician.

SEX, GENDER AND PAIN

As we noted in the definitions given earlier (Box 6.1), sex refers to the biological dimensions of being female or male, whereas gender denotes the broader social role aspects within a given society. The importance of a gender perspective is its explicit recognition that the meaningfulness of any differences between women and men in their thoughts, emotions or behaviours cannot be fully understood without understanding biological, sociological, political and cultural mechanisms (Unruh 1996b).

Sex differences in the prevalence of pain

In the past 10 years, increased attention has been given to sex and gender differences in the experience of pain (Unruh 1996a). There is increasing evidence of sex differences in the physiological risk of pain for women and men (Berkley 1997). Women are at greater risk for a variety of recurrent and chronic pains such as headache, migraine, facial pain, abdominal pain and musculoskeletal pain (Le Resche 1999, Unruh 1996a). The difference in prevalence rates for a variety of pains becomes noticeable with puberty and may be influenced by the menstrual cycle. Only small sex differences in the prevalence of back pain are reported in epidemiological studies and overall back pain may be more strongly related to occupational factors than to the sex of the individual (de Girolamo 1991, Unruh 1996a).

It is also possible that there are sex differences in the experience of pain related to disease. Men with osteoarthritis report more pain from the the disease than do women, independent of the severity of the disease or treatment (Davis 1981). Young men have more pain with sickle cell disease, but by age 35 women and men have similar occurences of sickle cell pain (Baum et al 1987). However, women report more pain than men when they have multiple sclerosis or metastatic cancer (Cleeland et al 1994, Moulin et al 1988, Warnell 1991).

In addition to these problems, women and men are vulnerable to sex-specific pains. Women have pain related to the normal processes of the menstrual cycle and childbirth. Approximately 80% of women under the age of 50 years who have menstrual pain, report moderate to unbearable pain (Taylor & Curran 1985). Labour is rated as more painful than back pain, cancer, phantom limb pain, postherpatic neuralgia, toothache or arthritis (Melzack et al 1981). In addition, women may have pain due to miscarriage, ectopic pregnancy and a variety of other pathological problems of the reproductive structures (Unruh 1996a).

Men do not have a regular non-pathological pain. However, many men experience circumcision, typically performed in infancy but in some societies in later childhood, and often conducted without analgesia or anaesthesia (Schoen & Fischell 1991). There are also a variety of other painful conditions that are specific to the male anatomy, such as varicoceles or testicular pain due to trauma or infection (Nocks 1992). An important difference between women and men is the much greater probability that pain in a man will be associated with injury or disease as an acute pain, which may be resolved by treatment of the underlying condition (Unruh 1996a).

Special issues concerning sex and gender differences in pain experience

Biological and psychosocial factors are both important in explaining sex and gender differences in pain experience. Sex differences in hormones, brain chemistry, metabolism and physical structures contribute to differences in prevalence rates (Unruh 1996a). Biological sex differences are particularly apparent for problems such as migraine. The prevalence of migraine increases dramatically for girls with the onset of puberty and decreases with menopause, although rates continue to be higher for women than men (Unruh 1996a). The risk of occurrence of migraine is also higher for women the day before and the first few days of menstruation. Women have more nausea, vomiting, unilateral numbness and tingling with migraine but men are more likely to have a visual aura preceding migraine (Celentano et al 1990, Rasmussen 1993, Stewart & Lipton 1993). Men have a higher prevalence rate than women for episodic and chronic cluster headaches

which are characterized by severe unilateral pain lasting 15–180 minutes in clusters of attacks (Nappi & Russell 1993) and headache with sexual activity (Lance 1993, Silbert et al 1991).

There are also important environmental factors that influence women's and men's risk for experiencing pain (Messing 1998). Men are often employed in work that requires large body movements, twisting and straining of the body, and the moving, lifting and pushing of large weights (e.g. construction, maintenance, agriculture and the fishery). Such work places men at greater risk than women for sudden, acute musculoskeletal and back injury. Some women are also employed in similar types of work, or work with related requirements, such as nursing. Many more women have low-paying sedentary and repetitive work, or work that requires considerable standing and rapid movement of small loads (e.g. secretaries, computer programmers and operators, cashiers, factory employees). Such work places women at greater risk for progressive soft-tissue injuries. This type of work probably contributes to the higher rates of carpal tunnel syndrome, and upper back and neck pain. Women are more likely to be employed in such work than men. Fifteen to seventeen percent of medical secretaries have almost constant neck or shoulder pain (Kamwendo et al 1991). Working with office machines five or more hours per day significantly increases risk for neck and shoulder pain.

In addition to biological and environmental factors, gender differences that influence social roles and expectations of women and men as partners, parents, caregivers, employers and employees influence the way women and men are socialized to think about, respond to and cope with painful experiences. Women and men construct a meaning of the pain as threatening or harmful, rather than as challenging in different ways (Unruh et al 1999). Threat appraisal of pain is influenced more strongly for women than men by the extent to which pain interferes with daily activities. Girls and women are also more expressive or communicative about pain (Unruh 1999, Unruh & Campbell 1999), whereas boys and men are expected to be more stoic in response to pain (Unruh & Campbell 1999). Although there are many ways in which women and men cope in a similar way with pain, there are also several noteworthy differences that are likely related to socialization process and difference in pain experiences.

Women are more likely to catastrophize in response to experimentally induced pain and dental pain (Sullivan et al 1999) but gender differences in catastrophizing have not been reported in chronic pain

(Vienneau et al 1999). Although catastrophizing is thought to be predictive of pain disability and poor coping (Bennett-Branson & Craig 1993, Turner & Clancy 1986), it may be adaptive for women and may be important in obtaining timely assistance and support for the management of pain (Sullivan et al 1999).

Women are also more likely to use a variety of coping strategies to manage pain, to use more social support, and to seek more healthcare services (Unruh 1997). Nevertheless, while women and men appear to have different risks for chronic pain and use different coping strategies, there are no significant differences in several recent studies with their adaptation to chronic pain (Strong et al 1994, Turk & Okifuji 1999).

It is important to note that there is sufficient evidence to suggest that psychological factors may be inappropriately used to explain the causation of pain for women (Unruh 1996a). The tendency to psychologize women's pain problems is often quite vexing. In addition, there is some evidence that in some settings the sex of the client may lead to inadequate intervention for pain. Physicians may prescribe less pain medication for women than they would for men, and nurses may administer fewer opioids and more sedatives for women (Calderone 1990, Faherty & Grier 1984, Lack 1982, McDonald 1994). Beyer et al (1983) found that significantly more codeine was prescribed for men and boys following open heart surgery. Women and girls were prescribed more acetaminophen (paracetamol), a weaker analgesic.

Cleeland et al (1994) reported that, while all clients in a national survey of people were undermedicated for pain due to metastatic cancer, women were given significantly less medication than men. While these studies demonstrate a disadvantage to women, several studies also indicated greater difficulties in the adequacy of pain management for men (Bond 1971, Bond & Pilowski 1966, Pilowski et al 1969). In these studies, women received the most powerful analgesics for pain due to cancer, even though women and men made similar requests for pain.

Unfortunately, there is very little research about whether the sex of the client has an impact on the nature and quality of the rehabilitation service that women and men receive for pain. However, Mudrick (1989) reported that when women and men received rehabilitation services, women were less likely to receive services that would facilitate employment. Communication, diagnosis and treatment for pain can all be influenced by the client's gender (Grace 1995).

Lastly, there is some suggestive evidence that what men say about how they respond to pain may depend on the sex of the person who is asking. For example, in experimental research, men report lower pain ratings if the experimenter is an attractive female (Levine & De Simone 1991). Unruh et al (1999) found that men were significantly less likely to tell a male interviewer that they cried, moaned or sought comfort for a recent pain experience.

Guidelines for considering sex and gender issues in assessment and management

Research in this area has not advanced sufficiently to make more than general recommendations at this point. Women are more likely to examine the psychological, environmental and behavioural aspects of their pain experiences. However, just because women are often more at ease with examining these aspects of pain, does not mean that their pain has a psychological cause. Men may have difficulty identifying psychological, environmental and behavioural contributors to their pain. A comprehensive assessment of all factors is important for women and men.

Occupational therapists and physiotherapists should also be attentive to the possibility that bias may exist within the healthcare team about the pharmacological and the rehabilitative management of pain for women and men.

RACE AND PAIN

There is very little useful research concerned with race and pain. It is difficult also to separate race from culture; a racial group may not only have unique biological features but may also have important distinctive cultural traditions. Differences due to race may be influenced in part by cultural issues associated with race. For example, Woodrow et al (1972) in a study of 41 119 subjects aged 20–70 years found that Caucasians tolerated more pain than did people of Oriental background with people of Black background in the middle. The administered pain was experimentally induced pressure pain. Pain tolerance might have been influenced by cultural attributes of being Caucasian, Oriental or Black and willingness or unwillingness to report or to tolerate more pain in an experimental setting. Response to experimental pain may be also be very different from response to other forms of pain.

Prevalence of pain by race

There have only been isolated epidemiological studies of the relationship between race and prevalence of pain. In a national survey of pain in the USA, Sternbach (1986) reported that Whites were more likely than Blacks or Hispanics to experience back pain, muscle pain and joint pain. However, White women had less menstrual and premenstrual pain than did Black or Hispanic women. Stewart et al (1996) reported that in the USA, the prevalence of migraine is highest among Caucasians, followed by African Americans and Asian Americans. Within each racial group, women also reported higher prevalence of migraine than did men. There were also some differences in associated symptoms. African Americans had less nausea or vomiting with migraine but they reported more severe pain. The authors concluded that while differences in socioeconomic status, diet and symptom-reporting may have contributed to these different prevalence rates, race-related differences in genetic vulnerability to migraine was a more likely explanatory factor.

There may also be differences by race in experience of procedural pain. Faucett and Levine (1994), in a study of acute postoperative dental pain, found that people of European descent reported significantly less severe pain than people of Black American or Latino descent. Men also reported less severe pain irrespective of racial group. Such differences may be related to sociocultural influences on pain reporting but they may also involve sex and racial differences in an endogenous pain-modulating system which mediates the response to opioids (Faucett & Levine 1994). Nevertheless, other studies of procedure-related pain have not found any racial differences (Flannery et al 1981, Weisenberg et al 1975).

It is unknown whether there are racial differences in risk for pain in association with different diseases. However, sickle cell disease, which is often extremely painful, is found primarily among Black Africans.

Special issues concerning pain and race

Unfortunately, race may affect pain experience in another way. Racism can interfere with adequate pain management. This problem may be best understood by examining the problem of sickle cell pain. Sickle cell disease is characterized by anaemia, delayed secondary sexual characteristics, shortened lifespan and episodes of severe pain (Schechter 1999). In the USA it affects more than 50 000 people and is among the most prevalent genetic diseases (Sickle Cell Disease Guideline Panel 1993). A variety of pains are associated with this disease, but the primary pain is associated with unpredictable and relentless vaso-occlusive episodes (Schechter 1999). The pain is described as an unending, gnawing or chewing pain (Schechter et al 1993). In English-speaking countries, most clients with this disease are African and most health professionals whom they will see are Caucasian (Shapiro 1993). Often these clients tend to be socioeconomically disadvantaged (Schechter 1999); they are often poorer and less well educated. Schechter (1999) points out that historically the attitude of health providers towards this client group has been negative and distrustful, with significant concerns about opioid addiction and potential opioid diversion. Health professionals overestimate the risk of addiction in this client population and assess the risk as much higher than for clients with other chronic health problems (Waldrop & Mandry 1995).

Schechter (1999) argued that the lack of research attention to sickle cell pain and effective interventions to manage it, and the inappropriate medications used for this pain, is in part due to the ethnoracial disparity between healthcare providers and clients in this case. As a result, a cycle of undertreatment occurs (Schechter et al 1988). Providers distrust their clients and typically provide inadequate analgesia. In turn, clients who continue to have pain may become manipulative and melodramatic to obtain adequate analgesia, which is then used as further evidence for opioid addiction and support for undertreatment.

There are few pain problems in which racial (and socioeconomic) factors can be so easily implicated to have a role in the inadequacy of pain management. Occupational therapists and physiotherapists should consider matters of racism that may affect healthcare delivery in their own region and be attentive to personal attitudes and biases that may interfere with providing a client-centred service.

Guidelines concerning assessment and intervention for pain in different racial groups

There is so little research concerned with pain and race that only suggestive guidelines can be presented. It is extremely important to avoid coming to wrong conclusions about a client's experience of pain on the basis of that person's race. Biological differences may place some groups at greater risk for different kinds of pain but more research is needed to determine if this is so. Race is also often associated with culture, which in turn may influence sociocultural expectations about how women and men think about, respond to and manage pain. Often these expectations about pain are unknown or open to misinterpretation if one does not come from the same racial group. It is important that occupational therapy and physiotherapy assessments and interventions for pain are sensitive and respectful of these racial and cultural perspectives.

PAIN AND PEOPLE WITH SPECIAL NEEDS

Problems such as cerebral palsy, spina bifida, muscular dystrophy, cognitive delays, aphasia, Alzheimer's disease, dementia and others difficulties may affect communication, as well as motoric or behavioural expression of pain. In some situations, the problems will be congenital in nature (e.g. cerebral palsy), whereas other difficulties appear later in life (e.g. dementia) or are the secondary consequences of disease or injury (e.g. stroke).

Prevalence of pain

People with severe cognitive and communication impairments have a greater risk of pain because of the nature of their difficulties or challenges, and the consequent risk of unrecognized and poorly managed pain (Collignon et al 1995, Giusiano et al 1995, McGrath et al 1998, Sengstaken & King 1993). They may require more invasive and more frequent procedures, and they may have secondary problems such as cramping of muscles, bone deformities and contractures, that are themselves painful (Broseta et al 1990, Hoffer 1986, Ireland & Hoffer 1985). In addition, approximately 25–65% of people with cerebral palsy develop scoliosis secondary to this condition, and this deformity may also be painful (Majd et al 1997).

Recently, Schwartz et al (1999), in a study of 62 adults with cerebral palsy, found that 67% reported one or more pains of more than 3 months' duration and for the majority the pain occurred on a daily basis. The pain was most often in the lower limbs and back and for 53% of the respondents, the pain was moderate to severe in intensity. This study was the first to examine the extent of pain in this population.

Special issues concerning pain in people with special needs

Until very recently, little has been known about the pain experience of children or adults with special needs. The overwhelming assumption has been that individuals with these difficulties have neurological impairments that reduce their capacity to feel pain. However, the existing research (Collignon et al 1995,

Schwartz et al 1999), while limited, is demonstrating that except for the occasional individual who may have some insensitivity to pain, severe cognitive and communication impairments do not appear to reduce the capacity to feel pain (Hadden 2000). For example, Cornu (1975) and Jonsson et al (1977) found that there were no significant differences in the pain threshold of adult research participants with or without dementia. In a study of response to venepuncture, participants with lower cognitive abilities had lower heart rate responses when they saw the syringe and a greater decrease in heart rate during the procedure (Porter et al 1993). Farrell et al (1996) suggested that these changes might be due to a lack of preparedness and greater alarm.

A major hindrance to understanding pain experience in this population and ensuring appropriate management is the difficulty in pain assessment. The self-report measures which are currently available are often very difficult for people with severe cognitive and communication impairments to use. LaChapelle et al (1999) found that 35% of a sample of people with intellectual disabilities were unable to give a valid self-report of pain for an intramuscular injection. Ferrell and Ferrell (1993) noted that 17% of 112 nursing home residents with mild to moderate cognitive impairment were unable to use at least one of five pain measures. Parmalee et al (1993) and Brody and Kleben (1983) excluded 22.5% and 34% of their research samples respectively, due to severe communication problems that interfered with completion of measures. Fanurik et al (1998) found that only 21% of a sample of children aged 8–17 years with borderline or mild cognitive impairment were able to understand and provide a meaningful rating of pain using a 0–5 numerical scale.

Behavioural measures are a better alternative for the measurement of pain in people who have cognitive impairments. LaChapelle et al (1999) measured pain using a self-report and an observational measure in a sample of 40 adults with intellectual disability who were having a routine influenza vaccination. Although 35% of the sample were able to provide self-report, the observational measure appeared to be a more sensitive and valid measure of the pain. Nevertheless, existing behavioural measures may not be useful if the individual has severe motoric disabilities that generate abnormal behaviour patterns or reduce the capacity for voluntary movement. For example, problems such as spasticity, reduced muscle tone, paralysis, athetoid movement and so on, can make behaviour difficult to understand. Health professionals who are not intimately familiar with the person with such impairments may have difficulty recognizing any of these behaviours as related to pain (Camfield et al 1997, Farrell et al 1996, McGrath et al 1998).

Recently, researchers have argued that the involvement of caregivers is critical to help health professionals identify behaviours that are related to pain for a person with severe impairment, to ensure more accurate assessment of pain (McGrath et al 1998). Research is currently underway to develop individualized pain measures for clients with special needs based on the vocalizations and behaviours caregivers use to determine whether the person is in pain (Breau et al 2001).

Guidelines for pain assessment and intervention for people with special needs

There is still a great deal that remains to be known about the pain experience of people with special needs. It is important to challenge ideas that children and adults with special needs do not feel pain, and reduce the risk that pain will go unrecognized and untreated, or inadequately treated. It is also essential for occupational therapists and physiotherapists who work in this area to be attentive to emerging research that will provide more information about pain assessment and management in the coming years, and more practical guidelines.

In the meantime, therapists should assume that every client with special needs is capable of feeling pain. Caregivers should be involved in helping to identify idiosyncratic pain behaviours, to guide intervention options, and to help determine whether these interventions have been effective in relieving pain. Involvement of family is particularly important to ensure that the family knows what is being done to help their family member.

As mentioned in Chapter 4, in Canada, a father killed his daughter, a 10-year-old child with cerebral palsy, because he could no longer endure her ongoing pain and suffering. Actions such as this one are a very sad reflection on our current difficulty to adequately assess and manage pain in people with special needs.

Many of the strategies that are used to manage pain may need modification to be useful for a person with special needs. For example, relaxation is very difficult for someone who has limited muscular control, but focusing on deep breathing combined with cognitive imagery may be very effective.

Medication requirements may also be different depending on the client's specific problem. Martin et al (1997) in a retrospective chart review found that children with Down's Syndrome received more morphine per kg per hour following surgery for congenital heart disease than other children. Unfortunately, because there was no measure of pain in this study, it is not possible to know on what basis these children were given more morphine.

CONCLUSION

Most people will experience headaches, back pain, musculoskeletal pain and abdominal pain at least once in their lifetime. Pain research and pain management programs are primarily concerned with pain in adulthood. Consequently, pain in childhood and pain in the elderly is often misunderstood. The influence of gender and race on pain experience are also not well understood.

Misconceptions about the impact of age and gender can hinder the adequacy of the services clients receive. Misconceptions about age and gender may also intersect with attitudes about culture and poverty and pain experience. In addition, although pain in infancy, childhood and adolescence has gained much more attention in the past 15 years and has challenged many strongly-held misconceptions, progress has remained slow in examining the needs of the elderly.

Attention to gender in pain research is relatively recent. Very little is currently known about the way that race or a client's special needs might affect pain experience. Nevertheless, increasing research in these areas will improve our understanding of the relationships between race, special needs and pain.

Study questions/questions for revision

1. What are five unique features of pain in infants and young children?
2. How might gender differences in pain experience affect the needs of men and women when they have pain?
3. What biases are commonly held about pain in the older person?
4. What are some of the adaptations that can be made to intervention programmes for the elderly client?
5. How does race potentially hinder the adequacy of pain management for some clients?
6. Why should caregivers be involved in providing pain management for clients with special needs?

ACKNOWLEDGEMENT

Portions of the section on sex, gender and pain first appeared in Unruh A 1996 Pain 65: 123–167

REFERENCES

Ambuel B, Hamlett K W, Marx C M, Blumer J L 1992 Assessing distress in pediatric intensive care environments: the COMFORT scale. Journal of Pediatric Psychology 17: 95–109

Anand K J S, McGrath P J 1993 An overview of current issues and their historical background. In: Anand K J S, McGrath P J (eds) Pain in Neonates. Elsevier, Amsterdam, pp 1–18

Arena J G, Hannah S L, Bruno G M, Meador K J 1991 Electromyographic biofeedback training for tension headache in the elderly: a prospective study. Biofeedback and Self-Regulation 16: 379–390

Balagué F, Dutoit G, Waldburger M 1988 Low back pain in schoolchildren: an epidemiological study. Scandinavian Journal of Rehabilitation Medicine 20: 175–179

Baum K F, Dunn D T, Maude G H, Serjeant G R 1987 The painful crisis of homozygous sickle cell disease: a study of risk factors. Archives of Internal Medicine 147: 1232–1234

Bennett-Branson S M, Craig K D 1993 Postoperative pain in children: developmental and family influences on spontaneous coping strategies. Canadian Journal of Behavioural Science 25: 355–383

Berde C B 1998 Gender differences in CRPSI/RSD in children and adolescents. Paper presented at the NIH Gender and Pain Conference, April 7–8 1998. Bethesda, Maryland

Berde C B, Collins J J 1999 Cancer pain and palliative care in children. In: Wall P D, Melzack R (eds) Textbook of Pain, 4th edn. Churchill Livingstone, New York, pp 967–989

Berkley K J 1997 Sex differences in pain. Behaviour and Brain Science 20: 371–380

Beyer J E 1984 The Oucher: a user's manual and technical report. The Hospital Play Equipment, Evanston, Illinois

Beyer J E, Knott C B 1998 Construct validity estimation of the African-American and Hispanic versions of the Oucher Scale. Journal of Pediatric Nursing 13: 20–31

Beyer J E, DeGood D E, Ashley L C, Russell G A 1983 Patterns of postoperative analgesic use with adults and children following cardiac surgery. Pain 17: 71–81

Bieri D, Reeve R A, Champion G D, Addicoat L, Ziegler J B 1990 The faces pain scale for the self-assessment of the severity of pain experienced by children: development, initial validation, and preliminary investigation for ratio scale properties. Pain 41: 139–150

Bond M R 1971 Pain in hospital. The Lancet i: 37

Bond M R, Pilowsky I 1966 Subjective assessment of pain and its relationship to the administration of analgesics in patients with advanced cancer. Journal of Psychosomatic Research 10: 203–208

Breau L M, McGrath P J, Camfield C, Finley G A 2001 Preliminary validation of an observational pain checklist for cognitively impaired, non-verbal persons. Developmental Medicine & Child Neurology, in press

Brody E M, Kleban M H 1983 Day to day mental and physical health symptoms of older people: a report of health logs. Gerontologist 23: 75–85

Broseta J, Garcia-March G, S'andrez-Ledesma M J, Anaya J, Silva I 1990 Chronic intrathecal baclofen administration in severe spasticity. Stereotactic and Functional Neurosurgery 54–55: 147–153

Brown J, Ritchie J 1990 Nurses' perceptions of parent and nurse roles in caring for hospitalized children. Children's Health Care 19: 28–36

Burton A K, Clarke R D, McClune T D, Tillotson K M 1996 The natural history of low back pain in adolescents. Spine 21: 2323–2328

Buskila D, Press J, Gedalia A, Klein M, Neumann L, Boehm R, Sukenik S 1993 Assessment of nonarticular tenderness and prevalence of fibromyalgia in children. Journal of Rheumatology 20: 368–370

Calderone K 1990 The influence of gender on the frequency of pain and sedative medication administered to post-operative patients. Sex Roles 23: 713–725

Camfield C, McGrath P, Rosmus C, Campbell M A 1997 Behaviors used by caregivers to determine pain in non-verbal, cognitively impaired children. Paediatric Child Health 2 (Suppl A): 8

Campbell M A, McGrath P J 1997 Use of medication by adolescents for the management of menstrual discomfort. Archives of Pediatric and Adolescent Medicine 151: 905–913

Cautela J R, Groden J 1978 Relaxation: a comprehensive manual for adults, children, and children with special needs. Research Press, Champaign, Illinois

Celentano D D, Linet M S, Stewart W F 1990 Gender differences in the experience of headache. Social Science and Medicine 30: 1289–1295

Chambers C T, Reid G J, McGrath P J, Finlay G A, Ellerton M L 1997 A randomized trial of a pain education booklet: effects on parents' attitudes and postoperative pain management. Children's Health Care 26: 1–13

Chan W Y, Dawood M Y, Fuchs F 1979 Relief of dysmenorrhea with prostaglandins synthetase inhibitor ibuprofen: effect on prostaglandin levels in menstrual fluid. American Journal of Obstetrics 135: 102–108

Choinière M, Melzack R, Girard N, Rondeau J, Paquin M-J 1990 Comparison between patients' and nurses' assessment of pain and medication efficacy in severe burn injuries. Pain 40: 143–152

Cleeland C, Gonin R, Hatfield A K, Edmonson J H, Blum R H, Stewart J A, Pandya K J 1994 Pain and its treatment in outpatients with metastatic cancer. New England Journal of Medicine 330: 592–596

Cohen F L 1980 Postsurgical pain relief: patients' status and nurses' medication choices. Pain 9: 69–78

Collignon P, Giusiano B, Porsmoguer E, Jimeno M T, Combe J T 1995 Difficultés du diagnostic de la douleur chez l'enfant polyhandicapé. Annales de Pédiatrie 42: 123–126

Cornu F 1975 Perturbations de la perception de la douleur chez les dements degeratifs. Journal de Psychologie Normale et Pathologique 72: 81–96

Cunningham N 1993 Moral and ethical issues in clinical practice. In: Anand K J S, McGrath P J (eds) Pain in Neonates. Elsevier, Amsterdam, pp 255–273

Davis M A 1981 Sex differences in reporting osteoarthritic symptoms: a sociomedical approach. Journal of Health and Social Behavior 22: 298–311

Davis M A 1988 Epidemiology of osteoarthritism. Clinics of Geriatric Medicine 4: 241–255

de Girolamo G 1991 Epidemiology and social costs of low back pain and fibromyalgia. Clinical Journal of Pain 7(Suppl. 1): S1–S7

Donovan M, Dillon P, McGuire L 1987 Incidence and characteristics of pain in a sample of medical-surgical inpatients. Pain 30: 69–78

Eland J M, Anderson J E 1977 The experience of pain in children. In: Jacox A K (ed) Pain: A Sourcebook for Nurses and Other Health Professionals. Little Brown, Boston, pp 246–250

Faherty B S, Grier M R 1984 Analgesic medication for elderly people post-surgery. Nursing Research 33: 369–373

Fanurik D, Koh J L, Harrison R D, Conrad T M, Tomerlin C 1998 Pain assessment in children with cognitive impairment: an exploration of self-report skills. Clinical Nursing Research 7: 103–124

Farrell M J, Katz B, Helme R D 1996 The impact of dementia on pain experience. Pain 67: 7–15

Faucett J, Levine J 1994 Differences in postoperative pain severity among four ethnic groups. Journal of Pain and Symptom Management 9: 383–389

Fearon I, McGrath P J, Achat H 1996 'Booboos': the study of everyday pain among young children. Pain 68: 55–62

Ferrell B A 1991 Pain management in elderly people. Journal of the American Geriatric Society 39: 64–73

Ferrell B A 1996 Overview of aging and pain. In: Ferrell B R, Ferrell B A (eds) Pain in the Elderly. IASP Press, Seattle, pp 1–10

Ferrell B A, Ferrell B R 1993 Pain assessment among cognitively impaired nursing home residents. Journal of the American Geriatric Society 41: SA25

Ferrell B R, Ferrell B A 1996 An international perspective on pain in the elderly. In: Ferrell B R, Ferrell B A (eds) Pain in the Elderly. IASP Press, Seattle, pp 119–130

Finley G A, McGrath P J 1998 Measurement of pain in infants and children. IASP Press, Seattle

Finley G A, McGrath P J, Forward S P, McNeill G, Fitzgerald P 1996 Parents' management of children's pain following 'minor' surgery. Pain 64: 83–83

Fitzgerald M 1993 Development of pain pathways and mechanisms. In: Anand K J S, McGrath P J (eds) Pain in Neonates. Elsevier, Amsterdam

Flannery R B, Sos J, McGovern P 1981 Ethnicity as a factor in the expression of pain. Psychosomatics 22: 39–50

Foley K 1994 Pain in the elderly. In: Hazzard W R, Bierman E L, Blass J P, Ettinger W H Jr, Halter J B (eds) Principles of Geriatric Medicine and Gerontology. McGraw-Hill, New York

Gaffney A 1993 Cognitive development of pain. In: Schechter N L, Berde C B, Yaster M (eds) Pain in Infants, Children and Adolescents. Williams & Wilkins, Baltimore

Gauvain-Piquard A, Rodary C, Rezvani A, Rezvani A, Lemerle J 1987 Pain in children aged 2–6 years: a new observational rating scale elaborated in a pediatric oncology unit – preliminary report. Pain 31: 177–188

Giusiano B, Jimeno M T, Collignon P, Chau Y 1995 Utilization of a neural network in the elaboration of an evaluation scale for pain in cerebral palsy. Methods of Information in Medicine 34: 498–502

Goodenough B 1998 Growing pains. Pediatric Pain Letter 2: 38–41

Grace V M 1995 Problems of communication, diagnosis, and treatment experienced by women using the New Zealand health services for chronic pain: a quantitative analysis. Health Care for Women International 16: 521–535

Hadden K L 2000 Pain in children with severe cognitive and communication impairment. Pediatric Pain Letter 4(1): 2–5

Harkins S W 1996 Geriatric pain. Pain perceptions in the old. Clinical Geriatric Medicine 12(3): 435–459

Henzl M R, Massey S, Hanson F W, Buttram V C, Rosenwaks Z, Pauls F D 1980 Primary dysmenorrhea: a therapeutic challenge. Journal of Reproductive Medicine 25: 226–235

Hester N K 1979 The pre-operational child's reaction to immunization. Nursing Research 28: 250–255

Hilgard J R, Le Baron S 1984 Hypnotherapy of pain in children. Kaufman, Los Altos, California

Hirschfeld S, Moss H, Dragisic K, Smith W, Pizzo P A 1996 Pain in pediatric human immunodeficiency virus infection: incidence and characteristics in a single-institution pilot study. Pediatrics 98: 449–452

Hoffer M M 1986 Management of the hip in cerebral palsy. Journal of Bone and Joint Surgery 68: 629–631

Ireland M L, Hoffer M M 1985 Triple arthrodesis for children with spastic cerebral palsy. Developmental Medicine and Child Neurology 27: 623–627

Jay M S, Durant R H, Shoffitt T, Linder C W 1986 Differential response by adolescents to naproxen sodium therapy for spasmodic and congestive dysmenorrhea. Journal of Adolescent Health Care 7: 395–400

Jonsson C O, Malhammar G, Waldton S 1977 Reflex elicitation thresholds in senile dementia. Acta Psychiatrica Scandinavica 55: 81–96

Kabela E, Blanchard E B, Appelbaum K A, Nicholson N 1989 Self-regulatory treatment of headache in the elderly. Biofeedback and Self-Regulation 14: 219–228

Kamwendo K, Linton S J, Moritz S U 1991 Neck and shoulder disorders in medical secretaries. Part 1: Pain prevalence and risk factors. Scandinavian Journal of Rehabilitation Medicine 23: 127–133

Kee W G, Middaugh S J, Pawlick K L 1996 Persistent pain in the older patients: evaluation and treatment. In: Gatchel R J, Turk D C (eds) Psychological Approaches to Pain Management: a Practioner's Handbook. Guilford Press, New York, pp 371–402

Keefe F J, Beaupré P M, Weiner D K, Siegler I C 1996 Pain in older adults: a cognitive–behavioural perspective. In: Ferrell B R, Ferrell B A (eds) Pain in the Elderly. IASP Press, Seattle, pp 11–19

Klein J R, Litt I F 1981 Epidemiology of adolescent dysmenorrhea. Pediatrics 68: 661–664

Kujala U M, Taimela S, Erkintalo M, Salminen J J, Kaprio J 1996 Low-back pain in adolescent athletes. Medical Science, Sports Medicine 28: 165–170

Kujala U M, Taimela S, Oksanen A, Salminen J J 1997 Lumbar mobility and low back pain during adolescence: a longitudinal three-year follow-up study in athletes and controls. American Journal of Sports Medicine 25: 363–368

Kuttner L 1988 Favorite stories: a hypnotic pain-reduction technique for children in acute pain. American Journal of Clinical Hypnosis 30: 289–295

LaChapelle D L, Hadjistavropoulos T, Craig K D 1999 Pain measurement in persons with intellectual disabilities. Clinical Journal of Pain 15: 13–23

Lack D Z 1982 Women and pain: another feminist issue. Women & Therapy 1: 55–64

Lance J W 1993 Miscellaneous headaches associated with a structural lesion. In: Olesen J, Tfelt-Hansen P, Welch K M A (eds) The Headaches. Raven Press, New York, pp 609–617

Leboeuf-Yde C, Kyvik K O 1998 At what age does low back pain become a common problem? A study of 29 424 individuals aged 12–41 years. Spine 23: 228–234

LeResche L 1999 Gender considerations. In: Crombie I K, Croft P R, Linton S J, LeResche L, Von Korff M (eds) Epidemiology of Pain. IASP Press, Seattle

Levine F M, De Simone L L 1991 The effects of experimenter gender on pain report in male and female subjects. Pain 44: 69–72

Levy M, Kewitz H, Altwein W, Hillebrand J, Eliakim M 1980 Hospital admissions due to adverse drug reactions: a comparative study from Jerusalem and Berlin. European Journal of Clinical Pharmacology 17: 25–31

Majd M E, Muldowny D S, Holt R T 1997 Natural history of scoliosis in the institutionalized adult cerebral palsy population. Spine 22: 1461–1466

Martin J, Macnab A J, Scott C S, Gakhal B 1997 Do Down's Syndrome children require more morphine following cardiac surgery? Pediatric Child Health 2 (Suppl A): 21

McDonald D D 1994 Gender and ethnic stereotyping and narcotic analgesic administration. Research in Nursing & Health 17: 45–40

McGrath P A 1990 Pain in Children: Nature, Assessment and Treatment. Guilford Press, New York

McGrath P J, Finley G A 1999 Chronic and recurrent pain in children and adolescents. Progress in Pain Research and Management, Vol. 13. IASP Press, Seattle

McGrath P J, Unruh A M 1987 Pain in Children and Adolescents. Elsevier, Amsterdam

McGrath P J, Unruh A M 1993 Social and legal issues. In: Anand K J S, McGrath P J (eds) Pain in Neonates. Elsevier, Amsterdam, pp 295–320

McGrath P J, Unruh A M 1999 Measurement and assessment of paediatric pain. In: Wall P D, Melzack R (eds) Textbook of Pain, 4th edn. Churchill Livingstone, New York, pp 371–384

McGrath P J, Johnson G, Goodman J, Schillinger J, Dunn J, Chapman J 1985 The CHEOPS: a behavioral scale to measure post operative pain in children. In: Fields H L, Dubner R, Cervero F (eds) Advances in Pain Research and Clinical Management. Raven Press, New York, pp 395–402

McGrath P J, Cunningham S J, Lascelles M J, Humphreys P 1990a Help yourself: a program for treating migraine headaches. Patient Manual and Audiotape. Ottawa University Press, Ottawa

McGrath P J, Cunningham S J, Lascelles M J, Humphreys P 1990b Help yourself: a program for treating migraine

headaches. Professional Handbook. Ottawa University Press, Ottawa

McGrath P J, Humphreys P, Keene D, Goodman J T, Lascelles M A, Cunningham S J, Firestone P 1992 The efficacy and efficiency of a self-administered treatment for adolescent migraine. Pain 49: 321–324

McGrath P J, Rosmus C, Camfield C, Campbell M A, Hennigar A 1998 Behaviours caregivers use to determine pain in non-verbal, cognitively impaired individuals. Developmental Medicine & Child Neurology 40: 430–343

Melzack R, Taenzer P, Feldman P, Kinch T 1981 Labour is still painful after prepared childbirth training. Canadian Medical Association Journal 125: 357–363

Messing K 1998 One-eyed Science: Occupational Health and Women Workers. Temple University Press, Philadelphia

Middaugh S J, Woods S E, Kee W G, Harden R N, Peters J R 1991 Biofeedback-assisted relaxation training for chronic pain in the aging. Biofeedback and Relaxation 16: 361–377

Middaugh S J, Kee W G, King S R, Peters J R, Herman K 1992 Physiological response of older and younger pain patients to biofeedback-assisted relaxation training. Biofeedback and Self- Regulation 17: 304–305

Morrison J C, Ling F W, Forman E K, Bates G W, Blake PG, Vecchio T J Linden C V, O'Connell M J 1980 Analgesic efficacy of ibuprofen for treatment of primary dysmenorrhea. South Medical Journal 73: 999–1002

Moulin D E, Foley K M, Ebers G C 1988 Pain syndromes in multiple sclerosis. Neurology 38: 1830–1843

Mudrick N R 1989 The association of roles and attitudes with disability among midlife women and men. Journal of Aging Health 1: 306–327

Naish J M, Apley J 1950 Growing pains: a clinical study of non-arthritic limb pains in children. Archives of Diseases in Childhood 26: 134–140

Newcomer K, Sinaki M 1996 Low back pain and its relationship to back strength and physical activity in children. Acta Paediatrica 85: 1433–1439

Nishikawa S T, Ferrell B A 1993 Pain assessment in the elderly. Clinical Geriatric Issues in Long Term Care 1: 15–28

Nappi G, Russell D 1993 Tension-type headache, cluster headache, and miscellaneous headaches: clinical features. In: Olesen J, Tfelt-Hansen, Welch K M A (eds) The Headaches. Raven Press, New York, pp 577–584

Nocks B N 1992 Erectile dysfunction and pain in the male genitalia. In: Aronoff G M (ed) Evaluation and Treatment of Chronic Pain, 2nd edn. Williams & Wilkins, Baltimore, pp 302–312

Oates J D L, Snowdon S L, Jayson D W H 1994 Failure of pain relief after surgery. Anesthesia 49: 755–758

Olness K, Gardner G G 1988 Hypnosis and Hypnotherapy with Children, 2nd edn. Grune & Stratton, Philadelphia

Pahor M, Guralnik J M, Wan J Y, Ferrucci L, Penninx B W, Lyles A, Ling S, Fried L P 1999 Lower body osteoarticular pain and dose of analgesic medications in older disabled women: the Women's Health and Aging Study. American Journal of Public Health 89: 930–934

Parmelee P A, Smith B, Katz I R 1993 Pain complaints and cognitive status among elderly institution residents. Journal of the American Geriatric Society 41: 517–522

Phillips S 1995 The social context of women's health: goals and objectives. Canadian Medical Association Journal 152: 507–511

Pilowsky T, Manzcp C H B, Bond M R 1969 Pain and its management in malignant disease. Psychosomatic Medicine XXXI: 400–404

Popp B, Portenoy R K 1996 Management of chronic pain in the elderly: Pharmacology of opioids and other analgesic drugs. In: Ferrell B R, Ferrell B A (eds) Pain in the Elderly. IASP Press, Seattle

Porter F L, Miller J P, Morris J, Berg L 1993 Pain in aging: attention, cognitive performance, perception and physiologic response. Proceedings of the VII IASP World Congress on Pain: 99

Rasmussen B K 1993 Migraine and tension headache in a general population: precipitating factors, female hormones, sleep pattern and relation to lifestyle. Pain 53: 65–72

Ross D M, Ross S A 1988 Childhood pain: current issues, research and management. Urban & Swarzenberg, Baltimore,

Ruhrah J 1925 Pediatrics of the Past. Paul B Hoeber, New York

Salmon P, Manyande A 1996 Good patients cope with their pain: postoperative analgesia and nurses' perceptions of their patients' pain. Pain 68: 63–68

Schanberg L E, Lefebvre J C, Keefe F J, Kredich D W, Gil K M 1997 Pain coping and the pain experience in children with juvenile chronic arthritis. Pain 73: 181–189

Schechter N L 1999 The management of pain in sickle cell disease. In: McGrath, P J, Finley G A (eds) Chronic and Recurrent Pain in Children and Adolescents. Progress in Pain Research and Management, Vol. 13: 99–114

Schechter N L, Berrien F B, Katz S M 1988 The use of patient controlled analgesia in adolescents with sickle cell pain crisis: a preliminary report. Journal of Pain and Symptom Management 3: 109–113

Schechter N L, Berde C B, Yaster M (eds) 1993 Pain in Infants, Children and Adolescents. Williams & Wilkins, Baltimore

Schoen E J, Fischell A A 1991 Pain in neonatal circumcision. Pediatrics 30: 429–432

Schwartz L, Engel J M, Jensen M P 1999 Pain in persons with cerebral palsy. Archives of Physical Medicine and Rehabilitation 80: 1243–1246

Sengstaken E A, King S A 1993 The problems of pain and its detection among geriatric nursing home residents. Journal of the American Geriatric Society 41: 541–544

Shapiro B S 1993 Management of painful episodes in sickle cell disease. In: Schechter N L, Berde C B, Yaster M (eds) Pain in Infants, Children, and Adolescents. Williams & Wilkins, Baltimore, pp 385–410

Shapiro B S, Dinges D F, Orne E C, Bauer N, Reilly L B, Whitehouse W G, Ohene-Frempong K, Orne M T 1995 Home management of sickle cell-related pain in children and adolescents: natural history and impact on school attendance. Pain 61: 139–144

Sickle Cell Disease Guideline Panel 1993 Clinical practice guidelines for sickle cell disease: screening, diagnosis, management and counselling in newborns and infants. AHCPR Pub No 93-0562. Agency for Health Care Policy and Research, Public Health Service, US Department of Health and Human Service, Rockville

Silbert P L, Edis R H, Stewart-Wynne E G, Gubbay S S 1991 Benign vascular sexual headache and exertional headache: interrelationships and long-term prognosis. Journal of Neurology, Neurosurgery and Psychiatry 54: 417–421

Sternbach R A 1986 Pain and 'hassles' in the United States: findings of the Nuprin Pain Report. Pain 27: 69–80

Stevens B, Johnston C C, Petryshen P, Taddio A 1996 Premature infant pain profile: development and initial validation. Clinical Journal of Pain 12: 13–22

Stewart W F, Lipton R B 1993 Societal impact of headache. In: Olesen J, Tfelt-Hansen, Welch K MA (eds) The Headaches. Raven Press, New York, pp 29–34

Stewart W F, Lipton R B, Liberman J 1996 Variation in migraine prevalence by race. Neurology 47: 52–59

Strong J, Ashton R, Stewart A 1994 Chronic low back pain: towards an integrated psychosocial assessment model. Journal of Consulting and Clinical Psychology 69: 1058–1063

Sullivan M J L, Tripp D A, Santor D 2001 Gender differences in pain and pain behavior: the role of catastrophizing. Cognitive Therapy & Research, 24: 121–134

Szfelbein S K, Osgood P F, Carr D B 1985 The assessment of pain and plasma beta-endorphin immunoactivity in burned children. Pain 22: 173–182

Taddio A, Goldbach M, Ipp M, Stevens B, Koren G 1995 Effect of neonatal circumcision on pain response during vaccination in boys. The Lancet 345: 291–292

Taddio A, Stevens B, Craig K, Rastogi P, Ben-David S, Shennan A, Mulligan P, Koren G 1997 Efficacy and safety of lidocaine-prilocaine cream for pain during circumcision. New England Journal of Medicine 336: 1197–1201

Taddio A 1999 Effects of early pain experience: the human literature. In: McGrath P J, Finley G A (eds) Chronic and Recurrent Pain in Children and Adolescents. Progress in Pain Research and Management, Vol. 13: 57–74

Taimela S, Kujala U M, Salminen J J, Viljanen T 1997 The prevalence of low back pain among children and adolescents: a nationwide, cohort-based questionnaire survey in Finland. Spine 22: 1132–1136

Tarbell S E, Cohen T, March J L 1992 The Toddler-Preschool Postoperative Pain Scale: an observational pain scale for measuring postoperative pain in children aged 1–5. Preliminary report. Pain 50: 273–280

Taylor H, Curran N M 1985 The Nuprin Pain Report. Louis Harris and Associates Inc, New York

Teasell R W 1997 The denial of chronic pain. Pain Research & Management 2: 89–91

Teasell R W, Merskey H 1997 Chronic pain disability in the workplace. Pain Research & Management 2: 197–205

Teperi J, Rimpela M 1989 Menstrual pain, health and behaviour in girls. Social Science and Medicine 29: 163–169

Thompson E N 1997 Back pain: bankrupt expertise and new directions. Pain Research & Management 2: 195–196

Turk D C, Okifuji A 1999 Does sex make a difference in the prescription of treatments and the adaptation to chronic pain by cancer and non-cancer patients? Pain 82: 139–148

Turner J A, Clancy S 1986 Strategies for coping with chronic low back pain. Relationship to pain and disability. Pain 24: 355–362

Unruh A M 1992 Voices from the past: ancient views of pain in childhood. Clinical Journal of Pain 8: 247–254

Unruh A M 1996a Gender variations in clinical pain experience. Pain 65: 123–167

Unruh A M 1996b The influence of gender on appraisal of pain and pain coping strategies. Interdisciplinary PhD Thesis. Dalhousie University, Halifax, Nova Scotia

Unruh A M 1997 Why can't a woman be more like a man? Behavioral and Brain Sciences 20: 467–468

Unruh A M, Campbell M A 1999 Gender variation in children's pain experience. In: McGrath P J, Finley G A (eds) Chronic and recurrent pain in children and adolescents. Progress in Pain Research and Management, Vol. 13: 199–241

Unruh A M, McGrath P J 2000 Pain in children: psychosocial issues. In: Melvin J, Wright F V (eds) Rheumatological Rehabilitation, Vol. III

Unruh A M, Ritchie J A 1998 Development of the Pain Appraisal Inventory: psychometric properties. Pain Research and Management 3: 105–110

Unruh A M, McGrath P J, Cunningham S J, Humphreys P 1983 Children's drawings of their pain. Pain 17: 385–392

Unruh A M, Ritchie J A, Merskey H 1999 Does gender affect appraisal of pain and pain coping strategies? Clinical Journal of Pain 15: 31–40

Vienneau T L, Clark A J, Lynch M E, Sullivan M J L 1999 Catastrophizing, functional disability, and pain reports in adults with chronic low back pain. Pain Research & Management 4: 93–96

von Baeyer C L 1997 Presence of parents during painful procedures. Pediatric Pain Letter 1: 56–59

von Baeyer C L, Baskerville S, McGrath P J 1998 Everyday pain in three-to-five-year-old children in day care. Pain Research and Management 3: 111–116

Waldrop R D, Mandry C 1995 Health professionals perceptions of opioid dependence among patients with pain. American Journal of Emergency Medicine 13: 529–531

Warnell P 1991 The pain experience of a multiple sclerosis population: a descriptive study. Axon 26–28

Weisenberg M, Kreindler M L, Schachat R, Werboff J 1975 Pain anxiety and attitudes in Black, White and Puerto Rican patients. Psychosomatic Medicine 37: 123–135

Woodrow K M, Friedman G D, Siegelaub A B, Collen M F 1972 Pain tolerance: differences according to age, sex, and race. Psychosomatic Medicine 34: 548–556

Assessing pain

SECTION CONTENTS

7

Pain assessment and measurement

*Jenny Strong   Jennifer Sturgess
Anita M. Unruh   Bill Vicenzino*

OVERVIEW

In earlier chapters, we discussed the multifaceted and all-encompassing experience of pain. It is not enough to ask, 'How intense is your pain on a 0–10 scale?' A therapist must carefully assess the multidimensional aspects of the pain phenomenon to develop a comprehensive programme with the patient. In this chapter, we will provide the beginning pain therapist with knowledge about pain assessment and measurement.

An overview of models and methods of assessing and measuring pain will be given. Broad, interdisciplinary models of pain assessment will be described, as well as profession or discipline-specific models. In particular, the occupational therapy model of occupational performance will be used as a guide to assessment by the occupational therapist, and the acute pain and orthopaedic models will be used to guide assessment by the physiotherapist. The interrelated but distinct categories of impairment, disability and handicap (as expressed in the WHO model), or impairment, activity and activity limitation, participation and participation limitation (WHO 1999) and their application to pain measurement will be outlined (see Box 7.1).

Specific tools for measuring aspects of pain will be described. For each measure, utility, reliability and validity will be addressed. As a patient's function is a particular concern for occupational therapists and physiotherapists, the measurement of function will be covered in detail. In conjunction with undertaking pain measurement for treatment, outcome measurement for determining therapy efficacy will also be reviewed. Lastly, we will consider other factors that may influence outcomes in the assessment and measurement of pain.

Learning objectives

At the end of this chapter, students will be able to:

1. Understand the differences between pain assessment and pain measurement.
2. Understand the reasons for evaluating pain in patients.
3. Describe the types of pain evaluation commonly used.
4. Describe some of the most commonly used pain-measurement tools.
5. Understand how assessment of pain needs to vary for different patients.
6. Understand occupational therapy or physiotherapy approaches to pain assessment and measurement.

SOME IMPORTANT ISSUES ON THE MEASUREMENT OF PAIN

There is a plethora of literature about the measurement of pain experience. There are many measurements available and many more are being developed and tested. How does one decide what measures are suitable for a particular setting? There are three important considerations. The measure must have clinical utility. It must be reliable, and it must be a valid measure of that aspect of pain for which it is intended. We will briefly discuss these three considerations before we discuss types of measures, and then measures for each of the three components of pain (description, response, impact).

Box 7.1 Key terms defined

In 1980, the World Health Organization (WHO) published the International Classification of Impairments, Disabilities and Handicaps (ICIDH) to help classify the consequences of injuries and diseases and their implications for people. This taxonomy provides a useful framework for considering the functional difficulties faced by the patient with chronic pain. Harper and his colleagues (1992) utilized the ICIDH to develop a functional taxonomy of impairments, disabilities and handicaps associated with low back pain. In 1999 an updated draft document (ICIDH-2) was published (WHO 1999). The concept of impairment was retained but concepts of disability and handicap were revised as noted in the definitions given below.

Impairment – Impairment is an objective, structural limitation which can be measured with a reasonable degree of accuracy and uniformity (Vasuderan 1989, Waddell & Main 1984, WHO 1980, 1999). It may relate to psychological, anatomical or physiological structures.

Disability or activity limitations – The World Health Organization (1980) defined disability as a restriction or lack of ability to perform an activity in the manner considered normal. The new WHO classification focuses on activity rather than disability. It defines activity as 'the performance of a task or action by an individual' and activity limitations as 'difficulties an individual may have in the performance of activities' (WHO 1999 p 14). Determining disability or activity limitation is complex. Jette's definition cited by Verbrugge (1990) as 'a gap between a person's capability and the environment's demand' is useful for therapists. The definition notes the importance of the need for a fit between the person and

the environment and the need to assess both components to fully understand activity limitations. Disability may be physical mental, or social.

Handicap or participation restrictions – Handicap is the extent to which the impairment and disability impinge on a person's normal vocational and social and family roles (WHO 1980). ICIDH-2 defines participation as 'an individual's involvement in life situations' (WHO 1999 p 14), and participation restrictions as 'problems an individual may have in the manner or extent of involvement in life situations' (WHO 1999 p 14).

Reliability – Reliability is the extent to which a measurement is consistent, that is, it measures the same way each time it is used even if some conditions have varied (the person administering it, the situation).

Validity – Validity is the extent to which a measurement actually measures what it claims to measure.

Function – Function is the output of active life-skills based on precursor physical abilities (e.g. range of motion, strength, grip, gait) and psychosocial abilities (e.g. temperament, self-concept, organizational ability).

Self-efficacy – Self-efficacy is the belief in one's ability to successfully perform particular behaviours which are needed to produce particular outcomes (Bandura 1977, Council et al 1988, Jensen et al 1991, Strong 1995).

Pain behaviours – Pain behaviours are overt manifestations of pain and suffering, such as grimacing, limping, avoiding activity, moaning.

Clinical utility

Clinical practice is often pragmatic or local in style, and may seem not to exactly match the theory on which a measure is based. Often, the primary consideration is that pain measurement must be clinically helpful to the setting in which it will be used. Most therapists find that there is a limit to the available time for assessment and measurement. Clinically useful measurement is therefore parsimonious; short, efficient measurements collecting the maximum, useable information are preferred. For this reason, in order to be comprehensive and parsimonious, it is advisable to aim for only one measurement tool from each of the three dimensions (description of the pain, responses to the pain, impact of pain) unless more measurement is essential.

The usefulness of the measures we incorporate into our practice depends on the quality of their reliability and the validity. Measures about which the reliability and validity is unknown may provide quantitative information, they may be in common usage, and may even be accepted by insurance companies, but they do not provide us with an accurate and confident assessment of the patient's pain experience. We do not really know that they measure what they claim to measure.

Reliability of pain measures

Reliable measures of pain provide consistent results from one time of use to the next. To illustrate, a reliable thermometer will give the same temperature from one hour to the next in a static thermal state. If there is much fluctuation in the temperature readings in the static thermal state, then the thermometer is not reliable. Of course, if circumstances change, such as the patient develops a fever, we would expect a reliable thermometer to measure this change. This property of a measurement tool is termed its responsiveness to change (Guyatt et al 1987). A reliable measure of pain also will provide similar information from one time to the next unless the pain changes (i.e, intrarater reliability). The measure will also give the same results, or very close to the same, if two different therapists administer the measure (i.e. interrater reliability).

Data on the reliability of an instrument may be context-specific. For example, the reliability may have been obtained in a population that may have specific characteristics (i.e. demographic, specific pain conditions or normal), which limits its use to that population. This is an issue that the therapist who is using reliability data of an instrument should take into consideration.

How does the reliability of a pain measure relate to clinical usage for therapists? In selecting the most appropriate assessment or battery of assessments to use for any particular patient, the aim is to balance the need for psychometrically reliable data against the need for a measurement tool which can be administered efficiently. It may be that the most reliable measurement tool is very long and the patient has a short attention span, or requires so many other evaluations that a long one is impractical. In many clinical situations, the time available for completing an assessment is short. The measures that are used need to use time efficiently. The utility of a measurement is also limited by its complexity. In some situations, the most effective way to assess the quality of pain would be the McGill Pain Questionnaire (MPQ) (Melzack 1975), but if the patient speaks little English or any of the languages into which the MPQ has been translated, then a visual analogue scale will be more useful. Jensen et al (1999) have recently shown that a simple, single 0–10 pain intensity rating has sufficient reliability and validity for use with patients with chronic pain, especially in research involving large sample sizes. When working with smaller sample sizes or when wanting to detect changes in pain intensity in individual patients, composites of 0–10 ratings (e.g. current, worst, least and average pain) may be preferable.

Validity of pain measures

A pain measure is valid if the measure truly measures what it is supposed to measure and not something else. Knowing exactly what some pain measures are measuring may be more contentious than one would expect. The Pain Drawing (Parker et al 1995), for instance, may not simply describe areas where patients feel pain of various types. Sometimes anatomically and physiologically impossible distributions of pain are selected. Does the Pain Drawing describe the location of pain or does it measure something else, like psychological distress? In fact, it has been proposed that scoring systems for the pain drawing may be used to assess psychological distress, but efforts to do this have met with equivocal success (Parker et al 1995). Unusual drawings may convey psychological distress but they may also mean an unusual pain distribution.

When a measure is being developed, we worry first about the content validity of the measure but overall if the measure is not reliable then it cannot be valid. A measure that provides inconsistent outcomes is giving information about something other than what it is intending to measure.

Types of pain measures

The distinction between categories of pain measures and their strengths and limitations will be assisted by completion of the Reflective exercise 7.1.

Self-report

As suggested in the Reflective exercise, there are three types of pain measures: self-report measures, observational measures, and physiological measures (see Box 7.2). The first type is 'self-report'. The person with the pain provides the information to complete the measure about the pain. Self-report measures are used in many ways. They often involve rating pain on some kind of metric scale. A therapist might ask the patient to rate the worst pain, the least pain, and the average pain in the past week. Diaries are another way to gain a prospective, subjective view of a patient's pain if the pain is persistent or chronic. It is a helpful way to measure the impact of the pain on the patient's life. Diaries can be relatively structured with the necessary information to record prepared in a format that is completed at regular intervals. Ratings of pain intensity, levels of rest and activity, and current mood and emotional or affective states can also be recorded.

Self-report is considered the gold standard of pain measurement because it is consistent with the definition of pain. Pain is a subjective experience. But, the dilemma of self-report measures is exactly that subjective nature. They are based on the patient's perception

---

Box 7.2   Types of pain measures

1. Self-report measures (e.g scales, drawings, questionnaires, diaries)
2. Observational measures (e.g. measure of behaviour, function, range of motion)
3. Physiological measures (e.g. heart rate, pulse)

---

of her or his pain and that perception may be influenced by other factors. To illustrate, the rating that you give about the severity of your migraine in Reflective exercise 7.1 is useful only to the extent that the therapist believes that you have given an honest response.

There has been controversy about the validity of self-report data; some work has shown the level of pain reported by patients with chronic pain was unrelated to their self-report of physical disability (Patrick & D'Eon 1996). The dilemma here is that we intuitively expect that the extent of disability should be proportionately related to the severity of the pain. When they are not related in this way, we are inclined to argue that the patient's self-report of pain intensity is exaggerated and invalid. This may be so, but actual physical performance and perceived level of physical performance may be two entirely different constructs, each of which is valid clinical information about a patient with chronic pain. Lastly, self-report measures rely on the person's ability to communicate about pain. Self-report is not possible for infants, young children, or people with special needs that impair communication.

Observational measures

Observational measures are another method of pain measurement. Observational measures usually rely on a therapist, or someone well known to the patient, completing an observational measure of some aspect of pain experience, usually related to behaviour or activity performance. Observational measures can be useful to corroborate the self-reports given by the patient. They are also very useful to identify other areas of concern, particularly measurement of function and ergonomic factors that may exacerbate or cause work-related pain.

The subjective components may help in determining which type of treatment programme is most appropriate for which type of patient with pain (Strong et al 1994). Nevertheless, observational measures may be relatively expensive as a technique since they require observation time. They may also be less sensitive to

---

Reflective exercise 7.1

Imagine that you have a severe migraine. Your roommate has never had migraines. She observes that you are listening to some quiet music while you are trying a relaxation strategy on your bed. Suppose that we want to measure how bad your migraine might be. We could ask you.

- What factors might influence the rating that you give?

Another alternative would be to ask your roommate to complete an observational pain measure.

- How accurate do you think her measurement of your pain would be?

A third way might be to record your pulse or rate of breathing.

- Do you think these measures would tell us anything about the severity of your migraine?

the subjective and affective components of the pain experience.

In research, observational measures have been shown to be most accurate for acute pain since pain behaviour tends to habituate as pain becomes more chronic (McGrath & Unruh 1999). There is also no behaviour that is an indicator of pain and nothing else. Clutching the abdomen may be due to pain but it might also be a spasm of nausea. To know what the behaviour signifies one may need to ask the person and that is back to self-report.

Lastly, observational measures appear to be a more objective measure of the patient's pain but they do reflect the therapist's objective *and* subjective measurement of the patient's pain. The roommate's observational measurement of your migraine in Reflective exercise 7.1 may be affected by her or his inexperience with migraines and the observation that you are lying down and appear to be relaxing.

Physiological measures

The third category of pain measurement is physiological. Pain can cause biological changes in heart rate, respiration, sweating, muscle tension and other changes associated with a stress response (Turk & Okifuji 1999). These biological changes can be used as an indirect measure of acute pain, but biological response to acute pain may stabilize over time as the body attempts to recover its homeostasis. For example, your breathing or heart rate may have shown some small change at the outset of your migraine if the onset was relatively sudden and severe, but over time these changes were likely to return to before migraine rates even though your migraine persists. Physiological measures are useful in situations where observational measures are more difficult. For example, observational measures can be used to measure pain in infants but physiological measures have provided important information about post-surgical pain in neonates (Anand & McGrath 1999).

In summary, self-report measures are considered the gold standard of pain measurement. After all, only you know how bad that migraine really is. Your roommate's measurement is also useful but her measurement is indirect. It is still very important to note here that all three categories of measures have some degree of error. They provide a part of the picture of the patient's pain experience but they do not have 100% accuracy. In the next sections, we discuss the various measures that can be used to obtain a description of the pain, responses to the pain, and the impact of pain on the person's life.

ASSESSMENT OF PAIN

Assessment of pain before intervention is important to ensure that the therapist and the pain team has a complete picture of the patient's needs and areas of difficulty. Although the words assessment and measurement are related and they are often used interchangeably, their meaning is somewhat different. Assessment is the broader examination of the relationship between different components of the pain experience for a given patient, whereas measurement is the quantification of each component. Sometimes therapists measure components without an assessment framework, with the result that the information gathered may have minimal usefulness in determining whether an intervention programme was useful for the patient. Deciding what to measure depends on the therapist's assessment model and the assessment model depends on the therapist's practice frame of reference.

Assessment of an individual patient's pain and its ramifications on that patient's life is an important task for occupational therapists and physiotherapists. In addition to the frame of reference used by the therapist, the type of assessment used may be influenced by the nature of the treatment facility and the referral request. The therapist needs to remember that there are differing reasons for performing an assessment of a patient's pain status. These different assessment rationales may not be mutually exclusive and may also assume importance at different stages in the patient's time with pain. A patient who is referred to a therapist for a resting splint and will be discharged shortly, to be followed by another therapist in the community, will be assessed differently from another patient who may be seen over many weeks. For many years, occupational therapists have utilized a biopsychosocial model in their pain assessment (e.g. Milne 1983). Physiotherapists on the other hand have tended to rely on a biomedical model. Physiotherapists have recently been urged to utilize a more comprehensive, psychosocial assessment model in their practice (Strong 1999, Watson 1999).

Assessment can be used to help with diagnosis; to assist in defining goals for clinical intervention and management; to help in evaluating the effectiveness of a treatment programme; to provide a picture of a patient's functional ability despite pain; and to provide data for insurance, compensation and pension claims. If assessment of pain is to occur repeatedly for one patient, it is likely to follow the order just listed, that is, it will be for diagnostic (or exploratory) reasons first, and then to help in making treatment goals more precise and relevant.

In chronic pain, the WHO classifications of impairment, disability (activity and activity limitation), and handicap (participation and participation limitation) are particularly important. Assessment of impairment may be judged by pain intensity, disability by self-care, ambulation and endurance deficits, and handicap by deficits in vocational, social or familial roles (Patrick & D'Eon 1996).

As noted previously, a therapist will usually assess a patient's pain using the most appropriate model or frame of reference for the situation. The frame of reference focuses the assessment and in turn determines what questions must be answered through measurement. In many cases a purely biomedical approach to pain assessment may be insufficient (Vlaeyen et al 1995), because it will focus on biological measurement and exclude other psychological and environmental factors. A biopsychosocial model is often advocated (Turk 1996). This model will lead to assessment that considers interaction between biological, psychological and social components in pain experience and will determine exactly what factors within each should be measured.

Several other factors determine which model or frame of reference is most appropriate for pain assessment. These factors include acuteness or chronicity of the pain, provision of intervention as a team member or sole pain therapist, a rehabilitation focus to the service, involvement of compensation, and difficulties that might complicate assessment (such as a cognitive impairment or lack of fluency in the primary language spoken at the service). Psychological, social, and demographic factors have been found to be crucial in influencing the development of chronicity of pain (Polatin & Mayer 1996) and so these areas need to be included in assessment protocols.

It is essential to remember that the information gathered in an assessment of the patient's pain must be used to the best ends. While this may sound self-evident, it is surprisingly common for the purpose of assessment information to be poorly considered. The effect is then to have not enough information, too much information for the context in which it is to be used, or information which is not specific enough to the particular individual. If the information is important as an outcome measure, then it is essential that the measures used at the outset are relevant to the goals of the intervention programme and can be measured again at discharge.

In order to safeguard against these pitfalls and ensure that relevant and adequate information is obtained, the therapist needs to follow the cardinal rules of data-gathering with patients:

- Ensure there is some initial time spent to establish a collaborative relationship by getting to know the person and her or his individual situation.
- Where possible, allow for the patient to expand on formal assessment items, and to elaborate on her or his responses.
- Actively listen to the patient's information, and notice signals which suggest that the patient would like to talk further (e.g. hesitations, rushing over a certain aspect, comments such as 'but you don't need to hear more about that').
- Try to understand the implications for the patient's lifestyle and quality of life as much as possible.
- Remember the information.

Experienced therapists will find in the pain literature a variety of assessment models that can be used to gather information about a patient's pain. For example, Jamison (1996) proposed a model of assessment with seven categories – pain intensity, functional capacity, mood and personality, pain beliefs and coping, medication monitoring, adverse effects and psychosocial history. Woolf and Decosterd (1999) recently advocated an interview-based assessment of the patient's pain which is similar to one previously advocated by physiotherapists (Maitland 1987). It comprises aspects of pain such as:

- Is the pain spontaneous or evoked?
- What is the nature and intensity of the stimulus if the pain is evoked?
- What is the quality of the pain?
- What is the pain distribution?
- Is the pain continuous or intermittent?
- What is the pain intensity?
- A clinical assessment.

Although there are important distinctions between different assessment models, in general, there are three essential components of pain assessment that will need to be considered for most patients with pain. These components are: description of the pain, responses to the pain, impact of pain on the person's life.

In the next section, we will examine the various measures which can be used for each of these three components. Each component has a range of sub-categories and for each sub-category there are usually a number of measurement tools or styles of measurement available. Many of these measures are summarized in the Tables which are included in this chapter.

Measurement of the description of the pain

Measures which describe pain are usually self-report in style. They are typically in the form of questionnaires, rating scales, visual analogue scales and drawings. Pain can be described in terms of its intensity (i.e. how much pain), its quality (e.g. if it is burning, aching, dull, sharp, etc), and its location on the body.

In gathering a description of the pain from a patient, several purposes are served. A baseline description of the pain allows for comparison of changes. Ideally, pain should be monitored for some time before treatment commences, and then during treatment and at the end of treatment. The brief scales, such as the numerical rating scale, have been used daily for up to 2 weeks in chronic pain programmes and the results averaged to increase the reliability of the assessment. Although this amount of assessment will provide a baseline to truly compare to changes following intervention, it is rather more than is achievable or desirable in most clinical contexts. There is considerable evidence that self-report of pain intensity is both reliable and valid (Jamison 1996).

Numeric scales

The numeric rating scale is the most popular, but visual analogue and verbal rating scales are also well used (Jamison 1996). In a study to examine the validity of a number of commonly used measures of pain intensity, the 11-point box scale emerged as the most valid compared to a linear model of pain (Jensen et al 1989). The box scale was also accurate to score. However, this study was of patients with postoperative (i.e. acute) pain. Earlier research had suggested that the numerical rating scale was best for use with chronic pain patients (Jensen et al 1986). Strong et al (1991) also found the box scale to be one of two preferred pain intensity measures for use with patients with chronic low back pain, along with the visual analogue scale in a horizontal orientation. A number of assessments for use in gathering a description of the patient's pain are listed in Table 7.1, while Figure 7.1 illustrates some of these pain intensity measures.

Visual analogue scales

Visual analogue scales are simply a 10-cm line with 'stops' or 'anchors' at each end. The line may be horizontal or vertical. The patient is asked to mark the line at a point corresponding to the severity of his/her pain. End-point descriptors are 'none' and 'severe' or similar phrases. Visual analogue scales (VAS) have been said to be sensitive, simple, reproducible and universal (i.e. can be understood in many situations where there are cultural or language differences to the assessor) (Huskisson 1983).

In a recent study it was shown that a mark above 3 cm on a 10-cm scale would include 85% of patients who had rated their pain as moderate on a four-point categorical scale, and 98% of patients who reported severe pain (Collins et al 1997). While this means a rating above 3 cm is going to be fairly reliable at including patients with severe pain, it will also include patients with pain that is moderate or less. This finding highlights the fact that, while the VAS may usefully compare a patient to themselves over time, it is less reliable to compare individuals to each other.

Table 7.1 Commonly used pain evaluations for describing pain

Assessment	Style	Psychometric status	Utility
Visual Analogue Scales including vertical, horizontal and numbered scales	Self report – there are a number of types, eg vertical,horizontal, plastic thermometer style	The accuracy of scoring on the 10-cm line is often questionable	Measure pain intensity Quick, able to be repeated regularly, and do not require complex language Useful in cancer pain
McGill Pain Questionnaire (MPQ) Also has short form (MPQ- SF)	Self-report 20 sets of adjectives to select one in each relevant category Short-form has 15-item adjective checklist and two scales for pain intensity	Total score and dimension scores Well-established reliability and validity Some problems with difficulty level of words used	Measures quality of pain – three dimensions affective, evaluative, sensory Widely used in clinical research
Pain Drawing (various protocols)	Self-report by drawing areas and types of pain with symbols on front and back outlines of the human body	Rating scales which have been developed for pain drawings have poor validity	Identifies location of pain perceived by client High face validity for patients

Visual Analogue Scale (Horizontal)

No pain ————————————————————| Pain as bad
as it could be

Numeric Rating Scale

Please indicate on the line below the number between
0 and 100 that best describes your pain.
A zero (0) would mean 'no pain' and a one hundred (100)
would mean 'pain as bad as it could be'.

Please write only one number. _____

Box Scale

If a zero means 'no pain', and a ten (10) means 'pain as bad as it
could be', on this scale of 0Ð10,what is your level of pain?
Put an 'X' through that number.

0	1	2	3	4	5	6	7	8	9	10

Verbal Rating Scale

( ) No pain
( ) Some pain
( ) Considerable pain
( ) Pain which could not be more severe

Behavioural Rating Scale

( ) No pain
( ) Pain present, but can easily be ignored
( ) Pain present, cannot be ignored, but does not interfere with everyday activities
( ) Pain present, cannot be ignored, interferes with concentration
( ) Pain present, cannot be ignored, interferes with all tasks except taking care of
basic needs such as toileting and eating
( ) Pain present, cannot be ignored, rest or bedrest required

Figure 7.1 Pain intensity measures.

The VAS line may be horizontal or vertical, however clinical evidence is often that the horizontal version is preferred. Patients with back pain have been known to misinterpret a vertical line as their spine and then place a mark on the line to describe the location of their pain, rather than to indicate its intensity.

There are variations of the VAS currently being used, such as the Visual Analogue Thermometer (Choinière & Amsel 1996) and the Pain-O-Meter (Gaston-Johansson 1996). These are somewhat more sophisticated plastic instruments designed to reduce some of the measurement error which can occur with the VAS if copies are used. If the line is not exactly 10 cm long, then the reliability of the measured score is questionable. In other variations of the VAS, the length of the line has been varied, and the descriptors have been altered so that the construct measured is pain sensation or pain affect (Price & Harkins 1987).

The VAS and similar instruments are useful in the measurement of cancer pain, because of their brevity. Measurement of cancer pain needs to be brief because tolerance of lengthy assessment may be poor in very ill people (Ahles et al 1984). The pain may change frequently requiring measurement to be frequent. Therefore a measurement which is quick to administer but remains reliable over many times is desirable.

The pain drawing

The pain drawing has been used as a simple way to gain a graphic representation of where the patient feels pain. While this may sound like a straightforward procedure, two important aspects of the pain drawing may differ widely from setting to setting: the instructions on how to complete the pain drawing, and the scoring (if any) and interpretation of the pain drawing. A pain drawing consists of outline drawings of the human body, front and back, on which the patient indicates where the pain is by shading the painful area (Margolis et al 1986), or by indicating the type of pain (e.g. pins and needles, aching) by symbols (Ransford et al 1976). Margolis et al (1986, 1988) developed a scoring system based upon the total body area in pain (see Fig. 7.2 for Margolis pain drawing and scoring system).

Ransford et al (1976) developed a detailed scoring system to screen for psychological disorders, whereby a patient's graphic representation of their pain which is physiologically impossible may indicate problems. As a result of this feature, various methods of scoring or rating pain drawings in order to suggest level of psychological distress have been attempted (Ransford et al 1976, Parker et al 1995). These rating scales have poor reliability. However, used without a scoring system, the pain drawing can be a useful tool to assist in clinical reasoning, giving as it does useful information about the location and distribution of the patient's pain. *bt have already*

McGill Pain Questionnaire

The McGill Pain Questionnaire (MPQ) (Melzack 1975) includes a numerical intensity scale, a set of descriptor words and a pain drawing. Patients are asked to indicate, from 20 groups of adjectives, descriptors of their present pain. Patients are restricted to using only one word from each group. These adjectives tap the sensory (categories 1–10), affective (categories 11–15) and evaluative (category 16) dimensions of a person's pain.

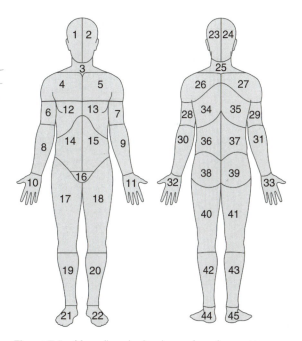

Figure 7.2 Margolis pain drawing and scoring system. The body was divided into 45 areas. A score of 1 was assigned if the patient indicated that pain was present and a score of 0 if pain was absent, for each area. Weights were assigned to each area equal to the percentage of body surface they covered. Reprinted from Pain 24, Margolis et al, pp. 57–65. © 1986, with permission from Elsevier Science.

A miscellaneous class (categories 17–20) of words was also described. Quantitative scores which can be derived from the MPQ are the 'number of words chosen', the 'pain rating index total', the 'pain rating index sensory', the 'pain rating index affective' and the 'pain rating index evaluative'. The MPQ is multidimensional, but its focus is still pain description. It is probably the most widely used pain evaluation measure. More recently, Melzack (1987) developed the short-form MPQ. The original MPQ adjectives and the short-form MPQ are illustrated in Figures 7.3 and 7.4.

While many researchers have utilized the MPQ in a highly quantitative way (for example, Lowe et al 1991, Strong et al 1989), its primary value for clinicians is to identify qualitative features of a person's pain experience, and to detect less than dramatic, more subtle clinical changes. From the words chosen, the therapist can also get an idea of unexpected features of a person's pain. For example, if a patient endorsed the adjective 'cold' as a descriptor of their low back pain, this would be unusual. Alternatively, for a patient with

Name: _____ Date: _____

What does your pain feel like?

Some of the words I will read to you describe your **present** pain. Tell me which
words best describe it. Leave out any word group that is not suitable.
Use only a single word in each appropriate group Ð the one that applies **best**.

1	2	3	4
1 Flickering	1 Jumping	1 Pricking	1 Sharp
2 Quivering	2 Flashing	2 Boring	2 Cutting
3 Pulsing	3 Shooting	3 Drilling	3 Lacerating
4 Throbbing		4 Stabbing	
5 Beating		5 Lancinating	
6 Pounding			

5	6	7	8
1 Pinching	1 Tugging	1 Hot	1 Tingling
2 Pressing	2 Pulling	2 Burning	2 Itchy
3 Gnawing	3 Wrenching	3 Scalding	3 Smarting
4 Cramping		4 Searing	4 Stinging
5 Crushing			

9	10	11	12
1 Dull	1 Tender	1 Tiring	1 Sickening
2 Sore	2 Taut	2 Exhausting	2 Suffocating
3 Hurting	3 Rasping		
4 Aching	4 Splitting		
5 Heavy			

13	14	15	16
1 Fearful	1 Punishing	1 Wretched	1 Annoying
2 Frightful	2 Gruelling	2 Blinding	2 Troublesome
3 Terrifying	3 Cruel		3 Miserable
	4 Vicious		4 Intense
	5 Killing		5 Unbearable

17	18	19	20
1 Spreading	1 Tight	1 Cool	1 Nagging
2 Radiating	2 Numb	2 Cold	2 Nauseating
3 Penetrating	3 Drawing	3 Freezing	3 Agonizing
4 Piercing	4 Squeezing		4 Dreadful
	5 Tearing		5 Torturing

Figure 7.3   The McGill pain questionnaire adjectives (from Melzack 1975, with kind permission from Professor R Melzack).

phantom limb pain to endorse the words stabbing, burning and constant is entirely expected. Jerome and his colleagues (1988) also suggest that attention be given to the specific words chosen by patients on the MPQ rather than concentrating on the total scores obtained. The reliability and validity of the MPQ are well established and were reviewed in Melzack and Katz (1994).

Comprehensive measurement of pain description, using several methods, allows the patient to feel they

Short-Form McGill Pain Questionnaire Ronald Melzack

Patient's name: _____   Date: _____

		None	Mild	Moderate	Severe
1	Throbbing	0) __	1) __	2) __	3) __
2	Shooting	0) __	1) __	2) __	3) __
3	Stabbing	0) __	1) __	2) __	3) __
4	Sharp	0) __	1) __	2) __	3) __
5	Cramping	0) __	1) __	2) __	3) __
6	Gnawing	0) __	1) __	2) __	3) __
7	Hot-burning	0) __	1) __	2) __	3) __
8	Aching	0) __	1) __	2) __	3) __
9	Heavy	0) __	1) __	2) __	3) __
10	Tender	0) __	1) __	2) __	3) __
11	Splitting	0) __	1) __	2) __	3) __
12	Tiring-exhausting	0) __	1) __	2) __	3) __
13	Sickening	0) __	1) __	2) __	3) __
14	Fearful	0) __	1) __	2) __	3) __
15	Punishing-cruel	0) __	1) __	2) __	3) __

VAS   No pain |—————————————| Worst possible pain

PPI

0	No pain	__
1	Mild	__
2	Discomforting	__
3	Distressing	__
4	Horrible	__
5	Excruciating	__

Figure 7.4   The short-form McGill pain questionnaire adjectives (from Melzack 1987, with kind permission from Professor R Melzack).

have fully communicated the way their pain feels to them, and so contributes to them feeling understood. A thorough evaluation can be valuable in the establishment of the therapeutic relationship. As a note of caution, there is a fine line to be negotiated between the patient feeling well-understood and feeling over-assessed and intruded upon. For this reason, measurement tools which are relatively brief yet efficient are often most suitable.

Measurement of responses to pain

A person's response to pain is very personal, based on physiology, personality, previous life experiences, family and culture. How someone responds to pain is often demonstrated by behavioural and psychological reactions or changes, and it is these features which therapists need to understand (Flaherty 1996). Therefore, aspects such as depression and illness behaviour are valuable components of a comprehensive pain assessment. Table 7.2 lists some of the available measures in this domain.

There is some evidence that a person's fears or beliefs about the source of their pain or possibility of re-injury can influence their responses to pain and their course of recovery (Main & Watson 1996). Fear-avoidance beliefs probably arise from the patient's experience of physical activity and pain, but can be altered by cognitive and affective factors (Waddell et al 1993). In an effort to completely understand the patient's perspective, and to understand what influ-

Table 7.2 Commonly used evaluations for pain responses

Assessment	Style	Psychometric status	Utility
Fear-avoidance beliefs questionnaire	Self-report 16 items on a single page	Only the initial study so far, however this showed good test-retest reliability, and a relatively stable 2-factor structure	To measure fear-avoidance beliefs about work and physical activity, specifically for patients with low back pain
Movement and pain predictions cale (MAPPS)	10 items on a 10-point rating scale with sequential drawings of particular movements	Correlations between 7 of the self-efficacy responses and actual movement	Assesses self-efficacy expectations, pain response expectancies and the reason for not completing a movement
Survey of Pain Attitudes-Revised (SOPA-R)	Self-report (57 items) 5-point Likert scale	Internal consistency, discriminant validity, construct validity, and factor structure are all adequate	Assesses seven beliefs which may affect long-term adjustment to chronic pain Is of most value for chronic low back pain
The Gauge	Self-report 27 items on a 1–10 point Likert scale	Has shown good internal consistency and test-retest reliability Convergent validity supported	Assesses the person's confidence in their ability to do a range of basic activities at home, without help
Illness Behaviour Questionnaire			Seven scales to assess abnormal illness behaviour in chronic pain and other conditions where the patient's response may appear discrepant to the physical pathology. This is widely used
Coping Strategies Questionnaire	Self-report		To determine the use of cognitive and behavioural coping strategies used to deal with pain This is widely used
Pain Beliefs and Perceptions Inventory	Self-report Has 16 items	Some debate about whether it has 3 or 4 valid sub-scales	This tool has some usage, but not as broadly as the SOPA-R
Pain Self-Efficacy Questionnaire (PSEQ)	Self-report on a 10-item questionnaire, using a 7-point scale	Internal consistency and test-retest reliability acceptable	Developed specifically for chronic pain
		Support for construct and concurrent validity	To rate confidence in performing activities despite pain

ences their behaviour, some of these attitudes and beliefs need to be evaluated (Strong et al 1992).

There are two measures of fears or beliefs about pain that have good reliability and validity, and may be useful to occupational therapists and physiotherapists. The Survey of Pain Attitudes (Revised) (SOPA-R) (Jensen & Karoly 1991, Jensen et al 1987), in its most recent version, assesses seven beliefs which possibly influence long-term adjustment for people with chronic

pain. The subscales of the SOPA-R measure the extent to which patients believe they can control their pain: they are disabled by their pain, they are damaging themselves and should avoid exercise, their emotions affect their pain experience, medications are appropriate, others, especially family, should be solicitous, and there is a medical cure for their problem (Jensen & Karoly 1991). More recently, a further revision has been made of the SOPA-R, to provide a shorter version for clinical use: the SOPA-B (brief) (Tait & Chibnall 1997). This 30-item version of the SOPA assesses the subscales of solicitude, emotionality, cure, control, harm, disability and medication.

Another tool, the Pain Beliefs and Perceptions Inventory (PBPI), examines patients' beliefs on the stability of pain over time, to what extent they see pain as a mystery, and how much they are to blame for their pain (Williams & Thorn 1989). More recent work with the PBPI has supported the existence of four rather than three scales across a number of patient groups (Herda et al 1994, Morley & Wilkinson 1995, Williams et al 1994). Using the four-scaled version of the PBPI may provide a simple yet clinically useful gauge of the patient's beliefs about pain as mystery, self-blame, pain permanence and pain constancy (Williams et al 1994). A scoring key and some normative data are contained as appendices in the article by Williams et al (1994). Both the SOPA-R and the PBPI have strengths, however the psychometric properties of the SOPA-R are stronger, and it may be useful for a broader range of patients than the PBPI (Strong et al 1992).

Another important concept that is related to beliefs is pain appraisal. Not all pains worry people. Some pains such as sports-related pains are appraised as challenging. Other pains, such as pain from a burn, are appraised as highly threatening because they cause obvious harm. Still other pains such as childbirth may be appraised as highly threatening because of the pain severity, but also as highly challenging because labour is usually perceived as normal and produces a child. The Pain Appraisal Inventory (Unruh & Ritchie 1998) is a measure of threat and challenge appraisal. The measure is applicable to many types of pain and has strong evidence of reliability and validity.

Related to attitudes and beliefs about pain is the concept of self-efficacy, or sense of confidence about ability to do certain activities. A self-efficacy expectation, combined with an outcome expectation (i.e. the belief that a particular behaviour will result in a certain outcome) may influence a person's avoidance of, or participation in, an activity (Bandura 1977). In relation to pain, it has been proposed that self-efficacy beliefs may explain in part the variability between a patient's skill level and their performance outside the treatment setting (Gage & Polatajko 1994, Strong 1995).

Several ways of measuring self-efficacy in relation to pain have been developed. The most useful are the Movement and Pain Prediction Scale (MAPPS) (Council et al 1988), the Pain Self-Efficacy Questionnaire

(PSEQ) (Nicholas 1994) and the Self-Efficacy Gauge (Gage et al 1994).

On the MAPPS, each of 10 simple movements are shown by five sequential drawings of the movement. Patients score how far they think they could go in the movement (self-efficacy), the pain at each stage (pain-response expectancies) and the reason they couldn't complete a movement (Council et al 1988). Seven of the self-efficacy responses significantly correlated with actual movement performance. The PSEQ is a 10-item Likert-type questionnaire, designed specifically for chronic pain, where patients are asked to rate their confidence in performing activities despite pain. It has supportive validity and reliability research (Nicholas 1994). The PSEQ is shown in Figure 7.5. The Self-Efficacy Gauge (Gage et al 1994) is also a questionnaire, with 27 items. Patients rate their degree of confidence to complete certain activities without help. See Figure 7.6 for the Self-Efficacy Gauge. It was developed by an occupational therapist for use with patients with a variety of disorders, including pain conditions, where occupational performance was affected.

A number of assessments are commonly used to measure psychological aspects of a person which may arise from, or help stimulate, certain responses to pain. The Beck Depression Inventory (Beck et al 1961) is widely used to evaluate the level of depression associated with chronic pain. It is considered extremely reliable for both clinical and research use. Its use however is restricted, and so is not useful for occupational and physical therapists, although therapists need to understand its value and the information it provides about patients.

The Minnesota Multiphasic Personality Inventory (MMPI) (Hathaway & McKinley 1942) has also been used to gain a picture of the personality profile of the patient with chronic pain. Different profiles have been associated with different patterns of pain responses (Keefe 1982). Chronic pain patients may exhibit certain personality traits, but they are rarely significantly psychopathological, therefore tests such as the Rorschach (which can tease out personality structure) are usually not appropriate. Measures of 'reactive emotional stress' are more suitable (Jamison 1996). The MMPI is never used by physiotherapists or occupational therapists, but may be a component of the complete pain assessment battery used by the team. Main et al (1991) and Main and Spanswick (1995a) have suggested that there exist other more focused measures to assess psychological functioning and responses to pain than the MMPI. For example, Etscheidt et al (1995) have shown that the West-Haven Yale Multidimensional Pain

Name: ———————————————— Date: ————————————————

Please rate how **confident** you are that you can do the following things **at present** despite the pain. To indicate your answer circle one of the numbers on the scale under each item, where 0 = not at all confident and 6 = completely confident.
For example:

Not at all confident   0   1   2   ③   4   5   6   Completely confident

Remember, this questionnaire is not asking whether or not you have been doing these things, but rather how confident you can do them at present, **despite the pain.**

1. I can enjoy things, despite the pain

    Not at all confident   0   1   2   3   4   5   6   Completely confident

2. I can do most of the household chores (e.g. tidying up, washing dishes, etc.) despite the pain.

    Not at all confident   0   1   2   3   4   5   6   Completely confident

3. I can socialise with my friends or family members as often as I used to do, despite the pain.

    Not at all confident   0   1   2   3   4   5   6   Completely confident

4. I can cope with my pain in most situations.

    Not at all confident   0   1   2   3   4   5   6   Completely confident

5. I can do some form of work, despite the pain.
    (Work includes housework, paid and unpaid work.)

    Not at all confident   0   1   2   3   4   5   6   Completely confident

6. I can still do many of the things I enjoy doing, such as hobbies or leisure activity, despite the pain.

    Not at all confident   0   1   2   3   4   5   6   Completely confident

7. I can cope with my pain without medication.

    Not at all confident   0   1   2   3   4   5   6   Completely confident

8. I can still accomplish most of my goals in life, despite the pain.

    Not at all confident   0   1   2   3   4   5   6   Completely confident

9. I can live a normal lifestyle, despite the pain.

    Not at all confident   0   1   2   3   4   5   6   Completely confident

10. I can gradually become more active, despite the pain.

    Not at all confident   0   1   2   3   4   5   6   Completely confident

Figure 7.5 Pain self-efficacy questionnaire (from Dr. Michael Nicholas, Pain Management Centre, St. Thomas' Hospital, London, with kind permission).

I'd like to know whether you can do everyday activities without the help of another person. It is **okay** if you carry out an activity with the use of something such as a cane or a wheelchair. Please read each question carefully. Circle the number that is closest to your level of confidence (sureness) that you can do the activity. 1 means that you are not at all confident (sure) that you can do the activity without the help of someone else. 10 means that you are completely confident (sure) that you can do the activity without the help of another person.
While it is important for us to know the answer to as many questions as possible please feel free to skip a question if answering it would make you feel uncomfortable.

How confident (sure) am I that I can:	Not at all confident (sure)								Completely confident (sure)	
1. Walk one block?	1	2	3	4	5	6	7	8	9	10
2. Write?	1	2	3	4	5	6	7	8	9	10
3. Feed myself?	1	2	3	4	5	6	7	8	9	10
4. Look after my family?	1	2	3	4	5	6	7	8	9	10
5. Wash myself?	1	2	3	4	5	6	7	8	9	10
6. Climb a flight of stairs?	1	2	3	4	5	6	7	8	9	10
7. Remember the things that I need to remember?	1	2	3	4	5	6	7	8	9	10
8. Get to the bathroom in time?	1	2	3	4	5	6	7	8	9	10
9. Concentrate on something difficult?	1	2	3	4	5	6	7	8	9	10
10. Walk up or down a hill?	1	2	3	4	5	6	7	8	9	10
11. Stand for 5 minutes?	1	2	3	4	5	6	7	8	9	10
12. Dress myself?	1	2	3	4	5	6	7	8	9	10
13. Sign my name?	1	2	3	4	5	6	7	8	9	10
14. Drink from a cup?	1	2	3	4	5	6	7	8	9	10
15. Do the things I like to do?	1	2	3	4	5	6	7	8	9	10
16. Enjoy myself?	1	2	3	4	5	6	7	8	9	10
17. Make my needs known to others?	1	2	3	4	5	6	7	8	9	10
18. Get out of bed?	1	2	3	4	5	6	7	8	9	10
19. Make it through the day without a nap?	1	2	3	4	5	6	7	8	9	10
20. Do the things I usually do with other people?	1	2	3	4	5	6	7	8	9	10
21. Do my usual share of household jobs?	1	2	3	4	5	6	7	8	9	10
22. Get into a car?	1	2	3	4	5	6	7	8	9	10
23. Move around my home safely?	1	2	3	4	5	6	7	8	9	10
24. Have enough energy to do things I like to do?	1	2	3	4	5	6	7	8	9	10
25. Get into the bathtub?	1	2	3	4	5	6	7	8	9	10
26. Walk one mile?	1	2	3	4	5	6	7	8	9	10
27. Have sex?	1	2	3	4	5	6	7	8	9	10

Figure 7.6   Self-efficacy gauge (from Gage et al 1994, with kind permission).

Inventory can provide information about chronic pain patients who might require further psychological assessment, and it is a much briefer assessment than the MMPI.

The adjustment of the patient with chronic pain, or ability to manage with pain, may be measured using such measures as the Coping Strategies Questionnaire (Rosenstiel & Keefe 1983, Robinson et al 1997b) or the Illness Behaviour Questionnaire (IBQ) (Pilowsky & Spence 1983). These measures concern cognitive and behavioural coping strategies that patients can use to help them manage their pain. Both positive and negative adjustment strategies are covered. For example, two strategies assessed in the Coping Strategies Questionnaire are diverting attention and catastrophizing. The Pain Catastrophizing Scale (Sullivan et al 1995) measures catastrophizing in more depth and may be particularly useful to gain more information about coping, for patients who are having substantial difficulty managing pain. Catastrophizing is linked with disability and depression. At present it is unknown whether catastrophizing can be changed to more positive coping. However, positive coping strategies are unlikely to be effective in improving coping with chronic pain without support of a coping-skills training program (Rosenstiel & Keefe 1983). The case example in Box 7.3 illustrates the coping strategies a patient with low back pain following a work injury may exhibit.

Recently, the clear demonstration of bias effects in some of these self-report measures has called into question their reliability when used in cases where over-reporting of poor adjustment may affect financial decisions (Robinson et al 1997a). The same study highlighted the difficulty for clinicians and researchers in interpreting results when many of these self-report scales used for chronic pain have no in-built mechanisms for identifying faking or social desirability responses. However, there is potential clinical value in having illness behaviour defined by the presence of psychological symptoms rather than the absence of physical symptoms (Main & Spanswick 1995b). Main and Spanswick (1995b) have also reported that the Illness Behaviour Questionnaire may differentiate neurosis from conscious exaggeration.

Clinical observation of responses to pain are also valid methods of assessment. These are typically taken while the patient is involved in assessment or treatment activities. Pain behaviours which may have been initiated by nociception may persist long after the time of healing, due to positive consequences of these behaviours (Keefe & Dolan 1986). Fordyce (1976) has described pain behaviours as comprising both verbal

---

Box 7.3   Case example

Mr B was a 52-year-old man who had had a work injury when he fell 5 feet from a ladder in the storeroom and landed on the concrete floor below. He immediately went home to bed, the next day visiting his GP and reporting that he was in agony. Plain X-rays revealed no significant findings, and his GP prescribed him bed-rest and regular panadol. Two weeks later he was still unable to work, and the GP sent him to a physiotherapist. Had he been asked to complete the Coping Strategies Questionnaire, his results on the Coping Strategies Questionnaire at this stage might look like:

- Diverting attention from his pain: 4/36
- Reinterpreting pain sensations: 0/36
- Catastrophizing: 28/36
- Ignoring pain sensations: 0/36
- Praying/hoping: 14/36
- Coping self-statements: 8/36
- Using behavioural coping: 8/36.

Such a profile is not inconsistent in an acute-injury pain situation, where the anticipated outcome is pain resolution. The pain can seem an awful, overwhelming thing, but the person will have faith in the doctor or physiotherapist to give pain relief and cure the pain. At this stage, it would be highly unlikely that the patient would be diverting attention from his pain problem. Should the pain continue unresolved, and the individual be one of the 10% of the population to develop a chronic pain problem, the persistence of coping strategies as endorsed above may make rehabilitation difficult.

---

and nonverbal methods of communication. They include such behaviours as grimacing, moaning, bracing, total body stiffness and verbal complaints (Fordyce 1976). All formal assessment is supplemented by clinical observation and to a certain extent interpretation is based on experience. The aim is to establish a realistic level of distress, which may not be simply related to numbers of obvious pain behaviours. Patients with chronic pain may, unintentionally, use a lot of learned pain behaviours to signal their pain. However, the distress may actually be psychological at the predicament in which they find themselves, rather than a direct function of presently-felt pain. A number of scoring systems can be used, ranging from the original system developed by Keefe and Block (1982) or the Pain Behavior Checklist (Kerns et al 1991).

Keefe and Block (1982) developed a behavioural observation system for use with patients with chronic low back pain. The tool requires the patient to sit, stand, walk, and/or recline for a number of short periods, during which time the patient is videotaped. The videotape is then analysed for the frequency with which the patient uses guarding, bracing, rubbing, grimacing and sighing pain behaviours. Development work with the tool pointed to the validity of this system for measuring a patient's pain. In the clinical setting, more unstructured observations of pain behaviours may be utilized.

Measurement of the impact of pain

Both occupational therapists and physiotherapists have an all-encompassing interest in the patient's best function – whether that is the greatest possible range and strength of high-quality movement, or the ability to manage as large a proportion as possible of the daily tasks that she or he wishes to perform. It follows, therefore, that the third level of pain evaluation commonly carried out is to measure functional status, level of activity, disability and other similar constructs.

A patient's function can be assessed in many different ways. The choice of assessment method will depend on such factors as the age of the patient (an 80-year-old man is unlikely to be assessed for return to work), the extent to which the pain has impacted to date (a patient who was bedridden and is now mobilizing will require a different measure to one who has always been mobile but limited in full range), and whether the assessment is occurring in a hospital, a clinic or home environment. There are eight potentially sequential steps which can be used in part or in full to assess function (Strong et al 1994a):

1. Ask the patient to tell you about their activities.
2. Complete an Activities of Daily Living checklist.
3. Observe performance on tasks.
4. Have the patient complete an activity diary.
5. Staff observe activity level of the patient.
6. Use of an automated measure of activity time.
7. Measurement of physical capacity.
8. A functional capacity evaluation.

There is considerable evidence that a daily activity diary is both reliable and valid when assessing daily activity patterns (e.g. uptime/downtime, pill-taking, mood, pain) for chronic pain patients in their home environment (Follick et al 1984). However, when self-report of uptime (i.e. time spent upright and moving rather than resting) is compared to that of an automated measuring device, there has been a significant under-report of uptime by patients (White & Strong 1992). Abdel-Moty et al (1996) observed that both patients with chronic low back pain and healthy volunteers, when asked to self-predict their ability to stair-climb and squat and then to do the activities,

showed significant under-reporting of their physical abilities. They recommended the use of both self-report and actual functional performance. The authors of this chapter also advocate such a combined approach. Keeping a diary of activity can be useful if a structured recording system is used, and if patients are instructed to make entries relatively frequently throughout the day. Memory factors may impinge on accuracy. Some clinicians feel that such a focus on activities and pain is not particularly helpful. It is, however, a frequent practice in many chronic pain facilities.

A number of measures to ask patients how pain is affecting their lifestyle have been devised. Table 7.3 lists many of these. It may also be measured by the number of activities which are still able to be enacted and enjoyed, which might be measured by something such as the Human Activity Profile (Fix & Daughton 1988). The Oswestry Low Back Pain Disability Questionnaire (ODQ) (Fairbank et al 1980) is one of the most frequently used. There are ten sections in which the patient marks one category which most accurately describes his limitations in sitting, standing, walking, lifting, having sex, socializing, sleeping, doing personal care and travelling. One item gauges pain intensity. A possible score out of 50 is obtained, and this is converted to a percentage (Fairbank et al 1980). Recent review of the ODQ has shown it to have good face validity, and some evidence of factorial and criterion-related validity, and some sensitivity to change (Fisher & Johnston 1997). These features, combined with its brevity, make it a very usable assessment of lifestyle effects for patients with low back pain.

The Sickness Impact Profile (SIP) (Bergner et al 1981) is a questionnaire with 136 items to be self-completed or administered by interview. It was designed to provide a measure of health status that is behaviourally based (Bergner et al 1981). The SIP was designed to be used with various populations, not only those in chronic pain, and is able to demonstrate change in health status over time and between groups. There have been some recent developments in trying to select items for specific use with low back pain patients, and thus create a shorter questionnaire specifically for this population (Stratford et al 1993b).

Disability, as defined earlier in this chapter, is difficult to measure. The Pain Disability Index (PDI) (Tait et al 1987, 1990) is a self-report measure which asks patients to rate how much the pain prevents them from doing, or doing as well as previously, in seven areas of functioning. It measures voluntary (work, social) activities and obligatory (self-care) activities. The PDI is a valid and reliable tool, with a high

Table 7.3 Commonly used evaluations for impact of pain

Assessment	Style	Psychometric status	Utility
Short-Form health survey (SF-36)	Self-report	This has excellent validity and reliability	Designed to measure health status Has eight scales: limitations in physical activities, limitations in social activities, limitations in usual role activities, bodily pain, mental health, limitations in roles due to emotional problems, vitality, general health perceptions
Daily Activity Diary	Self-report	There is some support for reliability and validity of the diary for chronic pain patients at home	Monitors activity type and duration for each hour or 1/2 hour Also monitors pain intensity and medication intake Creates a structured record
Human Activity Profile (HAP)	Self-report, up to 94 items	Included a chronic pain sample in normative sample Norms are provided for different age and gender groups	Can be used to help determine the effect of physical impairment on human daily activity

internal consistency and valid factor structure (Grönblad et al 1993, 1994, Strong et al 1994). It can be used with all types of pain and is quick to administer. Studies are still needed to ascertain its sensitivity to clinical change.

Impact of pain on a person's life can also be assessed by behavioural assessment – by measuring the patient's ability to perform actual tasks which are the same as or related to everyday life tasks. Harding et al (1994), for example, developed a battery of measures for assessing the physical functioning of patients with chronic pain. These types of assessment can be expensive, and have, in the past been relatively unreliable. However, more recent measurements have become more reliable. For example, Harding et al (1994) found that a 5-minute walking test, 1-minute standing-up test, 1-minute stair-climbing test and endurance for holding the arms horizontal test were reliable, valid and useful.

Multidimensional assessment of pain

In keeping with the approaches which stress a holistic view of patients, and of management techniques for pain, there are also some assessments which are multidimensional in nature. These assessments have been designed to gather as much data as possible in the one evaluation, although different professionals may be responsible for actually conducting various parts of the assessment procedure. Such assessments have the advantage of keeping a primary focus on the whole of the patient, rather than medical or therapy sub-specialties.

There are a number of multidimensional pain assessments, each of which is somewhat different in approach and style (see Table 7.4). The most well known is probably the McGill Pain Questionnaire (MPQ), through which the patient quantifies pain in three dimensions – sensory, affective and evaluative. While the MPQ gives a useful breakdown of sensory and affective components of pain, it may not be a true multidimensional assessment. It was reported earlier in this chapter as a tool to measure the description of a person's pain.

The West Haven–Yale Multidimensional Pain Inventory (WHYMPI), or the MPI as it is more commonly known, was developed from a cognitive–behavioural viewpoint to:

Examine the impact of pain on the patients' lives, the responses of others to the patients' communications of pain, and the extent to which patients participate in common daily activities (Kerns et al 1985 p 345).

The three parts to the inventory are nevertheless quite brief to administer, and are psychometrically sound. It contains 12 scales. The MPI is designed to be used with behavioural and psychological assessment strategies. Although it is multidimensional, this is only in relation to the patient's subjective pain experience in a range

Table 7.4   Multidimensional pain evaluations

Assessment	Style	Psychometric status	Utility
Integrated Psychosocial Assessment Model (IPAM)	Self-report	Preliminary support	This is a set of six tools, which in combination evaluate pain intensity, disability, coping strategies, depression, attitudes to pain, and illness behaviour It provides an overall picture of psychosocial adjustment in relation to chronic pain
McGill Pain Questionnaire	Self-report 20 sets of words describing pain experience from which client selects those relevant	Considerable support for basic structure, reliability, and validity	Used to assess the quality of pain in three dimensions: affective, evaluative, sensory
Multidimensional Pain Inventory (WHYMPI)	Self-report 61 items in three scales	This is well tested for reliability and is psychometrically strong Items fall into 12 subscales	Measures interference with activity, social support, pain severity, self-control, negative mood, response of significant others, ability to engage in activities, e.g. chores, social activity
Multiperspective Multidimensional Pain Assessment Protocol (MMPAP)	Physical examinations by two physicians plus client's subjective self-report	Has been shown to be reliable and valid in initial studies Test–retest reliability is acceptable Is a standardized protocol	Used mostly for assessing patients with chronic pain for treatment and to measure outcomes Can predict future employment of disability applicants

of contexts. Clinically, it is useful to gain the patient's view of her or his pain feeling, how supportive their spouse is, and how limited in activity the patient is. The MPI is sensitive to change following treatment.

The Integrated Psychosocial Assessment Model was developed by Strong (1992) for use with chronic pain patients in a clinical setting. It is a relatively new tool, which relates to a model of pain evaluation. Rather than designing a new assessment, Strong has used a complementary range of existing measures, which cover various aspects of the psychosocial experience of pain. This array of measurement tools, which cover pain intensity, pain disability, coping strategies, depression, attitudes to pain and illness behaviour, provides an integrated picture of patients, with similar profiles emerging in both Australia and New Zealand (Strong et al 1995). However, more work on the clinical utility of the assessment model is currently ongoing.

The fourth multidimensional assessment tool is the Multiperspective Multidimensional Pain Assessment Protocol (MMPAP) (Rucker & Metzler 1995). It is a combination of physical examinations by physicians and self-report by the patient with pain. The MMPAP

was designed to be of value for assessing applicants for disability pensions, and has been shown to successfully predict employment status (Rucker & Metzler 1995, Rucker et al 1996). The major domains assessed by the MMPAP are pain dimensions, medical information, mental health status, social support networks, functional limitations and abilities and rehabilitation potential.

Assessment and measurement of pain in patients from special populations

While pain is something which affects individuals in an idiosyncratic way, there are some populations of people with special features as a whole, who must be considered when evaluating pain. Infants and children, older people, and people with cognitive or physical impairments or other special needs often have more difficulty communicating about pain. The difficulty in communicating about pain places these individuals at greater risk for problems in pain management. We examined these issues in Chapter 6, 'Pain across the lifespan', and provided suggestions about assessment and measurement for these special populations.

OCCUPATIONAL THERAPY OVERVIEW

How an occupational therapist works with patients with pain, and specifically how he or she assesses them, will depend on the practice setting. If the occupational therapist is part of a multidisciplinary team, she will contribute a component of the overall picture of the pain. Often this will relate to the patient's performance system, habituation system or volitional system, as described by the model of human occupation (Kielhofner 1995). Guisch (1984) demonstrated an application of the model of human occupation to the patient with chronic pain. In other situations, for example if the therapist is working in a sole practice or in a rural or remote area, then he will not be part of a team dedicated to pain, and therefore will need to build as complete a picture of the patient's pain as possible by his own assessment.

Many of the measures an occupational therapist will use have already been discussed. However, the conceptualization of the results of these measures and the overall assessment will allow the therapist to consider what the patient is able to do (performance system); how these abilities and capacities affect management of roles and aspects of lifestyle which are important to the patient (habituation system); and how interests, goals, attitudes, coping strategies, self-esteem, self-efficacy and affective status impact on managing as rewarding a lifestyle as possible on a day-to-day and longer-term basis (volitional system). Assessments specific to occupational therapists include the Occupational History (Kielhofner et al 1986, Moorehead 1969), the Role Checklist (Oakley 1982, cited in Barris et al 1988), the Activity Diary (Fordyce et al 1984), the Occupational Performance History Interview (Kielhofner et al 1988a, 1988b), and the NPI Interest Checklist (Matsutsuyu 1969). The latter chiefly assesses the volitional subsystem, while the others provide information relevant to the habituation subsystem.

Another occupational therapy measure is the Canadian Occupational Performance Measure (COPM) (Law et al 1998). The COPM in an individualized measure that is used by occupational therapists to detect changes over time in the patient's self-perception of her or his occupational performance in the areas of self-care, productivity and leisure. It can be used in any area of practice, including pain. Research and discussion about the reliability, validity and utility of the COPM is acceptable or better depending on the patient sample, and summarized in the COPM manual. For a complete view of the occupational therapist's role, the reader is referred to the earlier book by Strong (1996).

PHYSIOTHERAPY OVERVIEW

Depending on the situation, physiotherapists are called upon to provide pain-management across a broad spectrum of conditions and special client groups (e.g. cardiothoracic and medical conditions, sports and orthopaedic injuries, neurology, gynaecology, paediatrics and geriatrics). This overview pertains only to pain assessment and measurement in acute musculoskeletal pain and orthopaedic models of physiotherapy practice.

The context in which the therapist is working will determine the extent to which he or she is able or required to perform an assessment and measurement of musculoskeletal pain. In an acute situation in which the injury has just occurred, only an abbreviated assessment is possible. The therapist is required to perform a general scan of body systems to ensure that the condition is isolated to the musculoskeletal system and that there are no other injuries requiring prioritization. The aim is then to identify the structures that have been injured and the extent to which they have been injured. The approach in the therapist's rooms is different in that the physiotherapist is able to perform a more comprehensive assessment of the client's condition. This also allows for the measurement of appropriate aspects of the musculoskeletal pain state.

In the clinical setting, it would be expected that the physiotherapist's evaluation of the client's condition involve an interview and a physical examination. In the interview, the therapist completes a body-chart, which is in essence a mapping of the extent of symptoms (i.e. area of pain). Each symptom is described in terms of its constancy (i.e. is it intermittent or constant), nature (i.e. the client is provided the opportunity to use their descriptors), and the intensity of severity of the symptoms (by using a visual analogue scale). In cases of persistent or chronic pain, the therapist may use an MPQ to further describe the client's pain experience. The factors that aggravate and ease the symptom(s) are also determined. These factors are described in both qualitative and quantitative terms, as they frequently form the basis of outcome measures on which the efficacy of the intervention is gauged.

A history of the current condition is also taken, noting the mechanism of injury, severity of initial symptoms, any treatment and its effects, as well as the progress of the condition since its inception. In addition, the therapist will elucidate the presence of other non-musculoskeletal conditions that may be responsible for the symptoms experienced by the client, requiring referral to the appropriate healthcare practitioner.

Following the interview a physical examination usually takes place. The physical examination can be compartmentalized for description sake into three different sections, the order of their description herein not indicating their order of importance or order in the physical examination. One section usually involves an examination of the symptom-aggravating factor(s) that were elucidated in the interview. During this part of the examination the therapist develops an understanding of the relationship between symptomatology and the aggravating factor(s). The other two sections of the physical examination evaluate and measure the impairments in the musculoskeletal system, as well as developing an understanding of the impact of such impairments on function. An example of some of the measurements of physical impairments and dysfunction have been reported by several authors (Daniel 1988, Jull 2001, Lephart 1991, 1992, Richardson et al 1999, Stratford & Balsor 1994, Stratford et al 1987, 1993a, Wilk et al 1994). The findings of the interview and the preliminary findings of the physical examination itself will guide the extent of the physical examination.

Increasingly, physiotherapists are being encouraged to assess and measure the psychosocial impact of the musculoskeletal condition, especially when involved in the management of complex regional pain syndromes (Simmonds et al 2000). In their management of these chronic pain states, physiotherapists, as a function of their concern and care for the client's wellbeing, take into account psychosocial issues such as altered mood states, education level, anxiety, work dissatisfaction, medicolegal compensation and fear of re-injury or pain.

FACTORS THAT MAY INFLUENCE ASSESSMENT AND MEASUREMENT OUTCOMES

Social desirability

Social desirability is the need to obtain approval by responding in a way which is culturally acceptable, and is recognized as a factor which may affect the quality of information provided by a patient during many types of assessment. Social desirability factors may affect self-report of pain dimensions. Deshields et al (1995) found that patients with chronic pain who are more sensitive to social desirability report less psychological distress, but greater pain, than patients who were less sensitive to social desirability. That is, they seem to respond to a set which says it is acceptable to acknowledge physical pain, but not psychological distress.

Therapists need to be sensitive to the possibility of patients giving answers they see as socially desirable. The development of a good therapeutic relationship with the patient, which promotes honest communication, is invaluable. Being able to let patients know that you can see their strengths and capabilities, despite their physical or psychological distress, will encourage them to report accurately. At the same time, being able to accept that the patient's pain is real and distressing will help minimize the patient's need to exaggerate pain. An overall demeanour from the therapist which suggests that the pain is a real problem, but that there is likely to be a future time when pain will be more manageable and less disabling, may also encourage more hopefulness.

Compensation

There is a tendency to assume that patients who stand to be compensated for their trauma and pain will be less accurate in their self-report of pain and disability, and more extreme in their demonstrated pain behaviours. To what extent compensation complicates pain assessment and intervention is a vexing question, and research in the area has, in the past, produced equivocal results. This important issue was considered more fully in Chapter 4.

Memory problems

Patients with chronic pain often report memory problems, and various reports in the literature support this clinical impression. It has sometimes been assumed that the memory difficulties are related to medication patients may be taking. However, Schnurr and MacDonald (1995) found that memory complaints were not related to medication, and that, even though memory complaints were associated with depression in chronic pain patients, depression was not a full explanation.

In assessing patients' pain profiles it may therefore be worthwhile to keep in mind the possibility of disturbances in memory. Patients may under- or overreport their pain, or be unreliable recorders within a diary. Any memory disturbance can create a feeling of anxiety, and an assessment which is structured to minimize the need for memory will be less anxiety-provoking.

Therapist attitudes

The appraisals and attitudes of the therapist to pain in general, and pain in a particular patient, can be very influential on the quality of therapy provided. Attitudes held by a therapist may be predominantly unconscious, and therefore the therapist will not be aware of acting from a basis which may compromise a patient's treatment. As noted in Chapters 4 and 6, gender, culture, age, etc, may influence the patient's experience of pain; these factors may also impact upon the therapist and their attitudes and behaviours.

It would seem that being female, older of a non-Anglo-Saxon background and/or of a lower socioeconomic class may place a patient at a disadvantage in seeking management of pain, probably because of unconscious attitudes and beliefs held by health professionals. However it is possible, as a therapist, to adapt aspects of your clinical practice to counteract the possibility of unwitting bias. Rainville et al (1995) published a survey of health professionals' attitudes towards people with pain. It is a useful examination of one's own stereotypes and prejudices.

Acknowledging that there can be a problem goes a long way towards reducing the problem. Reviewing your own attitudes will be helpful. This can be achieved by: reflection; considering your personal experience of pain prior to working as a therapist; seeking feedback from a trusted colleague; or establishing guidelines for practice and comparing your performance across different patients. For each patient, the assessment must be thorough and the patient's view considered as the primary source of information. Use of an interpreter, of the appropriate gender if sensitive areas are to be discussed, may be needed. All assessments chosen should be age- and culture-appropriate wherever possible.

CONCLUSION

In this chapter, we discussed the many issues that a physiotherapist or occupational therapist needs to consider in the assessment and measurement of a patient's pain. The underlying premise is that some sort of formal evaluation should be made of the patient's pain. The selection of appropriate measurement tools, while far from an easy task, can be guided by using an assessment model which considers a description of the patient's pain, the responses of that person to the pain, and the impact of the pain on a person's life.

Therapists should choose measures which have acceptable validity and reliability and are manageable in the clinical setting. Therapists need to be attentive to patients, to listen to their words, to observe their behaviours and abilities, and to integrate such information to help with clinical decision-making.

Study questions/questions for revision

1. What dimensions of the patient's pain problem should be measured by the occupational therapist and the physiotherapist?
2. What are the differences between pain assessment and pain measurement?
3. Name one measure of pain quality, and describe the type of data it yields about the patient's pain?
4. Identify three reasons why therapists need to obtain self-report data on a patient's pain?
5. What is a reliable measure of a patient's pain intensity?
6. How would you measure the functional implications of a patient's pain?

ACKNOWLEDGEMENTS

Part of this chapter was published in 'Manual Therapy' 1999, 4: 216–220 (Strong 1999).

REFERENCES

Abdel-Moty A R, Maguire G W, Kaplan S H, Johnson P 1996 Stated versus observed performance levels in patients with chronic low back pain. Occupational Therapy in Health Care 10: 3–23

Ahles T A, Ruckdeschel J C, Blanchard E B 1984 Cancer-related pain – II. Assessment with visual analogue scales. Journal of Psychosomatic Research 28: 121–124

Anand K J S, McGrath P J 1999 Pain in Neonates. Elsevier, The Netherlands

Bandura A 1977 Self-efficacy: toward a unifying theory of behavioral change. Psychological Review 84: 191–215

Barris R, Oakley F, Kielhofner G 1988 The role checklist. In: Hemphill B J (ed) Mental Health Assessment in Occupational Therapy: an integrative approach to the evaluation process. Slack, Thoroughfare

Beck A T, Ward C H, Mendelson M, Mock J, Erbaugh J 1961 An inventory for measuring depression. Archives of General Psychiatry 4: 5651–5671

Bergner M, Bobbitt R A, Carter W B, Gilson B S 1981 The Sickness Impact Profile: development and final revision of a health status measure. Medical Care 19: 787–805

Choinière M, Amsel R A 1996 Visual Analogue Thermometer for measuring pain intensity. Journal of Pain and Symptom Management 11: 299–311

Collins S L, Moore R A, McQuay H J 1997 The visual analogue pain intensity scale: what is moderate pain in millimetres? Pain 72: 95–97

Council J R, Ahern D K, Follick M J, Kline C L 1988 Expectancies and functional impairment in chronic low back pain. Pain 33: 323–331

Daniel D M, Stone M L, Riehl B, Moore M 1988 A measurement of lower limb function: The one leg hop for distance. American Journal of Knee Surgery, 1988. 1(4): 211–214

Deshields T L, Tait R C, Gfeller J D, Chibnall J T 1995 Relationship between social desirability and self-report in chronic pain patients. Clinical Journal of Pain 6: 189–193

Etscheidt M A, Steger H G, Braverman B 1995 Multidimensional pain inventory profile classifications and psychopathology. Journal of Clinical Psychology 51: 29–36

Fairbank J C T, Couper J, Davies J B, O'Brien J P 1980 The Oswestry Low Back Disability Questionnaire. Physiotherapy 66: 271–273

Fisher K, Johnston M 1997 Validation of the Oswestry Low Back Pain Disability Questionnaire, its sensitivity as a measure of changes following treatment and its relationship with other aspects of the chronic pain experience. Physiotherapy Therapy and Practice 13: 67–80

Fix A J, Daughton D M 1988 Human Activity Profile: professional manual. Psychological Assessment Resources Inc, Odessa, Florida

Flaherty S A 1996 Pain measurement tools for clinical practice and research. Journal of the American Association of Nurse Anesthetists 64: 133–140

Follick M J, Ahern D K, Laster-Wolston N 1984 Evaluation of a daily activity diary for chronic pain patients. Pain 19: 373–382

Fordyce W E 1976 Behavioural Methods for Chronic Pain and Illness. Mosby, St Louis

Fordyce W E, Lansky D, Calsyn D A, Shelton J L, Stolov W C, Ruck D L 1984 Pain measurement and pain behaviour. Pain 18: 53–69

Gage M, Polatajko H J 1994 Enhancing occupational performance through an understanding of perceived self-efficacy. American Journal of Occupational Therapy 48: 452–461

Gage M, Noh S, Polatajko H J, Kaspar V 1994 Measuring perceived self-efficacy in occupational therapy. American Journal of Occupational Therapy 48: 783–790

Gaston-Johansson F 1996 Measurement of pain: the psychometric properties of the Pain-O-Meter, a simple, inexpensive pain assessment tool that could change health care practices. Journal of Pain and Symptom Management 12: 172–181

Grönblad M, Napli M, Wennerstrand P, Järvinen E, Lukinmaa A, Kour J P 1993 Intercorrelation and test-retest reliability of the Pain Disability Index (PDI) and the Oswestry Disability Questionnaire (ODQ) and their correlation with pain intensity in low back pain patients. Clinical Journal of Pain 9: 189–195

Grönblad M, Jarvinen E, Hurri H, Hupli M, Karaharju E O 1994 Relationship of the Pain Disability Index (PDI) and the Oswestry Disability Questionnaire (ODQ) with three dynamic physical tests in a group of patients with chronic low-back and leg pain. Clinical Journal of Pain 10: 197–203

Guisch L R 1984 Occupational therapy for chronic pain: a clinical application of the model of human occupation. Occupational Therapy in Mental Health 4: 59–73

Guyatt G, Walter S, Norman G 1987 Measuring change over time – assessing the usefulness of evaluative instruments. Journal of Chronic Diseases 40(2): 171–178

Harding V R, Williams C de C A, Richardson P H, Nicholas M K, Jackson J L, Richardson I H, Pither C E 1994 The development of a battery of measures for assessing physical functioning of chronic pain patients. Pain 58: 367–375

Harper A C, Harper D A, Lambert L J, Andrews H B, Lo S K, Ross F M, Straker L M 1992 Symptoms of impairment, disability and handicap in low back pain: a taxonomy. Pain 50: 189–195

Hathaway S R, McKinley J C 1942 A multiphasic personality schedule (Minnesota): III The measurement of symptomatic depression. Journal of Psychology 14: 73–84

Herda C A, Siegerisk K, Basler H-D 1994 The Pain Beliefs and Perceptions Inventory: further evidence for a 4-factor structure. Pain 57: 85–90

Huskisson E C 1983 Visual analogue scales. In: Melzack R (ed) Pain Measurement and Assessment. Raven Press, New York

Jamison R N 1996 Psychological factors in chronic pain assessment and treatment issues. Journal of Back & Musculoskeletal Rehabilitation 7: 79–95

Jensen M P, Karoly P 1991 Control beliefs, coping efforts, and adjustment to chronic pain. Journal of Consulting & Clinical Psychology 59: 431–438

Jensen M P, Karoly P, Braver S 1986 The measurement of clinical pain intensity: a comparison of six methods. Pain 27: 117–126

Jensen M P, Karoly P, Huger, R 1987 The development and preliminary validation of an instrument to assess patients' attitudes towards pain. Journal of Psychosomatic Research 31: 393–400

Jensen M P, Karoly P, O'Riordan E F, Bland F, Burns R S 1989 The subjective experience of acute pain. Clinical Journal of Pain, 1989; 5: 153–159

Jensen M P, Turner J A, Romano J M 1991 Self-efficacy and outcome expectancies: relationship to chronic pain coping strategies and adjustment. Pain 44: 263–269

Jensen M P, Turner J A, Romano J M, Fisher L D 1999 Comparative reliability and validity of chronic pain intensity measures. Pain 83: 157–162

Jerome A, Holroyd K A, Theofanous A G, Pingel J D, Lake A E, Saper J R 1988 Cluster headache pain vs other vascular headache pain: differences revealed with two approaches to the McGill Pain Questionnaire. Pain 34: 35–42

Jull G 2001 Deep cervical flexor muscle dysfunction in whiplash. Journal of Musculoskeletal Pain, *In press*

Keefe F J 1982 Behavioral assessment and treatment of chronic pain: current status and future directions. Journal of Consulting & Clinical Psychology 50: 896–911

Keefe F J, Block A R 1982 Development of an observation method for assessing pain behaviour in chronic low back pain patients. Behaviour Therapy 13: 363–375

Keefe F J, Dolan E 1986 Pain behavior and pain coping strategies in low back pain and myofascial pain dysfunction syndrome patients. Pain 24: 49–56

Kerns R D, Turk D C, Rudy T E 1985 The West Haven-Yale Multidimensional Pain Inventory (WHYMPI). Pain 23: 145–156

Kerns R D, Haythornthwaite J, Rosenberg R, Southwick S, Giller E L, Jacob M C 1991 The Pain Behaviors Checklist (PBCL): factor structure and psychometric properties. Journal of Behavioral Medicine 14: 155–167

Kielhofner G 1995 A model of human occupation: theory and application, 2nd Edn. Williams & Wilkins, Baltimore

Kielhofner G, Henry A 1988a The use of an occupational history interview in occupational therapy. In: Hemphill B J (ed) Mental Health Assessment in Occupational Therapy: an integrative approach to the evaluation process. Slack, Thoroughfare

Kielhofner G, Henry A 1988b Development and investigation of the occupational performance history interview. American Journal of Occupational Therapy 42: 489–498

Kielhofner G, Harlan B, Bauer D, Maurer P 1986 The reliability of a historical interview with physically disabled respondents. American Journal of Occupational Therapy 40: 551–556

Law M, Baptiste S, Carswell A, McColl M A, Polatajko H, Pollock N 1998 Canadian Occupational Performance Measure, 3rd edn. CAOT Publications ACE, Ottawa, Ontario

Lephart S M, Perrin D H, Fu F H, Minges K 1991 Functional performance tests for the anterior cruciate ligament insufficient athlete. Athletic Training 26(1): 44–45

Lephart S C, Perrin D H, Fu F H, Gieck J H, McCue F C, Irrgang J J 1992 Relationship between selected physical characteristics and functional capacity in the anterior cruciate ligament-insufficient athlete. Journal of Orthopaedic and Sports Physical Therapy 16(4): 174–181

Lowe N K, Walker S N, MacCallum R C 1991 Confirming the theoretical structure of the McGill Pain Questionnaire in acute clinical pain. Pain 46: 57–62

Main C J, Spanswick C C 1995a Personality assessment and the MMPI. 50 years on: do we still need our security blanket? Pain Forum 4: 90–96

Main C J, Spanswick C C 1995b 'Functional overlay' and illness behaviour in chronic pain: distress or malingering? Conceptual difficulties in medico-legal assessment of personal injury claims. Journal of Psychosomatic Research 39: 737–753

Main C J, Watson 1996 Guarded movements: Development of chronicity. Journal of Musculoskeletal Pain 4: 163–170

Main C J, Evans P J D, Whitehead R C 1991 An investigation of personality structure and other psychological features in patients presenting with low back pain: a critique of the MMPI. In: Bond M R, Charlton J E, Woolf C J (eds) Proceedings of the VIth World Congress on Pain. Pain Research and Clinical Management. Elsevier, Amsterdam, pp 207–217

Maitland G 1987 The Maitland concept: Assessment, examination and treatment by passive movement. In: Twomey L, Taylor J (eds) Physical Therapy of the Low Back. Churchill Livingstone, New York

Margolis R B, Tait R C, Krause S J 1986 A rating system for use with patient pain drawings. Pain 24: 57–65

Margolis R B, Chibnall J T, Tait R C 1988 Test-retest reliability of the pain drawing instrument. Pain 33: 49–51

Matsutsuyu J 1969 The interest checklist. American Journal of Occupational Therapy 23: 368–373

McGrath P J, Unruh A M 1999 Measurement of paediatric pain. In: Wall P D, Melzack R (eds) Textbook of pain, 4th edn. Churchill Livingstone, New York, pp 371–384

Melzack R 1975 The McGill Pain Questionnaire: major properties and scoring methods. Pain 1: 277–299

Melzack R 1987 The short-form McGill Pain Questionnaire. Pain 33: 191–197

Melzack R, Katz J 1994 Pain measurement in persons in pain. In: Wall P D, Melzack R (eds) Textbook of pain, 3rd edn. Churchill Livingstone, New York, pp 337–351

Milne J M 1983 The biopsychosocial model as applied to a multidisciplinary pain management programme. Journal of New Zealand Association of Occupational Therapists 34: 19–21

Moorhead L 1969 The occupational history. American Journal of Occupational Therapy 23: 329–338

Morley S, Wilkinson L 1995 The pain beliefs and perceptions inventory: a British replication. Pain 61: 427–433

Nicholas M 1994 Pain self-efficacy questionnaire (PSEQ): preliminary report. Unpublished paper, University of Sydney Pain Management and Research Centre, St. Leonards

Parker H, Wood R L R, Main C J 1995 The use of the pain drawing as a screening measure to predict psychological distress in chronic low back pain. Spine 20: 236–243

Patrick L, D'Eon J 1996 Social support and functional status in chronic pain patients. Canadian Journal of Rehabilitation 9: 195–201

Pilowsky I, Spence N D 1983 Manual for the Illness Behaviour Questionnaire, 2nd edn. University of Adelaide Department of Psychiatry, Adelaide

Polatin P B, Mayer T G 1996 Occupational disorders and the management of chronic pain. Orthopedic Clinics of North America 27: 881–890

Price D D, Harkins S W 1987 Combined use of experimental pain and visual analogue scales in providing standardized measurement of clinical pain. Clinical Journal of Pain 3: 1–8

Rainville J, Bagnall D, Phalen L 1995 Health care providers' attitudes and beliefs about functional impairments and chronic pain. Clinical Journal of Pain 11: 287–295

Ransford A O, Cairns D, Mooney V 1976 The Pain Drawing as an aid to the psychologic evaluation of patients with low-back pain. Spine 1: 127–134

Richardson C, Jull G, Hodges P, Hides J 1999 Therapeutic Exercise for Spinal Segmental Stabilisation. Scientific basis and practical techniques. Churchill Livingstone, Edinburgh

Robinson M E, Myers C D, Sadler I J, Riley J L, Kvaal S A, Geisser M E 1997a Bias effects in three common self-report pain assessment measures. Clinical Journal of Pain 13: 74–81

Robinson M E, Riley J L, Myers C D, Sadler I J, Kvaal S A, Geisser M E 1996b. The Coping Strategies Questionnaire: a large sample, item level factor analysis. Clinical Journal of Pain 13: 43–49

Rosenstiel A K, Keefe F J 1983 The use of coping strategies in chronic low back pain patients: relationship to patient characteristics and current adjustment. Pain 17: 33–44

Rucker K S, Metzler H M 1995 Predicting subsequent employment status of SSA disability applicants with chronic pain. Clinical Journal of Pain 11: 22–35

Rucker K S, Metzler H M, Kregel J 1996 Standardization of chronic pain assessment: a multiperspective approach. Clinical Journal of Pain 12: 94–110

Schnurr R F, MacDonald M R 1995 Memory complaints in chronic pain. Clinical Journal of Pain 11: 103–111

Simmonds M, Harding V, Watson P, Claveau Y 2000 Physical therapy assessment: Expanding the model. In: Devor M, Rowbotham M, Wiesenfeld-Hallin (eds) Proceedings of the 9th World Congress on Pain. IASP Press, Seattle, pp 1013–1029

Stratford P, Levy D, Gauldie S, Levy K, Miseferi D 1987 Extensor carpi radialis tendonitis: A validation of selected outcome measures. Physiotherapy Canada 39(4): 250–255

Stratford P, Levy D, and Gowland C 1993a Evaluative properties of measures used to assess patients with lateral epicondylitis at the elbow. Physiotherapy Canada 45(3): 160–164

Stratford P, Solomon P, Binkley J, Finch E, Gill C 1993b Sensitivity of Sickness Impact Profile items to measure change over time in a low-back pain patient group. Spine 18: 1723–1727

Stratford P W and Balsor B E 1994 A comparison of make and break tests using a hand-held dynamometer and the Kin-Com. Journal of Orthopaedic and Sports Physical Therapy 19(1): 28–32

Strong J 1992 Chronic low back pain: towards an integrated psychosocial assessment model. Unpublished PhD thesis, The University of Queensland, Brisbane, Australia

Strong J 1995 Self-efficacy and the patient with chronic pain. In: Schacklock M (ed) Moving in on Pain. Butterworth-Heinemann, Melbourne

Strong J 1996 Chronic Pain: the Occupational Therapist's Perspective. Churchill Livingstone, Edinburgh

Strong J 1999 Assessment of pain perception in clinical practice. Manual Therapy 4: 216–220

Strong J, Cramond T O'R, Maas F 1989 The effectiveness of relaxation techniques with patients who have chronic low back pain. Occupational Therapy Journal of Research 9: 184–192

Strong J, Ashton R, Chant D 1991 Pain intensity measurement in chronic low back pain. Clinical Journal of Pain 7: 209–218

Strong J, Ashton R, Chant D 1992 The measurement of attitudes towards and beliefs about pain. Pain 48: 227–236

Strong J, Ashton R, Large R G 1994a Function and the patient with chronic low back pain. Clinical Journal of Pain 10: 191–196

Strong J, Ashton R, Stewart A 1994b Chronic low back pain: toward an integrated psychosocial assessment model. Journal of Consulting and Clinical Psychology 62: 1058–1063

Strong J, Large RG, Ashton R, Stewart A 1995 A New Zealand replication of the IPAM clustering model. Clinical Journal of Pain 11: 296–306

Sullivan M J L, Bishop S R, Pivik J 1995 The Pain Catastrophizing Scale: development and validation. Psychological Assessment 7: 524–532

Tait R C, Chibnall J T 1997 Development of a brief version of the Survey of Pain Attitudes. Pain 70: 229–235

Tait R C, Pollard A, Margolis R B, Duckro P N, Krause S J 1987 The Pain Disability Index: psychometric and validity data. Archives of Physical Medical Rehabilitation 68: 438–441

Tait R C, Chibnall J T, Krause S 1990 The Pain Disability Index: psychometric properties. Pain 22: 73–77

Turk D C 1996 Biopsychosocial perspective on chronic pain. In: Gatchel R J, Turk D C (eds) Psychosocial Approaches to Pain Management: a practitioner's handbook. Guilford Press, New York, pp 3–32

Turk DC, Okifuji A 1999 Assessment of patients' reporting of pain: an integrated perspective. Lancet 353: 1784–1788

Unruh A M, Ritchie J A 1998 Development of the Pain Appraisal Inventory: psychometric properties. Pain Research and Management 3, 105–110

Vasuderan S V 1989 Clinical perspectives on the relationship between pain and disability. Neurological Clinics 7: 429–439

Verbrugge L M 1990 Disability. Rheumatic Disease Clinics of North America 16: 741–761

Vlaeyen J W S, Kote-Snijders A M K, Boeren R G V, van Eek H 1995 Fear of movement/(re)injury in chronic low back pain and its relation to behavioural performance. Pain 62: 363–372

Waddell G, Main C J 1984 Assessment of severity in low-back disorders. Spine 9: 204–208

Waddell G, Newton M, Henderson I, Somerville D, Main C J 1993 A fear avoidance beliefs questionnaire (FABQ) and the role of fear-avoidance in chronic low back pain and disability. Pain 52: 157–168

Watson P J 1999 Psychosocial assessment. Physiotherapy 85: 533–535

White J, Strong J 1992 Measurement of activity levels in patients with chronic low back pain. Occupational Therapy Journal of Research 12: 217–228

Wilk K E, Romaniello W T, Soscia S M, Arigo C A, Andrews J R 1994 The relationship between subjective knee scores isokinetic testing and functional testing in the ACL reconstructed knee. Journal of Orthopaedic and Sports Physical Therapy 20(2): 60–73

Williams D A, Thorn B E 1989 An empirical assessment of pain beliefs. Pain 36: 351–358

Williams D A, Robinson M E, Geisser M E 1994 Pain beliefs: assessment and utility. Pain 59: 71–78

Woolf C J, Decosterd I 1999 Implications of recent advances in the understanding of pain pathophysiology for the assessment of pain in patients. Pain Supplement 6: S141–S147

World Health Organization 1980 International Classification of Impairments. Disabilities and Handicaps. WHO, Geneva

World Health Organization 1999 ICIDH-2 International Classification of Functioning and Disability Beta-2 Draft Full Version. WHO, Geneva

Managing pain

8

Generic principles of practice

Anita M. Unruh
Katherine Harman

OVERVIEW

In other chapters of this book, specific assessment and intervention approaches are examined. In this chapter, generic (see Box 8.1) principles of practice are presented that are important to the way in which assessment, intervention and discharge are approached with clients. We base these principles and their discussion on our practice and research experience.

Box 8.1   Key terms defined

Generic – Generic refers to the general applicability of something to a group. We use the term here to indicate that these principles are not of more importance to one profession than another. They are relevant to occupational therapists and physiotherapists, and may indeed have applicability for all health professions concerned with pain.

Baseline – The term baseline refers to measurement that is taken before intervention. Baseline measures provide a point of comparison when these measures are completed after intervention.

Evidence-based practice – Evidence-based practice is the use of research findings in conjunction with clinical knowledge, clinical reasoning and input from clients to make decisions about interventions that are the most effective for clients (Egan et al 1998, Law & Baum 1998).

Addiction – Drug-seeking behaviour to achieve a psychological high (McGrath & Unruh 1987).

Pseudoaddiction – Drug-seeking behaviour to obtain pain relief rather than a psychological high (Weissman & Haddox 1989).

Learning objectives

At the end of this chapter, students will have an understanding of:

1. Generic principles of practice for clients with pain.
2. Application of these principles to occupational therapy and physiotherapy.

PRACTICE PRINCIPLES

All practice is governed by a set of values and theoretical assumptions that are specific to individual professions. There are other, generic principles that guide the way in which practice should be conducted by all health professionals to ensure that a client or patient is most likely to achieve his or her aims. Treatment of all clients with pain requires attention to these basic principles but they become especially important for the client with chronic pain for whom intervention is more complex. These principles are summarized in Box 8.2.

BELIEVE THE CLIENT'S DESCRIPTION OF THE PAIN AND SUFFERING

As has been discussed in earlier chapters, many clients with chronic pain have to face and cope with the doubt of others that their pain complaint is legitimate. Unless there is compelling evidence to the contrary, when

---

Box 8.2 Generic principles of practice

- Believe the client's description of her or his pain and suffering.
- Treat acute pain aggressively.
- Always assess the client's pain and its impact on daily life before planning intervention.
- Avoid 'leaps to the head' to explain the client's pain.
- Determine whether the primary goal of intervention is pain reduction or improvement in function.
- Incorporate evidence-based decision-making into practice.
- Combine medical, pharmacological, cognitive–behavioural, occupational and physical strategies
- Understand and correct misconceptions about the use of pain medication and addiction risks.
- Recognize that a positive response to a cognitive–behavioural intervention does not mean that the client's pain has a psychological cause.
- Help the client to make long-term lifestyle changes.
- Involve the client's family whenever possible.
- Recognize dual responsibilities and obligations.
- Create a positive therapeutic milieu.
- Conduct an ethical practice.
- Participate in research, education and professional pain associations.

---

describing the pain and suffering a client must be believed. It is extremely difficult to form a collaborative partnership and expect to achieve goals that will be meaningful to the client if her or his concerns are doubted. The client's own views about the pain are an important and essential component of assessment and intervention. Conclusions drawn by members of the healthcare team are a reflection of a broad understanding of the nature of pain, the impact of pain on daily life, and the variability of the pain experience. A comprehensive assessment is vital to ensure that all factors contributing to the client's pain and disability are considered in developing an effective intervention plan.

TREAT ACUTE PAIN AGGRESSIVELY

Enduring acute pain has no physiological or psychological advantage to the person. Untreated or inadequately treated pain may lead to destabilization of sick children (Unruh & McGrath 2000), and in extreme cases, such as surgical pain in neonates, may increase mortality (Anand & Hickey 1987). Liebeskind (1991) argued that untreated pain may interfere with immune function, and there is evidence that painful events may sensitize people, neurophysiologically and psychologically, to experience pain more easily in future pain episodes (Grunau et al 1994, Harman 2000, Taddio et al 1995).

Many clinicians and researchers believe that more aggressive and timely intervention of acute pain would go a long way to preventing the onset of chronic pain or at least reducing the extent of the disability that is often associated with chronic pain. At present, there is only suggestive research rather than conclusive evidence to justify this belief, but the evidence is mounting that persistent pain causes physiological (Liebeskind 1991) and psychological harm (Wall 1999). Fear of pain and fear of the consequences of pain increase anxiety, and anxiety focuses the client's attention on the pain (Wall 1999), increasing the risk of disability and handicap if acute pain persists. There is no known contraindication to providing aggressive and timely intervention for acute pain.

There are two phases of aggressive treatment: the acute pain incident, and acute pain that is becoming chronic. The type of pain would clearly need to be taken into account. However, appropriate pharmacological strategies, combined with physical therapies and possibly short-term use of assistive devices may be helpful. If the acute pain becomes chronic or if repeated episodes are likely, then continuation of these strategies combined with cognitive–behavioural interventions may be very important (see Chapter 9).

Relaxation to reduce muscle tension and promote stress reduction aids in the reduction of the pain cycle. In addition, pacing with short but frequent rests may be beneficial. Focus on a challenge appraisal of pain, use of positive self-statements, and reduction of catastrophizing may be key. Education about the nature of the pain may ensure that the client has a realistic appraisal of his or her pain. A high threat appraisal that is based on inadequate information may impair coping with pain (Unruh & Ritchie 1998, Unruh et al 1999). Early intervention with family may be helpful to encourage appropriate support and to reduce excessive dependency. Timely assessment of ergonomic factors, particularly those related to the client's primary occupation, is important. Above all, reduction of waiting lists for intervention is needed.

ALWAYS ASSESS THE PAIN AND ITS IMPACT ON DAILY LIFE BEFORE PLANNING INTERVENTION

It can be tempting to begin immediately with an intervention but, without an adequate assessment of the pattern of pain and its impact on daily life prior to treatment, it is not possible to determine if an intervention has any beneficial effect. Many clinics with a rehabilitation programme will conduct baseline assessments on admission to the programme. These measures may be brief, primarily providing screening information, or they may be more detailed. In a multidisciplinary programme, each profession will administer another set of measures that are specific to the goals and objectives of that profession. The team will then collectively review the findings.

Chapter 7, 'Assessment and measurement of pain', provides a detailed discussion about models and measures that are relevant to occupational therapists and physiotherapists. Therapists should be familiar with the initial assessment materials that are used in their setting and use the baseline information that is relevant to their professional perspective. In some cases (and in particular with a complex pain presentation), the information provided in the initial assessment may not be detailed enough to guide intervention in a specific area. Whether acute or chronic, baseline levels of function are important to determine appropriate intervention and measure the efficacy of treatment. Baseline measures that are relevant to the goals of occupational therapy or physiotherapy are also important to provide outcome information about the degree of success or resolution on completion of the therapy programme. A daily diary tracking pain during a week may provide a comprehensive view of the variability of the client's pain and its relationship to function, activity and sleep (Jensen & McFarland 1993).

By understanding the impact of pain on a client's daily life, the practitioner is able to measure change in a meaningful way. As discussed in Chapter 7, pain is much more than intensity. Measures of the impact of pain on daily living will capture changes in pain that affect function. Assessments and measures should also be repeated at predetermined points during intervention and at discharge, to guide intervention and readiness for discharge.

AVOID 'LEAPS TO THE HEAD' TO EXPLAIN THE PAIN

Patrick Wall (1984) criticized the tendency for practitioners and researchers to jump to psychological explanations to account for pain when there is little or no evidence of tissue damage. Many clients with persistent pain will present with psychological, environmental and behavioural problems that exacerbate the pain, resulting in a complex clinical picture (see Chapter 4). If these problems become severe they may interfere with managing the pain. These difficulties require attention. However, in most instances, there is no evidence that they are the *cause* of the pain (Wall 1999). Indeed it is more likely that as pain persists and controls the quality of everyday life, psychological, environmental and behavioural difficulties will occur and will contribute to maintaining pain. For this reason, splitting pain into either a physical or a psychological problem is unlikely to be productive. All factors that may contribute to the persistence of pain should be considered in a comprehensive assessment and multidisciplinary intervention. A diagnosis of psychologically caused pain on the basis of negative evidence (no apparent tissue damage) is not logically justifiable. A diagnosis can only be based on positive evidence or the cause must be considered as unknown.

Remember that attributing psychological causation to the pain is different from recognizing the important contributory role of psychological factors. Attributing psychological causation is often perceived to be blaming the person for the pain, even if it is not intended to be perceived this way, by the client. Perceptions of blame typically lead to further mistrust of health professionals and feelings of alienation for the client, thereby blocking the potential for a collaborative therapeutic relationship.

Avoiding leaps to psychological causal explanations in the absence of identifiable pathology does not mean that contributing psychological issues should be ignored. Indeed, ignoring psychological aspects of pain, and focusing solely on physical or pharmacological treatments may cause further harm by perpetuating chronic pain, suffering and disability. Clients often benefit from explanation about the interactional relationship of psychological and physiological factors in maintaining pain, and the way in which the mind can be used to influence, control and change pain perception.

DETERMINE THE PRIMARY GOAL OF INTERVENTION: PAIN REDUCTION OR IMPROVEMENT IN FUNCTION

The primary goal of most intervention strategies will be either pain reduction or improvement of function. If the primary goal of intervention is pain reduction, then strategies will be directed towards determining the source of the pain and relieving it. Pharmacological approaches (prescription and non-prescription medications) and physical strategies (e.g. thermal agents, TENS, biofeedback, exercise, stretching and massage) may be used to reduce pain. Interventions for pain reduction may also have a secondary impact on improving function. To illustrate, a client whose pain medication provides substantial pain relief will likely have secondary improvement in function unless other important factors support disability. If family members, or other factors, reinforce dependency and disability, then a client whose pain has been effectively reduced may still have substantial disability, unless interventions for improvement of function are also used. In addition, excessive rest or reliance on medication may reduce pain but at the cost of increased disability and dependency.

If the primary goal of intervention is disability reduction, then ergonomic assessment of the home and workplace, cognitive–behavioural strategies, pacing, work simplification and other interventions may be more appropriate. If disability is exacerbated by excessive pain behaviour and poor coping then operant conditioning principles to reduce the focus on pain may be helpful (Fordyce et al 1985). Operant behavioural methods are focussed specifically on disability reduction:

Behavioural methods for treating pain problems (chronic pain behaviours) are not intended to 'treat pain' in the traditional sense, in which this implies directing attention to sources and mechanisms of noxious stimuli generating injury signals which lead to 'pain'. Behavioural pain methods do not have as their principal objective the modification of nociception, nor the direct modification of the experience of pain, although it very frequently happens that both are influenced by these methods. Rather, behavioural methods in pain-treatment programmes are intended to treat excess disability and expressions of suffering. . . . The goal is to render chronic pain patients functional again and as normal in behaviour as possible (Fordyce et al 1985 p 115).

As Fordyce et al (1985) suggested, interventions for disability reduction help to modify the client's appraisal of pain. Reappraisal of pain in a more positive direction may result in a higher level of activity (Unruh & Ritchie 1998). Reappraisal may then be associated with pain reduction. The pain reduction may be quite modest in comparison to disability reduction. If incorrectly used however, operant behavioural strategies may repress pain complaints and behaviours, without any impact on disability or pain reduction. In such cases, the client may feel more isolated and unable to obtain assistance for pain.

Cognitive–behavioural strategies may reduce stress and improve mood with an associated reduction in pain (Bradley 1996, McCaffery & Beebe 1989). These strategies can be effective in shifting attention away from the pain, and in doing so may enable the client to become more fully engaged in her or his activities or occupations. They may also help the client to feel more in control of the pain without changing or reducing the actual pain. The overall goal of cognitive–behavioural strategies is disability reduction.

Determining the primary goal of intervention can be difficult for the client and healthcare team. They may have different perspectives about intervention goals. Often the client's priority will be pain reduction, whereas the team's primary concern may be disability reduction. These differences need to be considered before effective progress can be made. Focusing on disability reduction means accepting to some extent that the pain is chronic. It also means examining environmental and psychological factors that may contribute to pain, and changing their influence. These changes often affect the roles and habits of someone's lifestyle and they are not easy to change in a meaningful way without the client's recognition that the problem will require this type of long-term management.

If the client has not been given an explanation of the difference between pain reduction strategies and disability reduction strategies, she or he may also misinterpret the therapist's intentions. For example, if the therapist proposes cognitive–behavioural interventions for disability reduction and the client is expecting interventions more appropriate to pain reduction, then the client may interpret the therapist's proposal of cognitive–behavioural interventions as an indicator that the therapist believes the pain is all psychological, or even not really present at all. Open discussion will avoid such misunderstandings and will ensure that the client has a better understanding of the purpose of cognitive–behavioural interventions, and other disability-reduction strategies.

Agreement on the primary goal is necessary for the client and therapist to make decisions about therapeutic options that will be most optimal for the client. The client's needs and goals need to be considered along with the nature of the pain, and the degree of disability and handicap.

INCORPORATE EVIDENCE-BASED DECISION-MAKING INTO PRACTICE

Over the past decade there has been tremendous pressure to incorporate evidence-based decision-making into all healthcare practice. Evidence-based practice incorporates evidence of the effectiveness of interventions from research (quantitative and qualitative) with information about the client's needs and goals, and the therapist's clinical experience. Clients have critical knowledge about their own needs and intervention preferences. Professional experience is very important to ensure that interventions which may be beneficial but have been insufficiently examined in research are included in future research. Many interventions have been examined in research but the quality of the research may be variable. The methodological strength of the research is an important consideration to ascertain the degree of evidence. An intervention that has positive benefit with minimal or no harm in repeated randomized controlled trials, has stronger evidence of effectiveness than an intervention that has not been researched in this way. Qualitative research provides limited evidence of effectiveness for comparison by groups but does yield valuable information about programme or treatment effectiveness that is important for planning meaningful interventions (Ritchie for individual clients 1999).

The process of using evidence-based decision-making can be intimidating for clinicians that are unfamiliar with this process. There are five basic steps (Box 8.3) to developing an evidence-based practice (Flemming 1998, Stewart 1999, Westmorland 1998).

The process may appear to be daunting but there are a variety of resources available to occupational therapists and physiotherapists to assist them in developing an evidence-based practice. Some of these resources are listed in Box 8.4.

In addition, many graduate and undergraduate professional education programmes include required or elective courses on evidence-based practice. Continuing education workshops or courses in this area may also be offered via professional associations.

Box 8.3 Five steps to developing an evidence-based practice

1. Develop a focused question based on the client context, the specific intervention and the expected outcomes of the intervention.
2. Collect evidence from the literature that is relevant to the question(s). Identification of databases and relevant search words are important at this step to ensure success in article retrieval.
3. Critically analyse the validity, reliability and generalizability of the research retrieved.
4. Integrate the evidence with clinical experience and client needs, to develop an intervention programme.
5. Evaluate the programme.

Box 8.4 Evidence-based resources for occupational therapists and physiotherapists

Occupational therapy
- Canadian Journal of Occupational Therapy 1998, 65, special issue on evidence-based practice
- Canadian Association of Occupational Therapists, (1999) Joint position statement on evidence-based occupational therapy
- Evidence-Based Practice column in Occupational Therapy Now (newsletter of the Canadian Association of Occupational Therapy)
- Letts et al (1999) A programme evaluation workbook for occupational therapists: an evidence-based practice tool
- Occupational Therapy Evidence-based Practice Research Group (1999) at McMaster University, Canada (completed a critical review of the effectiveness of cognitive–behavioural interventions for people with chronic pain, review available from the website: http://www.fhs.mcmaster.ca/rehab)

Physiotherapy
- Cole et al (1994) Physical rehabilitation outcome measures
- McIntyre et al (1999) Canadian physiotherapy research and evidence-based practice initiative in the 1900s
- Straker (1999) A hierarchy of evidence for informing physiotherapy practice
- Vanderkooy et al (1999) A clinical effort toward maximizing evidence-based practice

Occupational therapy and physiotherapy
- Helewa & Walker (2000) Critical evaluation of research in physical rehabilitation: towards evidence-based practice

---

One of the difficulties that many busy therapists experience with evidence-based practice is the time needed to read research and assess the quality of the evidence that is provided. There are several organizations that have taken on responsibility for providing timely, evidence-based information for health professionals. One of the most influential is the Cochrane Collaboration. The Cochrane Collaboration is an international network of people and organizations with a commitment to fostering evidence-based practice through the preparation, dissemination and application of systematic reviews of any healthcare intervention (Hayes & McGrath 1998, Pollock 1998, Snider 1999, Stewart 1999).

A Cochrane group conducts a thorough search for all experimental and non-experimental research that is pertinent to the intervention. The studies are evaluated and the outcomes of the best studies are examined to determine potential recommendations. Any Cochrane review is updated as new research becomes available, to ensure that new information about an intervention is taken into consideration in the evaluation of the intervention. The Cochrane Library is an electronic database of completed reviews. It can be accessed through most university libraries, and many hospital libraries.

Therapists should know what level of evidence currently exists for the effectiveness of any interventions or strategies that are considered with the client. It should be accepted practice to discuss this evidence with the client. Clients may choose options for which there is little, if any evidence of effectiveness, but should do so knowing that this is the case. Monitoring progress with attention to both positive and negative effects is particularly important in such cases, for several reasons. Evidence of effectiveness will be dependent on the identification of positive benefits for the client. Secondly, the absence of research information about possible negative effects indicates that the risk remains unknown. The temptation in this circumstance may be to focus on possible positive benefits but harm is also possible and should be considered.

COMBINE MEDICAL, PHARMACOLOGICAL, COGNITIVE–BEHAVIOURAL, OCCUPATIONAL AND PHYSICAL STRATEGIES

Because causal and contributory factors of chronic pain are multimodal, successful treatment is likely to combine multiple intervention strategies. Pharmacological approaches are frequently necessary to keep pain at a manageable level, but they are best combined with other strategies that increase function and activity and

reduce suffering (Polatin 1996). Physical strategies such as heat or cold packs, TENS units and massage may be particularly useful for acute pain and exacerbations of chronic pain (Gross et al 1996, Harding et al 1998, Minor et al 1989, van der Heijden et al 1997). Changes in diet, exercise, and posture may improve overall health and reduce lifestyle factors that contribute to the pain. Modification of work and living environments may reduce factors that aggravate pain or place the client at risk for injury. Cognitive–behavioural strategies such as cognitive restructuring help to alter the way the client has constructed a meaning of pain and may support use of more optimal coping strategies (Bradley 1996). Biofeedback and relaxation therapy will reduce underlying muscle tension and stress, and may improve sleep (Arena & Blanchard 1996, Kerr 2000). Supportive group therapy may help clients to feel less isolated with their difficulties (Diamond & Coniam 1997, Keefe et al 1996).

The existing research on the effectiveness of interventions for chronic pain support the use of multidisciplinary clinics in which comprehensive interdisciplinary assessment and multiple intervention approaches are utilized (Becker et al 2000, Flor et al 1992, Mason et al 1998, Russo & Brose 1998). The benefit may be that the client has a variety of strategies to use to manage the variability of pain on a day-to-day basis. Combined interventions may also have an overall synergistic effect.

Providing multiple interventions requires a multi-disciplinary pain team. Pharmacotherapy and medicine assure that nociceptive activation is kept at a manageable level for the client. Physiotherapy is used to reduce pain perception and improve physical fitness (strength and flexibility), posture, work and living environments. Occupational therapy is used to enable clients to have meaningful and productive occupations despite pain. Psychologists focus on appraisal, coping and pain behaviours.

Often these professions work together in educational and supportive client groups to improve the client's understanding about pain and its effects on daily life, and to teach and reinforce the use of different intervention strategies. All of these professions contribute to improvement in health and reduction of factors that contribute to the pain.

CORRECT MISCONCEPTIONS ABOUT PAIN MEDICATION AND ADDICTION RISKS

Pharmacological strategies are discussed in detail in Chapter 16, and also in Chapter 15. Pain medication has a very important role in the management of pain but many clients have difficulty knowing how to use medication to obtain the most optimal relief. Reduction of pain has physiological and psychological benefit. Decreasing pain promotes healing. It is also likely to reduce the onset of anxiety, depression and suffering that frequently occur with persistent pain. If the pain is an acute pain, then effective use of pain medication may also reduce the possibility that the pain will become a more chronic problem.

If pain can be managed without medication, in such a way that the client can continue to live a meaningful and productive life, then pain medication is unnecessary. But if a client is spending considerable portions of a day using cognitive–behavioral and physical interventions to keep the pain at bay, with little time to be engaged in meaningful occupations, then pain medication will be extremely useful (McCaffery & Beebe 1989). The client will have more time to do what is important in his or her life. Clients should not take medication for pain if the medication is not helpful or if the medication has substantial side-effects, unless side-effects can be controlled and are offset by the degree of benefit. Periodic reassessments of medications are often necessary.

Clients should be careful not to combine pain medication with other drugs, including herbal remedies, without the knowledge of their physician. They should use pain medication together with other pain management strategies (e.g. relaxation, pacing, biofeedback, TENS, hypnosis, imagery) to achieve maximum benefit. Often a client will need explicit information about the benefits of using these strategies together rather than as an either/or alternative.

Use and misuse of pain medication

A person's decision-making about the use of medication involves questions about how to take medication, side-effects, and 'moral' issues that concern the acceptability of taking pain medication. It is useful for clients and professionals alike to be aware of these issues, most of which involve some degree of conflict and a need to develop a balance between opposing issues.

The client is often directly responsible for taking any recommended or prescribed pain medication unless she or he is a child, disabled or in hospital. If the medication is available over-the-counter, then the client may use her or his own opinion about the extent to which package directions will be followed. Even when the physician provides a prescription for pain medication with instructions about how to use the medica-

tion, many clients do not take their medication in the way that it has been prescribed. In some cases, if the physician is not a pain specialist, the client may also have been given inaccurate information about the role of the medication and the way in which the medication should be taken. Inevitably, clients use their own decision-making process. Clients will consider:

- What should I take?
- When should I start?
- How much should I take?
- Which prescription can I manage without?
- Would the medication work better if I combine it with other medications?

Answers to these questions are based on the client's beliefs about pain and pain medication, advice from family, friends, and coworkers, advertisements and instructions from health professions. Pain intensity, other related symptoms, side-effects of medication, personal characteristics and other methods used to relieve pain also influence decision-making about pain medication (Purdy et al 1997).

This decision-making may not result in using medication in a way that will produce the most effective pain relief. To illustrate, although many adolescent girls experience substantial menstrual pain (Unruh & Campbell 1999), they do not appear to take over-the-counter medication according to package instructions (Campbell & McGrath 1997).

Concern about the side-effects is important because many medications should be taken in such a way as to prevent or minimize side-effects. However, one side-effect that is often ignored is the one due to errors of omission when medications are not taken (personal communication, June 2000, Frank New). The side-effects of not taking medication may be continued pain with increased disability and suffering. Such side-effects (due to not taking pain medication) are easier to ignore because they appear to be 'internal' and less tangible, whereas side-effects of medication are more tangible and clearly linked to an 'external' factor, the medication. The client must be attentive to potential side-effects of using medication, and at the same time recognize that not using medication may also have side-effects.

Some clients will be extremely reluctant to use pain medication, even if the pain is moderate or severe. They may believe that taking medication is 'giving in' to pain, that taking pain medication shows weakness in character, or that taking medication is in some way a crutch. The client may be afraid that if medication is taken too soon, then the medication will no longer be effective if the pain becomes more severe. In addition, clients often fear that taking medication for pain will result in addiction. This fear may be applied to non-steroidal anti-inflammatory medications as well as opioid analgesics and other medications used for pain.

Any of these beliefs may mean that the client takes pain medication primarily when she or he is feeling desperate about the severity of the pain. If the medication was not designed to be effective for severe pain, then the medication is likely to have less effect or to be ineffective. The client may then increase the dose or combine the medication with some other drug. The client may also seek out multiple physicians in the search for a drug that will provide more pain relief. These behaviours are unlikely to achieve adequate pain control, particularly if the client continues to take medication in a haphazard approach that does not reduce the cycle of increasing pain.

Using multiple medications may cause drug interactions or side-effects. Excessive use of some medications may exacerbate pain through rebound effects. This haphazard and ineffective use of pain medication also increases the probability that the client will be considered by others to be addicted to pain medication. The problem is better described as misuse of pain medication that may be due to an inadequate understanding of how to use medication to achieve effective pain relief.

In hospital, a person who is receiving inadequate or irregular doses of medication may begin 'clock-watching', focusing on the pain with marked concern about the availability of pain medications (Cherny & Portenoy 1999, Twycross 1999). It also encourages the client to consider pain medication as the primary approach to pain relief rather than as one component of a comprehensive approach. This problem is more accurately described as pseudoaddiction (Weissman & Haddox 1989); the person's behaviour may well be indicative of poorly controlled pain rather than drug addiction. As noted by Cherny and Portenoy (1999), increasing the dose to provide adequate pain relief eliminates these behaviours and usually distinguishes the patient from the true addict.

Family members may share some of the client's erroneous beliefs about pain medication. Family members may then dissuade the client from taking pain medication, or in the case of parents or caregivers of an elderly or disabled family member, may not give the medication or give it only if the pain is severe. As an illustration, Finley et al (1996) found that even when parents recognized that their children had moderate or severe pain following day surgery, and were given explicit instructions about giving pain medication, parents provided inadequate pain medication for the child at home. Family members may also contribute to misuse of medication by encouraging the client to try other drugs.

Pain medications should be taken as prescribed (if they were properly prescribed). Studies have shown that medications are most effective at lower levels of pain (Coderre & Melzack 1987). As mentioned earlier, severe peaks of pain should be avoided by careful design of an overall intervention plan incorporating medical, physical, cognitive–behavioural, occupational and dietary interventions. Some types of medication (e.g. antidepressants) work better with a constant level of the medication in the bloodstream. These drugs need to be taken even when there is no pain. A client who does not understand this issue might stop using the medication when the pain improves, only to start again because the pain has returned.

Any client taking opioids for pain should increase fibre and fluid intake and activity level, to reduce the risk of constipation associated with opioids. NSAIDs should be taken with food to prevent gastric irritation. COX-2 inhibitors have significantly less gastric irritation. An occupational therapist or physiotherapist who becomes aware that the client has symptoms that may be related to medication side-effects (discussed in more detail in Chapters 15 and 16), must report these problems to the team, and should encourage the client to speak with her or his physician.

Addiction

Many clients will have fears about addiction. Addiction is often confused with physical tolerance and physical dependence, both of which are physiological processes.

Physical tolerance is the need for increased doses of medication to achieve the same pain relief. Much of the research about tolerance was done with people with drug addictions. However, extensive research of people with cancer on long-term opioid therapy has shown that physical tolerance does not occur when opioids are taken for pain (Twycross 1999). The primary reason for increasing the dose of the medication is progression of the disease rather than tolerance to the drug (Brescia et al 1992).

Physical dependence is the occurrence of symptoms such as sweating or jitteriness, if the pain medication is suddenly withdrawn. Physical dependence can be prevented by gradual tapering off of the medication rather than its abrupt withdrawal. The occurrence of physical dependence is not evidence of addiction. Addiction to pain medication is demonstrated by drug-seeking behaviour to achieve a psychological high from the drug, rather than to obtain pain relief.

It may be helpful to explain to clients that pain appears to act like a sponge that soaks up the opioid to relieve pain. Unless the client has a prior history of drug or alcohol addiction, most clients with pain are not at risk for developing an addiction to pain medication. Clients should worry less about addiction and worry more about using pain medication in the way that it has been prescribed by a pain specialist. Any client who experiences a psychological high due to pain medication (euphoria that is separate from happiness associated with feeling free of the pain) should report this sensation to the physician. A person with pain who has a history of addiction may still be treated with opioids for pain but will need very careful monitoring (McCaffery & Beebe 1989, Twycross 1999).

Pain medication and chronic non-malignant pain

Pharmacological treatment of chronic non-cancer pain is discussed in Chapter 16. Opioids are an important part of pain management for cancer pain. They are still controversial for use in chronic non-cancer pain, although clinical experience and some controlled studies do support that opioids can be used for the management of this type of pain (Fuchs & Gamsa 1997, Portenoy 1990, 1996, Twycross 1999). Opioids can be just as effective for non-malignant pain, but chronic pain can persist for many years. The health consequences of long-term opioid use are unknown.

Guidelines have been developed for the use of opioids for chronic non-malignant pain but they are not yet generally agreed upon. The guidelines include expectations that the use of opioids is time-limited, contingent on the client's meeting of agreed-upon goals, and include periodic random blood samples (Gourlay & Cherry 1991). Other considerations include the use of alternative treatments that have failed, objective evidence of benefit from the use of opioids for the client, and specific assessment of side-effects.

Pain medication and palliative care

People who are receiving palliative care, and their families, may have many of the beliefs and fears about medication that have been previously discussed. In addition, poorly managed pain for a person who is terminally ill may increase the risk of suicide, and may raise questions about euthanasia and physician-assisted suicide as discussed in Chapter 1.

Information about pain medication, side-effects and their management should be provided for the client and the family. The side-effect of not taking pain medication must also be considered due to the potential for increased distress and suffering. Often, after the initial dose of opioids, clients become much more tolerant of side-effects such as respiratory depression, so that larger doses are unlikely to cause the same medical risk (personal communication, Frank New, June 2000).

Sometimes, clients and families fear that using opioids will hasten death. However, appropriate use of opioids in palliative care prolongs life, because the person is free of pain, has improved rest and sleep, increased appetite and strength, and is able to concentrate on being better-involved with increased physical activity (Twycross 1999). In some countries, clients' concerns may be related to fear that medications may be increased to hasten death rather than to reduce pain (Twycross 1999). Such fears can only be addressed by open and honest discussion between the client, family and healthcare team (Saunders & Platt 1999).

Therapists should consider the complex ethical and humanitarian aspects of pain management in this area. A person who is terminally ill should not die in pain. Appropriate pain management must be provided to ensure that the client can spend valuable time engaged in activities that bring some enjoyment and peace to this stage of life. A client must be a full participant in any decision-making about the use of pain medication.

Pro re nata (PRN) administration of medication

PRN is a common approach to medication administration for the person in hospital. PRN administration means that pain medication is given to the patient when she or he requests medication. The problem with the PRN approach is that receipt of medication is dependent on the patient's capacity to bring himself to the nurse's attention. He must then convince the nurse that he is in sufficient pain to warrant pain medication. This process leaves the patient and the nurse vulnerable to potential biases and problems of communication about pain. Decisions may be complicated by stereotypes about how the patient's age, sex, race, ethnicity, or socioeconomic class might affect pain behaviour and pain complaints. In addition, patients often assume that the nurse will bring medication when it is necessary, without the patient requesting it, and may not realize that they must initiate the process by requesting pain medication. The patient may be reluctant to trouble the nurse, and may feel that he should put up with the pain unless he becomes desperate about it.

Another serious problem is that PRN administration is not effective in breaking the pain cycle; it does not eliminate severe peaks in pain. Long intervals between allowable PRN doses (3–6 hours) are not pharmacologically logical, and impose periods of unnecessary pain. Providing sufficient medication at regular intervals maintains a steady level of medication in the bloodstream and reduces increasing severity of pain and break-through pain, thereby encouraging a person to develop and maintain her or his activity level rather than relying excessively on rest for symptom relief. The PRN approach has been sharply criticized by many researchers and health professionals (McCaffery & Beebe 1989).

RECOGNIZE THAT POSITIVE RESPONSE TO COGNITIVE–BEHAVIOURAL INTERVENTION DOES NOT MEAN THE PAIN HAS A PSYCHOLOGICAL CAUSE

Unfortunately, sometimes the interpretation of a positive clinical response to a cognitive–behavioural intervention is that the client's problem is of psychological origin. For example, it may be concluded that if a client's pain is reduced by relaxation training, then her or his pain was caused by stress. If operant conditioning results in a decrease in a client's pain behaviour, then the client's pain may be regarded as being due to a need for attention. A positive response to a psychological intervention does not mean that the pain was only psychological, any more than a positive response to a pharmacological intervention means that the client's pain was only organic. To illustrate, many people experience some pain from an injection. One person may choose to use a local anaesthetic to reduce this pain. Another person may use distraction to reduce the pain. In both cases, these very different approaches may have a positive effect on the pain. The cause of the pain, the injection, is the same.

Neither the client's behaviour nor her or his response to treatment provides definitive information about the cause of pain. A positive response to treatment can be attributed to many interacting factors. When one thing changes, the entire system behaves differently.

CONSIDER LONG-TERM LIFESTYLE CHANGES

There are three important aspects to preparing a client to make life-long changes: readiness to change psychologically, physical preparedness, and acceptance of pain as potentially a long-term issue. Someone whose pain has become chronic may have seen many different health practitioners, tried many interventions and had many disappointments. This client may have difficulty believing that the pain can be reduced or that quality of life will improve. Feelings of hopelessness, mixed with fears and beliefs that changes in behaviours and activities might cause increased pain reduce psychological readiness.

Making long-term lifestyle changes is dependent on readiness to adopt a self-management approach that is not ultimately dependent on health professionals. Dependency on life-style changes and possible need to continue with regular use of pain management strategies may engender concerns about loss of autonomy or self-control. Accepting some degree of dependency with willingness to change may be part of psychological readiness. Recent research in this area has produced a measure of psychological readiness and is beginning to elucidate intervention strategies that may support readiness (Jensen et al 2000, Keefe & Caldwell 1997, Kerns & Rosenberg 2000, Kerns et al 1997).

The physical fitness of someone in chronic pain is usually quite poor, as a good deal of time may have been spent avoiding movements, or causing re-injury by incorrect movement. Such experiences increase fear of movement and tension, and reduce the tolerance of pain. Clients who experience mild increased pain with interventions need to be reassured that this pain is not causing further damage. Physiotherapists and occupational therapists must attend to all of these issues to remove them as obstacles to interventions, particularly interventions that may require long-term lifestyle changes.

Unfortunately, chronic pain often reoccurs for many clients who appear to have recovered from pain. Von Korff and Saunders (1996), who reviewed outcome studies of the course of back pain in primary care, found that the majority of clients with back pain have recurrent pain rather than a single episode of acute or chronic pain. Clients tend to show considerable improvement during the first 4 weeks of treatment but up to 75% continue to have at least mild pain when they complete a treatment programme. At 1-year follow-up, approximately 33% have intermittent pain that is of moderate or severe intensity. Re-occurrence is not a sign of the client's lack of compliance or psychological problems. Nor is re-occurrence an indicator of the failure of treatment.

It may be very helpful for clients to be taught to think of using some intervention strategies preventatively. For example, relaxation may be helpful for current pain, but continued regular use may help reduce the likelihood of re-occurrence. Modification of work and home environments to reduce pain hazards will have current and future benefit. Maintaining an active lifestyle and keeping a positive outlook are important to insure that a beneficial effect is maintained and to reduce the probability of re-occurrence of pain.

INVOLVE THE CLIENT'S FAMILY WHENEVER POSSIBLE

Identifying the client's family is not always straightforward. The family structure may be the traditional nuclear family structure (parents with or without children) but structures can be quite complex. Sometimes children may have two nuclear families, if the biological parents have divorced and established new families. The family may include extended family (parents, grandparents, siblings, and so on). The partners may be homosexual. Sometimes a person's friend is the most significant source of trusted advocacy and support. It is most useful to identify the family from the client's perspective.

Therapists are sometimes unsure of whether to involve the family in their work with the client. If the client is a child, sometimes having a parent present may make the situation worse. The same concern may also exist if a partner has an overly solicitous spouse. Family members are often very concerned about helping the client but they are unsure about how to do so. They may worry that if a client does too much, then further injury or tissue damage may occur. Consequently, families may provide too much assistance and have low expectations from clients, particularly early in the onset of pain.

As pain persists, families may also become increasingly frustrated and even resentful even though they still want to be helpful. Families may be struggling with their own sense of loss and disappointment because of changes within the family. Roles and responsibilities in the family may change. The family may feel that much of their time together is dominated by the problem of pain. Families may also worry about the future and what it holds for them, particularly if there have been role changes in paid employment or financial difficulties. As a result, considerable interpersonal stress can occur among family members.

Families can benefit considerably from intervention that reduces the stress of living with the problem of chronic pain (Kerns & Payne 1996). The family requires sufficient information about the family member's pain and how they can best help. They may have misconceptions about its nature and what can be expected. Often, the family will be uncertain about how much assistance is really helpful for the client. The family may very well be assuming more responsibility than is necessary and the client may benefit from more support and encouragement to resume some tasks.

The family and client may need guidelines about when to talk about pain and when to put pain aside. Ignoring comments about pain may cause the family member to feel more isolated and may increase complaining. On the other hand, giving excessive attention is fatiguing for family members and may increase the client's level of disability. Scheduling a daily 15-minute period to ask and talk about pain provides an opportunity for comfort and support that can be mutually satisfying.

Family members often need help about planning activities. Frequently pain is unpredictable in its onset. The family needs an agreement about whether it is acceptable for them to carry on with a planned outing even if the affected family member is unable to go due to unexpected exacerbation of pain.

Family members may also need to have a better understanding of the nature of the client's pain. Family members may have had few opportunities to ask health professionals about the client's pain. They may doubt its legitimacy. They may have fears about underlying causes. They may be concerned about the client's mental health. Some couples may experience sexual difficulties because of pain. Information about alternative positioning, use of pillows or other strategies may be helpful. In some cases, family members may benefit from counselling or family therapy if other problems, such as marital stress or other preexisting psychosocial problems, compound the difficulty in adjusting to chronic pain.

There is some evidence that involvement of the family is helpful. Children prefer to have a parent present for interventions that may be painful (von Baeyer 1997). However, unless therapists actively involve parents and provide them with some guidance about what help would be beneficial, the actual presence of the parent may not be supportive (von Baeyer 1997).

In some instances, the client may prefer not to involve the family. It is difficult to involve family if the family does not want to be involved in the client's program. These wishes should be respected, but family involvement may need to be discussed again at a later date if their involvement would be important to recovery from pain. Sometimes family are uncomfortable with one-to-one intervention and show more interest in educational programmes intended for families. If family problems are long-standing then intensive family therapy may be necessary.

RECOGNIZE DUAL RESPONSIBILITIES AND OBLIGATIONS

Occupational therapists and physiotherapists in many countries adopt a client-centred perspective as a basis for practice. A client-centred practice places the client and his or her needs, concerns and preferences, at the centre of assessment and intervention (Gerteis et al 1993, Law 1998). The therapist has a responsibility and an obligation to provide services that are meaningful and relevant to the client. On the other hand, a therapist is also an employee. Professional obligations towards the client may conflict with the expectations of the employer.

This dilemma can be considerable for therapists who work with people experiencing chronic pain. To illustrate, a client-centred therapist will assume that clients with pain are truthful about their pain and its ramifications on daily life. Nevertheless, the therapist may feel an onus to be alert to clients whose pain complaints are influenced by compensation issues or litigation. Other therapists may be urged to identify clients who are malingerers and do not have a legitimate pain problem that necessitates intervention. These concerns are influenced by a need to insure that compensation funds and costly pain services are not provided for clients who would be better served by some other approach. In some settings, therapists may be asked to complete an assessment for an employer or may be requested to give a copy of the report to the employer. The therapist may be required to provide evidence in a legal context about the client's assessment and progress in therapy.

These competing perspectives mean that therapists can at times be in a conflict of interest because they may be weighing assessment strategies and intervention options in the direction of the employer or insurer's needs, rather than the needs of the client. As Merskey (1999) argued:

The best interests of an insurance company lie in getting the insured person back to health and strength, and in establishing that the insured person will receive treatment directed to her employability. That, too, is in the interest of the insured. Nevertheless, patients are more interested than insurance companies in relieving pain, but in order to satisfy the companies, clinics have to provide programmes which offer to remove disability rather than necessarily remove pain. In fact one aim is often sacrificed for the sake of another. The considerable popularity of behavioural programmes in the USA may have something to do with the need to talk to insurance companies in terms which encourage them to provide funds for treatment of the affected individuals (Merskey 1999 p 941).

These problems may be more prevalent for occupational therapists and physiotherapists who work in return-to-work or work-hardening programmes with third party payers such as insurance companies or compensation boards.

The problem is not resolved by choosing one or the other perspective. Therapists need to be attentive to the dilemma on a client-by-client basis. It is not helpful, and can be destructive and counter-therapeutic, to suspect all clients with pain of potential malingering.

Therapists must be careful to identify whether the primary client is the company or the person with pain, particularly since patients are likely to assume that they are the client. It must be clear to all parties what information will be disclosed, to whom and under what conditions.

CONDUCT AN ETHICAL PRACTICE

Some ethical issues concerning pain management were addressed in Chapter 1 and also earlier in this chapter. In addition, therapists must recognize the inherent imbalance of power between a therapist and a client. The therapist is typically perceived as an expert with specialized knowledge about pain. Therapists, and other health professionals, have considerable influence and power in determining access to interventions, and other factors involved in compensation and litigation. In addition, occupational therapists and physical therapists, as well as the pain team, will obtain considerable personal information about the client and her or his daily life. In many chapters of this text, we identified misconceptions and biases that can interfere with providing effective assessment and intervention for pain. The subjectivity of pain and its multidimensional nature, along with the economic and political environment in which intervention for pain occurs, increases the possibility that some clients may be harmed more than helped by the health service that they receive.

On the other hand, the client has the power to implement suggestions in a careful and considered way, or not, with the decision influenced by many factors including the quality of the client–therapist relationship. The therapist is relatively powerless in actually implementing suggestions.

Therapists must work towards a collaborative therapeutic relationship with their clients, that recognizes the rights and responsibilities of each person. It is also very important for therapists to be reflective of their own personal biases about people in pain, particularly vulnerable clients who may come from a racial, ethnic or socioeconomic class that is different from the therapist, or clients who may have special needs that require more time and care to form an accurate assessment and intervention plan. Therapists should ensure that their assessments about all clients are supported by reliable and valid evidence, and that their proposed interventions are in collaboration with the client and are in his or her best interests.

Ethical dilemmas, when they occur, are difficult to manage alone. Consultation and discussion with others is often helpful to clarify ethical issues. Such discussion must be open to diverse points of view in order to have the most comprehensive understanding of all perspectives. Professional bodies can also clarify standards of professional practice that would apply to specific situations. Institutions may also have ethics committee that can provide advice and assistance.

DO NOT CAUSE HARM

Clients can be harmed by wasting time and financial resources on interventions that are not effective or helpful. Therapists must also be attentive to the possibility of causing pain or injury unintentionally through interventions. Some pain may be due to reactivation of physical activity if the client has become deconditioned. Such pain should be explained to the client. Safety considerations for interventions are discussed in Chapters 9 to 16. Injury, pain due to interventions may increase the client's fear and anxiety about recovery and may impair the client–therapist relationship (Madjar 1998).

PARTICIPATE IN RESEARCH, EDUCATION AND PROFESSIONAL PAIN ASSOCIATIONS

Pain is a very common but complex problem. Our understanding of pain is continually evolving. Remaining current in this field is essential for a conscientious therapist who is committed to providing the best possible care for clients. Therapists can ensure that their understanding of pain is current through research, continuing education, and involvement in professional associations.

Research

Occupational therapists and physiotherapists must remain cognizant of pain research and use this research to inform practice. Some pain research will be published in occupational therapy, physiotherapy or rehabilitation journals. Other papers will appear in speciality journals concerned with children, ageing, women's health, or journals focused on clients with specific problems. There are also many pain-specific journals including 'Pain', the 'Clinical Journal of Pain', the 'Journal of Pain', the 'Journal of Pain and Symptom Management', 'Pain Research & Management', the 'European Journal of Pain', and others. Taking time to read the professional pain literature will expose the reader to new and often controversial ideas that have implications for the provision of care.

As more occupational therapists and physiotherapists pursue graduate education, they are also becoming active researchers in pain and other fields. Participating in research as principal investigators, co-investigators, or collaborators in pain research is essential to ensure that issues relevant to rehabilitation are considered in research plans.

Some assessments, measures and interventions used by occupational therapists and physiotherapists have not been adequately examined in research. For example, there is little published data in peer-reviewed journals about the reliability and validity of many of the functional capacity evaluations used in work-hardening settings. Some interventions are not sufficiently evaluated, and their degree of effectiveness for clients with varying problems is often unknown. Research in these areas is essential to provide the knowledge needed for evidence-based decision-making. Reliance on other health professionals to conduct such research is likely to mean that rehabilitation research relevant to physiotherapy or occupational therapy will be scant. In addition, occupational therapists and physiotherapists have a great deal to contribute to broader interdisciplinary areas of research that will advance our understanding and care for people with pain.

Education and other professional activities

Ensuring that occupational therapists and physiotherapists are consumers of research is one way of ensuring delivery of quality care. Another way is through participation in pain-related associations and conferences.

The International Association for the Study of Pain (IASP) is a multidisciplinary body of people representing more than 20 professions and more than 90 countries. Members of IASP receive 15 issues of 'Pain' yearly. In addition, they receive the IASP Newsletter and Clinical Updates (newsletter). The IASP

Newsletter provides information about the business and affairs of the association, timely issues in pain, upcoming meetings and recent pain publications. Clinical Updates are focused on the practitioner and provide research summaries with clinical implications. A November 1998 issue of Clinical Updates focused on physical therapy for chronic pain (Harding et al 1998). IASP organizes a World Pain Congress every 3 years (2002 in San Diego, California and 2005 in Sydney, Australia). Many countries have a national pain society that is affiliated with IASP, and these societies commonly hold yearly conferences.

There are also several Special Interest Groups (SIGs) affiliated with IASP. SIGs are multiprofessional and focused on a particular area of concern. At present the following SIGs exist: Pain in Childhood, Pain and the Sympathetic Nervous System, Clinical-Legal Issues in Pain, Rheumatic Pain, Systematic Review in Pain, Placebo, and, Sex, Gender, and Pain. Plans are also currently underway to establish a SIG in rehabilitation issues.

IASP frequently sponsors international and interdisciplinary task-forces or ad hoc committees to examine and address particular areas of concern. The outcomes of these groups are usually published in the IASP Newsletter, or as books. This work typically involves an international and interdisciplinary group of people. The work of a task-force or committee is approved by the IASP Council before publication. These publications provide timely and important information, but occasionally they can be controversial. For example, the publication, 'Back Pain in the Workplace' (Fordyce 1995) is the result of a task-force on this topic. This document has been severely criticized for primarily reflecting a behavioural perspective and ignoring considerable research that was contrary to the position of the task-force (Teasell 1997, Teasell & Merskey 1997, Thompson 1997). The report was not supported by the Canadian Pain Society. Nevertheless, this document and the critical papers that have been written about it provide an invaluable source of critical reflection and debate about an extremely important clinical problem, back pain.

At present, occupational therapists remain a small group of 19 members in IASP. However, the number of physiotherapists has increased dramatically in the last few years and is now approximately 200 members. Increasing participation by occupational therapists and physiotherapists in the work of IASP and its

---

Box 8.5 Contact information for IASP

International Association for the Study of Pain
909 Northeast 43rd Street, Suite 306
Seattle, WA 98105
USA
Telephone: +1-206-547-6409
Fax: +1-206-547-1703
Website: http://www.halcyon.com/iasp
Email: IASP@locke.hs.washington.edu

---

related organizations, conducting workshops and participating in presentations will ensure that issues of relevance and concern to occupational therapists and physiotherapists, and their clients, will be addressed. It is important that occupational therapists and physiotherapists become visible and contributing players in the generation of new knowledge and information about the care for people with pain. More information about IASP and its affiliates can be obtained by post, telephone, fax, email or the internet (see Box 8.5).

CONCLUSION

Occupational therapists and physiotherapists have different roles and responsibilities in their work with clients who have pain. Nevertheless, there are areas of overlap and shared obligations. There are also generic principles of practice that are common to both professions and indeed may have relevance for other members of a pain team. In this chapter, we reviewed these principles and the rationale on which they are based.

Study questions/questions for revision

1. Why is it important for the family to be involved in the client's care?
2. What are some of the beliefs and fears associated with pharmacological management of pain?
3. What are the hallmarks of evidence-based practice?
4. Why is long-term lifestyle change important for the client with pain?
5. How might aggressive management of acute pain be of benefit for the client?

ACKNOWLEDGEMENTS

The authors express their appreciation to Ms Jennifer Landry (occupational therapist) and Drs Allen Finley (anaesthesiologist), Patrick McGrath (psychologist), Frank New (psychiatrist), and Stephan Schug (anaesthesiologist) for their critical reviews of this chapter.

REFERENCES

Anand K J S, Hickey P R 1987 Pain and its effects in the human neonate and fetus. New England Journal of Medicine 317: 1321–1329

Arena J G, Blanchard E B 1996 Biofeedback and relaxation therapy for chronic pain disorders. In: Gatchel R J, Turk D C (eds) Psychological Approaches to Pain Management: a practitioner's handbook. Guildford Press, New York, pp 179–130

Becker N, Sjogren P, Bech P, Olsen A K, Eriksen J 2000 Treatment outcome of chronic non-malignant pain patients managed in a Danish multidisciplinary pain centre compared to general practice: a randomised controlled trial. Pain 84: 203–211

Bradley L A 1996 Cognitive–behavioral therapy for chronic pain. In: Gatchel R J, Turk D C (eds) Psychological Approaches to Pain Management: a practioner's handbook. Guildford Press, New York, pp 131–147

Brescia F, Portenoy R, Ryan M, Krasnoff L, Gray G 1992 Pain, opioid use, and survival in hospitalized patients with advanced cancer. Journal of Clinical Oncology 10: 149–155

Campbell M A, McGrath P J 1997 Use of medication by adolescents for the management of menstrual discomfort. Archives of Pediatric Adolescent Medicine 151: 905–913

Canadian Association of Occupational Therapists 1999 Joint position statement on evidence-based occupational therapy. Canadian Journal of Occupational Therapy 66: 267–272

Cherny N I, Portenoy R K 1999 Practical issues in the management of cancer pain. In: Wall P D, Melzack R (eds) Textbook of Pain, 4th edn. Churchill Livingstone, Edinburgh, pp 1479–1522

Coderre T J, Melzack R 1987 Cutaneous hyperanalgesia: contributions of the peripheral and central nervous systems to the increase in pain sensitivity after injury. Brain research 404: 95–106

Cole B, Finch E, Gowland C, Mayo N 1994 Physical Rehabilitation Outcome Measures. Canadian Physiotherapy Association, Toronto

Diamond A, Coniam S 1997 The Management of Chronic Pain, 2nd edn. Oxford University Press, Oxford

Egan M, Dubouloz C-J, von Zweck C, Vallerand J 1998 The client-centred evidence-based practice of occupational therapy. Canadian Journal of Occupational Therapy 65: 136–143

Finley G A, McGrath P J, Forward S P, McNeill G, Fitzgerald P 1996 Parents' management of children's pain following 'minor' surgery. Pain 64: 83–87

Flemming K 1998 Asking answerable questions. Evidence-Based Nursing 1(2): 36–37

Flor H, Fydrich T, Turk D C 1992 Efficacy of mulidisciplinary pain treatment centres: a meta-analytic review. Pain 49: 221–230

Fordyce W E (ed) 1995 Back pain in the workplace. IASP Press, Seattle

Fordyce W E, Roberts A H, Sternbach R A 1985 The behavioral management of chronic pain: a response to critics. Pain 22: 112–125

Fuchs P N, Gamsa A 1997 Chronic use of opioids for nonmalignant pain: a prospective study. Pain Research & Management 2: 101–107

Gerteis M, Edgman-Levitan S, Daley J, Delbanco T L (eds) 1993 Through the Patient's Eyes. Understanding and promoting patient centered care. The Jossey-Bass Health Series, San Francisco

Gourlay G K, Cherry D 1991 Response to controversy corner: 'Can opioids be successfully used to treat severe pain in nonmalignant conditions?'. Clinical Journal of Pain 7: 347–349

Gross A R, Aker P D, Goldsmith C H, Peloso P 1996 Conservative management of mechanical neck disorders. A systematic overview and meta-analysis. Online Journal of Current Clinical Trials, Doc No 200–201: 34457

Grunau R V E, Whitfield M F, Petrie J H, Fryer E L 1994 Early pain experience, child and family factors, as precursors of somatization: a prospective study of extremely premature and full-term children. Pain 56: 353–359

Harding V R, Simmonds M J, Watson P J 1998 Physical therapy for chronic pain. Pain Clinical Updates VI(3): 1–4

Harman K 2000 Neuroplasticity and the development of persistent pain. Physiotherapy Canada 52: 64–71

Hayes R, McGrath J 1998 Evidence-based practice: The Cochrane Collaboration and occupational therapy. Canadian Journal of Occupational Therapy 65: 144–151

Helewa A, Walker J M 2000 Critical Evaluation of Research in Physical Rehabilitation: towards evidence-based practice. WB Saunders Company, Philadelphia

Jensen M, McFarland D 1993 Increasing the reliability and validity of pain intensity measurement in chronic pain patients. Pain 55: 195–203

Jensen M P, Nielsen W R, Romano J M, Hill M L, Turner J A 2000 Further evaluation of the pain stages of change questionnaire: the transtheoretical model of change useful for patients with chronic pain? Pain 86: 255–264

Keefe F J, Caldwell D S 1997 Cognitive behavioral control of arthritis pain. Medical Clinics of North America 81: 277–290

Keefe F J, Beaupré, Gil K M 1996 Group therapy for patients with chronic pain. In: Gatchel R J, Turk D C (eds) Psychological Approaches to Pain Management: a practitioner's handbook. Guildford Press, New York, pp 259–281

Kerns R D, Payne A 1996 Treating families of chronic pain patients. In: Gatchel R J, Turk D C (eds) Psychological Approaches to Pain Management: a practitioner's handbook. Guildford Press, New York, pp 283–304

Kerns R D, Rosenberg R 2000 Predicting responses to self-management treatments for chronic pain: application of the pain stages of change model. Pain 84: 49–55

Kerns R D, Rosenberg R, Jamison R N, Caudill M A, Haythornwaite J 1997 Readiness to adopt a self-management approach to chronic pain: the Pain Stages of Change Questionnaire (PSOCQ). Pain 72: 227–234

Kerr K 2000 Relaxation techniques: a critical review. Critical Reviews in Physical and Rehabilitation Medicine 12: 51–89

Law M (ed) 1998 Client-centered occupational therapy. Slack, Thorofare, New Jersey

Law M, Baum C 1998 Evidence-based occupational therapy. Canadian Journal of Occupational Therapy 65: 131–135

Letts L, Law M, Pollock N, Stewart D, Westmorland M, Philpot A, Bosch J 1999 A programme evaluation workbook for occupational therapists: an evidence-based practice tool. Canadian Association of Occupational Therapy, Ottawa, Ontario

Liebeskind J C 1991 Pain can kill. Pain 44: 3–4

Madjar I 1998 Giving comfort and inflicting pain. International Institute for Qualitative Methodology, Edmonton, Alberta

Mason L W, Goolkasian P, McCain G A 1998 Evaluation of multimodal treatment program for fibromyalgia. Journal of Behavioral Medicine 21: 163–178

McCaffery M, Beebe A 1989 Pain – clinical manual for nursing practice. CV Mosby, St. Louis

McGrath P J, Unruh A M 1987 Pain in Children and Adolescents. Elsevier, Amsterdam

McIntyre D L, McAuley C A, Parker-Taillon D 1999 Canadian physiotherapy research and evidence-based practice initiative in the 1990s. Physical Therapy Reviews 4: 127–137

Merskey H 1999 Pain and psychological medicine. In: Wall P D, Melzack R (eds) Textbook of Pain. Churchill Livingstone, Edinburgh, pp 929–949

Minor M A, Hewett J E, Webel R R 1989 Efficacy of physical conditioning exercise in patients with rheumatoid arthritis or osteoarthritis. Arthritis & Rheumatism 32: 1397–1405

Occupational Therapy Evidence-based Practice Research Group 1999 The effectiveness of cognitive–behavioural interventions with people with chronic pain. A critical review of the literature. Available at http://fhs.mcmaster.ca/rehab

Polatin P B 1996 Integration of pharmacotherapy with psychological treatment of chronic pain. In: Gatchel R J, Turk D C (eds) Psychological Approaches to Pain Management: a practioner's handbook. Guildford Press, New York, pp 305–328

Pollock N 1998 The Cochrane Collaboration. Canadian Journal of Occupational Therapy 65: 168–170

Portenoy R K 1990 Chronic opioid pain in nonmalignant pain. (Review) Journal of Pain & Symptom Management 5: S46–62

Portenoy R K 1996 Opioid therapy for chronic nonmalignant pain. Pain Research & Management 1: 17–28

Purdy A, McGrath P J, Cambell M A, Hennigar A W 1997 Decision-making in patients using sumatriptan. Headache 37: 327

Ritchie J E 1999 Using qualitative research to enhance the evidence-based practice of health care providers. Australian Journal of Physiotherapy 45: 251–256

Russo C M, Brose W G 1998 Chronic pain. Annual Reviews of Medicine 49: 123–133

Saunders C, Platt M 1999 Pain and impending death. In: Wall P D, Melzack R (eds) Textbook of Pain, 4th edn. Churchill Livingstone, Edinburgh, pp 1113–1122

Snider L 1999 Practice makes perfect. Occupational Therapy Now March/April: 11–12

Stewart D 1999 Evidence for occupational therapy – the process of critical review. Occupational Therapy Now July/August: 17–19

Straker L 1999 A hierarchy of evidence for informing physiotherapy practice. Australian Journal of Physiotherapy 45: 231–233

Taddio A, Goldbach M, Ipp M, Stevens B, Koren G 1995 Effects of neonatal circumcision on pain response during vaccination in boys. Lancet 1(345): 291–292

Teasell R W 1997 The denial of chronic pain. Pain Research & Management 2: 89–91

Teasell R W, Merskey H 1997 Chronic pain disability in the workplace. Pain Research & Management 2: 197–205

Thompson E 1997 Back pain: bankrupt expertise and new directions. Pain Research & Management 2: 195–196

Twycross R G 1999 Opioids. In: Wall P D, Melzack R (eds) Textbook of Pain, 4th edn. Edinburgh, Churchill Livingstone, pp 1187–1214

Unruh A M, Campbell M A 1999 Gender variations in children's pain experiences. In: McGrath P J, Finley G A (eds) Chronic and Recurrent Pain in Children and Adolescents. IASP Press, Seattle

Unruh A M., McGrath P J 2000 Pain in children: psychosocial issues. In: Melvin J L, Wright F V (eds) Pediatric Rheumatic Diseases, Rheumatic Rehabilitation Series, Vol. 3. American Occupational Therapy Association, Bethseda, Maryland, pp 141–168

Unruh A M, Ritchie J A 1998 Development of the Pain Appraisal Inventory: psychometric properties. Pain Research and Management 3: 105–110

Unruh A M, Ritchie J A, Merskey H 1999 Does gender affect pain appraisal and coping strategies? Clinical Journal of Pain 15: 31–40

van der Heijden G J, van der Windt D A, de Winter A F 1997 Physiotherapy for patients with soft tissue shoulder disorders: a systematic review of randomised clinical trials. British Medical Journal 315: 25–30

Vanderkooy J, Bach B, Gross A 1999 A clinical effort toward maximizing evidence-based practice. Physiotherapy Canada 51: 273–279

von Baeyer C L 1997 Presence of parents during painful procedures. Pediatric Pain Letter 1: 56–59

von Korff M, Saunders K 1996 The course of back pain in primary care. Spine 21: 2833–2837

Wall P D 1984 Introduction. In: Wall P D, Melzack R (eds) Textbook of Pain, 1st ed. Churchill Livingstone, Edinburgh, pp 1–16

Wall P D 1999 Introduction. In: Wall P D, Melzack R (eds) Textbook of pain, 4th ed. Churchill Livingstone, Edinburgh, pp 1–16

Weissman D, Haddox J 1989 Opioid pseudoaddiction: an iatrogenic syndrome. Pain 36: 363–366

Westmorland M 1998 Five steps to developing an evidence-based practice. The National: The Newsletter of the Canadian Association of Occupational Therapists 15(1): 5–7

9

Psychologically based pain management strategies

Jenny Strong   Anita M. Unruh

OVERVIEW

Pain is often assumed to be a physical phenomenon, and to require chiefly physical methods of control. It may also seem that psychologically based management approaches would be best for clients who are thought to have psychologically based pain problems. However, as shown in Chapters 1, 4, 5, 6 and 8, other factors such as personality, environment, culture and personal history affect a person's experience and expression of pain. Pain is clearly a psychological and a physical phenomenon that benefits from intervention.

Attention to psychological management of pain should occur in association with physical management of pain. In fact, when one thinks about it, a therapist cannot conduct any intervention without at the same time doing something that has a psychological impact. A beneficial impact is more likely if the application is guided by an understanding of psychologically based management strategies. An occupational therapist or physical therapist who provides a physical modality or an assistive device to a client, without some background consideration of psychological aspects, may not be providing the best available intervention for the client. Psychological aspects of intervention are important for all clients, including those whose pain is caused by obvious tissue damage such as clients with an acute strain after a sporting injury, clients with pain following surgery or in association with other medical procedures, or clients with pain due to disease.

In Chapter 4 of this book, the psychological, behavioural and environmental dimensions of the pain experience were explained. This chapter will focus on an in-depth description of psychologically based management strategies for pain, and the principles and concepts behind them. There are two important approaches to psychologically based pain management and both of these approaches are derived from behavioural theory:

- Operant conditioning
- Cognitive–behavioural therapy.

Other psychological approaches include:

- Psychotherapy
- Group therapy
- Hypnosis and imagery
- Biofeedback and relaxation
- Family therapy.

Some of these approaches are usually provided by psychologists, psychiatrists or social workers (e.g. hypnosis, psychotherapy and family therapy). Other approaches are incorporated by occupational therapists and physical therapists into broader pain management programmes (e.g. operant conditioning, cognitive–behavioural therapy, relaxation, group therapy). Relaxation and biofeedback are covered in detail in Chapter 15, and will not be discussed in this chapter. A number of specific skill areas of intervention by occupational therapists and physical therapists that require an appreciation of psychological principles will be outlined. Client education, goal-setting, self-esteem development, coping skills training, and self-efficacy development (see Box 9.1) will then be considered. Pacing, which is an important component of psychological strategies used by occupational therapists and physical therapists, is discussed in Chapter 15. This chapter will conclude by offering some guidelines about which strategies are most useful for particular types of pain.

Learning objectives

At the end of this chapter, students will:

1. Be aware of intervention strategies that will promote active client involvement in a pain management programme.
2. Understand the effects of conditioned learning on the establishment or maintenance of pain behaviours.
3. Understand the ways in which pain behaviours and illness behaviour are manifested.
4. Know the principles of an operant approach to pain management.
5. Know the principles of cognitive–behavioural pain management.
6. Understand how psychological approaches are affected by the therapist–client relationship.

PAIN BEHAVIOUR AND ILLNESS BEHAVIOUR

Pain behaviour and illness behaviour are common targets in a psychologically based pain management programme, because they exacerbate disability and suffering and can interfere with progress in regaining function and better quality of life for the client.

Pain behaviours can be categorized as:

- Verbal pain responses (moaning, sighing)
- Non-verbal pain behaviours (grimacing, rubbing, limping, wearing braces or splints)
- General activity level (sitting, lying down)
- Use of pain medications (Sanders 1996).

Most pain behaviours are an unconscious response to pain. If a person falls down some stairs, moaning and

---

Box 9.1 Key terms defined

Operant conditioning – a theoretical model that overt behaviour is significantly influenced by the consequences of the behaviour and the contexts in which the behaviour occurs (Sanders 1996).

Pain behaviours – a set of behaviours which people who have pain commonly use to signal to others that they are in pain and distressed.

Illness behaviour – the way symptoms are interpreted individually and acted upon idiosyncratically, according to a person's particular nature (Mechanic & Volkart 1960).

Abnormal illness behaviour – the persistence of inappropriate behaviours about one's health, in spite of having been given a clear explanation of the condition by a health professional (Pilowsky 1978).

Avoidance – the performance of a behaviour or strategy that postpones or averts the presentation of an aversive (unpleasant) event.

Fear of pain – the fear of pain has been neatly described by the Fear Avoidance model. 'The fear of any expected evil is worse than the evil itself' (Crombez et al 1999). Fear urges escape from the object of threat and instigates avoidance behaviour.

Fear of movement/re-injury – a fear of movement and physical activity that is wrongfully assumed to cause re-injury.

Self-efficacy – the belief, and the ability to act on the belief, that one has the capacity to positively influence the course of events in one's life.

sitting down would not be an unusual response. The behaviour is an expression of pain and inadvertently conveys to others that the person is in pain. Some behaviours, such as using splints or other aids or taking pain medication, are deliberate and may have been advised.

For most people, pain behaviours diminish as the pain becomes less intense, less upsetting and less disabling. The persistence of pain behaviours over a long period can occur due to inadvertent operant conditioning of the behaviours. In these instances, the pain behaviours themselves may contribute to disability. Operant conditioning is explained in the next section.

Illness behaviour is part of an individual's personal style that has been built up over years through the combination of the person's particular nature and experiences. Medical sociologists Mechanic and Volkart said:

Whether by reason of education, religion, class membership, occupational status, or whatever, some persons will make light of symptoms, shrug them off, and avoid seeking medical care; others will respond to the slightest twinges of pain or discomfort by quickly seeking such medical care as is available (Mechanic & Volkart 1960 p 870).

Illness behaviour can impact on pain in the following ways:

- How symptoms are perceived (e.g. this pain in my gut is unbearable)
- The evaluation of symptom importance (e.g. this pain means I have got cancer)
- Verbal and non-verbal behaviours (e.g. exaggerated limping)
- Self-treatment (e.g. lying down with a hot-water bottle)
- Consultation behaviours (e.g. visiting many doctors and other practitioners)
- Treatment compliance (e.g. giving little credence to a behavioural management programme)
- Usual roles and activities (e.g. not being able to maintain usual roles).

The work of Pilowsky, an Australian psychiatrist, has been instrumental in increasing our understanding of abnormal illness behaviour. Abnormal illness behaviour is the persistence of inappropriate behaviours in regard to one's health, despite having been given a clear and appropriate explanation and management plan by the doctor (Pilowsky 1978). Abnormal illness behaviour can interfere with a client's response to treatment, and may be associated with psychological distress. Illness behaviour refers to a person's thoughts, feelings and overt behaviours. Thus, when examining the illness behaviours of someone in pain,

the implications are that cognitive style and level of functioning need attention, as well as overt behaviours (Pilowsky 1994). Normal illness behaviour might be considered as the client undergoing the following:

1. the client Notices a symptom
2. the client Reports the symptom
3. the client Accepts the need for a particular investigation
4. the client Listens to the diagnosis and recommended treatment
5. the client Decides whether to accept the treatment recommendations
6. the client Complies with the treatment
7. the client Works to get better (Frank New, personal communication).

Abnormal illness behaviour occurs when the client exhibits a marked increase or decrease in these behaviours; for example if a client consults a further four orthopaedic surgeons requesting MRI scans of their lumbar spine after assessment by two surgeons indicates no demonstrable findings; or when a person with sudden, severe chest pain which does not cease at rest fails to seek medical assistance.

The following dimensions of abnormal illness behaviour are determined by the Illness Behaviour Questionnaire:

1. General hypochondriasis
2. Disease conviction
3. Psychological vs somatic concern
4. Affective inhibition
5. Affective disturbance
6. Denial
7. Irritability (Pilowsky & Spence 1981).

These dimensions need to be evaluated in many clients with chronic pain, and considered as an influence on the outcome of a pain management programme.

Waddell and his colleagues (1984) defined illness behaviour as, 'observable and potentially measurable actions and conduct which express and communicate the individual's own perception of disturbed health'. Illness is a composite of the physical problem, psychological distress, and illness behaviour, and exists in a social environment that can be very influential on how the illness is experienced. In examining the pattern of illness behaviours, Waddell et al (1984) suggested that the common feature of all inappropriate symptoms and signs is magnification. Indicators of such abnormal or inappropriate illness behaviour may be:

- A non-anatomical pain drawing
- Description of pain in terms of affective or evaluative words
- Non-dermatomal numbness
- Generalized rather than localized pain
- Superficial tenderness
- Lumbar pain with axial loading
- Regional sensory signs
- Regional motor signs (Waddell et al 1989 p 51).

FEATURES COMMON TO PSYCHOLOGICAL APPROACHES FOR PAIN MANAGEMENT

Turk and Holzman (1986) identified a number of features that are common in different psychological approaches used with people with pain. The seven features are:

- Reconceptualizing: the client is provided with an explanation of the pain which is compatible with the treatment modality or management strategy advocated, for example, using the Gate Control theory of pain to explain how transcutaneous nerve stimulation can close the gate at the spinal cord level.
- Instilling optimism and combating demoralization: by suggesting to clients that the new treatment you are proposing will help them in some way, for example, when recommending the client enter a group to learn new coping skills, giving an example of how a specific skill can help in daily life.
- Individualizing the treatment to suit the client's needs: when a client who is a school teacher is participating in a body mechanics class, applying the principles to particular activities this teacher will use in the classroom.
- Getting the client to play an active role in the treatment and accept some responsibility: asking the client to identify a daily activity of choice to use in a reconditioning programme.
- Having clients actively participate to acquire new skills: if an ongoing exercise programme is recommended for general fitness, having clients arrange for themselves to enrol at a local gym and participate in gym classes.
- Encouraging a client's self-efficacy: instead of telling the client that he can lift a 10 kg weight as part of the work routine, give him safe, supervised experiences of success in doing this task.
- Enable the client to acknowledge her or his successes: for example, if the client is discharged from a pain management programme walking independently and without adaptive equipment,

after coming in to the programme with a neck brace, elbow crutches and working splints, help the client to recognize this accomplishment as his own success rather than as the therapist's success.

Use of these features will enable physical therapists and occupational therapists to promote active involvement of clients in therapy. Harding and Williams (1998) also identified these features as important for physical therapy practice in pain management.

BEHAVIOURAL MODELS AND PSYCHOLOGICALLY BASED INTERVENTIONS

There are four primary behavioural models: the operant conditioning model (based on the work of Skinner 1953, 1989), the classical conditioning model (Pavlov 1927), the social learning model (Bandura 1969, 1986), and the cognitive–behavioural model (Cameron & Meichenbaum 1980). These models have been applied to many areas, including pain, to understand the relationships between behaviour, cognition and emotion, and to develop psychologically based interventions.

Operant conditioning has been used extensively in pain to explain and treat disabling pain behaviour. It is discussed in more detail in the next section. The classical conditioning model has been used to explain the relationship between fear, avoidance and pain, which was discussed in more detail in Chapter 7. The social learning model has been helpful in understanding how pain response and behaviour is influenced by the modelling of others and can be changed by positive modelling. Group therapy often utilizes a social learning model. The cognitive–behavioural model has been used extensively to develop cognitive–behavioural strategies of intervention. We will discuss operant conditioning and the cognitive–behavioural model in more detail because they are the most prevalent psychological models used in pain management.

Operant conditioning

There are three essential components of operant conditioning: positive reinforcement, negative reinforcement and punishment. If a behaviour is followed systematically by a reinforcer, then the subsequent rate of occurrence will tend to increase. A reinforcer may be positive or negative but in both cases the behaviour will tend to increase in response to the reinforcement. For example, a client's complaints of pain may be repeatedly followed by solicitous attention (positive reinforcement). If the attention is desirable to the person, then complaining of pain may continue. Solicitous attention is a positive reinforcer in this instance. On the other hand, a client may experience considerable criticism except when she or he complains of pain. In this case, complaints of pain are increased by a negative reinforcer, criticism.

Another example would be, if a person hangs out the washing (a task that is not enjoyed) and this activity result in painful muscle twinges and spasms (a negative reinforcer), then pain complaints may be increased because undesirable tasks could then be avoided. If complaints of pain are followed systematically by adverse consequences, in effect punished, then the behaviour often decreases. Timing of reinforcers is crucial, both in understanding how a pattern of behaviour develops, and in designing a programme to change it. Initially, reinforcers must immediately follow the behaviour if they are to be effective, but may follow less closely or more intermittently over time.

As is implied in the preceding discussion, operant approaches are used to reduce pain behaviours. In operant–behavioural terms, pain is thought of as an unpleasant experience that is signalled to others by pain behaviours. Pain behaviours may be verbal, non-verbal, or related to changes in activity. Medication use is also often considered as a pain behaviour in this model.

It is important to remember that some degree of pain behaviour is inevitable if one has pain. Pain behaviour that is excessive and contributes to disability is the primary concern. For example, one man came into the pain clinic wearing a neck collar, soft wrist splints, knee splints, used crutches and has a friend pushing his wheelchair behind him. His pain was described as 'total body pain' in the referral letter to the Pain Clinic. This person could be considered to have excessive pain behaviour.

Elton et al (1983) proposed a descriptive model of reinforcers of chronic pain. This model is illustrated in Figure 9.1. Figure 9.2 uses the model to illustrate the use of operant conditioning in chronic pain based on Mrs K (Box 9.2) (Mrs K's case was first published in Strong 1996, and is reprinted here with permission).

The ostensible precipitator of Mrs K's pain was an incident in which heavy furniture was lifted to vacuum the house. A second possible precipitator was the birth of Mrs K's grandchild. This event resulted in Mrs K's daughter having less available time to devote to her mother. Mrs K developed pain in her lower back along with left-sided sciatica. Mrs K was able to carry out her personal activities of daily living, but there was inhibition of her normal instrumental activities of daily living. Mrs K also avoided aversive situations such as car rides to the farm on weekends, because she found the pain intolerable. She became invalided by the pain.

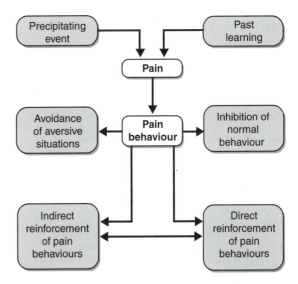

Figure 9.1 Reinforcement interactions maintaining chronic pain (from Elton et al 1983, Psychological control of pain. © Grune & Stratton, Sydney, with kind permission).

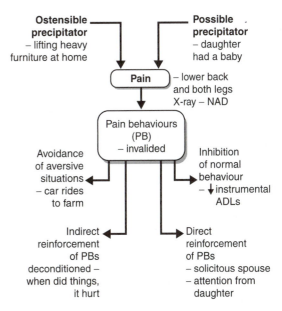

Figure 9.2 Operant conditioning in chronic pain in the case of Mrs K.

Direct reinforcement of her pain behaviours came from the solicitousness of her spouse. Her daughter gave her increased solicitous attention, and her husband did not spend his weekends at the farm. Indirect reinforcement of her pain behaviours arose due to her rapid deconditioning, so that when she did attempt to do an activity, it hurt.

Box 9.2   Case example – Mrs K

Medical history
Mrs K, a 58-year-old woman developed low back pain and left-sided sciatica following a lifting injury at home 4 years prior to this hospitalization. 2 years ago, she had an L5–S1 disc excision. On this second presentation to hospital, she had low back pain with left-sided sciatica with radiation to the left buttock and left posterior thigh and posterolateral calf with radiation toward the ankle. There was an associated poorly localized paraesthesia in the calf and foot. Myelogram findings provided no significant evidence of disc protrusion.

Assessment
Performance system
Pain intensity. 8/10 on the Box Scale, where 0=no pain, and 10=worst possible pain. This was a high self-report of pain.
Functional ability/disability. Pain Disability index – 25/70. This was a low score.
Pain description. Words chosen on the McGill Pain Questionnaire (Melzack 1975) were burning, stinging, aching, miserable, radiating and drawing.

Volitional system
Survey of Pain Attitudes Revised (SOPAR)
SOPAR Solicitude 16/24
SOPAR Medical cure 22/24
SOPAR Emotional link 15/24
SOPAR Disability 5/16
SOPAR Medication 12/16
SOPAR Pain control 11/36.
These scores indicated a high belief in a medical cure, a belief that medication would help her pain, a need for solicitude and support, yet low disability from the pain. She also had a low belief that she could do anything to help control her pain.

Coping Strategy Questionnaire (CSQ)
CSQ Diverting attention 16/36
CSQ Reinterpreting pain sensations 8/36
CSQ Catastrophizing 14/36
CSQ Ignoring sensations 17/36
CSQ Praying/hoping 23/36
CSQ Coping self-statements 21/36
CSQ Increased behavioural activities 24/36
CSQ Pain control 3/6
CSQ Pain decrease 3/6.

Beck Depression Inventory (Beck et al 1961) 10/63. Kerns and Haythornthwaite (1988) suggest that a score between 0 and 9 indicates no depression, a score between 10 and 17 indicates mild depression, and a score greater than or equal to 18 indicates depression. Using these criteria, Mrs K might have been mildly depressed.

Illness Behaviour Questionnaire (IBQ). IBQ Denial 3 [as compared to an Adelaide General Practice sample mean score of 2.91, and an Adelaide Pain Clinic sample mean score of 3.88 (Pilowsky & Spence 1983)].

Self-efficacy MAPPS. 18/40, where 0=ability to move without limitation, and 40=total inability to do the movements. She reported all movements to be limited by pain.

Habituation system
Occupational roles. Married, lived in own home with husband. Was the primary home-maker. She had two grown children, both daughters, who were married and lived locally.

Interests. She reported few interests. She and her husband had a hobby farm, but she found it difficult to sit for the long drive to the farm at weekends.

Assessment summary
Mrs K described herself as having a minimal level of dysfunction due to the pain. Yet she reported a high level of pain. She was independent in all areas of ADL, particularly personal ADLs. It was in the areas of social activities and recreation that Mrs K expressed some limitations. Her physical mobility was fairly good, yet she did not perform some movements due to her fear of pain. She could sit for an hour without distress, and could stand for around 30 minutes.

Mrs K had a firm belief in a medical cure for her pain. She thought that medication would help her. She had a strong desire for solicitude, and a low belief in her own ability to manage her pain. She reported using many strategies to try and cope with her pain. She denied having any underlying problems – if it were not for her pain, all in her life would be fine. Her denial score was higher than for a sample of patients attending general practice facilities, but lower than a pain clinic sample.

In terms of life roles, now that her two daughters had married and left home. It seemed that Mrs K felt some sense of loss and rolelessness. It could be that Mrs K experienced pain more intensely due to her feelings of loss. It may be that the pain was a legitimate way to get attention and help. Such somatization of an emotional state is a frequently seen occurrence. The sum of these findings suggest that Mrs K might have been somatizing. She reported a high level of pain, for which she wanted medical help and support from her loved ones. Yet she was not particularly disabled by her pain. She felt she had little control over her pain. She had some role losses in her life, but denied she had any personal/emotional problems. Now that a comprehensive assessment had been made of Mrs K, her pain, her functioning, her volition and her habituation, a management programme which addressed her individual needs could be developed and implemented.

An operant behavioural programme must first identify what functional goals are appropriate for the client, and determine the appropriate reinforcers for desired and unwanted behaviours.

Principles of an operant behavioural programme include:

- The establishment of a treatment contract with the client (Gotestam & Bates 1979). This contract is negotiated between the client, therapist (and significant others). The establishment of such a contract makes explicit the rationale for the therapy, the problems to be worked on, the methods of therapy and the goals of the therapy (Gotestam & Bates 1979).
- The withdrawal, or at least rationalization, of medication, using regular scheduling of medication on a time-contingent basis. Slight reductions in medication are often made using this schedule (Fordyce 1976).
- The engagement of the client in an active program of physical activity based upon carefully prepared performance quotas. These quotas are below the client's observed tolerances for activity duration (such as sitting) and exercise repetitions.
- The use of positive reinforcement of clients for achieving performance quotas, with a gradual increase in quotas. Attention is focused on the client's successes.
- The use of extinction for pain behaviours, such as moaning, bracing, limping and so on, by ignoring pain complaints. In some cases, talking about pain is restricted to agreed-upon times that are of short duration (Keefe & LeFebvre 1994).

Physical activity and exercise has to be engaged in on a 'time-contingent' rather than 'pain-contingent' basis. Thus a baseline of activity tolerance is determined, and then a schedule of exercise or functional activity constructed which includes an increase in quota each day followed by a rest period. Rest is therefore continuously rewarding.

Positive attention of the therapist can also become a reward, and is separate from aspects of pain. Therapists ignore expressions of pain behaviours during the treatment using inattention to extinguish pain behaviour during treatment. Ideally, the gains in exercise or functional behaviour tolerance also are accompanied by improved fitness and mobility, and therefore provide a positive buffer against pain and suffering.

In addition to the above, operant behavioural programs teach clients a number of behavioural coping strategies such as relaxation, with or without biofeedback, and pacing. The reader is referred to Chapter 15 for a full discussion of relaxation and pacing techniques.

In summary, operant conditioning is important in the perpetuation of disability associated with chronic pain, particularly sick-role and avoidance behaviour (Fordyce 1976). An understanding of operant conditioning will avoid the inadvertant reinforcement of pain behaviours, and provide a framework to actively reduce pain behaviour. Unfortunately, many behaviours which are intended to convey caring concern (such as asking 'how is your pain today?' 'is that better?', etc) can increase attention to the pain and maintain pain behaviours. Pain management programmes based on operant conditioning are designed to 'treat excess disability and expressions of suffering' (Fordyce et al 1985 p 115), and not to eliminate or reduce pain intensity.

Safety considerations

Acceptance of a client into an operant behavioural therapy programme only occurs after careful assessment of the client, with all active 'curative' medical treatment, such as surgery, considered and completed. Clients who have pain due to malignancy would be excluded from an operant behavioural programme. Additionally, elderly frail clients with osteoporotic fractures would not be suitable for such programmes. While pain behaviours by clients are 'ignored' and not responded to positively by therapists, they are nonetheless carefully monitored to ensure no concomitant morbidity arises during the exercise/activity programme.

Careful management by the treating physician is necessary if drug withdrawal is part of the programme, with careful observation for problems with withdrawal, especially when clients have been on a combination of analgesics and benzodiazepines.

Recommended application and current evidence

Operant behavioural programmes are typically used with clients with chronic pain of non-cancer origin, such as non-specific low back pain. Slater et al (1997) evaluated the clinical significance of individually delivered, 8-hour operant behavioural treatment provided to 17 clients with back pain of non-cancer origin. A matched comparison group of clients attending an orthopaedic clinic was used in the study. Forty-seven percent of clients who had the operant behavioural treatment showed clinically significant improvement on at least one of the outcome measures of pain, disability and depression, as compared to none of the comparison group. However, the difference was not statistically significant.

Lindstrom, a physiotherapist, and her colleagues (1992) found that clients with subacute low back pain, who participated in a randomized prospective clinical trial of graded activity, utilizing an operant conditioning paradigm, returned to work significantly earlier than did the participants in the control group.

Linton (1982, 1986) provided early evidence supporting the effectiveness of operant behavioural programmes for clients with chronic non-cancer pain. In reviewing five studies that employed operant techniques, he concluded that operant programmes were successful in increasing activity levels, and decreasing medication consumption, and were probably effective in improving mood and pain levels. Turner and Chapman (1982) also provided support for such programmes. A recent Cochrane Review of behavioural treatment for chronic low back pain (van Tulder et al 2000) concluded that this treatment was effective but that it was still unknown what types of clients benefited most from what type of behavioural treatment. It should be noted that in this review, behavioural treatments referred to modification of environmental contingencies and cognitive processes. In other words, the positive effect may be for operant approaches when they are used in combination with other cognitive–behavioural strategies.

In behavioural terms, increasing compliance with treatment in the short term requires:

- Giving instructions with guided performance and shaping if necessary
- Helping the client work out how to fit the activities into the daily routine, rather than leaving it to the client to work it out alone
- Providing positive feedback from therapist and family members.

An example of an occupational therapy programme using operant principles used by Cardenas et al (1986), was described by Strong et al (1996 p 61) and is reprinted here with permission:

Cardenas et al (1986) reported on the use of a behavioural program with a 37-year-old woman with chronic pain and hysterical right arm paralysis. In occupational therapy, the client was helped to set goals for the use of her arm, and baseline data on her arm and hand function were obtained. The client then began a daily hand-exercise program, which contained a number of step-wise increments. As each increment or quota was attained, the client was praised. It was reported that after 1 month, the client had attained normal hand function scores, and therapy ceased.

Since one of the goals of operant behavioural programmes is to decrease pain behaviour, withdrawal of attention when pain behaviour occurs is used to extinquish pain behaviour; assessment of pain is used infre-quently. Too-frequent assessment of pain may reinforce pain behaviours. Establishing goals of functional change that are closely linked to limitations caused by pain would be a better alternative. Assessment is then focused on functional change rather than pain. This point does not mean that pain should never be assessed; the assessment of pain becomes secondary to the focus on functional change.

Typically, pain management programmes rarely use pure behavioural approaches, instead incorporating aspects into a more comprehensive package. A weakness of the behavioural approach is its failure to recognize that humans are thinking, feeling, hoping individuals. Treatment programmes that include attention to the cognitive component of human behaviour, as well as its conditioned components, are becoming more prevalent. This is what makes cognitive–behavioural programmes so intuitively appealing and successful.

Cognitive–behavioural approach

The cognitive–behavioural approach was applied to pain by Turk and colleagues (Holzman et al 1986). It is the most widely endorsed psychological approach to pain management and is commonly applied in interdisciplinary pain clinics. Papers by Harding and Williams (1998), Kendall and Thompson (1998) and Strong (1998) have described the use of cognitive–behavioural methods by occupational therapists and physiotherapists working with patients with pain.

Principles of the cognitive–behavioural approach

Cognitive–behavioural approaches to pain management are based on the assumptions that a client's thoughts, feeling, beliefs and behaviours are important, and that behavioural strategies such as graded practice and relapse prevention are important therapy procedures. The strength of the approach lies in the acknowledgment that clients (and therapists) bring to therapy their own attitudes, beliefs, hopes and fears, and that these can help and/or hinder treatment outcomes.

Turk and Meichenbaum (1994 p 1338) identified five assumptions of the cognitive–behavioural approach:

1. Individuals are active processors of information and not passive reactors.
2. Thoughts (e.g. appraisals, expectancies, beliefs) can elicit and influence mood, affect physiological processes, have social consequences and can also serve as an impetus for behaviour; conversely,

mood, physiology, environmental factors and behaviour can influence the nature and content of thought processes.

3. Behaviour is reciprocally determined by both the individual and environmental factors.
4. Individuals can learn more adaptive ways of thinking, feeling, and behaving.
5. Individuals should be active collaborative agents in changing their maladaptive thoughts, feelings and behaviours.

Using a cognitive–behavioural framework, therapists are seen as 'educators, coaches and trainers' (Turk & Meichenbaum 1994). This role fits comfortably with the goals of the occupational therapist and physical therapist.

A cognitive–behavioural therapy programme will:

1. Assist the client to see their problem with pain as manageable, not overwhelming (reconceptualizing).
2. Help the client understand the need to be actively involved with treatment and making links between the programme components and their problem.
3. Instruct the clients in ways to convert unhelpful thoughts into positive thoughts.
4. Teach clients specific coping skills.
5. Anticipate problems which may arise so the client is prepared with strategies for set-backs, and thus feels active and resourceful rather than passive and helpless (Jamison 1996, Turk & Meichenbaum 1994, Turk & Rudy 1988).

Cognitive–behavioural therapy allows the therapist and client to develop a shared understanding of the therapeutic situation. Therapy involves:

1. Assessment of the client.
2. Reconceptualization of the client's situation as requiring active management on their part rather than waiting for something to be done for their pain by someone else.
3. Acquisition and rehearsal of skills already held, and new skills, such as positive-thinking strategies, relaxation, conditioning exercises, etc.
4. Setting goals. A structured set of goals towards some closer approximations of this state can be devised.
5. Specifying steps to achieve these goals, which can include smaller, interim goals and new abilities that need to be mastered.
6. Treatment generalization and maintenance, which can be worked on by setting progressively more functional goals, by attendance at community-based support groups rather than therapy centres, by setting times for review of maintained rather than improved function (Turk & Meichenbaum 1994).

Safety considerations

No adverse side-effects from cognitive–behavioural treatment are known (Turk & Meichenbaum 1994). As with an operant behavioural approach, a cognitive–behavioural programme is only initiated following careful assessment of the client's pain. If such programmes are not carefully conducted, the possibility of clients 'failing' and being further disillusioned may exist.

While programmes are typically used with clients with chronic pain of non-cancer origin, cognitive–behavioural strategies can be used for disease-related pain. Golden and Gersh (1990) used cognitive–behavioural strategies with clients with cancer (e.g. using coping self-statements to help manage pain). These strategies have also been used successfully with many different types of pain experienced by children and adolescents (McGrath & Unruh 1987). A cognitive–behavioural programme does not preclude the use of a comprehensive pharmacologically based pain management programme.

Recommended applications and current evidence

The cognitive–behavioural approach has been well validated by numerous studies and a number of meta-analyses (Flor et al 1992, Morley et al 1999, Morley et al 1999). Turk and Meichenbaum (1994) reported that over 100 studies have shown the effectiveness of cognitive–behavioural treatment for clients with chronic pain. There is now level I evidence to support the efficacy of cognitive–behavioural treatment programmes for clients with chronic pain (Morley et al 1999).

A critical review of cognitive–behavioural approaches for chronic pain by an occupational therapy evidence-based practice research group (Law et al 1999) noted that while cognitive–behavioural therapies have positive outcomes when compared with no interventions, the nature of the cognitive–behavioural intervention and the outcomes used to measure success vary considerably from study to study.

A number of related psychological constructs important to occupational therapists and physical therapists should be mentioned including expectancy and self-efficacy, fear of pain and re-injury, and coping. These constructs are an important part of a cognitive–behavioural programme.

SKILL DEVELOPMENT AREAS

Expectancy and self-efficacy

Accuracy of past prediction of potential pain from a certain activity leads a client to have a degree of expectancy about what may produce or increase pain for them. Prediction in general becomes more accurate with experience, however, those who predict an event to be less aversive than it turns out to be are more guarded in attempting that experience again (Cipher & Fernandez 1997).

For example, if a client decides he can now mow the lawn, and collapses in agony when he has finished mowing the 700 square metre block, he may be unlikely to attempt such an activity again. The dilemma for the clinician is how to increase the accuracy of prediction of pain by the client, so that they are able to be involved in more activities and able to plan ways to cope with the level of pain they will experience, in order to achieve the pleasure or satisfaction of the activity they wish to do.

It is useful here to work with the client to establish how many metres he can comfortably push the mower currently (X metres). Once this baseline is established, suggest to the client that he then sets up a mowing schedule for a week where, at the same time each day, he mows X plus one more metre each day, and then review his progress at the end of that week. If he can comfortably mow X plus 7 metres of grass, then suggest a further gradual increase. This way, the client is assisted to work within his pain barrier, and develop a sense of satisfaction at having met his goals.

Self-efficacy expectations are beliefs that a person has that he or she can successfully perform a particular behaviour (Bandura 1977, 1982, Jensen et al 1991). Outcome expectations are beliefs that the person has that a particular behaviour will result in a particular outcome (Bandura 1977). These two expectancies may differ, as a person may believe that a particular action may result in a given outcome, and yet not believe that he or she can do that action. Self-efficacy beliefs may go some way towards explaining the variability between a client's skill level and his or her performance outside the clinic (Gage & Polatajko 1994, Strong 1995).

Bandura's (1977) model of self-efficacy posits that performance accomplishments, vicarious experience, verbal persuasion and emotional arousal can all modify a client's self-efficacy expectations. Performance accomplishments are things which occupational therapists and physical therapists set up daily in client therapy sessions, such as giving clients the opportunity to succeed in doing an activity such as walking up a flight of stairs or sitting in the car for a 1-hour journey. Through such accomplishments, the client gains feelings of mastery and success. Performance accomplishments are particularly relevant for therapists:

> If we, as therapists, provide experiences for clients to successfully achieve activities, be it using their arm to complete a parenting task independently and without pain escalation (when previously they had guarded their arm for 6 months due to sympathetically maintained pain), or be it successfully completing a walked obstacle course (when they had been 'confined' to a wheelchair at hospital admission), then self-efficacy for these and other tasks is likely to be enhanced (Strong 1995 p 102).

Therapists can also utilize vicarious experience to help clients gain an enhanced sense of competence. This can be achieved by using the group process, whereby clients meet and see and hear about others performing activities they thought they would never do again because of pain. Another powerful method can involve getting a previous client who has graduated from a pain programme to come back to provide a relevant role-model for successful coping.

Furthermore, verbal methods for enhancing self-efficacy are typically incorporated into cognitive–behavioural programmes, whereby clients are told that they can learn to successfully cope with their pain. Similarly, most pain management programmes will use techniques such as relaxation to try and reduce emotional arousal and avoidance behaviour of clients (see Chapter 15).

Goal-setting

For many clients with chronic pain, the uppermost goal is 'to get rid of this pain'. This is especially so for clients for whom the pain has been a constant companion for years. It can be very helpful for therapists to help the clients to re-establish valued life-goals. Occupational therapists may do this in their work with clients by using such tools as the Canadian Occupational Performance Measure (Law et al 1994), or the Role Checklist (Oakley 1982, cited in Barris et al 1988). The Role Checklist assists the client to explore their current life roles and the value of each of those roles, their previous life roles and the value each role had for the client, and their future desired roles.

Completing the assessment with the occupational therapist can greatly assist the client to look beyond his desire for pain relief to other things of importance in his life. For example, a previous valued life role of a client with low back pain and arachnoiditis may have been as a cricket fast bowler. If such an activity was incompatible with the client's current physical status, the therapist may help the client to examine other related activities which may offer similar opportunities for belonging to a team, being a competitive creature, and enjoying cricket, such as in sport administration, scoring or coaching.

It is important for the therapist to assist the client in arriving at goals that may be achievable, and to help the client identify sub-goals along the way. This is important in enhancing the client's self-efficacy, and their willingness to continue working in partnership with you as therapist. It is best to help clients avoid early and significant failures, as these do little to bolster self-esteem or self-efficacy.

Fear of pain and re-injury

Another factor to be considered in psychological responses to pain and psychological approaches to pain management is the fear of pain. In the last 5 years or so, increasing attention has been given to the role of fear-avoidance and fear of pain in the determination of outcome after low back injury. Gordon Waddell, a British orthopaedic surgeon, and his colleagues commented, 'fear of pain and what we do about it may be more disabling than pain itself' (Waddell et al 1993). Pain-related fear and the fear of movement and subsequent re-injury are being seen as a possible factor in the low correlation between pain intensity and resultant disability.

Developed by Lethem et al (1983) the fear-avoidance model has been found useful in terms of assessing clients along a continuum of adaptive/non-adaptive responses to pain. A key concept in this model is the way individuals deal with the fear of pain, using either confrontation or avoidance. A confrontation response will lead to a reduction/abolition of fear, and cognitive and/or behavioural avoidance will lead to the maintenance/exacerbation of fear.

Recent literature is highly supportive of the important contribution which fear of pain, and fear of re-injury has upon client outcome. For example, Crombez et al (1999) found that pain-related fear was a better predictor of disability than pain intensity and negative affect in 104 clients with chronic low back pain seeking rehabilitation/pain clinic treatment. In a similar vein, Klenerman et al (1995), in examining the prediction of chronicity in clients following an acute attack of low back pain, found that fear-avoidance was most important in determining outcome.

Physical therapists and occupational therapists can assist clients to cognitively re-appraise the feared movement, and to learn that such movement will not result in tissue injury and increased pain.

Coping

One of the oft-mentioned goals of pain management programmes for clients with pain of non-cancer origin is to teach people how to cope with pain (see Reflective exercise 9.1). It is therefore important for physical therapists and occupational therapists to have some familiarity with the coping construct. Jensen and his colleagues (1991) provided a useful review of the literature related to coping with chronic pain.

Coping has been defined as intentional efforts to deal with the negative impact of a particular stressor (Jensen et al 1991, Lazarus 1993). Around one-third of people with pain in one study reported that pain was the main stressor in their lives (Turner et al 1987). Hence, ways to cope with pain are important for many people. In our examination of coping strategies used by people with chronic back pain, we found that a variety of physical, behavioural and cognitive strategies were used (Large & Strong 1997, Strong & Large 1995). Such coping strategies needed to be situation-specific.

Implications for therapy are that clients need to develop a wide repertoire of coping strategies for successful adjustment to pain. Therapists would do well to ask clients about their typical way of dealing with life stressors, so as to help in the match between coping preference and coping strategies. For example, a client who has always used action-oriented coping, such as getting out of the house or doing an enjoyed

---

Reflective exercise 9.1

Take a few moments to think about how you cope best when stressed.

- Do you get busy, trying not to think of the stressor?
- Do you become quiet and retreat into your own thoughts to focus on the stressor, and to develop a plan of action?
- Do you seek out a friend to discuss the issue with and get support from?
- Do you rush into action to deal with the stressor head on?

Having reflected on your usual personal coping style, remember the last time you went to have an injection or to have blood withdrawn by venepuncture, or to the dentist to have a procedure like a filling or an extraction.

- Was the situation stressful to you?
- What did you do to cope?
- Did you cope well?
- If you used a particular strategy, is it a strategy you often use to cope with other stressful situations or is it a situation-specific strategy just for this situation?
- What made you adopt this particular strategy?

task such as gardening when stressed, is unlikely to derive as much benefit from a cognitive strategy like reinterpreting pain sensations. An action-oriented strategy such as taking a shower may be more helpful for that client.

Catastrophizing in response to pain is one coping strategy that is consistently associated with poor outcomes (Turk & Rudy 1992). Catastrophizing can be typified by a statement such as, 'when I feel pain, it overwhelms me and I know it is going to get more and more unbearable'. Turk and Rudy (1992) suggested that attention to helping clients reduce the use of such negative coping strategies might be more effective than focusing on the acquisition of positive coping strategies. Our work suggests that emphasis be given to both an increase in the use of positive adaptive strategies and a decrease in negative catastrophizing strategies. The case example in Box 9.3 illustrates the application of a cognitive–behavioural approach.

Using a cognitive–behavioural approach, the occupational therapist might first address Mrs D's faulty belief about her spinal fusion. The therapist could give Mrs D information on what a fusion is and how it was done, using models of the spine, the client's own X-rays, and discussion. Some pain clinics, such as the Auckland Regional Pain Service, ensure that a radiologist provides an expert, individualized information session to explain the consequences of a procedure such as a fusion (McCallum & Large, personal communication). This session contributes enormously to the abandonment of faulty beliefs. The therapist could also focus attention on Mrs D's behaviour, and with medical consultation, provide activities that would enable Mrs D to use her back without causing damage.

Group therapy

Several therapists have described the value of the use of groups for people with chronic pain (e.g. Herman &

Box 9.3 Case example – Mrs D

Mrs D was a 58-years-old woman who had a decompression laminectomy and L5–S1 fusion 2 years before referral to the pain service. Since returning home from hospital after the surgery, Mrs D, formerly an active housewife, did little except lie on her bed, and sit in her lounge chair to watch television. She did not shop, in case someone bumped her and damaged the fusion. She also did not do many of her former activities because she believed that if she bent her back, her fusion would snap. As a result of this faulty belief, she did not do any activities which involved bending.

Baptiste 1981, 1990, Subramanian 1991, Weinstein 1990). Most chronic pain management programmes utilize groups for service delivery, education, and support, with individual sessions as needed. The group is a vehicle for learning that one is not alone in having a pain problem, and for learning to deal with pain in a supportive, understanding environment. As noted by Weinstein (1990 p 63):

Groups help to ameliorate the social isolation and alienation common to pain sufferers, who can now openly share their feelings of anger, helplessness, and loss of control in a socially supportive setting.

In such an environment, learning about changing behaviours can be more successful. Such groups usually have some clearly defined behavioural expectations which help to promote a safe environment for members (Weinstein 1990). Respect for confidentiality, regular attendance, and acceptable ways of dealing with pain behaviours are discussed at the outset of the group. Therapists need to be familiar with group dynamics, group process, leadership styles, group development, norms, and termination. A useful text here for occupational therapists is Cole (1998).

Client education

A large part of the success or failure of the rehabilitation process for clients with chronic pain depends upon providing appropriate information and intervention that is relevant to the client's needs and concerns. It is not at all unusual to hear health professionals saying, 'But I told Mr Patient that. Why didn't he do what I told him?'. Appropriate education is critical to enable the client to be an active participant in his or her rehabilitation rather than a passive recipient of care. Good education is not telling a client what to do, but teaching the client and helping him or her to learn new approaches. Lorig (1996) defined patient education as: 'any set of planned, educational activities designed to improve patients' health behaviours and/or health status' (p xiii). The purpose of such education is to assist clients to maintain and improve their own health (Lorig 1996). Kate Lorig's 1996 book on patient education is a useful practical resource for therapists wanting to further develop their patient-education skills.

Self-esteem building

Self-esteem refers to:

The evaluation which an individual makes and customarily maintains with regard to himself [herself]: it expresses the attitude of approval or disapproval, and indicates the extent to which the individual believes himself [herself] to be capable, significant, successful and worthy. In short, self-esteem is a *personal* judgement of worthiness, that is expressed in the attitudes the individual holds towards himself [herself] (Coopersmith 1967 p iv).

Many clients with chronic pain have low self-esteem, viewing themselves as failures. If one thinks about the 'typical' client with back pain seen in a pain clinic, it will be a man in his mid-40s, who is in a long-term relationship, with 2 children. His occupation typically often involves manual work such as lifting, carrying heavy loads and driving machinery. His back pain will typically have begun at work, and his current functional status will preclude him from working. For someone with a partner and children, important life goals would be providing income to support the family, putting the children through school, playing some sport with the kids, and being an active part of a family unit. These goals are often difficult for clients, and subsequently clients might begin to despair, and feel like they are letting down the family. Self-esteem can plummet, and clients may not be able to see ways to improve their self-esteem.

In therapy, clients can be helped to regain self-esteem. Therapists can work with clients to identify their current strengths, and to acknowledge these strengths. Therapy plans can then be developed which look at realistic ways to accomplish other valued goals (refer back to the goal setting and self-efficacy sections). Successful accomplishment of tasks and activities is a powerful booster of self-esteem. This is why the engagement of the client in activities and exercises by the occupational therapist or physiotherapist is such a useful part of the rehabilitation process for clients with chronic pain.

It may also be important to help clients learn to use positive self-talk. For example, instead of a client saying, 'I am never going to be able to work as a plant operator again', encourage them to focus on the positives and say, 'I have some good knowledge about machines that I might be able to use as a technical college instructor'. The amount of assistance a client needs in this area needs to be determined by careful therapist assessment.

Psychotherapy

Psychotherapy is not used by physical therapists or occupational therapists unless they have acquired recognized postgraduate training. Psychotherapy may be helpful for clients who continue to suffer with chronic pain despite the use of other interventions (Grzesiak et al 1996). Psychotherapy is usually integrated with the use of other cognitive–behavioural, medical and pharmacological strategies. Interested readers are referred to Pilowsky (1994) for a brief introduction to the area.

Hypnosis

Hypnosis is a condition of altered attention in an individual, achieved by an induction process (Elton et al 1983). Hypnosis may help by altering the pain sensations, by directing the person's attention away from the pain, or by suggesting pain relief (Elton et al 1983). Specialized training in hypnosis is needed, it is not a technique used by physical therapists and occupational therapists and so will not be covered further in this chapter. Detailed coverage on this topic can be found in Spanos et al (1994) and Stanley (2000).

INCORPORATING PSYCHOLOGICALLY BASED PAIN MANAGEMENT INTO INTERDISCIPLINARY WORKING

The cognitive–behavioural approach is often used within a multidisciplinary or interdisciplinary perspective. Interdisciplinary pain management programs provide more benefits than management by one discipline or profession (Flor et al 1992). Goals of interdisciplinary programmes include:

- Reduction of pain intensity
- Increased physical functioning
- Proper use of medication
- Improvement of sleep, mood, and interaction with others
- Return to work or to normal daily activities (Jamison 1996).

Psychologically based strategies that are incorporated into an interdisciplinary programme may include all or some of the following:

- Education
- Relaxation training
- Group therapy
- Family therapy
- Exercise
- Vocational counselling
- Cognitive–behavioural treatment.

ISSUES TO CONSIDER

Therapists need to consider when they should incorporate different psychological approaches in their management of people with pain. They also need to be conscious of the quality of the therapist–client relationship. The context within which therapy is delivered may have an impact upon these issues. Therapists also need to be able to recognize when to refer clients to other professionals.

Indications for use of particular methods

Cognitive–behavioural approaches have wide acceptance by therapists, and can be selected in most cases. Within this approach, the relative balance of different components can be adjusted to suit individuals. For instance, some clients may respond very well to the structured behavioural component, and less to supportive group cognitive therapy. Others may respond most to the group component.

There may be some common psychosocial problems associated with the chronic pain syndrome which require amelioration before the pain management process itself can be started. There is a powerful sense of loss associated with accepting that a chronic pain condition exists, and so the client may experience grief (Cohen 1995).

Grief due to the loss of health or wholeness may manifest as sadness, anger, or other emotion. The grief process can impede progress of therapy because the client concentrates on the loss, or ways to reverse it, and is unable to integrate the loss and move on. If the therapist is able to identify the grief process with the client, and provide support through an understanding therapeutic relationship, individual or group psychotherapy, then progress in pain management becomes possible. Sometimes individual or group therapy may be necessary before another pain management approach is successful.

Physical therapists and occupational therapists need to be able to identify when their clients require specialized psychological help, and to refer when appropriate. In some situations, the client's condition may be characteristic of a psychiatric disorder. Psychiatric aspects of chronic pain are discussed in more detail in Chapter 22.

Therapist–client relationship as a factor in interventions

There are a number of principles for managing a therapist–client relationship, which derive from understanding the constructs of learning theory, self-efficacy and expectancy effects described above. It is essential to remember that a therapist–client relationship may be friendly and relaxed, but should always be professional and goal-directed. The therapist input into the relationship needs to be considered rather than intuitive, and planned rather than reactive.

It is a principle of therapeutic communication to provide meaningful information, because information reduces anxiety. Information that is relevant to the client's needs and concerns is reassuring. In order to fill 'spaces' during therapy, or to respond to the client's distress about their pain, it may be tempting to offer bland reassurance. Such reassurance can increase anxiety.

The therapeutic relationship is a powerful influence on the client's motivation and active involvement in the therapeutic process and persistence with interventions. If the client has been using increasing pain as a gauge of when to stop activity, then motivation and persistence may be difficult to achieve. An approach that focuses on increasing exercise and function, rather than working to a pain limit, depends partially on the quality of the therapeutic relationship.

The client's viewpoint needs to be considered and actively canvassed to enable the client to have a more active lifestyle. Clients also require positive, and accurate, feedback about their performance. Compliance will be helped by a relationship which encourages open communication and clear goals. Compliance will be assisted by establishing a collaborative relationship with the client, and helping the client to analyse and solve her or his own problems in the pain management programme.

Nurturing self-efficacy is a therapist responsibility. The client must understand that improvement is the result of her or his own efforts, more than the efforts of the therapist. Flexibility on the part of the therapist is important. Being able to suggest methods of treatment outside the therapist's normal approach or theoretical preference, or to support the use of adjunct methods, if the client may benefit, is part of the role of a mature therapist. In this way, the direction of the therapeutic relationship remains firmly directed on the client's needs and preferences.

Therapeutic context

Occupational therapists and physical therapists should be cognisant of, and attuned to, the prevailing psychological practice model used in their facility. Interventions that are consistent with each other in their underlying assumptions are more likely to have a beneficial impact. Using approaches that are based on widely differing or controversial approaches may be confusing for the client and the team.

Referral to other health professionals

Some clients will require more specialized services, particularly if underlying psychological problems are severe. Referral to psychologists, psychiatrist or social workers in such instances should be considered.

CONCLUSION

Occupational therapists and physical therapists need to remember that a client's pain is both a physical and a psychological experience, and to plan their management accordingly. The two most prominent psychological approaches to pain management are the operant behavioural and cognitive-behavioural approaches. Aspects of both approaches can be utilised to make therapy more effective for clients with pain problems.

Study questions/questions for revision

1. What are the assumptions underlying operant behavioural approaches to pain?
2. What are the assumptions underlying behavioural therapy approaches to pain?
3. When working within an operant behavioural framework, would a therapist focus on pain reduction or functional gains?
4. What is a possible weakness of the operant behavioural approach?
5. What are the assumptions underlying a cognitive–behavioural perspective to pain?
6. What can the therapist do to promote active involvement of the client in therapy?
7. What methods could a therapist use to increase the client's sense of self-efficacy?
8. How would you approach treatment with a client if fear of re-injury was an important issue for the client?

ACKNOWLEDGEMENT

The authors express their appreciation to Dr Frank New (Psychiatrist) and Jennifer Sturgess (Occupational Therapist) for their assistance with this chapter.

REFERENCES

Bandura A 1969 Principles of behavior modification. Holt, Rinehart & Wilson, New York

Bandura A 1977 Self-efficacy: towards a unifying theory of behavioral change. Psychological Review 84: 191–215

Bandura A 1982 Self-efficacy mechanisms in human agency. American Psychologist 37: 122–147

Bandura A 1986 Social foundations of thought in action: a social cognitive theory. Prentice-Hall, Englewood Cliffs, New Jersey

Barris R, Oakley F, Kielhofner G 1988 The role checklist. In: Hemphill B J (ed) Mental Health Assessment in Occupational Therapy: an integrative approach to the evaluation process. Slack, Thoroughfare

Beck A T, Ward C H, Mendelson M, Mock J, Erbaugh J 1961 An inventory for measuring depression. Archives of General Psychiatry 4: 5651–5671

Cameron R, Meichenbaum D 1980 Cognition and behaviour change. Australia and New Zealand Journal of Psychiatry 14: 121–125

Cardenas D D, Larson J, Egan K J 1986 Hysterical paralysis in the upper extremity of chronic pain clients. Archives of Physical Medicine & Rehabilitation 67: 190–193

Cipher D J, Fernandez E 1997 Expectancy variables predicting tolerance and avoidance of pain in chronic pain clients. Behaviour Research Therapy 35: 437–444

Cohen M J 1995 Psychosocial aspects of evaluation and management of chronic low back pain. Physical Medicine and Rehabititation 9: 725–746

Cole M B 1998 Group Dynamics in Occupational Therapy. The theoretical basis and practice application of group treatment, 2nd edn. Slack, Thoroughfare

Coopersmith S 1967 The antecedents of self-esteem. Freeman and Co, San Francisco

Crombez G, Vlaeyen J W S, Huets P H T G, Lysens R 1999. Pain-related fear is more disabling than pain itself: evidence on the role of pain-related fear in chronic back pain disability. Pain 69: 231–236

Elton D, Stanley G, Burrows G (eds) 1983 Psychological control of pain. Grune & Stratton, Sydney

Flor H, Fydrich, T, Turk D C 1992 efficacy of multidisciplinary pain treatment centres: a metaanalytic review Pain 49: 221–230

Fordyce W E 1976 Behavioral Methods for Chronic Pain and Illness. Mosby, St Louis

Fordyce W E, Roberts A H, Sternbach R A 1985 The behavioral management of chronic pain: a response to critics. Pain 22: 113–125

Gage M, Polatajko H 1994 Enhancing occupational performance through an understanding of perceived self-efficacy. American Journal of Occupational Therapy 48: 452–461

Golden W L, Gersh W D 1990 Cognitive–behaviour therapy in the treatment of cancer clients. Journal of Rational-Emotive & Cognitive-Behavior Therapy 8: 41–51

Gotestam K G, Bates S 1979 Behavioral contracting – principles and practice. Behaviour Analysis Modification 3: 126–134

Gotestam K G 1980 A behavioral approach to drug abuse. Drug & Alcohol Dependence 5: 5–25

Grzesiak R C, Ury G M, Dworkin R H 1996 Psychodynamic psychotherapy with chronic pain problems. In: Gatchell R J, Turk D C (eds) Psychological Approaches to Pain Management: a practioner's handbook. The Guilford Press, New York, pp 148–178

Harding V R, Williams A C de C 1998 Activities training: integrating behavioral and cognitive methods with physiotherapy in pain management. Journal of Occupational Rehabilitation 8: 47–60

Herman E, Baptiste S 1981 Pain control: mastery through group experience. Pain 10: 79–86

Herman E, Baptiste S 1990 Group therapy: a cognitive behavioural model. In: Tunks E, Bellissimo A, Roy R (eds) Chronic Pain: psychosocial factors in rehabilitation, 2nd edn. Krieger, Melbourne

Holzman A D, Turk D C, Kerns R D 1986 The cognitive-behavioral approach to the management of chronic pain. In: Holzman A D, Turk D C (eds) Pain Management: a handbook of psychological treatment approaches. Pergamon Press, Elmsford, New York, pp 31–50

Jamison R N 1996 Psychological factors in chronic pain assessment and treatment issues. Journal of Back & Musculoskeletal Rehabilitation 7: 79–95

Jensen M P, Turner J A, Romano J M, Karoly P 1991 Coping with chronic pain: a critical review of the literature. Pain 47: 249–283

Keefe F J, LeFebvre S C 1994 Behaviour therapy In: Wall PD, Melzack R Textbook of Pain, 3rd edn, pp. 1367–1380. Churchill Livingstone, Edinburgh

Kendall N A S, Thompson B F 1998 A pilot programme for dealing with comorbidity of chronic pain and long-term unemployment. Journal of Occupational Rehabilitation 8: 5–26

Kerns Haythornthwaite 1988 Depression among chronic pain patients: cognitive–behavioural analysis and effect on rehabilitation outcome. Jownal of Consulting Clinical Psychology 5: 870–876

Klenerman L, Slade P D, Stanley I M, Pennie B, Reilly J P, Atchison L E 1995 The prediction of chronicity in clients with an acute attack of low back pain in a general practice setting. Spine 20: 478–485

Large R G, Strong J 1997 The personal constructs of coping with chronic low back pain. Pain 73: 245–252

Law M, Baptiste S, Carswell A, McColl M A, Polatajko H, Pollock N 1994. Canadian Occupational Performance Measure, 2nd edn. CAOT Publications Ace, Toronto, Ontario

Law M, Stewart D, Pollock N, Letts L, Bosch J, Westmorland M, Philpot A 1999 The Effectiveness of Cognitive–behavioural Interventions with People with Chronic Pain. A critical review of the literature by the Occupational Therapy Evidence-Based Practice Research Group (www-fhs.mcmaster.ca/rehab/ebp)

Lazarus R S 1993 Coping theory and research; past, present, and future. Psychosomatic Medicine 55: 234–247

Lethm J, Slade P D, Troup J D G, Bertley G 1983 Outline of a fear-avoidance model of exaggerated pain perception-I. Behavior Research Therapy 21: 401–408

Lindstrom I, Ohlund C, Eek C, Wallin L, Peterson L-E, Fordyce W E, Nachemson A L 1992 The effect of graded activity on clients with subacute low back pain: a randomised prospective clinical study with an operant-conditioning behavioral approach. Physical Therapy 72: 279–290

Linton S J 1982 A critical review of behavioral treatments for chronic benign pain other than headache. British Journal of Clinical Psychology 21: 321–337

Linton S J 1986 Behavioral remediation of chronic pain: a status report. Pain 24: 125–141

Lorig K 1996 Patient education: a practical approach, 2nd edn. Sage, Thousand Oaks, California

McGrath P J Unruh A M 1987 Pain in Children and Adolescents. Elsevier, Amsterdam

Mechanic D, Volkart E H 1960 Illness behaviour and medical diagnosis. Journal of Health & Human Behaviour 1: 86–94

Melzack R 1975 The McGill Pain Questionnaire: major properties and scoring methods. Pain 1: 277–299

Molloy A R, Blyth F M, Nicholas M K 1999 Disability and work-related injury: time for a change? Medical Journal of Australia 170: 150–151

Morley S, Eccleston C, Williams A 1999 Systematic review and meta-analysis of randomised controlled trials of cognitive behaviour therapy and behaviour therapy for chronic pain in adults, excluding headache. Pain 80: 1–13

Pavlov I P 1927 Conditioned Reflexes. Oxford University Press, London

Pilowsky I 1978 A general classification of abnormal illness behaviours. British Journal of Medical Psychology 51: 131–137

Pilowsky I 1994 Pain and illness behaviour: assessment and management. In: Wall P D, Melzack R (ed) Textbook of Pain, 3rd edn. Churchill Livingstone, Edinburgh, pp 1309–1319

Pilowsky I, Spence N 1981 Manual for the Illness Behaviour Questionnaire. University of Adelaide, Adelaide

Pilowsky I, Spence N 1981 Manual for the Illness Behaviour Questionnaire, 2nd Edn. University of Adelaide Department of Psychiatry, Adelaide

Sanders S H 1996 Operant conditioning with chronic pain: back to basics. In: Gatchell R J, Turk D C (eds) Psychological Approaches to Pain Management: a practioner's handbook. The Guilford Press, New York, pp 112–130

Skinner B F 1953 Science and Human Behavior. MacMillan, New York

Skinner B F 1989 Recent issues in the analysis of behavior. Charles E Merrill, Columbus, Ohio

Slater M A, Doctor J N, Pruitt S D, Atkinson J H 1997 The clinical significance of behavioural treatment for chronic low back pain: an evaluation of effectiveness. Pain 71: 257–263

Spanos N P, Carmanico S J, Ellis J A 1994 Hypnotic analgesia. In: Wall P D, Melzack R Textbook of Pain, 3rd edn. Churchill Livingstone, Edinburgh, pp 1349–1366

Stanley R 2000 Clinical hypnosis in the management of pain. Abstracts of The Progress of Pain Before, Betwixt & Beyond. Annual Scientific Meeting of the Australian Pain Society p 40

Strong J 1995 Self-efficacy and the client with chronic pain. In: Schacklock M (ed) Moving in on Pain. Butterworth Heinemann, Melbourne, pp 97–102

Strong J 1996 Chronic Pain Management: the occupational therapist's perspective. Churchill Livingstone, Edinburgh

Strong J 1998 Incorporating cognitive-behavioural therapy with occupational therapy: a comparative study of clients with low back pain. Journal of Occupational Rehabilitation 8: 61–71

Strong J, Large R G 1995 Coping with chronic low back pain: an idiographic exploration through focus groups. International Journal Psychiatry in Medicine 25: 361–377

Subramanian K 1991 Structured group work for the management of chronic pain: an experimental investigation. Social Work Practice 1: 32–45

Turk D C, Holzman A D 1986 Commonalities among psychological approaches in the treatment of chronic pain: specifying the meta-constructs. In: Holzman A D, Turk D C (eds) Pain Management: a handbook of psychological treatment approaches. Pergamon Press, New York, pp 257–267

Turk D C, Meichenbaum D 1994 A cognitive-behavioural approach to pain management. In: Wall P D, Melzack R (eds) Textbook on Pain, 3rd edn. Churchill Livingstone, Edinburgh, pp 1337–1418

Turk D C, Rudy T E 1988 A cognitive-behavioral perspective on chronic pain: beyond the scapel and syringe. In: Tollison C D (ed) Handbook of Chronic Pain Management. Williams & Wilkins, Baltimore, pp 222–236

Turk D C, Rudy T E 1992 Cognitive factors and persistent pain: a glimpse into Pandora's Box. Cognitive Therapy and Research 16: 99–122

Turner J, Chapman C R 1982 Psychological interventions for chronic pain: a critical review. I. Relaxation training and biofeedback. Pain 12: 1–21

Turner J A, Clancy S, Vitaliano P P 1987 Relationships of stress, appraisal and coping to chronic low back pain. Behaviour Research Therapy 25: 281–288

van Tulder M W, Ostelo R W J G, Vlaeyen J W S, Linton S J, Morley S J, Assendelft W J J 2000 Behavioural treatment for chronic low back pain (Cochrane Review). In: The Cochrane Library, Issue 3. Update Software, Oxford

Waddell G, Bircher M, Finlayson D, Main C J 1984 Symptoms & signs: physical disease or illness behaviour? British Medical Journal 289: 739–741

Waddell G, Pilowsky I, Bond M R 1989 Clinical assessment and interpretation of abnormal illness behaviour in low back pain. Pain 39: 41–53

Waddell G, Newton M, Henderson I, Somerville D, Main C J 1993 A Fear-Avoidance Beliefs Questionnaire (FABQ) and the role of fear-avoidance in chronic LBP and disability. Pain 52: 157–168

Weinstein E 1990 The role of the group in the treatment of chronic pain. Occupational Therapy Practice 1: 62–68

10

Physical treatments

Bill Vicenzino   Anthony Wright

OVERVIEW

This chapter covers the role of manual physical therapy treatment modalities such as mobilization, manipulation and to a lesser extent massage (see Box 10.1), in the management and control of pain. It will review the increasing body of knowledge that indicates that manual physical therapy treatments can exert pain relieving effects, which enable beneficial clinical outcomes in clients with a range of musculoskeletal pain disorders. The role of endogenous pain control systems in these clinically beneficial outcomes will be briefly discussed.

Manual therapy also appears to exert additional effects and confer benefits beyond those of direct pain control. For example, manual physical therapy has been shown to produce changes in functioning of the motor, articular and sympathetic nervous systems. These will be covered because there is preliminary evidence indicating that some of these additional effects may be related to the pain relieving effects.

Current best practice in physical therapy emphasizes the role of clinical reasoning skills in the management of musculoskeletal pain syndromes. In using their clinical reasoning skills, therapists interpret the presenting signs and symptoms in light of the relevant theoretical knowledge-base, before developing a treatment programme. Increasingly, practitioners are required to substantiate the treatment methods that they use in clinical practice. This requires an understanding of the evidence-base for the therapeutic approach being considered.

In terms of manual physical therapy the practitioner has a number of sources on which to base a decision. At the highest level of the evidence-base hierarchy there is the systematic review or meta-analysis of a number of randomized controlled trials. Should a specific meta-analysis not exist, usually because of a lack of sufficient trials, then individual clinical trials may form the basis of a decision. If there is no evidence

---

Box 10.1 Key terms defined

Mobilization and manipulation – Mobilization and manipulation are two terms that are used to differentiate two classes of manual physical therapy techniques applied to the joints of the body. Some of the differentiating features are that mobilizations are delivered in an oscillatory and repetitive fashion, whereas manipulations are often single thrusts of high velocity and low amplitude. Mobilization techniques may also involve sustained positions to compress or stretch intra-articular or peri-articular structures. The high-velocity manipulations are often associated with a joint noise (i.e. click, pop or crack) and are done at such speed that the client cannot control the technique. Mobilizations do not normally produce a joint noise and allow the client the ability to exert some control over the technique should it be required.

Massage – Massage has been said to come from the word 'mass' which is to touch in Arabic, from 'massein' which is to knead in Greek or from 'manus' which means hand in Latin. Massage is the mechanical manipulation of body tissues, usually the soft tissues (i.e. muscle and connective tissue). It can be self-administered or administered by a therapist and is most usually applied via the hand, but may also be applied by use of the foot, elbow, forearm or a variety of mechanical/electromechanical devices. Much has been written about the history of massage; its origins date back to recordings of massage as early as 8000 BC. A testament to its perceived value to society is that, despite a lack of scientific evidence to substantiate its effects and efficacy, it has endured and is popular today.

---

from these two sources the practitioner is then left with a number of presumably less satisfactory strategies. One is to look for evidence of sound scientific studies of the treatment approach (e.g. placebo-controlled, blinding of investigator and subjects). If this is lacking then single case studies, case series and clinical notes may provide some direction for the clinician, on which to base a therapeutic approach.

Should this evidence-based literature approach prove fruitless the practitioner is left to using his/her clinical reasoning skills to structure the treatment program. In this instance the practitioner will base decisions on the findings of the clinical examination and any related information from the scientific literature (e.g. anatomical, biomechanical, physiological and pathological). In terms of evidence-based practice this is deemed to be the least satisfactory situation, however while most treatments await further investigation it remains the basis of clinical practice in the management of musculoskeletal pain. It must be noted that the clinical reasoning-based approach to treatment selection is not only employed when there are none of the higher levels of evidence available. Rather it is necessary in all situations where a manual physical therapy treatment is being administered in the clinical setting.

The scope and nature of this chapter does not allow for a treatise of the clinical reasoning skills and the broad range of practical clinical skills, most of which require high levels of manual dexterity and skill, required by clinicians to adequately manage musculoskeletal pain. There are several authoritative texts and programs from which the reader can obtain more detailed insight into the clinical reasoning process in physical therapy.

This chapter will reflect the contemporaneous approach to clinical practice by first looking for evidence from the highest stratum of the evidence-base hierarchy. Characteristically, in manual physical therapy the quality of the clinical trials is poor and does not provide the practitioner with sufficient information on which to base a treatment approach. Therefore, this chapter will also review studies that have evaluated the clinical effects of manual physical therapy and outline the implications of such studies on our understanding of this treatment approach. This will provide the reader with a basis on which to proceed in using manual physical therapy in the management of musculoskeletal pain.

Learning objectives

At the end of this chapter the reader will have an understanding of:

1. The extent and quality of the evidence-base supporting the clinical efficacy of manual physical therapy.
2. The issues that need to be considered when judging the level of research-based evidence of manual physical therapy.
3. The pain relieving effects of manual physical therapy.
4. The effects of manual physical therapy beyond those of pure pain control but complementary to the clinical role of this treatment approach.
5. The proposed mechanism(s) by which manual physical therapy exerts its clinically beneficial effects.

META-ANALYSES AND RANDOMIZED CONTROLLED TRIALS

The clinical efficacy of manual therapy in the treatment of pain of spinal origin has attracted much interest over recent times. Such has been the interest in this topic that of all treatments for back pain, manipulation has been evaluated the most (Meeker 1996). The gold standard for investigating clinical efficacy of any health-related intervention has become the randomized controlled trial. It has been advocated in musculoskeletal clinical research (Deyo 1993). In systematic reviews of manual physical therapy, Koes et al (1996) identified 36 randomized clinical trials that compared this therapy with other treatments of low back pain and Hurwitz et al (1996) found 14 such studies of neck pain. The presence of such a number of clinical trials indicates that a structured review process such as a meta-analysis should be possible.

Meta-analysis consists of four steps as outlined in Box 10.2. Some of the fundamental features of the meta-analysis are that every attempt is made to access all of the available literature in a systematic and unbiased manner, and that once all available studies are obtained, they are organized into clinically meaningful groupings and analysed for quality and validity. Criteria taken from several recently reported scales against which the quality and validity of the randomized controlled trials are evaluated are listed and briefly explained in Table 10.1 (Gross et al 1996a, Koes et al 1991a). The quality and validity of the studies under structured review not only influence the clinical inferences that can be drawn from their results but also provide guidelines for future investigations of the therapeutic approach. Statistical pooling of the

---

Box 10.2 The process involved in conducting a structured review or meta-analysis

1. Identification of all relevant papers, usually by using computer-based search facilities as well as other search strategies (e.g. manual searches, direct communications)
2. Organization of the reported studies into clinically meaningful groupings
3. Assessment of the identified studies for quality and validity based on previously agreed criteria (see Table 10.1 for example)
4. Statistical pooling of the results of the studies in order to increase the power to detect differences between the manual therapy treatment and comparison treatments (e.g. other treatments, non-treatment control, or placebo)

(after Anderson et al 1992, Assendelft et al 1996, Naylor 1989, Shekelle 1996)

---

results of a number of studies by the confidence profile method of meta-analysis (Hurwitz et al. 1996), or similar procedures, provides an indication of the effect size of manual therapy and consequently the much sought-after answer to the question: does manual physical therapy work?

Overview of meta-analyses of mobilization and manipulative therapy

This section will deal with meta-analyses of neck treatment. The reader will explore the literature for meta-analyses of other areas of the body in the reflective exercises. There have been two comprehensive meta-analyses of clinical trials of manual therapy for neck pain conducted recently. One was conducted by the RAND Corporation in California (Hurwitz et al 1996) and the other by a Canadian group that was predominantly based at McMaster University (Aker et al 1996; Gross et al 1996a, 1996b, 1997), referred to herein as the McMaster study. Their results are presented as a means of identifying significant issues pertaining to research methodology that impact on the interpretation of the studies' results and also to determine whether manual therapy of the cervical spine works.

Hurwitz et al (1996) systematically reviewed the literature regarding manipulation and mobilization of the cervical spine and reported that there were 14 randomized clinical trials on this topic. Only three of these, of which two were of manipulation only and one combined manipulation and mobilization, were considered suitable for statistical pooling of treatment effects and subsequent reduction to a single numerical index of the pooled treatment effect.

The McMaster study conducted a meta-analysis study, in which the focus was conservative management of mechanical neck pain, which included manual therapy as well as rest, medication and other physical therapy modalities such as exercise therapy, collars and electrotherapy. This is a subtle, but nonetheless different approach to that of Hurwitz et al (1996). In the area of manual therapy they found eight studies in which manual therapy was combined with other conservative interventions. Five of these were suitable for the statistical pooling of effects. Three of these studies investigated mobilization and the other two included manipulation as well as mobilization. One of the studies (Jensen et al 1990) that was included in the computations was a headache trial. Hurwitz et al (1996) partitioned out the headache trials to a separate analysis.

Table 10.2 provides an overview of the studies that were considered by these two groups of researchers to

Table 10.1 An overview of study features and criteria, by which the quality and validity of a clinical trial of spinal treatment is evaluated Based on the quality scale of Koes et al (1991, 1996)

Study feature	Criteria	Description	Domain[1]
Study population	1. Homogeneity	Inclusion and exclusion criteria to ensure this	I
	2. Baseline comparability of groups	Includes the duration of complaint, outcome measure values, age, recurrence or history, referred symptomatology	V
	3. Randomization	Randomization schedule blinded so as to exclude bias	V
	4. Reason for loss of follow-up	Information about patients who dropped out should be followed up for each group (e.g. treatment, control, etc)	I
	5. Loss of follow-up	Expressed as a percentage of all randomized subjects	V
	6. Subject numbers	Number in smallest group immediately after randomization	P
Interventions	7. Description	Explicit description of the manual therapy treatment techniques and comparison interventions (e.g. duration, spinal levels, type of technique)	I
	8. Pragmatic study	Comparison intervention is an established treatment	I
	9. Co-interventions	Avoid or standardize other treatments (e.g. exercise, electrotherapy, medication)	V
Effect	10. Placebo-controlled	Comparison with a suitable placebo	I
	11. Therapist expertise level	Statement of educational qualifications, experience levels	I
	12. Patients blinded	Placebo study: blinding of subjects to placebo condition, evaluation of success of blinding process; Pragmatic study: subject naivety, assessment of naivety and success of procedure	V
	13. Outcome measures	Relevancy of measure, use of pain, global measurement of improvement, functional status, spinal mobility, use of drugs and medical services	I
	14. Blinded outcome measure	Blinding of therapist and subject to the outcome	V
	15. Adequate follow-up period	Follow-up should be immediately after treatment and at least 6 months later	I
Data management	16. Intention-to-treat analysis	When loss to follow up is < 10%: analyses on all randomized patients for main outcome measures, and on the most important points of measurement minus missing values, irrespective of non-compliance and co-interventions When loss to follow up is > 10%: intention-to-treat as well as an alternative analysis that accounts for missing values	V
	17. Presentation	Frequencies and descriptives for most important outcome measures presented for each group and each measurement time	I

[1]The critical review domain that is being evaluated is partitioned by study validity (V), the information needed for analysis of sensitivity and to assess generalizability (I) and the assessment of the precision of the quantitative estimate of the individual study (P) (Koes et al 1996)

be appropriate for the meta-analysis of manual therapy in neck pain. The pooled estimate of the effect size (expressed as mm on a 100-mm visual analogue scale) was 12.6 mm (95% confidence intervals: –0.15 mm and 25.5 mm) improvement in the Hurwitz et al (1996) study and 16.2 mm (95% confidence intervals: 6.9 mm and 23.1 mm) improvement in the McMaster study (1996). A remarkably similar result considering that only one study (see Koes et al in Table 10.2) was common to the calculation of the effect index in both reviews. This may be indicative of the robustness of the treatment effect.

The other interesting feature of these results is that only two studies (Howe et al 1983, Sloop et al 1982) investigated manipulation without mobilization and both studies were included in the Hurwitz et al (1996) study but not in the study by Gross et al (1996). Gross et al (1996) reported that they were unable to abstract the effect size from these two papers. Nonetheless, the results of the two meta-analyses indicate that both mobilization and manipulation appear to be efficacious in the treatment of neck pain in the short term (3–4 weeks). There is little evidence available to support any long-term influence on pain.

A number of authors have suggested that in view of the lack of a clearly superior clinical effect of cervical manipulative therapy over mobilization and the real, albeit low, risk of a significant adverse event from cervical manipulation, mobilization and not manipulation of the neck should be favoured in clinical practice (Barr 1996, Di Fabio 1999).

Judging the efficacy of manual therapy on the basis of the pooled estimates of treatment effect belies the variability in the standard of quality and validity of the clinical trials from which these estimates were derived. The quality score given to the clinical trials presented in Table 10.2 ranged from 33–77 (out of 100) points and the validity score ranged from 2–4 (out of 5) points on the McMaster scale. A study of high quality would be expected to rate in the high seventies (Hurwitz et al 1996). In terms of the quality scale scores, the large proportion of scores below 50 is similar in these studies of neck pain to those investigating low back pain, and suggests that caution should be used when interpreting the outcome of meta-analyses (now look at Reflective exercise 10.1).

Overview of meta-analyses of massage therapy

Massage therapy is frequently used in the management of pain, especially musculoskeletal pain states. Two recent meta-analyses have evaluated the available randomized controlled trials of massage therapy (Ernst 1998, 1999). Ernst (1999) systematically reviewed the literature pertaining to massage therapy as a monotherapy in the treatment of low back pain and reported that all of the four randomized controlled trials (Godfrey et al 1984, Hoehler et al 1981, Hsieh et al 1992, Konrad et al 1992) were burdened with major methodological flaws, such that no reliable evaluation of massage on low back pain could be made. Interestingly, massage therapy is frequently used as a control or passive treatment in the investigation of manipulative therapy or therapeutic exercise in spinal pain (Hsieh et al 1992, Kankaanpaa et al 1999, Konrad et al 1992, Manniche et al 1991, Nilsson 1995; Pope et al 1994, Werners et al 1999). The findings of these

---

Reflective exercise 10.1

- Obtain a randomized controlled trial of a manual physical therapy treatment of an area of your interest (e.g. low back pain, neck pain, shoulder or knee pain) and critically evaluate it against the criteria listed in Table 10.1. The following databases may facilitate the location of a suitable study:
  — MEDLINE (http://www.ncbi.nlm.nih.gov/entrez/query.fcgi?db=PubMed)
  — ISI Web of Science (http://wos.isiglobalnet.com)
  — Pedro (http://ptwww.cchs.usyd.edu.au/pedro/)
- Read one or more of the following meta-analyses and discuss their findings and the impact of such research on clinical practice and clinical research with an experienced clinician and academic of your discipline.

Note how manual physical therapy is often only one treatment approach that is evaluated and sometimes it is not included, indicating the lack of information regarding this modality:
  — Lumbar spine (Koes et al 1996)
  — Lateral epicondylalgia (Labelle et al 1992). As an additional part to the exercise seek out clinical trials of conservative treatment of this condition conducted since this meta-analysis (e.g. Pienimaki et al 1996)
  — General physical therapy (Beckerman et al 1993)
  — Shoulder (van der Heijden et al 1997) NB: read the follow-up discussions in the British Medical Journal (Saunders 1998, van der Heijden et al 1998)
- Alternatively find a meta-analysis or systematic review of your interest and do as requested in this exercise

Table 10.2 A summary of the randomized controlled trials that were used in calculating combined effect sizes for the meta-analyses of Hurwitz et al (1996) and the McMaster study (Gross et al 1996)

Treatment	Subject type	Quality score[1]	Validity score[2]	Included by	Outcome[3]
Manual therapy, physical modalities other than manual therapy, physician, placebo (Koes et al 1991a, 1992a, 1992b, 1993)	Non-specific neck pain (> 6 weeks) with reduced range of motion	73	4	Both	Effect size range: 0.1–0.6 depending on comparison
Manual therapy vs cold packs (Jensen et al 1990)	Post-traumatic headache (chronic: > 1 year)	52	3	McMaster Study (1996)	Effect size: 0.7
Manual therapy and diazepam (Sloop et al 1982)	Non-specific neck pain or cervical spondylosis without radiation (subacute to chronic: 1 month–30 years)	49	2	Hurwitz et al (1996)	18-mm improvement on visual analogue scale compared to 5 mm in diazepam
Mobilization vs collar and TENS (both had analgesics) (Nordemar & Thorner 1981)	Neck pain without radiation (acute: < 3 weeks)	44	3	McMaster Study (1996)	Effect size: 0.5
Rotation manipulations with and without Azapropazone (Howe et al 1983)	Neck and or upper limb pain (acute: < 4 weeks)	42	–	Hurwitz et al (1996)	68% of manipulation group and 6% of control reported improvement
Mobilization and physiotherapy vs rest and education (both had analgesics) (McKinney 1989, McKinney et al 1989)	Acute whiplash injury without fracture (acute: noted stated)	38	2	McMaster Study (1996)	Effect size: 0.6
Mobilization and physical therapies vs rest, collar and advice vs control (all had analgesics as well) (Mealy et al 1986)	Acute flexion–extension sprain without fracture, dislocation or symptomatic degenerative disease (acute: < 3 days)	33	3	McMaster Study (1996)	Effect size: 0.8

[1] Quality score out of 100 (Koes et al 1991b).
[2] McMaster validity score out of 5.
[3] Outcome of study represented as effect size when McMaster study. A positive effect size indicates reduction in pain or improvement in condition (Aker et al 1996). Note that McMaster study was unable to abstract the effect size from the study of Sloop et al (1982) and did not rate the Howe et al (1983) study. Effect size is calculated by dividing the mean difference between the treatment and control groups by the pooled standard deviation.

studies are mixed and seem to indicate that massage may have potential as a treatment of pain of spinal origin (Ernst 1999).

Massage therapy is frequently used in the treatment of delayed-onset muscle soreness, which is a common symptom following strenuous and unaccustomed athletic or physical activity. Ernst (1998) conducted a structured review of the literature concerning delayed-onset muscle soreness and found that there were seven randomized controlled trials, all of which suffered from serious methodological flaws. There is an urgent need to determine the efficacy of massage therapy in the treatment of pain of muscle and spinal origin. As there is difficulty in finding many studies of massage therapy, massage will not be discussed further herein. The reader is directed to the meta-analyses and databases mentioned above for further information about massage.

THE ROLE OF PLACEBO IN MANUAL PHYSICAL THERAPY RESEARCH

Placebo has historically been linked to the healing arts and literally means, 'I shall please' (Simmonds & Kumar 1994, Straus & Ammon Cavanaugh 1996, Wall 1994). Over the past few decades, placebo has had a somewhat chequered reputation, especially with reference to manual therapy. It has been ascribed as being the predominant underlying mechanism by which manual therapy produces pain relief (Curtis 1988, Farfan 1980), especially since manual therapy involves the laying on of hands.

Until recently, placebo has been viewed to have negative connotations (Oh 1991), partly because it has been conceptualized as a non-specific effect. The implication is that manual therapy treatment techniques have no intrinsically specific physiological basis. The placebo response is, however, much more complex, as has been canvassed in Chapter 5 (Ochoa 1993, Wall 1994). Notwithstanding this, the use of a suitable placebo control in the evaluation of any treatment is mandatory (Svedmyr 1979) and should be included in the study of manual physical therapy treatment techniques, especially in the treatment of chronic pain states (Ochoa 1993). The current information on placebo indicates that in the manual physical therapy research paradigm, the placebo condition should account for expectations of the patient, the behaviour and presentation of the therapist, and be similar in presentation but not in intended therapeutic effect to the manual therapy treatment technique.

PAIN RELIEVING EFFECTS OF MANUAL PHYSICAL THERAPY

Pain of musculoskeletal origin is a leading cause of health systems' expenditure in many countries and is the primary symptom that brings a patient to a manual therapy practitioner (Zusman 1984). The pain relieving effect of some manual physical therapy treatment techniques has been investigated in a limited set of circumstances (i.e. a limited number of treatment techniques, outcome measures and pain states). The following is a review of studies of the pain relieving effects of mobilization and manipulation. A brief summary of the literature is contained in Box 10.3.

Effects of mobilization on pain

The initial pain relieving effects of a number of mobilization treatment techniques have been investigated. This research has predominantly evaluated spinal treatment techniques such as the lateral glide, posteroanterior glide, sympathetic slump and combined movement techniques of the spine (Buratowski 1995, Giebel 1995, Slater & Wright 1995, Sterling et al 2000, Vicenzino 2000, Vicenzino et al 1996, 1998a, Wright & Vicenzino 1995, Zusman et al 1989). Except for Zusman et al (1989) all of these investigators conducted within-subjects experiments on the pain relieving effects of the treatment technique, placebo and a no-treatment control condition. Zusman et al (1989)

> **Box 10.3** Summary of findings from studies of the effects of mobilization and manipulation on pain
>
> **Mobilization**
> - Pain elicited during physical examination improves with mobilization but resting pain scores do not
> - Improvements in pressure pain threshold but not thermal pain threshold have been shown in asymptomatic and symptomatic subjects (chronic lateral epicondylalgia and neck pain)
> - Mobilization-induced hypoalgesia is not reversed by naloxone, indicating that it is probably a non-opioid mechanism.
>
> **Manipulation**
> - Equivocal effects on pain following manipulation
> - Pressure pain threshold increases with cervical manipulation (chronic neck pain) but not with lumbar manipulation (chronic low back pain)
> - Cutaneous pain tolerance (electrical stimulus) increases markedly (larger than pressure pain) with thoracic spine treatment
> - Plasma β-endorphin levels not elevated in 3 of 4 studies. However, 2 of these 3 studies did not measure pain relief

conducted a between-subjects study with the express intent of examining the effect of a naloxone or placebo saline injection on the pain relieving effects of the mobilization therapy. Some preliminary studies of the pain relieving effects of mobilization treatment techniques of peripheral joints have also been undertaken (McDonald 1995, O'Brien & Vicenzino 1998, Vicenzino & Wright 1995).

Vicenzino et al (1996, 1998) studied the pain relieving effects of the lateral glide treatment technique of the cervical spine in subjects who had chronic lateral epicondylalgia. A double-blind, placebo-controlled, repeated measures study design was utilized. The outcome measures that were used to measure pain relief were pain-free grip strength (Haker 1993, Stratford et al 1993), upper limb tension test 2b (Wright et al 1994, Yaxley & Jull 1993), and pressure and thermal pain thresholds (Vicenzino et al 1996, 1998a, Wright et al 1994). Thermal pain threshold is the only one of these outcome measures that is not reduced in lateral epicondylalgia (Vicenzino et al 1996, 1998a, Wright et al 1994). In all outcome measures except thermal pain threshold, the lateral glide treatment technique produced improvements that were significantly greater than placebo and control conditions (Vicenzino et al 1996, 1998a). Pain-free grip strength improved by approximately 12–30%, upper limb tension 2b exhibited approximately 22–43% improvement and pressure pain threshold underwent a 25–30% improvement.

The lateral glide and posteroanterior glide treatment techniques of the cervical spine have been shown to increase pressure pain threshold but not thermal pain threshold in normal asymptomatic subjects and in symptomatic subjects (Sterling et al 2000, Vicenzino et al 1995, 1998a, Wright & Vicenzino 1995). The lateral glide treatment technique raised pressure pain threshold by 24% over the lateral epicondyle in both asymptomatic and chronic lateral epicondylalgia subjects (Vicenzino 2000, Vicenzino et al 1995, 1998a). The posteroanterior glide treatment technique produced increases locally over the cervical spine in the order of 15% in asymptomatic subjects and 23% in subjects with chronic neck pain (Buratowski 1995, Sterling et al 2000).

The differential effect on mechanical and thermal pain thresholds in both symptomatic and asymptomatic subjects was viewed as preliminary evidence of a modality-specific effect of manual therapy, with potential implications on our understanding of the mechanisms subserving the effects of mobilization therapy (Vicenzino 2000). This sensory modality-specific effect is different to that found in a study of the effects of transcutaneous electrical nerve stimulation

on causalgia, in which an improvement of thermal but not mechanical pain was reported (Somers & Clemente 1996, 1998). There is evidence that the mechanical and thermal pain modulatory systems have different neuro-anatomical, pharmacological and physiological features (Kuraishi et al 1985, Sawynok 1989). Mechanical pain modulation preferentially involves noradrenergic nuclei and pathways, such as those found in the dorsolateral pons region, whereas thermal pain modulation is associated with serotonergic mechanisms involving the midline medullary structures such as the midline raphe nuclei (Giordano 1991). Chapter 3 provides further information on these mechanisms.

Apart from improving our understanding of the mechanisms of manual physical therapy, there is potentially a direct clinical benefit of this research. An improvement in the rationale underpinning physical therapy treatment selection would be possible if this sort of research was progressed. For example, certain treatment techniques with demonstrated modality-specific effects would be selected for the physical therapy management of musculoskeletal pain states that exhibit preferential dysfunction of the same sensory modalities (e.g. mechanical or thermal). That is, the selected treatment technique would match the pain condition being treated.

Zusman et al (1989) investigated the proposition that manual therapy-induced pain relieving effects were mediated by an endogenous pain control system that involves opioid peptides (Zusman et al 1989). In patients who had pain of spinal origin, naloxone was administered to 10 subjects and saline was administered as a placebo in another 11 subjects. Naloxone and saline were administered immediately following the treatment. An expert manipulative therapist delivered all treatments, which were described as consisting of a combination of combined movement mobilizations and manipulations (Edwards 1992, Zusman et al 1989). Naloxone reversal of the pain relieving effect of any intervention is viewed as a necessary but not the sole criterion in the classification of an opioid-mediated analgesia (Sawynok et al 1979). The outcome measure of pain relief was a visual analogue scale measurement of the pain experienced by the subject, elicited by the most symptomatic movement test during the combined movements part of the physical examination (Edwards 1992). There was an average improvement of the order of 50% from pretreatment pain levels following application of the treatment technique. Administration of naloxone and saline resulted in deterioration in pain levels of only 19% and 26%, respectively. Only the change following the saline condition was statistically significant. Several factors may have contributed to the acceptance of the null hypothesis (i.e. that naloxone had no effect on the treatment-induced hypoalgesia). They were the relatively small dose of naloxone that was used, the administration of the naloxone after the treatment and possibly the small sample size.

Vicenzino et al (2000) recently studied the effect of naloxone on the pain relieving effects of a lateral glide treatment technique of the cervical spine in subjects who had chronic lateral epicondylalgia. They used a double-blind placebo (saline)-controlled, repeated measures study design and reported similar findings to that of Zusman et al (1989). That is, the mobilization-induced hypoalgesia was not reversed by the administration of naloxone and appears not to involve an opioid-mediated endogenous pain control system (Vicenzino et al 2000). Further work is required to validate this interpretation of the data.

Investigation of mobilization-induced hypoalgesia is in its infancy and requires further attention. Future research should pay careful attention to the outcome measures and treatment techniques that are chosen, in particular in selecting clinically appropriate treatment techniques.

Effects of manipulation on pain

Not unlike mobilization, the effect of manipulation on pain has been investigated in a number of ways. These include the use of quantitative sensory testing (Boivie et al 1994) and visual analogue scales for pain. Additionally, the roles of the opioid-mediated endogenous pain inhibitory systems and to a lesser extent the non-opioid systems have also been evaluated.

Pressure pain threshold has been used as an objective measure of change produced by rotation manipulation (Cote et al 1994, Vernon et al 1990). Vernon et al (1990) studied the differences in effect between a rotation manipulation and mobilization of the cervical spine, in patients undergoing chiropractic treatment for chronic neck pain. Pressure pain thresholds at standardized paraspinal points about the manipulated segments were assessed by a blinded investigator before and after the application of the manipulation or control (mobilization) condition (Vernon et al 1990). A mean increase in pressure pain threshold of 45% following manipulation compared to no change following mobilization indicated that manipulation had a significant effect on nociceptive system function. The findings in the mobilization group may reflect patient selection criteria rather than a true treatment effect or lack thereof. That is, the subjects in this study were

undergoing chiropractic treatment immediately prior to participating in this study and may have identified that they had received the control condition. Especially when the investigators report that during the post-experiment questioning, all four control subjects (mobilization) described their treatment as not being 'real' (authors' classification), whereas all five treatment subjects identified a 'real' treatment (Vernon et al 1990). Although the investigator who took the threshold measurements was blind to the intervention, it is possible that the subjects' prior knowledge of manipulative therapy biased the outcome of the study. This could have been overcome by recruiting subjects who were naive to manipulation and mobilization therapy.

In a follow-up study, Cote et al (1994) investigated the effect of a rotation manipulation on pressure pain thresholds over standardized myofascial points in 30 patients with chronic low back pain. The control comparison was a sustained (3 seconds) passive flexion of the lumbar spine applied through the pelvis and lower limbs. Sixteen subjects experienced the manipulation and the remaining 14, the sustained position. Cote et al (1994) found no significant effect of treatment or control on pressure pain threshold. The standardization of points at which the pressure pain thresholds were measured, rather than measuring pressure pain threshold at the clinically relevant (i.e. the most tender and symptomatic) points, could have reduced the likelihood of demonstrating a positive effect for the manipulation. Furthermore, Cote et al (1994) and Vernon et al (1990) used markedly different rates of pressure application (i.e. by a factor of 10). This could have contributed to the differences between the studies because pressure pain threshold is sensitive to changes in rate of application of the pressure stimulus (List et al 1991, McMillan 1995).

Terrett and Vernon (1984) assessed the effect of a cross-bilateral, thoracic spine manipulation on paraspinal cutaneous pain tolerance levels in 50 male subjects (undergraduate chiropractic students) who were asymptomatic at the time of the study. An electrical stimulus (110 volts at 60 Hz) was used to detect a symptomatic paraspinal site in the thoracic spine at which electrically induced pain tolerance was measured before and after treatment. A no-treatment control group consisting of half the subject pool was used as a comparison for the treatment effect. Pain tolerance exhibited a significant increase (in the order of 140%) in the manipulation group and no change in the control group (Terrett & Vernon 1984). Detracting from these findings is the issue that all subjects (chiropractic students) were as reported by the authors, aware of spinal manipulation and all expected to receive a manipulation. This may have unduly influenced the subjects' pain tolerance, as well as the ability to draw inferences from the findings of this study to other settings.

The study by Terret and Vernon (1984) that used electrical stimulation as the outcome measure demonstrated far greater proportional increase in tolerance levels than did the study that found increases in pressure pain threshold (Vernon et al 1990). This may reflect a difference in the tests, either in the difference between tolerance and threshold tests or in the tissues which are accessed by the two stimuli (i.e. cutaneous tissues with electrical as compared to combined superficial and deep tissues with pressure stimuli). The spinal regions that were manipulated may also have contributed to the different outcomes.

Visual analogue scales have become an accepted means of measuring a client's perceived level of pain. The effect of spinal manipulation on perceived levels of pain has been evaluated (Cassidy et al 1992a, 1992b, Sanders et al 1990). Cassidy et al (1992b) found on average a 12-point improvement in pain on a 101-point scale in an uncontrolled pilot study of a series of 50 subjects with chronic neck pain. In a follow-up study in which manipulation ($n = 52$) was compared to a muscle energy mobilization technique ($n = 48$), Cassidy et al (1992a) found that manipulation accounted for a statistically significant mean improvement of 17%, compared to 11% with mobilization. Interestingly, the pre-treatment levels of perceived pain were about 7% higher in the manipulation group whereas the post-treatment pain levels were similar. It is possible that manipulation and mobilization procedures of the cervical spine are capable of producing a change in perceived pain that is limited by an effect ceiling (i.e. limits in pain reduction to a certain level) and this may have accounted for some of the difference between treatments.

The influence of a lumbar spine manipulation ($n = 6$), sham (light physical contact, $n = 6$) and control ($n = 6$) on perceived levels of pain as measured on a 5-point visual analogue scale was studied by Sanders et al (1990). A slight but significant reduction in pain occurred following manipulation but not following the sham or control conditions. In addition, these investigators reported that there were no concomitant changes in β-endorphin levels (Sanders et al 1990). The Sanders et al (1990) study was one of a number (Christian et al 1988, Richardson et al 1984, Vernon et al 1986) that have looked at the effect of manipulation on endogenous opioid levels. Interestingly it was the only one to measure and report perceived pain levels in an unambiguous manner.

Christian et al (1988) evaluated the effect of manipulation or sham in a group of 40 subjects (20 symptomatic (cervical or thoracic spine) and 20 asymptomatic) and found no treatment effect on β-endorphin levels. Richardson et al (1984) manipulated 20 healthy asymptomatic subjects and found that there were no significant pre- to post-treatment changes in endogenous opioid levels. The control group ($n = 11$) behaved similarly (Richardson et al 1984). The failure to measure pain relief by some appropriate measure (e.g. pain perception with visual analogue scales, quantitative sensory testing) limits the interpretation of these papers because these investigators did not demonstrate that the treatment technique produced pain relief. Documented pain relief in the presence of no increase in plasma levels of β-endorphin would provide more compelling evidence against the role of opioids in manipulation-induced hypoalgesia.

Contrary to the other studies into the role of opioid peptides in manipulation, Vernon et al (1986) reported small but significant increases in β-endorphin levels in a sham-controlled study of a single rotary manipulation of the cervical spine. Healthy asymptomatic subjects were used in this study, so it was not possible to elucidate the relationship of changes in circulating endogenous opioids and changes in function of the nociceptive system through the measurement of perceived pain with visual analogue scales. However, quantitative sensory testing could have been used to this end.

In summary, it would appear that manipulation does not increase the level of circulating opioid peptides as measured from blood samples but not cerebrospinal fluid. However, the evidence against a role for these neuropeptides in manual therapy is by no means conclusive. Two factors contribute to this conclusion: one is that the levels of circulating neuropeptide do not accurately reflect levels within the central nervous system and cerebrospinal fluid (Baker et al 1997, Spaziante et al 1990). Opioid-mediated analgesia following manipulation would probably occur at the spinal cord level and/or higher centres (Zusman et al 1989). The second factor relates to the rapid breakdown of these neuropeptides by non-specific peptidases (Barker 1991), potentially underestimating their levels at the time of measurement postmanipulation. In addition, caution has been recommended in the recovery and measurement of β-endorphin in plasma by immunological techniques, because of changes that occur in vitro (Sandin et al 1998). There still exists a need for well conducted experiments to further investigate the role of endogenous opioids in manipulation-induced pain relief.

EFFECTS OF MANUAL PHYSICAL THERAPY ON THE SYMPATHETIC NERVOUS SYSTEM

The relationship between the sympathetic nervous system and the nociceptive system provides an opportunity to study the role of endogenous pain control mechanism(s) in the pain relieving effects of manual physical therapy. A summary of some of the findings of the effects of manual physical therapy on the sympathetic nervous system is presented in Box 10.4.

Mobilization

Research into the effects of mobilization on the sympathetic nervous system has evaluated the lateral glide and posteroanterior glide techniques of the cervical spine, the sympathetic slump technique, the standard slump technique and the anteroposterior glide of the glenohumeral joint (Kornberg & McCarthy 1992, McDonald 1995, McGuiness et al 1997, Petersen et al 1992, Slater & Wright 1995, Slater et al 1994, Sterling et al 2000, Vicenzino 2000, Vicenzino et al 1998a, 1998b). The sympathetic nervous system functions that have been monitored are sudomotor function, cutaneous vasomotor function and cardiorespiratory function.

Grade III lateral glide and posteroanterior glide treatment techniques applied to the fifth cervical vertebra have been studied for their sympathetic nervous system effects. The sympathetic nervous system functions that were studied were the cutaneous sudomotor and vasomotor activity of hand glabrous skin, cutaneous vasomotor activity in the pileous skin of the elbow, heart rate, blood pressure and respiratory rate (McGuiness et al 1997, Petersen et al 1992, Sterling et al 2000, Vicenzino 2000, Vicenzino et al 1998a, 1998b). As in the pain studies of mobilization, these investigations utilized a randomized double-blind placebo-controlled, within-subjects study design. These studies have reported substantial increases in sudomotor activity, cutaneous vasomotor activity of glabrous skin, heart rate, respiratory rate and blood pressure, and a decrease in pileous skin cutaneous vasomotor activity, which are most likely indicative of a sympathoexcitatory response profile. These increases occurred during treatment, peaking towards the end of the application of treatment and were significantly greater than the effects of a placebo or control condition. They were of the order of 60–100% for sudomotor function, 20–35% for cutaneous vasomotor function, 35% for respiratory rate, and 15% for cardiac measures (McGuiness et al 1997, Petersen et al 1992, Sterling et al 2000, Vicenzino 2000, Vicenzino et al 1998a, 1998b).

Further work with the lateral glide treatment technique, involving confirmatory factor analysis modelling of the data, has elucidated relationships that may be important in explaining the mechanism of pain relief (Vicenzino 2000, Vicenzino et al 1998a, Wright 1995, Wright & Vicenzino 1995). The treatment-induced sympathoexcitatory effect was strongly correlated with the hypoalgesic effect (Vicenzino 2000, Vicenzino et al 1998a). In addition, the battery of tests of pain and those of sympathetic nervous system function were found to best represent a manual therapy-induced hypoalgesia and sympathoexcitation, respectively. Based on findings from the stimulation-produced analgesia and stress-induced analgesia paradigms of neurobiology research, the data from manual therapy research has been interpreted as evidence of the involvement of a descending pain inhibitory system in producing these effects.

Box 10.4 Summary of studies of the effects of mobilization and manipulation on the sympathetic nervous system

Mobilization
- Oscillatory mobilizations of the cervical spine produce sympathoexcitation
- Frequency of oscillation influences effects
- Sympathetic slump showed similar trends but much larger magnitude of effect
- Static slump stretch produced a different effect in the lower limbs
- Treatment technique, body region (pileous vs glabrous skin, upper vs lower limb) or (oscillatory vs sustained) may influence response
- The presence of symptoms does not appear to influence these effects
- Research characterized by use of control and placebo conditions, randomization of conditions, blinding the investigators and using naive subjects
- Treatment techniques were well described

Manipulation
- Manipulation-induced changes are characterized as being mixed and complex (i.e. could not be globally described as excitatory or inhibitory)
- Skin temperature changes were variable dependent to some extent on spinal level treated and possibly pre-existing conditions (e.g. upper limb paraesthesia)
- Research characterized by lack of placebo and control conditions in a significant number of studies, use of non-naive subjects, non-blind investigators in some studies, the treatment techniques were poorly described

The control site of this descending pain inhibitory system that is favoured at this stage is the periaqueductal grey region, most notably the lateral column of the periaqueductal grey (Vicenzino 2000, Vicenzino et al 1998a, Wright 1995, Wright & Vicenzino 1995). The lateral periaqueductal grey, when stimulated, produces a coordinated response in sensory, motor and sympathetic nervous systems, typically the response profile is one of analgesia, sympathoexcitation and motor excitation (Bandler & Keay 1996, Bandler & Shipley 1994). The findings of excitation across a broad spectrum of sympathetic nervous system functions, all of which have discretely different control sites in the rostral medulla (McAllen et al 1995), further points to the probable involvement of a coordinating mechanism at pontomedullary or midbrain levels in controlling the pain relieving effects of manual physical therapy (Vicenzino 2000, Vicenzino et al 1998a).

The frequency of oscillation of the treatment technique appears to influence the sympathetic nervous system response (Chiu & Wright 1996). Chiu and Wright (1996) demonstrated that a posteroanterior treatment technique applied at a 2-Hz oscillation produced a sympathoexcitatory effect, whereas the technique applied at 0.5 Hz did not. The lateral glide treatment technique of the cervical spine was applied at a rate of 1.3 Hz (Vicenzino et al 1999). The effect of changing rate of oscillation on its effects has not been studied.

The effects of two different neural mobilization techniques have also been investigated (Kornberg & McCarthy 1992, Slater & Wright 1995, Slater et al 1994). Slater and colleagues (1994, 1995) studied a unilateral posteroanterior mobilization (grade IV) applied to the thoracic spine (right T6 costovertebral joint), while the subjects were positioned in a long sit, slump-like position. Both asymptomatic and symptomatic (frozen shoulder) subjects were studied (Slater and Wright 1995, Slater et al 1994). The treatment technique produced significant and substantial (about 300%) increases in sudomotor activity and reduction in skin temperature at the hand but not in the symptomatic frozen shoulder, in a study of symptomatic subjects. This was interpreted in a similar vein to the cervical spine technique, that is, a sympathoexcitatory effect.

Kornberg and McCarthy (1992) studied a different type of neural mobilization technique to that of Slater and colleagues in that they used a sustained (7-seconds) slump stretching procedure (Butler 1991), which had been found to be efficacious in treating grade I (minor) hamstring tears (Kornberg & McCarthy 1992). A computerized infrared telethermographic system measured skin temperature changes over the proximal and mid-posterior thigh region, as well as proximal and distal-posterior leg region. A relative increase in skin temperature in the treated lower limb resulted from the treatment technique, whereas a slight reduction in skin temperature occurred on the control non-treated lower limb (Kornberg & McCarthy 1992). The authors interpreted these findings as a sympathoinhibitory effect of the slump stretch technique, which is different to those that were reported for the cervical spine treatment technique and sympathetic slump. The reasons for this different outcome have yet to be investigated but could involve factors such as measurement of cutaneous vasomotor activity over different and complexly controlled areas of pileous and glabrous skin, the body regions treated, as well as the method of skin temperature measurement. The type of mobilization technique, such as oscillatory vs sustained manoeuvres or joint vs neural-specific treatment techniques would also contribute to differences in results.

Chiropractic and osteopathic manipulation

The quest for knowledge of the effects of chiropractic and osteopathic manipulation on sympathetic nervous system function has attracted a reasonable level of research activity. This research activity can be categorized on the basis of the functions of the sympathetic nervous system that have been investigated, such as electrodermal activity, skin temperature and heart rate and blood pressure.

Electrodermal effects of manipulation have been evaluated in asymptomatic (Clinton & McCarthy 1993) and symptomatic (Ellestad et al 1988) subjects. Clinton and McCarthy (1993) studied the effect of a manipulation of the first rib, sham manipulation (soft-tissue thrust to the deltoid, i.e. placebo), a set-up for the unilateral manipulation and auditory shocks in 20 male chiropractic students who had an asymptomatic first rib 'fixation'. All procedures were delivered in the same experimental session. An increase in hand sudomotor activity was recorded in all conditions (i.e. no significant differences between conditions).

Ellestad et al (1988) measured skin resistance bilaterally 2 cm either side of the L2 spinous process, following a series of manipulations of the thigh muscles, pelvic, sacral, lumbosacral, thoracolumbar, thoracic spine and ribs, and cervical spine in one treatment session. Forty subjects, 20 with low back pain and 20 without low back pain, participated in the study. In each group of 20 subjects, 10 were treated by manipulation and 10 served as non-treatment controls. This study found a reduction in skin resistance (i.e. increase in skin conductance) following treatment in both low back pain and asymptomatic subjects who were treated (Ellestad et al 1988). There was no change in electrodermal activity in the non-treatment groups. It would seem that sudomotor activity is influenced by manipulative therapy but the type of manipulation may dictate the degree and nature of the engendered differences.

Changes in skin temperature have also been documented in two case-series studies of manipulation (Harris & Wagnon 1987, Kappler & Kelso 1984). Harris and Wagnon (1987) studied 196 patients attending a student chiropractic clinic for treatment of unspecified conditions. They measured changes in fingertip temperature using a skin-contact thermistor after the first manipulation that was administered to the patient in a single treatment period. No placebo or control conditions were used. Except for the spinal region to which they were applied, the treatment procedures were not described. The fingertip skin temperature did not significantly change when considering manipulations performed on all parts of the spine. However, there were significant effects when the spine was considered in terms of the sympathetic and non-sympathetic outflow regions. An increase of about 0.42°F (0.23°C) in fingertip temperature was observed when C1–7 and L4–5 were manipulated and a reduction of 0.25°F (0.13°C) when the thoracic spine and upper lumbar spine was treated (Harris & Wagnon 1987). It should be noted that these changes were relatively small and transient.

Kappler and Kelso (1984) investigated the effect on thermographically measured skin temperature of osteopathic manipulation in the treatment (one session) of 15 patients who had paraesthesia in one upper limb. The manipulation technique(s) that were applied to the T2–5 region were chosen by the therapist on a clinical basis (i.e. treatment technique was not standardized). No placebo or control conditions were employed. Of the 15 subjects, six were found to have abnormally reduced skin temperature in the upper limb and trunk before treatment. The treatment effect was a rapid increase in skin temperature (Kappler & Kelso 1984).

The studies by Harris and Wagnon (1987) and Kappler and Kelso (1984) highlight inadequacies of research into manipulative therapy that should be avoided in future work. The studies were uncontrolled for placebo responses and for potential bias on behalf of the clinician or patient. The time-course of improve-

ment or variability of the conditions being treated was not factored into the study design. That is, no information was gleaned from the cohort as to the change that would occur in the outcome measures over time if treatment were not applied.

The effect of manipulation on indicators of cardiovascular function such as heart rate and blood pressure in asymptomatic (McKnight & DeBoer 1988, Nansel et al 1991) and symptomatic (Rogers et al 1986, Yates et al 1988) subjects has also been investigated. An early study by McKnight and DeBoer (1988) studied the effect of cervical spine manipulation on systolic and diastolic blood pressure in 75 chiropractic students. All subjects were asymptomatic and normotensive. The student cohort was divided into two groups: a treatment group ($n = 53$) and non-treatment control group ($n = 22$). According to the authors, membership of the treatment group depended on the presence of a cervical spine subluxation which was deemed amenable to manipulation (McKnight & DeBoer 1988). This study demonstrated a small but statistically significant drop in blood pressure (mean reduction systolic = 2.8 mm Hg, diastolic = 2.6 mm Hg) in the treatment group but no significant change in the control group (mean reduction systolic = 1.6 mm Hg, diastolic = 0.2 mm Hg). In a further analysis of the data McKnight and DeBoer (1988) report that clinically meaningful changes in the order of 8–20 mm Hg were present only in 14 of the treatment group (26%) and one of the control group (5%). These findings suggest that treatment-induced cardiovascular effects are determined to some extent by the subject (i.e. cervical spine motion segment dysfunction in this study) and/or some other unidentified variable. Although a control group was used in this study no control for potential placebo effects was included.

Nansel et al (1991) investigated the differential effect of a manipulative thrust and sham manipulation (i.e. placebo = set up for manipulation to the point of applying high-velocity thrust) on heart rate, blood pressure and circulating levels of noradrenaline, adrenalin and dopamine. Twenty-four subjects (12 to each treatment condition) participated in the study. Outcome measures were taken before and after treatment at 5, 30, 60, 120 and 240 minutes. No effect on heart rate, blood pressure and circulating catecholamines by the manipulative thrust technique, beyond that attributable to the sham procedure, was evident in this study (Nansel et al 1991). These two studies provide conflicting evidence of the cardiovascular effects of manipulative therapy.

The literature pertaining to the sympathetic nervous system effects produced by manipulative procedures has demonstrated a complex response profile which appears to be in part determined by the spinal region being manipulated, the presence of pathology (symptomatic vs asymptomatic subjects), and the type of manipulative therapy technique. However, these inferences were marred by the lack of suitable control of potentially confounding or biasing factors, which characterize the majority of this research.

The effects of manual physical therapy on sympathetic nervous system function provide a further indication that this form of treatment influences the central nervous system and this may be linked to the ability of these treatments to produce pain relief. In particular the initial pain relieving effect of these treatments may be a predominantly neurophysiological phenomenon.

Box 10.5 Summary of studies of the effects of mobilization and manipulation on the motor system

Mobilization
- Improved activation of deep neck flexor muscles as measured by electromyography and staged pressure biofeedback testing following cervical mobilization

Manipulation
- Motor function studied in a number of ways: electromyographic activity and manual muscle tests. The latter showed no treatment effect
- Manipulation induces an initial increase in electrical activity of adjacent muscle, which was influenced by speed of force application but not the amount of force nor joint noise (i.e. the pop)

EFFECTS OF MANUAL PHYSICAL THERAPY ON THE MOTOR SYSTEM

Many clients attending musculoskeletal physiotherapy and occupational therapy clinics exhibit movement dysfunctions in conjunction with their pain. It appears that these movement dysfunctions involve a number of systems, such as the sensory, sympathetic and motor systems. Evidence of motor-system dysfunction following injury and pain of many body regions has come to light over the past 20 years, for example, at the knee, lumbar spine and cervical spine (Jull 2000, Jull & Richardson 2000, Richardson et al 1999, Suter et al 1998). The effect of manual physical therapy treatment techniques on the motor system has lagged behind. Not only would information about the effect of manual physical therapy treatment techniques on the motor system directly support such therapy in the treatment of movement dysfunction, but it would also contribute to our understanding of the underlying mechanisms of manual physical therapy.

The lateral periaqueductal grey-mediated descending pain inhibitory system produces concomitant analgesia and excitation in the motor and sympathetic nervous systems. If this system contributes to pain relief with manual physical therapy as hypothesized above then it may be possible to demonstrate enhanced motor function as a result of applying manual physical therapy techniques. A brief overview of the motor system effects of manual physical therapy is included in Box 10.5.

Mobilization

The effect of mobilization on direct measures of motor-system function has not been reported. However, there is some evidence that points to an initial excitatory effect in the motor system following treatment with a manual physical therapy treatment technique. A preliminary randomized controlled study of the effect of a posteroanterior mobilization treatment technique of the cervical spine on the activation pattern of the cervical flexor muscles during the craniocervical flexion test (Jull 2000) demonstrated a significant reduction of superficial neck-flexor activity (Sterling et al 2000). A reduction of superficial neck-flexor activity in the craniocervical flexion test indicates a facilitation of the deep neck flexors (Jull 2000). Such findings indirectly strengthen the model that suggests the pain relieving effects of manual therapy result from the treatment's ability to activate an endogenous pain inhibitory system, postulated to be located in the lateral periaqueductal grey region.

Manipulation

The effect of manipulation on the motor system has been evaluated in a number of ways, the most frequent being the measurement of reflex electromyographic activity of the muscles adjacent to the region being manipulated (Boesler et al 1993, Herzog 1995, Triano & Schultz 1990). Another way has involved measurement of the change in manual muscle tests (Haas et al 1994).

In a pilot study of cervical spine manipulation (transverse), Triano and Schultz (1990) evaluated the electromyographic responses of eight muscles (sternocleidomastoid, trapezius, semispinalis capitus and longus capitus, on the left and right sides) around the perimeter of the C2 vertebra being manipulated. The authors reported that muscle electrical activity between 18–54% of maximum voluntary exertion occurred during the application of the manipulation. These values were approximately 3–4-fold greater than the resting electrical activity in the sampled muscles before and after manipulation (Triano & Schultz 1990). The influence of movement artefact and crosstalk on the recorded levels of muscle activity was not considered except for a mention that movement artefact might explain the particularly high response in the semispinalis capitis muscle underlying the manipulator's hand. Manipulation of the cervical spine with its inherently mobile nature makes it difficult to control for the movement artefact in electrical muscle signals. The thoracic spine undergoes far less movement during manipulation, especially manipulations performed in prone lying, and appears to be a better model.

Herzog (1995) and Suter et al (1994) investigated a unilateral posteroanterior thrust of the T3, T7 and T9 vertebrae and the T3, T6 and T9 vertebrae, respectively. Fast and slow manipulations (e.g. pre-load to peak-load time of about 100–150 milliseconds and 2–4 seconds, respectively) of comparable force (at onset of electrical muscular activity) were compared (Herzog 1995; Suter et al 1994). Electromyographic activity of the contralateral paraspinal muscles was consistently observed within 50–100 milliseconds (Herzog 1995, and 50–200 milliseconds (Suter et al 1994) of the onset of the fast manipulation, whereas no increase in activity occurred during the slow manipulation. These findings in both fast and slow manipulations were independent of any concurrent joint sound. The speed of force application, but not the level of force or the presence of a joint sound, was critical in eliciting a muscle reaction (Herzog 1995, 1996; Suter et al 1994).

The preceding studies were conducted in asymptomatic subjects. Two studies of the motor effects of manipulative therapy in symptomatic subjects were found. Boesler et al (1993) studied the electromyographic activity of paraspinal lumbar muscles following one osteopathic treatment session in a group of 12 dysmenorrhoeic subjects. The manipulative therapy was not standardized (i.e. many techniques were used in many spinal regions) but a non-treatment control session was included in the experiment. Electrical muscle activity was measured during active extension from a prone position and during a movement from neutral standing into flexion and back to neutral standing position. Despite presenting no data on perceived pain, the authors claimed that manipulation produced reductions in electromyographic activity

that coincided with a reduction in low back pain. In addition, the electromyographic data were not normalized.

Thabe (1986) performed a study of 20 subjects who had acute upper cervical spine and sacroiliac joint dysfunction. The manipulation and mobilization techniques that were evaluated were not clearly described, the methodology was poor and the presentation of the results was barely rudimentary. For example, electromyographic activity of the muscles tested (mainly obliquus capitis muscle and multifidus muscle) was not normalized, the spinal dysfunctions were not described and several raw electromyographic traces were presented as the only results. This investigator reported that prior to manipulation there was continuous spontaneous activity in the segmental muscles of the dysfunctional motion segment and that the manipulation produced an immediate reduction in the spontaneous muscle activity, whereas mobilization, although producing a significantly lower electrical activity, did not have the same spontaneous effect (Thabe 1986). It must be emphasized that these results should be viewed with caution as they are based on studies that were methodologically poor and inadequately presented. Further study that uses sound experimental principles and methodology is required to investigate the effect of manual therapy on the motor system.

Tests of muscle strength are frequently used in the physical examination of musculoskeletal disorders (Hutchinson & Oxley 1995), so it is somewhat surprising that only one study was found that investigated the effects of manipulation on muscle strength. Haas et al (1994) conducted such a study in which they measured the effect of a high-velocity, low-amplitude manipulation, sham manipulation and a control non-treatment condition on a manual muscle strength test of the piriformis. They found that there was little influence exerted by the treatment, sham or control conditions on muscle strength (Haas et al 1994).

The influence of manipulative therapy on the motor system remains largely unknown at this stage. Research in this area to date highlights the need to carefully select outcome measures of motor system function that are sensitive to, and specific to, any manual therapy-induced changes.

EFFECTS OF MANUAL PHYSICAL THERAPY ON THE ARTICULAR SYSTEM

There is a substantial body of research that has investigated the biomechanical effects of manual physical therapy treatments on joints and other structures (Herzog 2000, Lee et al 1996, Vicenzino 2000). To date there have been few studies directly relating the biomechanical effects of manual therapies to their pain relieving effects, and the parameters of the techniques that are responsible for eliciting a pain relieving effect remain largely undefined. It is important to recognize that, as well as its pain relieving effects, manual therapy has mechanical effects that appear to play a role in the management of musculoskeletal pain.

CONCLUSION

The evidence-base for manual physical therapy is usually considered under two categories: one is clinical efficacy as determined by randomized controlled trials and the other is the study of its effects and mechanism(s) of action. The main question addressed by randomized clinical trials is: 'Does manual therapy work?', whereas the study of the effects and mechanisms of manual physical therapy deal with the questions: 'What does manual therapy do and how it does it do it?'.

Over recent times and particularly in response to socioeconomic concerns, there has been a preoccupation with randomized controlled trials as a means of providing valuable information such as number of treatments required, most efficacious treatment, and the costs to the community. This approach does not provide any insight into what the treatment does (i.e. its effects) and how or why the treatment works (i.e. its mechanisms of action) (Zusman 1992).

> **Reflective exercise 10.2**
>
> 1. How do the studies of the effects of manual physical therapy on pain and the motor, sympathetic and articular systems impact on:
>   - Clinical practice and the decision-making process?
>   - The findings from and the planning of randomized clinical trials of manual physical therapy?
>   - Research into manual physical therapy?
> 2. List the factors that might influence the effects of manual physical therapy on pain and the sympathetic, motor and articular systems. Highlight those that have some level of evidence to substantiate their role in the induced effects.
>
> How would these influence your treatment technique selection in the management of musculoskeletal pain?

Knowledge of the effects and mechanisms of physical therapy treatment techniques will facilitate the efficient planning of a treatment programme in the clinical situation by providing a scientifically based rationale. It will also provide opportunities for improvement of the treatment techniques. Most importantly it will lay the ground for clinically meaningful and valid randomized controlled trials.

The reader is asked to work through Reflective exercise 10.2 as a means of reviewing the material presented in this chapter and the associated literature-base and relating it to both clinical practice and much-needed clinical research.

REFERENCES

Aker P D, Gross A R, Goldsmith C H, Peloso P 1996 Conservative management of mechanical neck pain: systematic overview and meta-analysis. British Medical Journal 313: 1291–1296

Anderson R, Meeker W C, Wirick B E, Mootz R D, Kirk D H, Adams A 1992 A meta-analysis of clinical trials of spinal manipulation. Journal of Manipulative and Physiological Therapeutics 15: 181–94

Assendelft W J, Koes B W, van der Heijden G J, Bouter L M 1996 The effectiveness of chiropractic for treatment of low back pain: an update and attempt at statistical pooling. Journal of Manipulative Physiological Therapeutics 19: 499–507

Baker D G, West S A, Orth D N, Hill K K, Nicholson W E, Ekhator N N, Bruce A B, Wortman M D, Keck P E Jr, Geracioti T D Jr 1997 Cerebrospinal fluid and plasma beta-endorphin in combat veterans with post-traumatic stress disorder. Psychoneuroendocrinology 22: 517–529

Bandler R, Keay K A 1996 Columnar organization in the midbrain periaqueductal gray and the integration of emotional expression. Progress in Brain Research 107: 285–300

Bandler R, Shipley M T 1994 Columnar organization in the midbrain periaqueductal gray: modules for emotional expression? Trends in Neuroscience 17: 379–389

Barker R 1991 Neuroscience: an illustrated guide. In: Turner A (ed.) Ellis Horwood Series in Neuroscience. Ellis Horwood, New York, pp 285

Barr J 1996 Point of View: Manipulation and mobilization of the cervical spine. A systematic review of the literature. Spine 21: 1759–1760

Beckerman H, Bouter L M, Vanderheijden G, Debie R A, Koes B W, 1993 Efficacy of physiotherapy for musculoskeletal disorders – what can we learn from research? British Journal of General Practice 43: 73–77

Boesler D, Warner M, Alpers A, Finnerty E, Kilmore M 1993 Efficacy of high-velocity low amplitude manipulative technique in subjects with low-back pain during menstrual cramping. Journal of the American Osteopathic Association 93: 203–14

Boivie J, Hansson P, Lindblom U 1994 Touch, temperature, and pain in health and disease: mechanisms and assessments, Vol. 3. IASP Press, Seattle

Buratowski S 1995 The Effect of a Cervical Mobilisation on Pressure Pain Thresholds in Normals. Physiotherapy Department, University of Queensland, Brisbane, pp 70

Butler D 1991 Mobilisation of the Nervous System, Churchill Livingstone, Melbourne

Cassidy J D, Lopes A A, Yonghing K 1992a The immediate effect of manipulation versus mobilization on pain and range of motion in the cervical-spine – a randomized controlled trial. Journal of Manipulative and Physiological Therapeutics 15: 570–575

Cassidy J D, Quon J A, Lafrance L J, Yonghing K 1992b The effect of manipulation on pain and range of motion in the cervical-spine – a pilot-study. Journal of Manipulative and Physiological Therapeutics 15: 495–500

Chiu T, Wright A 1996 To compare the effects of different rates of application of a cervical mobilisation technique on sympathetic outflow to the upper limb in normal subjects. Manual Therapy 1: 198–203

Christian G, Stanton G, Sissons D, How H, Jamison J, Alder B, Fullerton M, Funder J 1988 Immunoreactive ACTH, β-endorphin, and cortisol levels in plasma following spinal manipulative therapy. Spine 13: 1411–1417

Clinton E, McCarthy P 1993 The effect of a chiropractic adjustment of the first rib on the electric skin response in ipsilateral and contralateral human forelimbs. Complementary Therapies in Medicine 1: 61–67

Cote P, Mior S A, Vernon H, 1994 The short-term effect of a spinal manipulation on pain/pressure threshold in patients with chronic mechanical low back pain. Journal of Manipulative and Physiological Therapeutics 17: 364–368

Curtis P 1988 Spinal manipulation: does it work? Occupational Medicine 3: 31–44

Deyo R A 1993 Practice variations, treatment fads, rising disability. Do we need a new clinical research paradigm? Spine 18: 2153–2162

Di Fabio R 1999 Manipulation of the cervical spine: risks and benefits. Physical Therapy 79: 50–65

Edwards B 1992 Manual of Combined Movements: their use in the examination and treatment of mechanical vertebral column disorders. Churchill Livingstone, Edingurgh

Ellestad S, Nagle R, Boesler D, Kilmore M 1988 Electromyographic and skin resistance responses to osteopathic manipulative treatment for low-back pain. Journal of the American Osteopathic Association 88: 991–997

Ernst E 1998 Does post-exercise massage treatment reduce delayed onset muscle soreness? A systematic review. British Journal of Sports Medicine 32: 212–214

Ernst E 1999 Massage therapy for low back pain: A systematic review. Journal of Pain and Symptom Management 17: 65–69

Farfan H 1980 The scientific basis of manipulative procedures. Clinics in Rheumatic Disease 6: 159–77

Giebel A 1995 The Effect of a Cervical Mobilisation Technique on Thermal Pain Thresholds in Normal Painfree Subjects. Physiotherapy Department, University of Queensland, Brisbane, pp 59

Giordano J 1991 Analgesic profile of centrally administered 2-methylserotonin against acute pain in rats. European Journal of Pharmacology 199: 233–236

Godfrey C, Morgan P, Schatzker J 1984 A randomized trial of manipulation for low-back pain in a medical setting. Spine 9: 301–304

Gross A R, Aker P D, Goldsmith C H, Peloso P 1996a Conservative management of mechanical neck disorders. A systematic overview and meta-analysis. Online Journal of Current Clinical Trials, Doc No 200–201

Gross A R, Aker P D, Quartly C 1996b Manual therapy in the treatment of neck pain. Rheumatic Disease Clinics of North America 22: 579–598

Gross A, Hondras M, Aker P, Peloso P, Goldsmith C 1997 Manual therapy for neck pain [protocol]: conservative management of mechanical neck disorders. Part one: manual therapy. In: Brooks P, Bosi-Ferraz M, de Bie R, Gillepsie W, Tugwell P, Wells G (eds), Musculoskeletal Module. The Cochrane Collaboration, Oxford

Haas M, Peterson D, Hoyer D, Ross G 1994 Muscle testing response to provocative vertebral challenge and spinal manipulation: a randomized controlled trial of construct validity. Journal of Manipulative and Physiological Therapeutics 17: 141–148

Haker E 1993 Lateral epicondylalgia: Diagnosis, Treatment and Evaluation. Critical Reviews in Physical and Rehabilitative Medicine 5: 129–154

Harris W, Wagnon J 1987 The effects of chiropractic adjustments on distal skin temperature. Journal of Manipulative and Physiological Therapeutics 10: 57–60

Herzog W 1995 Mechanical and physiological responses to spinal manipulative treatments. Journal of the Neuromusculoskeletal System 3: 1–9

Herzog W 1996 On sounds and reflexes. Journal of Manipulative and Physiological Therapeutics 19: 216–218

Herzog W 2000 The mechanical, neuromuscular and physiologic effects produced by spinal manipulation. In: Herzog W (ed) Clinical Biomechanics of Spinal Manipulation. Churchill Livingstone, New York, pp 191–207

Hoehler F, Tobis J, Buerger A 1981 Spinal manipulation for low back pain. Journal of the American Medical Association 245: 1835–1838

Howe D H, Newcombe R G, Wade M T 1983 Manipulation of the cervical spine – a pilot study. Journal of the Royal College of General Practitioners 33: 574–579

Hsieh C Y J, Phillips R B, Adams A H, Pope M H 1992 Functional outcomes of low back pain: comparison of four treatment groups in a randomized controlled trial. Journal of Manipulative and Physiological Therapeutics 15: 4–9

Hurwitz E L, Aker P D, Adams A H, Meeker W C, Shekelle P G 1996 Manipulation and mobilization of the cervical spine. A systematic review of the literature. Spine 21: 1746–1759

Hutchinson M, Oxley J 1995 Principles of assessment. In: Zuluaga M, Briggs C, Carlisle J, McDonald V, McMeeken J, Nickson W, Wilson D, Woolf L (eds) Sports Physiotherapy: The Science and Practice. Churchill Livingstone, Melbourne, pp 131–146

Jensen O K, Nielsen F F, Vosmar L 1990 An open study comparing manual therapy with the use of cold packs in the treatment of post-traumatic headache. Cephalalgia 10: 241–250

Jull G 2000 Deep cervical flexor muscle dysfunction in whiplash, Journal of Musculoskeletal Pain (*in press*)

Jull G A, Richardson C A 2000 Motor control problems in patients with spinal pain: A new direction for therapeutic exercise. Journal of Manipulative and Physiological Therapeutics 23: 115–117

Kankaanpaa M, Taimela S, Airaksinen O, Hanninen O 1999 The efficacy of active rehabilitation in chronic low back pain – Effect on pain intensity, self-experienced disability, and lumbar fatigability. Spine 24: 1034–1042

Kappler R, Kelso A 1984 Thermographic studies of skin temperature in patients receiving osteopathic manipulative treatment for peripheral nerve problems. Journal of the American Osteopathic Association 84: 126–127

Koes B W, Bouter L M, Knipshild P G, Van Mameren H, Essers A, Houben J P, Verstegen G M, Hofhuizen D M 1991 The effectiveness of manual therapy, physiotherapy and continued treatment by the general practitioner for chronic nonspecific back and neck complaints: design of a randomized clinical trial. Journal of Manipulative and Physiological Therapeutics 14: 498–502

Koes B W, Bouter L M, van Mameren H, Essers A H, Verstegen G M, Hofhuizen D M, Houben J P, Knipschild P G 1992a A blinded randomized clinical trial of manual therapy and physiotherapy for chronic back and neck complaints: physical outcome measures. Journal of Manipulative and Physiological Therapeutics 15: 16–23

Koes B W, Bouter L M, van Mameren H, Essers A H, Verstegen G M, Hofhuizen D M, Houben J P, Knipschild P G 1992b Randomised clinical trial of manipulative therapy and physiotherapy for persistent back and neck complaints: results of one year follow up. British Medical Journal 304: 601–615

Koes B W, Bouter L M, van Mameren H, Essers A H, Verstegen G J, Hofhuizen D M, Houben J P, Knipschild P G 1993 A randomized clinical trial of manual therapy and physiotherapy for persistent back and neck complaints: subgroup analysis and relationship between outcome measures. Journal of Manipulative and Physiological Therapeutics 16: 211–219

Koes B, Assendelft W, van der Heijden G, Bouter L 1996 Spinal manipulation for low back pain. An updated systematic review of randomized clinical trials. Spine 21: 2860–2871

Konrad K, Tatrai T, Hunka A, Vereckei E, Korondi I 1992 Controlled trial of balneotherapy in treatment of low-back-pain. Annals of the Rheumatic Diseases 51: 820–822

Kornberg C, McCarthy T 1992 The effect of neural stretching technique on sympathetic outflow to the lower limbs. Journal of Orthopaedic and Sports Physical Therapy 16: 269–274

Kuraishi Y, Hirota N, Satoh M, Takagi H 1985 Antinociceptive effects of intrathecal opioids, noradrenaline and serotonin in rats: mechanical and thermal algesic tests, Brain Research 326: 168–171

Labelle H, Guibert R, Joncas J, Newman N, Fallaha M, Rivard C 1992 Lack of scientific evidence for the treatment of lateral epicondylitis of the elbow: An attempted meta-analysis. Journal of Bone and Joint Surgery 74B: 646–651

Lee M, Steven G, Crosbie J, Higgs R 1996 Towards a theory of lumbar mobilisation – the relationship between applied manual force and movements of the spine. Manual Therapy 2: 67–75

List T, Helkimo M, Karlsson R 1991 Influence of pressure rates on the reliability of a pressure threshold meter. Journal of Craniomandibular Disorders 5: 173–178

Manniche C, Lundberg E, Christensen I, Bentzen L, Hesselsoe G 1991 Intensive dynamic back exercises for chronic low-back-pain – a clinical trial. Pain 47: 53–63

McAllen R M, May C N, Shafton A D 1995 Functional anatomy of sympathetic premotor cell groups in the medulla. Clinical and Experimental Hypertension 17: 209–221

McDonald R 1995 An investigation of the effects of peripheral mobilisation at the shoulder on range of motion, sympathetic nervous system activity and pressure pain thresholds in asymptomatic subjects: An impingement model. Physiotherapy Department, University of Queensland, Brisbane, pp 79

McGuiness J, Vicenzino B, Wright A 1997 The influence of a cervical mobilisation technique on respiratory and cardiovascular function. Manual Therapy 2: 216–220

McKinney L A 1989 Early mobilisation and outcome in acute sprains of the neck. British Medical Journal 299: 1006–1008

McKinney L A, Dornan J O, Ryan M 1989 The role of physiotherapy in the management of acute neck sprains following road-traffic accidents. Archives of Emergency Medicine 6: 27–33

McKnight M E, DeBoer K F 1988 Preliminary study of blood pressure changes in normotensive subjects undergoing chiropractic care. Journal of Manipulative and Physiological Therapeutics 11: 261–266

McMillan A S 1995 Pain-pressure threshold in human gingivae. Journal of Orofacial Pain 9: 44–50

Mealy K, Brennan H, Fenelon G C 1986 Early mobilization of acute whiplash injuries. British Medical Journal Clinical Research Edition 292: 656–657

Meeker W 1996 Point of View: Spinal manipulation for low back pain. An updated systematic review of randomized clinical trials. Spine 21: 2873

Nansel D, Jansen R, Cremata E, Dhami M S, Holley D 1991 Effects of cervical adjustments on lateral-flexion passive end-range asymmetry and on blood pressure, heart rate and plasma catecholamine levels. Journal of Manipulative and Physiological Therapeutics 14: 450–456

Naylor C D 1989 Meta-analysis of controlled clinical trials. Journal of Rheumatology 16: 424–426

Nilsson N 1995 A randomized controlled trial of the effect of spinal manipulation in the treatment of cervicogenic headache. Journal of Manipulative and Physiological Therapeutics 18: 435–440

Nordemar R, Thorner C 1981 Treatment of acute cervical pain: A comparative group study. Pain 10: 93–101

O'Brien T, Vicenzino B 1998 A study of the effects of Mulligan's mobilization with movement treatment of lateral ankle pain using a case study design. Manual Therapy 3: 78–84

Ochoa J 1993 Essence, investigation, and management of 'neuropathic' pains: Hopes from acknowledgement of chaos. Muscle and Nerve 16: 997–1007

Oh V M 1991 Magic or medicine? Clinical pharmacological basis of placebo medication. Annals of the Academy of Medicine, Singapore 20: 31–37

Petersen N, Vicenzino B, Wright A 1992 An evaluation of the influence of a grade III postero-anterior central vertebral pressure on sympathetic nervous system activity in the upper limb. Proceedings of the International Federation of Orthopaedic and Manipulative Therapists, Colorado, USA

Pienimaki T, Tarvainen T, Siira P, Vanharanta H 1996 Progressive strengthening and stretching exercises and ultrasound for chronic lateral epicondylitis. Physiotherapy 82: 522–530

Pope M H, Phillips R B, Haugh L D, Hsieh C Y J, Macdonald L, Haldeman S 1994 A prospective randomized 3-week trial of spinal manipulation, transcutaneous muscle stimulation, massage and corset in the treatment of subacute low-back-pain. Spine 19: 2571–2577

Richardson D, Kappler R, Klatz R, Tarr R, Cohen D, Bowyer R, Kistling G 1984 The effect of osteopathic manipulative treatment on endogenous opiate concentration. Journal of the American Osteopathic Association 84: 127

Richardson C, Jull G, Hodges P, Hides J 1999 Therapeutic Exercise for Spinal Segmental Stabilisation. Scientific basis and practical techniques. Churchill Livingstone, Edinburgh

Rogers F, Glassman J, Kavieff R 1986 Effects of osteopathic manipulative treatment on autonomic nervous system function in patients with congestive heart failure. Journal of the American Osteopathic Association 86: 122

Sanders G E, Reinert O, Tepe R, Maloney P 1990 Chiropractic adjustive manipulation on subjects with acute low back pain: visual analog pain scores and plasma beta-endorphin levels. Journal of Manipulative and Physiological Therapeutics 13: 391–395

Sandin J, Nylander I, Silberring J 1998 Metabolism of beta-endorphin in plasma studied by liquid chromatography electrospray ionization mass spectrometry. Regulatory Peptides 73(1): 67–72

Saunders L 1998 Physiotherapy for soft tissue shoulder disorders – Authors of systematic review misreported one trial that did give significant results. British Medical Journal 316: 555–556

Sawynok J 1989 The 1988 Merck Frosst Award. The role of ascending and descending noradrenergic and serotonergic pathways in opioid and non-opioid antinociception as revealed by lesion studies. Canadian Journal of Physiology and Pharmacology 67: 975–988

Sawynok J, Pinsky C, LaBella F 1979 Minireview on the specificity of naloxone as an opiate antagonist. Life Sciences 25: 1621–1632

Shekelle P 1996 Point of View: Spinal manipulation for low back pain. An updated systematic review of randomized clinical trials. Spine 21: 2872

Simmonds M J, Kumar S 1994 Pain and the placebo in rehabilitation using TENS and laser. Disability and Rehabilitation 16: 13–20

Slater H, Wright A 1995 An investigation of the physiological effects of the sympathetic slump on peripheral sympathetic nervous system function in patients with frozen shoulder. In: Shacklock M (ed) Moving in on Pain. Butterworth-Heinemann Adelaide pp 174–184

Slater H, Vicenzino B, Wright A 1994 'Sympathetic Slump': The effects of a novel manual therapy technique on peripheral sympathetic nervous system function. Journal of Manual and Manipulative Therapy 2: 156–162

Sloop P, Smith D, Goldengerg E, Dore C 1982 Manipulation for chronic neck pain: A double-blind controlled study. Spine 7: 532–535

Somers D, Clemente F 1996 Treatment of causalgia with nerve stimulation. Physical Therapy Reviews 1: 1–12

Somers D, Clemente F 1998 High-frequency transcutaneous electrical nerve stimulation alters thermal but not mechanical allodynia following chronic constriction injury of the rat sciatic nerve. Archives of Physical Medicine and Rehabilitation 79: 1370–1376

Spaziante R, Merola B, Colao A, Gargiulo G, Cafiero T, Irace C, Rossi E, Oliver C, Lombardi G, Mazzarella B 1990 Beta-endorphin concentrations both in plasma and in cerebrospinal fluid in response to acute painful stimuli. Journal of Neurosurgical Sciences 34: 99–106

Sterling M, Jull G, Wright A 2000 Cervical mobilisation: Concurrent effects on pain, sympathetic nervous system activity and motor activity in press

Stratford P, Levy D, Gowland C 1993 Evaluative properties of measures used to assess patients with lateral epicondylitis at the elbow. Physiotherapy Canada 45: 160–164

Straus J, Ammon Cavanaugh S 1996 Placebo effects: Issues for clinical practice in psychiatry and medicine. Psychosomatics 37: 315–326

Suter E, Herzog W, Conway P, Zhang Y 1994 Reflex response associated with manipulative treatment of the thoracic spine. Journal of the Neuromusculoskeletal System 2: 124–130

Suter E, Herzog W, De Souza K, Bray R 1998 Inhibition of the quadriceps muscles in patients with anterior knee pain. Journal of Applied Biomechanics 14: 360–373

Svedmyr N 1979 The placebo effect. Scandinavian Journal of Rehabilitation Medicine 11: 169

Terrett A C, Vernon H 1984 Manipulation and pain tolerance. A controlled study of the effect of spinal manipulation on paraspinal cutaneous pain tolerance levels. American Journal of Physical Medicine and Rehabilitation 63: 217–225

Thabe H 1986 Electromyography as tool to document diagnostic findings and therapeutic results associated with somatic dysfunctions in the upper cervical spinal joints and sacroiliac joints. Manual Medicine 2: 53–58

Triano J, Schultz A 1990 Cervical spine manipulation: applied loads, motions and myoelectric responses. Proceedings, 14th Annual Meeting of the American Society of Biomechanics, Miami

van der Heijden G, van der Windt D, de Winter A F 1997 Physiotherapy for patients with soft tissue shoulder disorders: A systematic review of randomised clinical trials. British Medical Journal 315: 25–30

van der Heijden G, van der Windt D, de Winter A F 1998 Physiotherapy for soft tissue shoulder disorders – Authors of systematic review misreported one trial that did give significant results – Reply. British Medical Journal 316: 556

Vernon H T, Dhami M S, Howley T P, Annett R 1986 Spinal manipulation and beta-endorphin: a controlled study of the effect of a spinal manipulation on plasma beta-endorphin levels in normal males. Journal of Manipulative and Physiological Therapeutics 9: 115–123

Vernon H T, Aker P, Burns S, Viljakaanen S, Short L 1990 Pressure pain threshold evaluation of the effect of spinal manipulation in the treatment of chronic neck pain: a pilot study. Journal of Manipulative and Physiological Therapeutics 13: 13–16

Vicenzino B 2000 Physiological correlates of manipulation induced hypoalgesia. Physiotherapy Department, University of Queensland, Brisbane, p 413

Vicenzino B, Wright A 1995 Effects of a novel manipulative physiotherapy technique on tennis elbow: a single case study. Manual Therapy 1: 30–35

Vicenzino B, Gutschlag F, Collins D, Wright A 1995 An investigation of the effects of spinal manual therapy on forequarter pressure and thermal pain thresholds and sympathetic nervous system activity in asymptomatic subjects: A preliminary report. In: Shacklock M (ed) Moving in on Pain. Butterworth-Heinemann, Adelaide, pp. 185–193

Vicenzino B, Collins D, Wright A 1996 The initial effects of a cervical spine manipulative physiotherapy treatment on the pain and dysfunction of lateral epicondylalgia. Pain 68: 69–74

Vicenzino B, Collins D, Benson H, Wright A 1998a An investigation of the interrelationship between manipulative therapy induced hypoalgesia and sympathoexcitation. Journal of Manipulative and Physiological Therapeutics 21: 448–453

Vicenzino B, Collins D, Cartwright T, Wright A 1998b Cardiovascular and respiratory changes produced by lateral glide mobilisation of the cervical spine. Manual Therapy 3: 67–71

Vicenzino B, Neal R, Collins D, Wright A 1999 The displacement, velocity and frequency profile of the frontal plane motion produced by the cervical lateral glide treatment technique. Clinical Biomechanics 14: 515–521

Vicenzino B, O'Callaghan J, Kermode F, Wright A 2000 The Influence of Naloxone on the Initial Hypoalgesic Effect of Spinal Manual Therapy. In: Devor M, Rowbotham M, Wiesenfeld-Hallinz (eds) Proceedings of the 9th World Congress on Pain, Vol. 16. IASP Press, Seattle, pp 1039–1044

Wall P 1994 The placebo and the placebo response. In: Wall P, Melzack R (eds) Textbook of Pain. Churchill Livingstone, Edinburgh, pp 1297–1308

Werners R, Pynsent P B, Bulstrode C J K 1999 Randomized trial comparing interferential therapy with motorized lumbar traction and massage in the management of low back pain in a primary care setting. Spine 24: 1579–1584

Wright A 1995 Hypoalgesia post-manipulative therapy: a review of a potential neurophysiological mechanism. Manual Therapy 1: 11–16

Wright A, Vicenzino B 1995 Cervical mobilisation techniques, sympathetic nervous system effects and their relationship to analgesia. In: Shacklock M (ed) Moving in on Pain. Butterworth-Heinemann, Adelaide, pp 164–173

Wright A, Thurnwald P, O'Callaghan J, Smith J, Vicenzino B 1994 Hyperalgesia in tennis elbow patients. Journal of Musculoskeletal Pain 2: 83–97

Yates R G, Lamping D L, Abram N L, Wright C 1988 Effects of chiropractic treatment on blood pressure and anxiety: a randomized, controlled trial. Journal of Manipulative and Physiological Therapeutics 11: 484–488

Yaxley G, Jull G 1993 Adverse tension in the neural system. A preliminary study in patients with tennis elbow. Australian Journal of Physiotherapy 39: 15–22

Zusman M 1984 Spinal pain patients' beliefs about pain and physiotherapy. Australian Journal of Physiotherapy 30: 145–151

Zusman M, Edwards B, Donaghy A 1989 Investigation of a proposed mechanism for the relief of spinal pain with passive joint movement. Journal of Manual Medicine 4: 58–61

Zusman M 1992 Central nervous system contribution to mechanically produced motor and sensory responses. Australian Journal of Physiotherapy 38: 245–255

11

Electrophysical agents in pain management

G. David Baxter   Panos Barlas

OVERVIEW

Electrophysical modalities of various types have been used for the alleviation of pain for well over two millennia: application of electroanalgesia predates the earliest written records (Walsh 1997). With contemporary technology has come convenience in application (see Box 11.1), and more widespread use of such modalities, indeed, it is difficult to find a physiotherapy department or rehabilitation unit without a range of electrotherapeutic devices.

Such agents may be broadly categorized into three main groups: thermal modalities which rely upon superficial heating or cooling of the tissues (usually via conductive methods), treatments based upon the direct application (i.e. using electrodes) of some form of electrical simulation to the patient, and finally, treatments based upon delivery of other forms of energy to the patient's tissues; apart from ultrasound, these are based upon electromagnetic energy. The three main groups of electrophysical agents are summarized in Box 11.2.

In the first group, treatment methods range from simple hot and ice packs to infrared lamps. So-called 'transcutaneous electrical nerve stimulation' (commonly abbreviated TENS, or sometimes TNS) is the most widely known (and employed) pain relieving treatment in the second group of modalities. While the terminology could arguably be applied to any form of electrical stimulation applied via surface electrodes (i.e. non-invasively, through the intact skin), its use is generally restricted to describe the application (commonly, but not exclusively, by the patient) of biphasic electrical stimulation over the course of peripheral nerves using small, battery-powered portable devices.

Another form of electrical stimulation commonly used for pain relief is so-called 'interferential therapy', based upon the application of two medium-frequency

---

Box 11.1 Key terms defined

Cryotherapy – Cryotherapy is a term used to describe the application of cold as a therapeutic modality. When used for pain management, cryotherapy is generally applied as an ice pack or vapocoolant spray.

Electrical stimulation/electrostimulation – At its simplest level, electrostimulation (sometimes abbreviated 'electrostim') refers to the application of electrical currents to the body to stimulate biological processes (e.g. stimulation of muscles to produce involuntary contractions). For pain relief, electrostimulation is typically applied with the objective of stimulating afferent activity in peripheral nerves, which will ultimately result in pain relief.

Electroanalgesia – Pain relief produced by means of electrical stimulation.

Electrophysical agent/electrophysical modality – A therapeutic agent or modality that is based upon the application of energy to the body: Such energy may be electrical, electromagnetic or thermal. Used as a more inclusive term than electrotherapy/electrotherapeutic (see below), which strictly only applies to the therapeutic use of electrical currents.

Electrotherapy – Although generally used to describe the therapeutic application of electrophysical agents (with the possible exception of superficial heating and cooling with packs), the term electrotherapy is literally the use of electrical currents as a means of treatment.

Infrared therapy – Infrared therapy (abbreviated to IR or IR therapy) is a term used to describe the use of infrared sources (typically lamps) for therapy.

Interferential therapy – A form of treatment based upon the application of two medium-frequency currents that 'interfere' within the tissues to produce a low-frequency current. Applied in this way, a low-frequency treatment can be provided without the problem of high skin impedence typically associated with electrostimulation at lower frequencies.

Laser therapy – Laser therapy (also termed low-intensity laser therapy, LILT, or low level laser therapy,

LLLT) is a term to describe the use of relatively low-power (athermal) laser and superluminescent sources, typically within the visible red and infrared spectra, as a form of therapy.

Microwave diathermy – The term diathermy refers to the therapeutic heating of tissues using electromagnetic radiation. Microwave diathermy means the application of electromagnetic radiation at microwave frequencies to cause deep tissue heating.

Shortwave diathermy – (See microwave diathermy above). Shortwave diathermy refers to the application of a 27.12 MHz electromagnetic field to cause deep tissue heating.

Skin testing – Skin testing is completed as a mandatory safety test prior to application of certain electrophysical agents. The latter principally include thermal (or potentially thermal) modalities, for which testing of hot and cold sensation (discrimination) is necessary, and electrostimulation for which sharp and blunt sensation is typically tested.

Thermal agent – Any electrophysical modality that is applied with the intention of producing measurable changes in tissue temperature is a thermal modality. While cryotherapy is by definition a thermal modality, the term is most commonly used to refer to heating techniques, i.e. hot packs, infrared therapy and diathermy.

Transcutaneous electrical nerve stimulation – The term transcutaneous electrical nerve stimulation (abbreviated TENS or TNS) in its widest sense refers to the application of electrical currents to stimulate nerves. However, the term is almost exclusively applied to the use of small, portable electrical stimulators to treat pain.

Ultrasound therapy – Ultrasound therapy (or therapeutic ultrasound, sometimes abbreviated US) is based upon the therapeutic application of 'sound' energy at frequencies beyond the human hearing capacity. A commonly used modality in physiotherapy, its effectiveness for the relief of pain is a matter of ongoing debate.

Box 11.2 Electrotherapeutic devices

Thermal modalities
- Heat
- Cold
- Infrared lamps

Electrical stimulation
- TENS
- Inferential therapy
- Other forms of electrical stimulation

Use of other forms of energy
- Diathermy
- Ultrasound
- Laser therapy

---

currents (in the kilohertz range) that 'interfere' within the patient's tissues to produce a low-frequency current, thus overcoming the impedance of the skin to the latter.

Other forms of electrical stimulation may also be used as pain relieving modalities. While some of these are based upon the stimulation of muscles (and thus are different in action to TENS), most are distinguished by the specific waveform produced by the relevant apparatus, which also frequently gives the modality (or device) its name, for example, so-called 'H-wave therapy'. The final group encompasses a range of modalities that are commonly described as electrotherapies, including diathermy (short-wave diathermy and microwave diathermy), ultrasound, and laser therapy.

Following a brief overview of principles of treatment and mechanisms of action, this chapter provides an account of the therapeutic use of the main agents falling within these three broad categories. For each of the modalities indicated, the principles of application are outlined, noting relevant safety considerations for use, after which the proposed mechanisms of action are described. Finally, a brief summary of recommended applications and current evidence is provided. Given the scope of the current text, and the limitations on space for what represents a single aspect of therapeutic pain management, it is not possible to provide a detailed account of application, related theory and discussion of the current evidence for all those electrophysical agents that may be used to effect pain relief. Rather, this chapter provides an overview for those modalities that find most popular application, at a level that should be accessible to all therapists. For more detailed accounts of any of the modalities, the reader is directed to one of the range of electrotherapy textbooks that is currently available (e.g. Kitchen & Bazin 1996, Lehmann 1982, Low & Reed 2000, Wadsworth & Chanmugan 1980).

Learning objectives

On completion of this chapter, the reader will, for the most commonly used electrophysical agents, have an understanding of:

1. The potential role of electrophyiscal agents in pain management, and principles of application.
2. The potential benefits, risks and relevant safety issues associated with the use of such agents.
3. Proposed mechanisms of action underlying the pain relieving effects of electrophysical agents reviewed here.
4. Current evidence to support the clinical application of these modalities.

PRINCIPLES OF TREATMENT

In most cases, electrophysical agents are used in conjunction with other treatment strategies as part of a comprehensive approach to the management of pain. None, with the possible exception of TENS in certain instances, should be regarded as a monotherapy, and their use should be planned to complement other interventions, whether these are exercise, manual therapy or standardized advice, etc.

It is also important to stress that, while electrophysical agents are inherently safe when used appropriately, most are potentially injurious if applied without due regard to accepted standards of good practice. These standards include use of appropriate treatment parameters and, in particular, observation of appropriate safety measures such as completion of mandatory tests and exclusion of patients with contraindications.

Electrophysical agents: mechanisms of action

Electrophysical agents are thought to produce pain-relieving effects by a variety of mechanisms, which can usefully be considered to operate at four main levels: peripheral, spinal segmental, supraspinal, or cortical (Walsh 1997). At the peripheral level, a range of physiological effects mediated by the application of the electrophysical agent may limit or reduce the noxious stimulus, or the response of peripheral nociceptors. The local effects of some modalities (principally thermal agents) include alterations in bloodflow (decreases in acute stage of injury, increases in subacute and chronic phase), reduction of production (or levels) of bradykinin and other algogenic substances and mediators, and finally the alteration or blocking of conduction in sensory afferents. This notwithstanding, there is also evidence for similar effects due to electrostimulation (Jansen et al 1989, Lundeberg 1993). The clinical significance of such findings is that electrostimulation can be used not only for the relief of pain, but also for the facilitation of healing (Lundeberg 1993).

At the spinal segmental level, electrophysical agents may effect pain relief by 'closing the pain gate' through the stimulation of large-diameter afferents, or by mediating the release of endogenous opiates which will attenuate the passage of nociceptive information through the dorsal spinal cord. At more rostral levels in the central nervous system, i.e. supraspinal and cortical levels, electrophysical agents applied at high intensities, or at the appropriate parameters, may stimulate descending inhibitory control mechanisms.

It has to be noted, however, that such effects are critically dependent upon the mode of application or parameters of stimulation. For electrostimulation in particular, the influence of frequency of stimulation upon opiate systems is well documented and supported by a wealth of experimental and clinical research (Han & Terrenius 1982, Johnson et al 1991, 1992, Thomas & Lundeberg 1994).

In the main, low-frequency (1–4 Hz) currents have the ability to stimulate endogenous mechanisms of analgesia that are dependent upon β-endorphin and the enkephalins, whereas high-frequency currents (40–200 Hz) seem to stimulate mechanisms which include dynorphin as the primary mediator of analgesia (Han & Wang 1992). With electrostimulation at higher frequencies ($\geq$ 200 Hz), the main neurotransmitters responsible for the observed analgesia seem to be serotonin (5HT) and noradrenaline (Han & Terrenius 1982, Han & Wang 1992). While there seems little reason for these effects not to be present with any type of electrostimulation typically used by the therapist, these effects have been noted only after the use of TENS and electroacupuncture (i.e. the delivery of an electical stimulus via an acupuncture needle). Similar findings have not been reported for other forms of electrical stimulation such as interferential therapy (IFT) or faradism (see later) and thus further work is required in these areas.

It has become apparent that electrostimulation is a potentially useful means of analgesia. The main factors that are able to affect its efficacy involve its use according to recommendations pertaining to the type of pain, and the parameters to use for stimulation. Current practice does not seem to address the issue of frequency, intensity and electrode placement as important considerations for the therapeutic outcome. Indeed, the research evidence seems concentrated around the issue of frequency. Very little has been reported with reference to electrode placement and intensity as factors likely to affect the therapeutic response.

It is also important to recognize placebo reactions as an important mechanism of action in any pain relieving therapy in routine clinical practice. Such effects are thought to be mediated by mechanisms operating at the higher levels of the nervous system. While placebo reactions are considered at length elsewhere (see Chapter 5), it is important to recognize here the potential reaction of patients to therapeutic devices incorporating high-tech control panels with impressive sounding names.

In summary, when applying electrophysical agents for the alleviation of pain, it is important for the therapist to understand not only the proposed mechanisms of action for the modality in question, but also, and just as importantly, how selection of treatment regime or stimulation parameters may influence production of the physiological effects and, in turn, the desired pain relief.

THERMAL MODALITIES: SUPERFICIAL HEAT AND COLD

The application of heat or cold as methods of treatment (or, indeed, for recreation) predates written records. While hot baths or ice packs are popular methods of therapy that are available to all, in therapy departments contemporary thermal modalities include hot packs, paraffin wax baths or bandages, radiant infrared and heating lamps, as well as ice massage and coolant sprays (e.g. Lehmann & de Lateur 1982, Palastanga 1988). In addition, a number of other modalities rely on tissue heating for their therapeutic effects; these include short wave and microwave diathermy and (depending upon the treatment intensities used), therapeutic ultrasound; these are considered further below. Nevertheless, while these latter modalities may represent significant technological advances over previously available heating or cooling agents (particularly in relation to control of temperature, and ease or convenience of application), the underlying physiological mechanisms of action of thermal modalities are invariable.

Notwithstanding the widespread availability and popular use of these modalities, it should be noted that therapeutic application of thermal agents represents one of the most common causes of patient injury (i.e. burns), and, associated with this, patient litigation. Therapists should therefore exercise particular care when applying such modalities, and ensure that relevant precautions are taken to minimise associated risks, particularly by ensuring that appropriate testing of sensation is completed in all cases prior to therapy.

Principles of application

In most cases, tissue heating or cooling as part of pain therapy is achieved by conductive heating: a 'hot' or 'cold' object is applied to the appropriate tissues and temperature change is primarily effected by conductive methods. Hot packs, ice packs and paraffin-wax bandages are the best examples of this type of application. Where infrared heating lamps are used, the primary mode of heating is through conversion of the radiant infrared energy to heat, by superficial absorption within the irradiated tissues.

Hot packs

Hot packs come in a variety of sizes, and are usually selected depending upon the site of proposed application. Packs are filled with a material that has a high specific heat capacity, allowing the pack to maintain its temperature over an extended period. While the majority of packs used in clinical practice are heated in a boiler or heating tank prior to application, some (including those now increasingly marketed for home use) may alternatively be heated in a standard domestic microwave oven. Apart from the convenience associated with the latter type of packs, their use also avoids the need for a hot water tank, with its associated safety considerations. Alternatively, electrical heating pads may also be used where these are available.

Regardless of which type is used, packs are only applied to areas of normal skin sensation. If a patient is unable to distinguish hot from cold, treatment is contraindicated (i.e. skin test is mandatory). The area of treatment should be carefully monitored and the patient appropriately briefed about the danger of burns and the need to inform the therapist immediately of any adverse effects or increase in painful sensations. The pack is applied directly to the area of pain or the associated lesion and left in situ for periods of 20–30 minutes. The area should be checked at intervals for the appearance of the expected redness or erythema.

Infrared therapy

Infrared therapy is delivered using a lamp that produces (wideband) infrared electromagnetic radiation (3000–5000 nm), which may be either luminous or non-luminous (i.e. radiation may be visible, emitting some visible red radiation, or invisible). Such lamps are usually floor-standing units, incorporating a mains-supplied base controller unit to regulate output, and a radiator and reflector on the end of an adjustable arm. As for heat packs, skin testing prior to infrared treatment is required in all cases. For treatment, the relevant anatomical area is exposed and the patient carefully positioned relative to the reflector of the treatment unit, to ensure that the incident infrared radiation strikes the target tissue perpendicularly, thus minimizing reflection.

Treatment times depend on a variety of factors, including the power output of the unit, although in most cases the treatment period will not exceed 20 minutes. While most physiotherapy departments will have at least one infrared unit, they are perhaps not as widely used as in previous years due to the relative ease of application of alternative forms of heating. For a more detailed discussion of infrared radiation, the reader is directed to one of the electrotherapy textbooks already indicated above (Kitchen & Bazin 1996, Wadsworth & Chanmugan 1980).

Ice packs

Ice packs may be prepared as required using a plastic bag or similar container, which is filled with ice produced by a machine. As is the case when using heat packs (see above), the area to be treated should be skin-tested before application of the ice pack. Some oil applied to the skin will reduce the likelihood of ice burns caused by rapid cooling. The pack is usually wrapped with a towel prior to application, and the patient briefed on the potential risk of ice burn and the need to inform the therapist of any increase in pain. Depending upon the tissue reaction, and the patient's tolerances, ice packs should be applied for up to 20 minutes in most cases. Alternatively, treatment can be performed using vapocoolant sprays, which are particularly popular in sports therapy as they provide an instantaneous form of cold therapy that can be relatively easily applied 'pitch side'. As the spray is an irritant, care needs to be exercised to avoid spraying open lesions, or accidentally spraying the eye, and to minimize any inhalation of the spray, e.g. in enclosed spaces.

Safety considerations

The primary and most obvious risk associated with thermal modalities is burning. To avoid this potential risk to patients, the area to be treated should be tested in all cases for thermal sensation (ability to distinguish hot from cold) prior to application, and the patient specifically warned of the risk of burning. In addition, the patient should be checked at regular intervals during treatment and provided with some means of attracting the therapist's attention if left unattended for any period. For cold therapy, it has been argued that thermal testing is of little practical benefit (Low & Reed 2000), nevertheless, testing in such circumstances would seem a sensible precaution, allowing the therapist to exercise extra vigilance if sensation is determined to be altered. If a patient reports a burn, the area should immediately be treated with cold water; in cases of 'ice burns', the area should be treated with warm water and then wrapped with towels.

The following may be regarded as routine contraindications to cold therapy:

1. Vasospasm (e.g. in Buerger's disease or where Raynaud's phenomenon is present)
2. Cold urticaria. In some cases, cold urticaria is limited to local reactions such as weal and erythema. Systemic reactions may include hypotension and tachycardia.

In addition to the above, care should be exercised when treating patients with cardiovascular diseases (including hypertension). In some rare instances, patients may present with cryoglobinaemia (sometimes associated with rheumatoid arthritis), which gives rise to local ischaemia in response to cold (Low & Reed 2000). The (minor) risks associated with use of vapocoolant sprays have already been indicated above.

The principal contraindications to therapeutic heating include:

1. Absence of skin sensation in the area to be treated.
2. Systemic or local vascular disorders, e.g. hypertension and arteriosclerosis respectively.
3. Local burn, wound or oedema.
4. Dermatological conditions, including dermatitis and eczema. These conditions may be exacerbated by heating, and particularly application of wax. In addition, heating should not be applied to areas of skin damage resulting from ionizing radiation (e.g. radiotherapy).
5. Acute febrile conditions. In the presence of fever, therapeutic heat is contraindicated.

Apart from the above, acute musculoskeletal injuries may be considered a contraindication to therapeutic heat, as heat may exacerbate the response to injury (especially the inflammatory response). Where infrared lamps are used, prolonged viewing of the source should be avoided, and the positioning of the reflector carefully considered to minimize the risk of it accidentally touching or falling on the patient.

Mechanisms of action

The primary physiological reactions to heat or cold are stimulation of peripheral nerve fibres, and localized alteration in bloodflow and metabolic activity (both of which are increased with heating and reduced with cooling). In the acute stage of injury, application of cold therapy will limit oedema formation and the release of algogenic substances (e.g. kinins and histamine). Short-term effects of cold therapy also include blocking of nerve-fibre activity, with the smallest-diameter fibres first affected, followed (after a period) by large-diameter fibres (Douglas & Malcolm 1955), the latter mediating the familiar experience of 'numbness' which accompanies tissue cooling. Such direct effects upon nerves in the area of damage will limit the initial afferent barrage of the dorsal horn and therefore serve to reduce nociception and thus pain.

The mechanisms underlying the pain relief associated with therapeutic heat are more complex (Lehmann & de Lateur 1982, Palastanga 1988, Low & Reed 2000). In the first instance, stimulation of cutaneous heat receptors will produce a pain relieving effect via spinal segmental mechanisms; such effects will be enhanced by the increase in local bloodflow. Increases in cell metabolism will further promote tissue repair, and thus help to resolve the initial injury and source of pain.

Other possible physiological effects of heating which might be relevant to pain relief include reduction of muscle spasm (Lehmann & de Lateur 1982) and increases in joint mobility resulting from enhanced collagen extensibility (Lehmann et al 1970). Such effects of heating can be particularly beneficial in the management of chronic musculoskeletal pain. Apart from the above, and in contrast to reactions to cold, application of heat produces well-recognized psychological reactions that can help to alleviate pain, including feelings of relaxation, warmth and sedation (Lehmann & de Lateur 1982).

Recommended applications and current evidence

Cold therapy is typically reserved for the immediate/early treatment of musculoskeletal injuries (e.g. ankle sprain, traumatic injury to muscle etc. Lehmann & de Lateur 1982, Low & Reed 2000, Palastanga 1988). Its ubiquitous application in such cases is reflected in the use of the acronym RICE (rest, ice, compression, elevation) to summarise the early management of musculoskeletal injuries. While most texts acknowledge such primary application, its potential efficacy in other painful conditions, including chronic arthralgia and perineal pain, has also been noted, although the paucity of supporting evidence from controlled clinical trials is also recognized (Ernst & Fialka 1994, Hay-Smith & Reed 1997, Palastanga 1988).

Therapeutic heat is widely used (by both patients and therapists) in the management of subacute and particularly chronic musculoskeletal pain of various aetiologies including low back pain, rheumatic pain and arthralgia. As part of routine therapy, therapeutic heat is typically used as a precursor to other interventions such as exercise and mobilizing techniques. Although declining somewhat in popularity, therapeutic heat remains a simple and effective means of pain alleviation.

ELECTRICAL STIMULATION

Transcutaneous electrical nerve stimulation

As already indicated, transcutaneous electrical nerve stimulation (TENS) is probably one of the most widely used (and known) forms of electroanalgesia (Pope et al 1995). It can be defined as the application of low-frequency, pulsed biphasic electrical currents, over the painful site or the course of peripheral nerves, for the relief of pain (Walsh 1997), using small battery-powered portable stimulators.

While typically provided to patients for home-use after initial assessment by a therapist or physician, in some countries TENS units are also now available from other sources, including pharmacists or via mail order outlets. TENS treatment is widely regarded by clinicians as (solely) a treatment for chronic pain, and is rarely considered for the management of acute pain, even though other forms of electrical stimulation are routinely applied. However, it is important to stress that the modality can be used effectively in most types of pain, regardless of whether the pain to be treated is acute or chronic in nature, although chronicity may be an important factor in selection of stimulation parameters.

Principles of application

TENS may be applied by a therapist as a part of routine management, as for other electrophysical agents, but is more typically given to the patient for self-application according to standardized instructions, after a detailed briefing and assessment of suitability. Most contemporary machines are battery-powered portable units which allow the therapist to set (essentially 'prescribe') the stimulation parameters on the TENS machine prior to patient issue. TENS units may be single or double channelled, with each channel comprising a pair of anode and cathode electrodes (typically made of carbon rubber or disposable gel-based material). TENS stimulation may be effectively applied to a variety of sites: the area of pain, over relevant nerve trunks or nerve roots, or, where indicated, to appropriate trigger or acupuncture points. The availability of dual channel units allows the simultaneous stimulation of two painful areas (e.g. bilateral arthralgia in rheumatoid arthritis), the treatment of larger areas of pain (e.g. low back pain), or for the simultaneous treatment of acupuncture points and painful area, or nerve root and nerve trunk, etc.

The electrostimulation parameters to be determined in prescribing TENS treatment are as follows:

1. **Pulse frequency** – this is the number of pulses delivered by the machine per second and is specified in Hertz. Typical ranges are from 2–250 Hz, with lower frequencies of < 10 Hz typically used (with higher intensities) for treatment of more chronic pain, and higher frequencies of around 100 Hz for treatment of subacute pain. The mechanisms underlying the action

of different ranges of frequencies (and combinations of parameters) are liable to be different (see below).

2. **Pulse duration** (also termed pulse width) – the duration of each pulse of electrical stimulation is measured in microseconds (μs). Typical values for this parameter range from 50–1000 μs. Shorter pulse durations are generally considered more comfortable by patients (as these pulses don't evoke muscle contractions), although longer pulse durations are considered useful in delivering more aggressive stimulation.

3. **Stimulation intensity** – intensity is usually controlled via a slider or wheel control and is (rarely) measured as electrical current in mA. Usually, devices have a scale of arbitrary units (e.g. 0–10) to facilitate some standardization of stimulation from one treatment to the next. This notwithstanding, it is important to stress that TENS stimulation intensity is assessed in terms of the patient's reported sensation. For so-called 'conventional TENS' treatment intensity should be increased until the patient first reports a tingling sensation, and then until this sensation is reported as 'strong but comfortable'. The patient's sensation should then be reassessed at regular intervals (2–3 minutes) and stimulation intensity increased as necessary to counter any adaptation (i.e. when the patient reports sensation as fading).

4. **Stimulation mode** – Walsh (1997) has described four basic modes of TENS stimulation that are essentially particular combinations of stimulation parameters (i.e. pulse duration, pulse frequency and intensity). Conventional TENS is the most commonly employed mode of stimulation and combines high-frequency (> 100 Hz) stimulation with relatively short pulse durations (50–100 μs) to produce a rapid-onset localized analgesia. Based upon the use of relatively low stimulation intensities, it is regarded as the most comfortable mode of TENS stimulation. 'Acupuncture-like TENS', in contrast, relies on application of high-intensity electrical stimulation (sufficient to effect muscle contractions) using a combination of low pulsing frequency (< 4 Hz) and longer duration pulses (> 200 μs). Such stimulation produces a longer lasting analgesia (but with a relatively longer latency to onset), than conventional TENS, however, due to the muscle contractions, some patients do not easily tolerate this form of stimulation. 'Brief/intense TENS' combines a high pulsing frequency (> 100 Hz) with long pulse duration (> 150 Hz), applied at the highest intensity that the patient can tolerate. This mode of TENS (as its names suggests) can only be applied for relatively short periods of time (10–15 minutes maximum), but can

operate as an effective counterirritant. Finally, so-called 'burst train TENS' is essentially a combination of conventional and acupuncture-like modes, with bursts of high-frequency stimulation (c. 100 Hz) delivered at a much lower frequency (< 4 Hz). This mode of stimulation, which was originally developed by Eriksson and Sjolund (1976), based upon observations with chronic pain patients using (needle) electroacupuncture, is more easily tolerated by patients than acupuncture-like TENS as described above.

5. **Site of treatment** – TENS may be applied directly to the painful area, or over the course of relevant nerve trunks or nerve roots supplying the painful area. Electrodes may also be applied over acupuncture or trigger points, depending upon the circumstances and the training of the therapist.

6. **Treatment regime** – TENS may be applied for extended periods of time, but stimulation periods (at a single site) are generally kept under 1 hour to limit skin irritation, and for convenience. Where home or patient use is prescribed, treatment can be applied 2–3 times a day if necessary, provided this regime is acceptable to the patient. Alternatively some have recommended extensive periods of stimulation (8–10 hours) to achieve best effects (Walsh 1997). Clinic use will of necessity be limited to days (and periods) of attendance.

Safety considerations

While TENS is considered a relatively safe modality, the following should be regarded as contraindications:

1. Treatment over the pregnant uterus. Although a contraindication for most electrophysical agents, it is important to stress that this does not preclude the use of TENS for the treatment of pregnant women at other anatomical sites.
2. Treatment of areas with abnormal or absent sensation. In such cases, the risk of skin irritation or (chemical) burns precludes TENS treatment. However, stimulation may be applied to proximate areas of intact sensation.
3. Application over the carotid sinus (anterior aspect of the neck).
4. Treatment of patients with cardiac pacemakers. While some have challenged the exclusion of these patients (Rasmussen et al 1988), it remains prudent to regard such patients as contraindicated.
5. Treatment of unreliable or incompetent patients (particularly where home use is being considered).
6. Direct treatment over the eyes or gonads.
7. Treatment of undiagnosed pain.

Beyond these situations, the therapist should also carefully assess skin reaction to treatment, as in a minority of cases, severe skin reactions may occur.

Mechanisms of action

The neurophysiological mechanisms underlying the pain relief achieved with the main modes of TENS stimulation are considered to be different (Low & Reed 2000, Bowsher 1988). in particular, manipulation of combinations of stimulation parameters is critical to the physiological effects of electrical stimulation (Johnson et al 1992, Kishioka et al 1994, Walsh 1997).

Conventional TENS, which is used to produce a rapid-onset localized analgesia, works mainly through segmental inhibition (or gating mechanisms), via direct stimulation of low-threshold, myelinated AB mechanoreceptive afferents, and the release in the central nervous system of opiates such as dynorphin (Han & Wang 1992).

In contrast, acupuncture-like TENS and burst train TENS are thought to effect pain relief through stimulation of the descending pain suppression systems (Chen & Han 1992). These opiate-mediated systems at spinal and supraspinal levels are initiated by selective stimulation of high-threshold thinly myelinated A-delta afferents. In addition, where TENS stimulation is applied over the course of a peripheral nerve at relatively higher frequencies (> 50 Hz), stimulation may also induce a localized block of conduction, specifically in nociceptive afferents. These afferents are more likely to fatigue in response to repeated stimuli.

Finally, and although poorly studied to date, TENS will also have a direct effect upon the autonomic nervous system (Han & Wang 1992, UvnasMoberg et al 1993), which may be of particular relevance in the treatment of so called 'sympathetically-maintained' pains, such as reflex sympathetic dystrophy (complex regional pain syndrome). This direct effect may offer some explanation for the beneficial effects of such stimulation on sleep patterns and blood pressure. Apart from such direct neurophysiological effects, TENS stimulation may also affect bloodflow, typically producing a localized vasodilation, which can be useful in the treatment of some types of (chronic) musculoskeletal or ischaemic pains (Lundeberg 1993).

Recommended applications and current evidence

TENS may be recommended for the non-pharmacological management of virtually any type of pain.

However, its typical application is for home/ patient self-use in chronic pain states, where its inherent simplicity and safety in routine use coupled with its recognized efficacy make it an indispensable tool for the therapist. Although most commonly used for the management of musculoskeletal and neurogenic pains of various aetiologies, it has also been recommended for the relief of a variety of other types of pains, including labour pain (Kaplan et al 1997), pain due to burns (Lewis et al 1990) and angina (Borjesson 1999, Orwin 1998), as well as for palliative care in the terminally ill (Urba 1996). Despite apparently wide application, the evidence for the clinical efficacy of TENS in some situations has been challenged by a number of authors (Carroll et al 1997, McQuay et al 1997).

Irrespective of the type of pain for which TENS is applied, in order to optimize analgesia, it is essential that the therapist should consider and design a protocol of application which will take into consideration the impact of factors such as frequency, intensity and duration of the stimulation upon the specific symptoms for which the patient is seeking relief. Despite the relative lack of evidence of effectiveness upon clinical conditions, experimental studies on animal and human models of experimental pain have consistently demonstrated TENS-induced analgesia.

Interferential therapy

Treatment using interferential currents is based upon the application of two different medium-frequency (i.e. kilohertz range) electrical currents to the skin surface, with the aim of producing a low-frequency current deep within the target tissues by interference of the two higher frequencies. This means of electrical stimulation was originally developed in the 1950s to avoid the high current intensities necessary to overcome skin impedance, which is higher with low-frequency electrical stimulation (Nelson & Currier 1991). Interferential therapy has been reported to be one of the most widely used electrotherapies in routine clinical practice in the UK (Pope et al 1995), and is the most commonly employed electrotherapy for the treatment of low back pain, its use surpassing even TENS (Foster et al 1999, Gracey et al 2001).

Principles of application

Interferential therapy (IFT) is usually delivered using two pairs of electrodes (i.e. four electrodes or 'quadripolar' technique), with each pair of electrodes providing one of the two medium-frequency currents.

While the therapy is typically applied using standard carbon-rubber electrodes, circular suction electrodes may also be used (in conjunction with a specialized vacuum unit) to enhance electrode–skin contact.

IFT treatment units comprise a base unit, which is generally mains-powered, and vary in sophistication from relatively simple devices providing limited user controls (e.g. intensity, timer and power units), to highly complex units allowing selection of preprogrammed treatment protocols incorporating variable frequency and waveforms.

More recently, a number of portable devices similar to TENS units have become available, although these devices provide a relatively limited range of stimulation parameters. The principal sites of application when used to treat pain are the painful area, or over associated nerve trunks or roots (spinal application).

The parameters to be determined when applying IFT are as follows:

1. **Pulsing frequency** – amplitude modulation frequency (AMF), also sometimes termed 'beat' frequency. The AMF results from the interference of the two medium frequency currents and will typically range from 2–250 Hz, based upon a carrier frequency of around 2000–4000 Hz. This frequency range is essentially identical to that for TENS, with lower frequencies of < 10 Hz typically used for treatment of more chronic pain, and higher frequencies of > 100 Hz for treatment of acute or subacute pain.

2. **Sweep frequency** – in contrast to TENS, interferential machines also permit the operator to vary the pulsing frequency over time, over a predetermined range. This 'range' is usually termed the sweep frequency, and is specified in Hz. To illustrate, the operator selecting a 'sweep' frequency of 20 Hz together with a base frequency of 50 Hz would result in a machine output which varied from 50–70 Hz over the selected treatment period. Alternatively, some machines will allow specification of 'base' and 'upper' frequencies, however the net result (in terms of output) will be the same. Most machines will also have a control to allow selection of the rate of change of frequency (i.e. the rate at which the frequency 'sweeps' from one extreme to the other), or the period over which a sweep-cycle occurs. The relevance of the sweep facility is unclear, as few studies have systematically assessed this parameter. This notwithstanding, it is likely that varying the frequency over time will stimulate a wider variety of nerve types than possible at a single frequency (particularly where sweep frequency is large), and will also limit the likelihood of nerve habituation (Low & Reed 2000,

Martin 1996). The precise relevance of length of sweep-cycle is similarly occult. However, it is apparent that shorter cycles (i.e. faster sweeps between the extremes of frequency) will result in a more intensive form of stimulation, while longer cycles will be more comfortable for the patient.

3. **Vector** – the interference pattern of the two medium-frequency currents in the tissue has been proposed to approximate a (two-dimensional) clover leaf. Some machines allow the operator to select an additional control known as 'rotating vector', 'scanning', 'dynamic interference' or 'vector sweep', etc. With this feature enabled, the device will systematically vary the current intensity to each pair of electrodes to effectively 'rotate' the area of interference within the tissues, thus stimulating a larger area of the target tissues.

4. **Stimulus intensity** – as with TENS, intensity is usually established on the basis of the patient's subjective report. For higher frequencies the stimulus intensity should be adjusted until the patient reports a 'strong but comfortable' sensation. For lower stimulus frequencies, stimulus levels will be less comfortable, particularly where muscle contraction is desired. Where sweep frequency is employed, the stimulus intensity should be carefully selected to ensure that the setting is appropriate across the frequency range.

5. **Electrode configuration** – the most usual electrode configuration is quadripolar, based upon the use of two pairs of electrodes, which are carefully placed to ensure that the area of interference overlaps the target tissue. For example, for treatment of a painfully arthritic knee joint, the electrodes would be placed above and below the knee, on the medial and lateral aspect of the joint, with each pair 'crossing' the joint. So-called bipolar technique can also be employed where appropriate. It is based upon the use of a single pair of electrodes, to which the controller unit delivers both medium-frequency currents. In such cases, the interference pattern occurs at the electrode level, and throughout the tissues lying between the two. Where this arrangement is used, stimulation, and thus treatment effects, will be more superficial than for quadripolar application. Thus, siting of electrodes needs to be carefully considered in respect of target tissue.

6. **Electrode type** – several types of electrodes may be used in interferential therapy. The most commonly seen are carbon rubber or metal, which may be covered with sponges that have been soaked in saline. Such electrodes come in a variety of sizes to suit the particular area to be treated, and are usually held in place via some form of bandaging. Alternatively,

vacuum suction units provided on some machines may also be used to attach specially designed rubber electrodes. Use of such vacuum units provide additional tissue stimulation by virtue of the negative pressure produced under the electrodes. Where suction is used, care needs to be exercised in the avoidance of tissue injury due to high levels of negative pressure under the electrodes. To limit such risks, most machines vary the level of suction during application.

7. **Site of treatment** – as with TENS, the primary sites for application of interferential therapy are directly to the painful area, or over the course of the relevant nerve trunks or nerve roots supplying the painful area. With quadripolar technique, and the use of larger electrodes, interferential currents can be effectively used to treat larger and deeper areas of tissue.

8. **Treatment regime** – in contrast to TENS, interferential therapy is typically applied for relatively limited periods of time, with stimulation periods (at a single site) usually kept under 30 minutes. Despite the appearance of smaller units to facilitate home or patient self-use, most interferential treatments will be applied by therapists during clinic attendance, and thus frequency of treatment will be limited to days of attendance.

A number of modern machines are based upon 'built-in' treatment programmes (sometimes up to 100 are provided) which are selected on the basis of condition or desired effect. Such programmes will comprise a set combination of the parameters described here.

Safety considerations

The safety considerations for interferential therapy are as already described above for TENS. In addition, where suction is to be used, care should be taken to ensure that the negative pressure does not cause injury or bruising.

Mechanisms of action

Apart from its claimed pain relieving effects, interferential currents may also be used to stimulate muscle contraction, and are claimed to increase bloodflow and promote tissue healing (De Domenico 1982, Martin 1996). While the evidence for the latter may be regarded as equivocal, if true, such putative effects would be useful in the management of a variety of conditions where nociceptive pain is the primary problem (e.g. pain in some types of wound, musculoskeletal injuries).

Where used specifically to relieve pain, interferential therapy is proposed to work in a similar fashion to TENS (see above), with higher frequencies primarily achieving effects via segmental inhibition, and lower frequencies by stimulation of descending control systems. Apart from such mechanisms that are common to TENS, the use of suction electrodes adds another form of sensory stimulation to complement that produced by the interferential treatments. The (rhythmically varying) negative pressure produces a 'massage-like' effect, which most patients describe as relaxing or soothing, and which additionally stimulates large-diameter afferents to enhance the inhibitory effects at spinal segmental levels.

Recommended applications and current evidence

As already indicated above, interferential therapy is one of the most commonly used modalities for the management of back pain (Foster et al 1999, Gracey et al 2001). However, despite a long history of application, and recommendation for routine use in physiotherapy (Belcher 1974, De Domenico 1982, Willie 1969), good evidence (i.e. from controlled clinical trials) for the analgesic efficacy of this modality is virtually non-existent (Low & Reed 2000, Martin 1996). Although evidence from trials on TENS-mediated analgesia may (with some caution and due recognition of the relevance of stimulation parameters) be extrapolated to support the potential effectiveness of interferential therapy in a variety of conditions, the additional benefit of IFT currents beyond that achieved with TENS has yet to be definitively established under controlled clinical conditions. For the time being, further discussion awaits the results of ongoing studies at a number of centres (e.g. The Northern Ireland Trial of Backpain Management using IFT and Manipulation, at the University of Ulster). In the meantime, studies using experimental laboratory pain would indicate potential benefits of IFT at appropriate stimulation parameters (Noble 2000, Stephenson & Johnson 1995).

Other forms of electrical stimulation

A wide variety of other forms of electrical stimulation currents have been reported as beneficial in the management of pain. These include, but are not limited to: long established (but declining) modalities such as faradic and sinusoidal currents, as well as novel electrostimulation modalities such as diadynamic currents, rebox, H-wave therapy, action potential stimulation and so-called transcutaneous spinal electroanalgesia. While space precludes a detailed analysis of each of these types of current, it useful to stress that detailed controlled investigations of the physiological and analgesic effects of such modalities is frequently lacking. Furthermore, in some cases, published reports claiming positive results for 'novel' therapies have been authored by developers or inventors and thus the objectivity of such reports, regardless of the intentions of the authors, would appear to be open to question. Pending more comprehensive investigation, there is little data to support the preferential use of such currents over simple TENS.

ELECTROPHYSICAL AGENTS USING ALTERNATIVE FORMS OF ENERGY

Laser therapy

The term laser therapy describes the use of electromagnetic energy in the visible or near-infrared spectra at sub-thermal intensities to stimulate tissue repair and wound healing processes, and to relieve pain (Baxter 1994). Alternative terminologies include low-level laser therapy, low-intensity laser therapy, cold laser therapy, or laser photobiostimulation, most of which are used to distinguish the therapy from high-intensity laser applications in medicine (e.g. as laser scalpels in surgery) and/or tissue interactions associated with higher irradiation intensities. Although it has long been a popular electrotherapeutic modality in routine clinical practice for the promotion of wound repair (e.g. Baxter et al 1991), its use as an analgesic agent has proved to be contentious in some quarters (Devor 1990).

Principles of application

Laser therapy is most commonly delivered using diode sources, which can be applied singly, or in the form of a multisource array, which may incorporate anything from two to over 100 diodes. While the former are most useful for treating points (e.g. over the course of nerves), arrays are more popular for treating more extensi e lesions or sites of pain. Alternatively, gas-based lasers of various types have also been successfully used for laser therapy. Such treatment units may incorporate helium–neon (He-Ne) lasers (producing visible red light in the milliwatt range), or higher powered carbon dioxide (CO_2) or neodymium–yttrium–aluminium garnet (Nd:YAG) sources (producing near-infrared radiation at outputs over a watt, but defocused to ensure intensities on the tissue surface are kept low).

Compared to alternative electrophysical agents, laser therapy is relatively safe, with the main danger arising from the potential ocular danger associated with highly collimated beams. The risk of burning with laser therapy systems is negligible, and for the diode-based systems most commonly used in therapy, effectively zero. Although the output powers used in treatment have been rising steadily over the last decade, the vast majority of therapeutic units are well within the upper limit for classification as Class IIIB laser systems (500 mW). It is important to remember that this limit applies to a single laser light source; the total power output of multisource arrays may be well over one watt.

When treating pain, laser therapy may be applied to a number of sites, either individually or in combination. These include the lesion or site of pain, any indicated acupuncture or trigger points, or over the course of relevant peripheral nerves or spinal nerve roots. During irradiation, the laser treatment head is applied to the skin overlying the target tissue (using so-called 'contact technique'), with the head held in firm contact using a firm pressure within the patient's tolerances. Treatment is defined in terms of the wavelength (expressed in nanometres, nm) and power output of the device (milliwatts, mW), and the dosage per point or area treated. The latter can be expressed in joules (J) for the energy applied (per point or as a total across multiple points), or more precisely as radiant exposure or energy density (in joules per square centimetre, $J\,cm^{-2}$). Apart from the above, laser radiation may also be pulsed, which has been argued as important to some physiological (and in turn clinical) effects of treatment. Typical ranges for the various parameters indicated are as follows:

1. Wavelengths are typically of 630–904 nm (although wavelengths for CO_2 and Nd:YAG systems are somewhat higher.
2. Power outputs range from several milliwatts up to the classification limit of 500 mW, although most systems in routine practice tend to fall between 5–200 mW. Outputs for diode arrays may be higher still.
3. Energy per point may vary from fractions of a joule to over 10 J. In musculoskeletal therapy, where treatment is applied through intact skin, energy would tend to be somewhat higher (i.e. > 1 J typically).
4. Continuous wave or pulsed mode may be employed. In the latter case, pulse repetition rates are typically kept low (i.e. < 100 Hz), although positive results have been reported at higher rates.

Safety considerations

The following should be regarded as the major contraindications to laser therapy (Baxter 1994):

1. The presence of active or suspected carcinoma (except possibly in hospice care where the ethical considerations will be different)
2. Direct irradiation of the eyes, given the potential ocular hazard from focusing the beam onto the retina. Goggles should be worn by patient and therapist to avoid the risk of accidental intrabeam viewing
3. Cognitive difficulties or unreliable patient
4. Increased sensitivity to light (i.e. where photosensitizing drugs are used)
5. Irradiation over the pregnant uterus.

While not regarded as absolute contraindications to treatment, care should also be exercised in the following situations:

1. Irradiation of the gonads
2. Treatment of patients with a history of epilepsy
3. Irradiation of areas of altered skin sensitivity.

It should be remembered that laser therapy is essentially an athermal modality and therefore can be applied in the early stage post injury or trauma.

Mechanisms of action

The principal (and best-understood) effects of laser irradiation are at the cellular level (Karu 1998). These effects provide the theoretical underpinnings for the cardinal application for this modality, treatment of delayed or compromised wound healing. Thus, similarly to ultrasound (see below), laser may help to achieve pain relief by promoting earlier resolution or healing of the underlying lesion. Beyond this, the putative mechanisms underlying the application of laser therapy as a specific pain relieving agent (as compared to its biostimulatory effects) are less well understood, which no doubt contributes to the controversy surrounding this particular application. Certainly any simplistic explanation in terms of segmental inhibition based upon the stimulation of large-diameter afferents is inherently flawed given the lack of any evoked neurophysiological effects or associated sensation during laser irradiation (Wu et al 1987), notwithstanding thermal sensations with irradiation using defocused CO_2 and Nd:YAG systems.

However, other possible (and more likely) mechanisms of action include direct effects upon conduction in peripheral nerves (Baxter et al 1994), selective suppression of activity in small-diameter nociceptive afferents as a result of laser irradiation (Wesselmann et al 1990), and alteration in metabolism of various endogenous opiate-like substances (Wedlock & Shephard 1996).

Evidence would also suggest that laser irradiation may selectively affect bloodflow, depending upon the underlying pathology or perfusion of the treated tissue. Findings of laser-mediated reductions in bloodflow (Lowe et al 1997), which are more marked in hyperaemia, coupled with the athermic nature of the modality (and, indeed its biostimulatory effects) would indicate its use in the very acute stages of injury, where the application of alternative electrophysical agents may not be appropriate.

Recommended applications and current evidence

Laser therapy has been reported to be effective in the treatment of pain of various aetiologies, including musculoskeletal, arthrogenic and neurogenic pain (Baxter 1994, Tuner & Hode 1999). Musculoskeletal pain is perhaps the most commonly treated type of pain, with reports of significant benefits in the treatment of a range of conditions from tendinopathies (England et al 1989), lateral epicondylitis (Simunovic et al 1998) to low back pain (Basford et al 1999). While positive reports predominate, the general standard of publications (and research) has been criticized by a number of authors, although it has been recognized that the quality of this research has been improving over recent years (e.g. Basford 1995). A recent criteria-based systematic review by de Bie and colleagues (1998) found some (limited) evidence to support the use of 904 nm laser in the treatment of tendinopathies and arthralgia of the knee. However, in other areas, there was insufficient evidence of benefit (e.g. for rheumatoid arthritis). While more extensive systematic reviews of this type have yet to be completed for other wavelengths, previous narrative or open reviews have suggested best evidence for pain relief in neurogenic pain conditions (including post-herpetic neuralgia), and where infrared wavelengths are used (see Baxter 1994, Walker 1988). Positive results have also been found to be associated with the use of relatively higher power and energy (dosage) levels.

Ultrasound

Ultrasound remains one of the most widely used electrophysical modalities in physiotherapy (ter Haar et al 1985). The principal indications for ultrasound are typically associated with the stimulation of repair processes (in chronic wounds and ulcers, as well as soft tissue injuries), rather than pain management per se. Indeed a number of standard texts on ultrasound have either overlooked or dismissed the potential pain relieving effects of the modality (Kahn 1987, Young 1996). Despite this, ultrasound has been reported as effective in a variety of painful conditions, including rheumatoid arthritis and other forms of arthrogenic pain (Clarke & Stenner 1976, De Preux 1952), herpes zoster/post-herpetic neuralgia (Jones 1984, Payne 1984) and low back pain (Patrick 1978).

In contrast to other 'electrotherapeutic' modalities, therapeutic ultrasound is based upon the application of sound energy to the tissues, rather than electromagnetic energy. This is an important factor in treatment, as sound waves are a longitudinal waveform, based upon the compression–rarefraction of a medium. Sound waves therefore cannot be propagated through a vacuum (unlike light), and as a consequence, application of ultrasound requires use of a coupling medium (usually water-based gels or water) to deliver the sound waves to the tissues (see below).

Principles of application

Ultrasound devices comprise a treatment head (incorporating a piezoelectric crystal), and a mains-powered base unit or controller. The frequency of the ultrasound energy emitted by a unit is fixed by the crystal in the treatment head, which operates via the reverse piezoelectric effect. The base unit or controller will typically allow selection of pulsed vs continuous modes of operation, as well as of output intensity, and also provide a timer and on–off switch. Ultrasound frequencies are within the megahertz range (i.e. millions of waves per second), typically being between 0.5 and 3 MHz, and as the name 'ultrasound' suggests, are too high to be heard by the unassisted human ear.

As already indicated, because of the relatively poor transmission of ultrasonic waves in air, some form of coupling agent is required for ultrasound treatment. The coupling agent may vary from water-based gels (e.g. for treating a painful muscle), or submersion of the affected body part in a water basin or tank (e.g. for treatment of arthritis in the small joints of the hand).

To limit the potential problems associated with unstable cavitation, standing wave formation, and excessive tissue heating (see below), the ultrasound treatment head is typically moved across the skin of the area to be treated during insonation, using a scanning or sweeping motion, or alternatively with a circular 'polishing' movement. Such movement has been argued to provide an additional 'massage-like' stimulation, which may enhance the pain relieving effect of the insonation.

Treatment intensities are typically in the region of 0.1–3 W cm^{-2}, with lower range (i.e. athermic) intensities being more popular in some countries (principally the UK) and the higher, heating intensities used more commonly in North America (Young 1996).

Treatment time is usually defined in relation to whether the condition is acute or chronic, and the size of the area to be treated, and can range from around 1–20 minutes, although treatment times of 2–10 minutes are most common. Given its potential thermal effects, patients should be skin-tested for hot and cold discrimination prior to application of ultrasound. In addition, therapeutic ultrasound may cause periosteal pain when applied close to bone, particularly around bony prominences where geometry may cause build up of energy, e.g. on epicondylar areas. Similar concentrations of energy by metal implants may also cause painful reactions or burning to tissue. All patients should therefore be screened for the presence of metal implants close to the proposed area of ultrasound treatment, and extra care taken when treating close to underlying bony areas.

Safety considerations

The following can be regarded as the major contraindications and precautions associated with ultrasound treatment (see Dyson 1988):

1. Compromised skin sensation (the patient should be tested for skin sensation)
2. 'Sensitive' areas: eye, cranium, stellate ganglion, gonads
3. Pregnant uterus
4. Active or suspected carcinoma, areas receiving radiation therapy
5. Vascular abnormalities (e.g. deep venous thrombosis), cardiac region in chronic disease
6. Boney prominences
7. Metal implants
8. Acute infections.

Mechanisms of action

The principal clinical effect of therapeutic ultrasound is the promotion of wound healing or tissue-repair processes. In cases where stimulation of repair mechanisms is the primary goal of treatment (whether in acute muscle tears, or in chronic ulceration), pain relief will occur concomitantly with progression of repair, that is, the patient's pain will reduce as healing progresses.

The two primary mechanisms by which therapeutic ultrasound affects tissue repair at non-thermal intensities are 'cavitation' (production of gas bubbles within the tissues), and 'acoustic streaming' (movement of tissue fluids and ions as a result of ultrasound). These physical effects of ultrasound produce in turn a variety of cellular events that include alteration of membrane permeability, increase in calcium uptake, and increased production of growth factors by macrophages (Dyson 1982, 1985, Mortimer & Dyson 1988, Young & Dyson 1990). This cascade of cellular responses initiated by insonation at non-thermal intensities ultimately leads to acceleration of wound healing or tissue repair, and, with this, reduction of pain.

Other physiological effects of ultrasound that are potentially relevant to pain relief include possible alteration of local bloodflow or oxygen tension (Dyson & Pond 1973, Hansen & Kristensen 1973, Hogan et al 1982, Rubin et al 1990) and peripheral neural function (Cosentino et al 1983, Hong 1991, Moore et al 2000). Apart from potential application for the alleviation of ischaemic muscle or limb pain (Hogan et al 1982), ultrasound-mediated increases in local bloodflow as a result of thermal effects of insonation may be beneficial when treating subacute or chronic musculoskeletal pain. In addition, evidence of altered nerve conduction following insonation (Hong 1991, Moore et al 2000) indicates the potential of direct neurophysiological effects upon peripheral nerve function, even if the precise relevance of such effects to pain relief is not entirely clear.

At relatively higher insonation intensities, thermal tissue reactions predominate as absorption of sound energy leads to heating of the tissue. The physiological effects produced by tissue heating (as already described above) represent an important mechanism of pain relief at higher ultrasound output levels. However, it must also be recognized that the risk of adverse events concomitantly increases with insonation intensity. Such adverse events (which can include production of high levels of free radicals and localized areas of tissue destruction) are principally associated with two potential effects of ultrasound, unstable cavitation, and standing wave formation. In the former instance, the (normally stable) gas bubble produced by ultrasound collapses and reforms, potentially causing high levels of localized damage in the process. Standing waves result from the interference of ultrasound energy reflected from a relatively dense surface within the tissue (e.g. bone) with the incident ultrasound beam to produce a 'fixed' wave, and in turn high concentrations of energy at focal points within the tissue. As with unstable cavitation, tissue damage is possible in such circumstances. While 'thermal' ultrasound intensities are commonly used in North America, elsewhere (and particularly in the UK), concern over such adverse reactions has led to routine use of much lower ultrasound power levels, and pulsed rather than continuous waveforms.

Apart from the above, it is also important to recognize the potential relevance of the associated 'mechanical' stimulation provided by the movement of the ultrasound head over the tissue during treatment. This 'massaging' of the tissue selectively stimulates low-threshold mechanoreceptors, and therefore increases large-diameter afferent activity, with consequent activation of spinal segmental mechanisms. Although not always recognized as a potential mechanism of pain relief by ultrasound, the pain relief reported for 'placebo' or sham insonation groups in controlled studies (see Van der Windt et al 1999, 2000) are highly suggestive of the potential benefits of the 'massaging' component of ultrasound therapy.

Finally, it should be noted that ultrasound has been used in conjunction with various gels (and sometimes creams) to help drive an active compound (e.g. an NSAID) into a target area of tissue. Such phono- or sono-phoresis has been investigated at a number of centres, with variable results for pain relief (Ciccone et al 1991, Shin & Choi, 1997, Klaiman et al 1998). This notwithstanding, it is important to remember that the mechanisms underlying any pain relief achieved with this therapy are as likely to be due to the drug, rather than any specific effects of ultrasound per se (Kanikkannan et al 2000).

Recommended applications and current evidence

As already indicated, ultrasound has been reported as effective in the management of a variety of painful conditions, including musculoskeletal (Clarke & Stenner 1976, De Preux 1952, Patrick 1978), and neurogenic pains (Jones 1984, Payne 1984). Nevertheless, recent reviews of the literature in this area have indicated only limited evidence for pain relieving effects of ultrasound, but recommended that further controlled clinical trials are necessary before more making more definitive pronouncements (Van der Windt et al 1999).

Shortwave and microwave diathermy

Apart from the use of direct superficial heating methods as already described above, diathermy using relatively high frequency electromagnetic currents to provide deeper tissue heating has been popular for several decades. The principal and most enduring form of this is so-called shortwave diathermy, based upon the use of a 27.12 MHz electromagnetic field. More recently, microwave diathermy based upon much higher frequencies of electromagnetic radiation (433.9, 915 or 2450 MHz) has also been introduced.

Principles of application

Shortwave diathermy is delivered using a machine that comprises a base unit (incorporating a mains supply module, frequency generator, amplifier as well as oscillator and resonator coils) and some form of applicator(s), which are typically mounted on the end of moveable arm(s). The therapy can be applied in one of several ways. Conductive methods use a pair of rigid electrodes, which are typically mounted on the ends of 'arms' to allow positioning either side of the treated area with an air gap, or a pair of plate electrodes that are applied through some insulating medium that provides space between the electrodes and the skin.

Inductive methods rely on the use of an insulated cable that is wrapped around the body part, or a 'coil' of such cable, either constructed on an ad hoc basis by the therapist, or incorporated within a single 'monode' treatment head. The selection of application method is crucial to the effectiveness of treatment, as the method determines the depth and site of maximum tissue heating. For example, so-called contraplanar application using a pair of rigid electrodes on either side of a limb will produce the deepest heating, however, in such cases most heating will take place in fatty tissue. In contrast, coplanar application, for example using two electrodes placed underneath the patient to treat a painful back, will predominantly heat (more superficial) muscle tissue. For a more detailed discussion of the relative merits of application methods, the reader is directed to Low and Reed (2000).

For microwave diathermy, treatment is applied using a device that has a base unit containing a special generator called a magnetron and its associated power supply and controller modules, attached to a treatment applicator incorporating a microwave antenna. The applicator (also termed an emitter) may be applied with an air gap or, depending on design, in contact with the skin, the therapist taking care to direct the emitter perpendicularly to the target tissue to limit reflection.

For both types of diathermy, the main treatment parameters (apart from mode and site of treatment) are time and intensity of treatment. Time of treatment for microwave diathermy is usually up to 20 minutes to allow sufficient temperature rise in deeper tissues, while for shortwave diathermy, treatment times of up to 30 minutes may be required.

Treatment intensity, rather like TENS, is determined by patient report rather than the arbitrary units provided on device controls. It has been suggested that a scale of patient descriptors can be effectively used to distinguish different intensities of heating using diathermy: i.e. 'just feel the warmth' corresponding to minimal perceptible heating, 'mild gentle warmth' for mild heating, and 'comfortable warmth' representing moderate heating intensities (Low & Reed 2000). In all cases, patients should be carefully briefed that even at its highest level, the heating should never feel uncomfortable, and that excessive heating above what is comfortable has no therapeutic benefit.

Safety considerations

The safety measures already outlined above for therapeutic heat apply equally to shortwave and microwave diathermy. In particular, it is useful to reiterate the potential of heating modalities to cause burns, and thus skin-testing together with warning the patient of such risks prior to application should be regarded as mandatory. In addition, the reliance on the patient to remain still and to report heating that is uncomfortable will preclude treatment for the uncooperative or incompetent patient.

Beyond this, the following may be regarded as contraindications to either form of diathermy:

1. **Implanted metal devices** – the therapist should check for internal metal devices in the area of treatment (e.g. fixators, pins, etc), as these devices will also cause field concentration and may therefore result in burns.
2. **Cardiac pacemakers** – the operation of pacemakers may be adversely affected by the electromagnetic field generated by shortwave diathermy devices, or potentially by microwave diathermy devices. Not only should these be recognized as a contraindication, but also suitable warning notices should be displayed where shortwave diathermy devices are used.
3. **Areas of active or suspected carcinoma**, as (deeper) heat treatment may stimulate further cancerous changes.
4. Treatment over or through the **pregnant uterus** should be avoided. This represents a standard contraindication for all electrotherapies.
5. **Vascular disorders** – ischaemic tissues should not be treated with diathermy, as the ischaemia will compromise the ability of the tissue to cope with

the heating. In such cases, application to proximal tissues may sometimes be beneficial. Treatment of areas of (recent) thrombosis should also be avoided, anaemorrhagic tissues (or potentially haemorrhagic areas) should not be treated with diathermy as this may exacerbate the loss of blood.

6. **Sites of infection** – treatment should not be applied to areas of infection, as treatment may stimulate the infection. Diathermy should not be applied in cases of fever.

In addition, when applying either form or diathermy, and especially for shortwave diathermy, the patient should be adequately undressed and the treatment area examined. In particular, synthetic materials that may cause the build-up of electrostatic charges or heat should be removed from the area. Clothes may also have metal fasteners, hooks or clips (e.g. bras, corsets, trousers or skirts) and thus these should be removed from the treatment field to avoid potential burns, as they will concentrate or reflect the electromagnetic energy and thus the heating effect of the treatment. Finally, given that diathermy will produce greatest heat in water, the patient's skin should be examined and if necessary dried before treatment is initiated.

Mechanisms of action

The physiological mechanisms underlying the pain relieving effects of diathermy are essentially as already described for therapeutic heating using hot packs and infrared lamps. However, it is important to recognize that the mechanisms by which shortwave and microwave diathermy produce tissue heating, and the depth of such heating (particularly for shortwave) is very different than for conductive methods (or indeed infrared).

The principal mechanism through which diathermy produces heating is the rapidly changing electromagnetic field, which produces an equally rapid 'to and fro' movement of charged ions within the treated tissues. For both types of diathermy, maximum heating will usually be in tissues with the highest water content, and especially muscle. When shortwave is applied using a contraplanar electrode arrangement, heating will be produced throughout the tissue being treated (and greatest in fatty tissue), although it must be stressed that in cases of monode application and for microwave diathermy, the depth of heating will be somewhat more limited, essentially to skin and superficial muscle.

Shortwave and microwave diathermy may be pulsed to avoid or reduce the heating effects of the electromagnetic radiation, and thus the risk of tissue burns or exacerbation of acute conditions. In such cases, the mechanisms underlying the claimed therapeutic benefits, at least in terms of pain relief, are unclear.

Recommended applications and current evidence

Similarly to the other forms of therapeutic heat already described above, diathermy is recommended for the management of a variety of musculoskeletal pains. However, given its relatively greater depth of effect, diathermy (and particularly shortwave when applied using contraplanar technique) may be more useful for the relief of pain associated with deeper-seated lesions and conditions. For example, microwave diathermy was found to be of benefit in arthralgia (Weinberger et al, 1989).

While there are few clinical trials of the analgesic efficacy of shortwave diathermy, the effectiveness of pulsed shortwave (also termed pulsed electromagnetic energy or PEME) has been assessed in a variety of painful conditions with variable (i.e. both positive and negative) results (Foley-Nolan et al 1990, Klaber Moffett et al 1996, Wagstaff et al 1986). While further research is indicated in this area before any more definitive pronouncements on efficacy are possible, it would appear that any analgesic effects may be critically dependent upon the treatment parameters employed (Low 1995).

CONCLUSION

Electrophysical modalities used in the management of pain principally include:

1. Thermal agents producing superficial heating or cooling of the tissues, using hot or cold packs

2. Electrical simulation, typically based upon the application of electrical currents to the peripheral nerves (principally TENS and IFT)
3. Treatments based upon electromagnetic radiation (including diathermy and laser therapy), or ultrasound at therapeutic levels.

This chapter has provided an overview of the principles underlying the treatment of pain with electrophysical agents, and the proposed mechanisms of action of these modalities. In addition, for each of the main modalities covered, the chapter has outlined the principles of application (including relevant safety considerations) and provided a brief summary of recommended applications and current evidence.

Knowledge of the material covered in this chapter will equip the therapist to understand the potential role of electrophysical agents in pain management and, ultimately, help to improve the care of the patient in pain.

Study questions/questions for revision

1. What are the main mechanisms by which thermal agents may modulate nociceptive information before it reaches the most rostral levels of the CNS?
2. Under what conditions would electrostimulation (e.g. TENS) be contraindicated for pain relief?
3. Identify which electrophysical modalities might be indicated for application in the management of low back pain in pregnancy.
4. By what mechanisms may therapeutic ultrasound alleviate subacute muscle pain?
5. What are the main indications for laser therapy for pain relief?

REFERENCES

Basford J R 1995 Low intensity laser therapy: still not an established clinical tool. Lasers Surgery Medicine 16: 331–342

Basford J R, Sheffield C G, Harmsen W S 1999 Laser therapy: a randomised controlled trial of the effects of low intensity N:YAG laser irradiation on musculoskeletal pain. Archives Physical Medicine and Rehabilitation 80: 647–652

Baxter G D 1994 Therapeutic lasers: theory and practice. Churchill Livingstone, Edinburgh

Baxter G D, Bell A J, Allen J M et al 1991 Low level laser therapy: current clinical practice in Northern Ireland. Physiotherapy 77: 171–178

Baxter G D, Walsh D M, Allen J M et al 1994 Effects of low intensity infrared laser irradiation upon conduction in the human median nerve in vivo. Experimental Physiology 79: 227–234

Belcher J 1974 Interferential therapy. New Zealand Journal of Physiotherapy 6: 29–34

Borjesson M 1999 Visceral chest pain in unstable angina pectoris and effects of transcutaneous electrical nerve stimulation (TENS): a review. Herz 24: 114–125

Bowsher D 1988 Modulation of nociceptive input. In: Wells P, Frampton V, Bowsher D (eds) Pain: Management and Control in Physiotherapy. Heinemann, London

Carroll D, Tramer M, McQuay H et al 1997 Transcutaneous electrical nerve stimulation in labour pain: a systematic review. British Journal of Obstetrics Gynaecology 104: 169–175

Chen X-H, Han J S 1992 All three types of opioid receptors in the spinal cord are important for 2/15Hz electroacupuncture analgesia. European Journal of Pharmacology 211: 203–210

Ciccone C D, Leggin B G, Callamara J J 1991 Effects of ultrasound and trolamine salicylate phonophoresis on delayed onset muscle soreness. Physical Therapy 71: 666–675

Clarke G R, Stenner L 1976 Use of therapeutic ultrasound. Physiotherapy 62: 185–190

Cosentino A B, Cross D L, Harrington R J et al 1983 Ultrasound effect on electroneuromyographic measures in sensory fibers of the median nerve. Physical Therapy 63: 1788–92

De Bie R A, de Vet H C W, Lenssen A F et al 1998 Efficacy of 904nm laser therapy in the management of musculoskeletal disorders: a systematic review. Physical Therapy Reviews 3: 59–72

De Domenico G 1982 Pain relief with interferential current. Australian Journal of Physiotherapy 28: 14–18

De Preux T 1952 Ultrasonic wave therapy in osteoarthritis of the hip joint. British Journal of Physical Medicine 15: 14–19

Devor M 1990 What's in a laser beam for pain therapy? Pain 43: 139

Douglas W W, Malcolm J L 1955 The effect of localised cooling on cat nerves. Journal of Physiology 130: 53

Dyson M 1982 Nontherapeutic cellular effects of ultrasound. British Journal of Cancer 45 (Suppl V): 165–171

Dyson M 1985 Therapeutic applications of ultrasound. In: Nyborg W L, Ziskin M C (eds) Biological Effects of Ultrasound. Churchill Livingstone, Edinburgh, pp 121–133

Dyson M 1988 The use of ultrasound in sports physiotherapy. In: Grisogono V (ed) Sports Injuries. Churchill Livingstone, Edinburgh

Dyson M, Pond J B 1973 The effect of ultrasound on circulation. Physiotherapy 59: 284–287

England S, Farrell A J, Coppock J S et al 1989 Low-power laser therapy of shoulder tendonitis. Scandanavian Journal of Rheumatology 18: 427–431

Eriksson M, Sjolund B 1976 Acupuncture-like electroanalgesia in TNS-resistant chronic pain. In: Zotterman Y (ed) Sensory Function of the Skin in Primates. Pergamon Press, Oxford

Ernst E, Fialka 1994 Ice freezes pain? A review of the clinical effectiveness of analgesic cold therapy. Journal of Pain Symptom Management 9: 56–59

Foley-Nolan D, Barry C, Coughlan R J et al 1990 Pulsed high frequency (27 MHz) electromagnetic therapy for persistent neck pains. Orthopedics 13: 445–451

Foster N E, Thompson K A, Baxter G D, Allen J M 1999 Management of nonspecific low back pain by physiotherapists in Britain and Ireland. Spine 24: 1332–1342

Gracey J, McDonough S, Baxter G D 2001 A questionnaire survey of physiotherapists treating patients with low back pain. Spine *in press*

Han J S, Terrenius L 1982 Neurochemical basis of acupuncture analgesia. Annual Reviews in Pharmacology and Toxicology 22: 193–220

Han J S, Wang Q 1992 Mobilization of specific neuropeptides by peripheral stimulation of identified frequencies. News in Physiological Sciences 7: 176–180

Hansen T I, Kristensen J H 1973 Effect of massage, shortwave diathermy and ultrasound upon ^{133}Xe disappearance rate from muscle and subcutaneous tissue in the human calf. Scandanavian Journal of Rehabilitation Medicine 5: 179–82

Hay-Smith E J, Reed M A 1997 Physical agents for perineal pain following childbirth: a review of systematic reviews. Physical Therapy Reviews 2: 115–121

Hogan R D, Burke K M, Franklin T D 1982 The effect of ultrasound on microvascular hemodynamics in skeletal muscle: effects during ischaemia. Microvascular Research 23: 370–379

Hong C Z 1991 Reversible nerve conduction block in patients with polyneuropathy after ultrasound thermotherapy at therapeutic dosage. Archives of Physical Medicine Rehabilitation 72: 132–137

Jansen G, Lundberg T, Kjartansson J, Samuelson U E 1989 Acupuncture and sensory neuropeptides increase cutaneous blood flow in rats. Neuroscience Letters 97: 305–309

Johnson M I, Ashton C H, Thompson J W 1991 An in-depth study of long term users of transcutaneous electrical nerve stimulation (TENS). Implications for clinical use of TENS. Pain 44: 221–229

Johnson M I, Ashton C H, Marsh V R et al 1992 The effect of transcutaneous electrical nerve stimulation (TENS) and acupuncture on concentrations of betaendorphin, met-enkephalin and 5HT in the peripheral circulation. European Journal of Pain 13: 44–51

Jones R J 1984 Treatment of herpes zoster using ultrasonic therapy. Physiotherapy 70: 94–96

Kahn J 1987 Principles and practice of electrotherapy, 3rd Edn. Churchill Livingstone, New York

Kanikkanan N, Kandimalla K, Lamba S S et al 2000 Structure-activity relationship of chemical penetration enhancers in transdermal drug delivery. Current Medicine Chemistry 7: 593–608

Kaplan B, Rabinerson S, Pardo J et al 1997 Transcutaneous electrical nerve stimulation (TENS) as a pain-relief device in obstetrics and gynaecology. Clinics Experiment Obstetrics Gynaecology 24: 123–126

Karu T 1998 The Science of Low Power Laser Therapy. Gordon & Breach/OPA, Amsterdam

Kishioka S, Miyamoto Y, Fukunaga Y et al 1994 Effects of a mixture of peptidase inhibitors (amastatin, captopril and phosphamidon) on met-enkephalin, β-endorphin, dynorphin (1-13) and electroacupuncture induced antinociception in rats. Japanese Journal of Pharmacology 66: 337–345

Kitchen S, Bazin S 1996 Clayton's Electrotherapy, 10th Edn. W B Saunders, London

Klaber Moffett J A, Richardson P H, Frost H et al 1996 Placebo controlled, double blind trial to evaluate the effectiveness of pulsed shortwave therapy for osteoarthritic hip and knee pain. Pain 167: 121–127

Klaiman M D, Shrader J A, Danoff J V et al 1998 Phonophoresis versus ultrasound in the treatment of common musculoskeletal conditions. Medical Sciences Sports Exercise 30: 1349–1355

Lewis S M, Clelland J A, Knowles C J et al 1990. Effects of auricular acupuncture-like transcutaneous electrical nerve stimulation on pain levels following wound care in patients with burns: a pilot study. Journal of Burn Care Rehabilitation 11: 322–329

Lehmann J F (ed) 1982 Therapeutic Heat and Cold. Williams & Wilkins, Baltimore

Lehmann J F, de Lateur B J 1982 Therapeutic heat. In: Lehmann J F (ed) Therapeutic Heat and Cold. Williams & Wilkins, Baltimore

Lehmann J F, Mastock A J, Warren C G et al 1970 Effect of therapeutic temperatures on tendon extensibility. Archives physical Medicine Rehabilitation 51: 481–487

Low J 1995 Dosage of some pulsed shortwave clinical trials. Physiotherapy 81: 611–616

Low J, Reed A 2000 Electrotherapy Explained, 3rd Edn. Butterworth Heinemann, Oxford

Lowe A S, Walsh D M, Baxter G D and Allen J M 1997 Low-intensity laser irradiation (830 nm) reduces skin blood flow in humans. Lasers in Medical Science 10: 245–251

Lundeberg T 1993 Peripheral effects of sensory nerve stimulation (acupuncture) in inflammation and ischemia. Scandinavian Journal of Rehabilitation Medicine (Suppl 29): 61–86

McQuay H J, Moore R A, Eccleston C et al 1997 Systematic review of outpatient services for chronic pain control. Health Technology Assessment 1: 1–135

Martin D 1996 Interferential therapy. In: Kitchen S, Bazin S 1996 Clayton's Electrotherapy, 10th Edn. W B Saunders, London, pp 306–315

Moore J H, Gieck J H, Saliba E N et al 2000 The biophysical effects of ultrasound on median nerve distal latencies. Electromyography and Clinical Neurophysiology 40: 169–180

Mortimer A J, Dyson M 1988 The effect of therapeutic ultrasound on calcium uptake in fibroblasts. Ultrasound Medicine Biology 14, 499–506

Nelson R M, Currier D P 1991 Clinical Electrophysiology, 2nd Edn. Appleton & Lange, California

Noble G 2000 Doctoral Thesis, University of Ulster, Jordanstown, UK

Orwin R 1998 A non-pharmacological approach to angina. Professional Nurse 13: 583–586

Palastanga N P 1988 Heat and Cold. In: Wells P, Frampton V, Bowsher D (eds) Pain: Management and Control in Physiotherapy. Heinemann, London

Patrick M K 1978 Applications of therapeutic pulsed ultrasound. Physiotherapy 64: 103–104

Payne C 1984 Ultrasound for postherpetic neuralgia. Physiotherapy 70: 96–97

Pope G D, Mockett S P, Wright J P (1995) A survey of electrotherapeutic modalities: ownership and use in NHS in England. Physiotherapy 81: 82–91

Rasmussen M J, Hayes D L, Vlietstra R E et al 1988 Can transcutaneous electrical nerve stimulation be safely used in patients with permanent cardiac pacemakers? Mayo Clinic Proceedings 63: 443–445

Rubin M J, Etchinson M R, Condra K A et al 1990 Acute effect of ultrasound on skeletal muscle oxygen tension, blood flow and capillary density. Ultrasound Medicine Biology 16: 271–7

Shin S M, Choi J K 1997 Effect of indomethacin phonophoresis on the relief of temperomandibular joint pain. Cranio 15: 345–348

Simunovic Z, Trobonjaca T, Trobonjaca Z 1998 Treatment of medial and lateral epicondylitis – tennis and golfer's elbow – with low level laser therapy. Journal of Clinical Laser Medicine & Surgery 16: 145–51

Stephenson R, Johnson M 1995 The analgesic effects of interferential therapy on cold-induced pain in healthy subjects: a preliminary report. Physiotherapy Theory Practice 11: 89–95

ter Haar G, Dyson M, Oakley, E M 1985 The use of ultrasound by physiotherapists in Britain. Ultrasound Medicine Biology 13: 659–663

Thomas M, Lundeberg T 1994 Importance of modes of acupuncture in the treatment of chronic nociceptive pain. Acta Anaesthesiologica Scandinavica 38: 63–69

Tuner J, Hode L 1999 Low Level Laser Therapy. Clinical Practice and Scientific Background. Prima Books, Grangesberg, Sweden

Urba S G 1996 Nonpharmacologic pain management in terminal care. Clinics in Geriatric Medicine 12: 301–311

UvnasMoberg K, Bruzelius G, Alster P et al 1993 The antinociceptive effect of non-noxious sensory stimulation is mediated partly through oxytocinergic mechanisms Acta Physiologica Scandinavica 149: 199–204

Van der Windt DAWM, Van der Heijden GJMG, Van den Berg S G M et al 1999 Ultrasound therapy for musculoskeletal disorders: a systematic review. Pain 81: 257–271

Van der Windt D A, Van der Heijden GJMG, Van den Berg S G M et al 2000 Ultrasound therapy for acute ankle sprains. Cochrane Database of Systematic Reviews 2: CD001250

Wadsworth H, Chanmugan A P P (1980) Electrophysical agents in physiotherapy. Science Press, Marrickville

Wagstaff P, Wagstaff S, Downey M 1986 A pilot study to compare the efficacy of continuous and pulsed magnetic energy (short wave diathermy) in the relief of back pain. Physiotherapy 72: 563–566

Walker J B 1988 Low level laser therapy for pain management: a review of the literature and underlying mechanisms. In: Ohshiro T, Calderhead R G (eds) Low Level Laser Therapy: a practical introduction. Wiley, Chichester

Walsh D M 1997 TENS: Clinical Applications and Related Theory. Churchill Livingstone, Edinburgh

Wedlock P M Shephard R A 1996 Cranial irradiation with GaAIAs laser leads to naloxone reversible analgesia in rab. Psychological Reports 78: 727–731

Weinberger A, Fadilah R, Lev A et al 1989 Treatment of articular effusions with local deep microwave hyperthermia. Clinic Rheumatology 8: 461–466

Wesselmann U, Rymer W Z, Lan S-F 1990 Effect of pulsed infrared lasers on neural conduction and axoplasmic transport in sensory nerves. In: Joffe S N, Atsumi K (eds) 1990 Laser Surgery: advanced characterisation, therapeutics and systems II. Progress in Biomedical Optics, SPIE Volume 1200. International Society for Optical Engineering

Willie C D 1969 Interferential therapy. Physiotherapy 55: 503–505

Wu W-H, Ponnudurai R, Katz J et al 1987 Failure to confirm report of light-evoked response to low-power helium-neon laser light stimulus. Brain Research 401: 407–408

Young S 1996 Ultrasound therapy. In: Kitchen S, Bazin S (eds) Clayton's Electrotherapy, 10th Edn. W B Saunders, London, pp 243–267

Young S, Dyson M 1990 Macrophage responsiveness to therapeutic ultrasound. Ultrasound Medicine Biology 16, 809–816

12

Alternative and complementary therapies

Anita M. Unruh
Katherine Harman

OVERVIEW

Conventional healthcare (see Box 12.1) does not always meet the needs of clients in pain. When clients continue to suffer despite treatment, many choose to explore alternative or complementary therapies (ACTs) to manage pain, and underlying illness or disease that may be associated with the pain. It can be difficult to draw the line between traditional physiotherapy, occupational therapy interventions and ACT. Indeed, physiotherapy and occupational therapy are essentially legitimized therapies that are complementary to conventional medicine.

ACTs are 'alternative' partly because they do not easily fit into a conventional healthcare model. They are often based on an understanding of human physiology that is unfamiliar to a conventional understanding of health. The mechanisms by which they may effect health are elusive, and most research evidence to demonstrate their effectiveness is weak. Possible harmful effects may have inadequate attention. Nevertheless, the use of ACTs appears to be on the increase.

In this chapter, we will discuss the attraction of ACTs, sources of information about these therapies, the possible benefits and risks associated with ACTs, and the extent of evidence for the more commonly used therapies for pain.

Occupational therapists and physiotherapists need to know how to find information about ACTs and determine their potential for positive effect or possible harm. Therapists also need to judge the complementarity of the client's choices with interventions used in physiotherapy or occupational therapy. A client may also ask the therapist for advice or direction about the use of ACTs.

Box 12.1 Key terms defined

Holistic – Holistic refers to a perspective that is focused on the whole person, rather than on the individual parts. The assumption of a holistic perspective is that individual components have an interactive synergy that makes up the whole.

Conventional healthcare – Conventional healthcare refers to theoretical approaches, diagnostic tests and intervention strategies, as used by health professionals and sometimes considered as 'Western medicine'. These professionals include occupational therapists, physiotherapists, nurses, social workers, dieticians, speech therapists, audiologists, psychologists and physicians. Conventional healthcare is also sometimes referred to as traditional or conventional medicine. We are using the term conventional because traditional is also sometimes used to mean folk medicine. We use the term 'healthcare' because it includes care provided by other health professionals as well as physicians.

Alternative or complementary – The terms alternative therapy and complementary therapy are often used interchangeably because they refer to the same strategies. However, these terms refer to the way in which these therapies are used. When used in conjunction with traditional health approaches, the term 'complementary' therapy is appropriate. A person with chronic low back pain may see a physiotherapist and a Reiki Master simultaneously. All parties should be aware of the different interventions being employed, to ensure that there are no contraindications to the therapy and to help determine the efficacy of each treatment. A person may reject conventional healthcare in favour of an 'alternative' therapy. For example, a person with a reoccurrence of cancer may decide to use naturopathy instead of chemotherapy or radiotherapy and rely only on naturopathy. In this example, naturopathy is used as an alternative, rather than as a complementary therapy. Alternative therapy may carry more risks if the rejected conventional treatment is known to have positive benefit.

We conclude the chapter with a discussion of implications for physiotherapists and occupational therapists.

Learning objectives

At the end of this chapter, readers will adopt a critical approach to learning about ACTs and will have an understanding of:

1. The differences between conventional healthcare practices and ACTs
2. The role of ACTs in the management of pain
3. The benefits and potential harm of these therapies
4. Some examples of common therapies used for pain
5. Implications for occupational therapists and physiotherapists.

WHAT ARE ALTERNATIVE/COMPLEMENTARY THERAPIES (ACTs)?

Alternative/complementary therapies refer to a broad range of philosophies, approaches and therapies that are usually developed and offered outside of traditional or conventional healthcare (National Center for Complementary & Alternative Medicine 1999a). They are heterodox therapies, that is, they may be considered to present unorthodox positions when contrasted with conventional medicine.

As noted in Box 12.1, ACTs are also sometimes referred to as 'holistic' therapies, because the approach addresses the physical, mental, emotional and spiritual needs of the person and places a greater emphasis on prevention than on treatment (National Center for Complementary & Alternative Medicine 1999a).

In the past, these therapies were not usually taught in medical or health-profession schools, and generally were not reimbursed by medical insurance provided by governments or insurance companies. However, the past decade has seen the inclusion of interventions such as acupuncture into physiotherapy and medical curricula, as well as in continuing education programmes.

As will become evident in the next section on ACTs used for pain, there is some overlap between conventional health interventions and alternative/complementary therapy. For example, hypnosis and visualization can be viewed as conventional healthcare as well as alternative/complementary care. There are several issues that determine whether an intervention might be considered as conventional or alternative. The appropriate classification depends on whether the intervention is used for a purpose that is considered legitimate in conventional healthcare or for an unusual purpose that is not generally accepted by conventional healthcare or delivered by someone not recognized for that specialty.

For example, hypnosis and visualization would be considered as conventional interventions for treatment of pain but alternative for treatment of enuresis. In some cases, therapies such as hypnosis and visualization might be considered as alternative even when they are used for pain, if the practitioner is not a person who is recognized as one of the conventional health professions. In this case, the alternative/complementary practitioner may be using a therapy such as hypnosis or visualization for pain somewhat differently from the way in which it would be used by a conventional health professional.

Other therapies may be largely considered as ACTs even when they are provided by conventional health professionals such as physiotherapists, occupational therapists or nurses (e.g. Alexander technique, Feldenkrais, therapeutic touch and others), because the underlying theoretical rationale is not widely understood or accepted in conventional healthcare. It may also be the case that although one professional group believes that the intervention is a legitimate form of conventional practice, that other health professionals do not have the same opinion.

Acceptance of different therapies as a legitimate component of conventional healthcare can also vary among countries and among institutions. If the effectiveness of an intervention is demonstrated in well-designed research and is matched by a correspondingly low risk of harm, then interventions gain more wide acceptance in conventional healthcare. As evidence-based practice becomes increasingly more important in conventional healthcare, the degree of evidence for effectiveness may be a key determining point of whether an intervention is considered as an ACT or as an acceptable part of conventional healthcare.

Categories of alternative/complementary approaches for pain

The most common ACTs used for pain include the following:

1. Mind–body approaches (e.g. cognitive–behavioural therapies such as visualization, relaxation, biofeedback, hypnosis, meditation)
2. Alternative medical systems (e.g. acupuncture)
3. Biologically-based therapies (e.g. herbal remedies, aromatherapy, bee stings)
4. Manipulative and body-based systems (e.g. body works, chiropractic, TENS)
5. Biofield therapies using metals (e.g. chelation, copper bracelets, coin rubbing) or based on energy fields (e.g. Reiki, therapeutic touch, vibrational medicine)
6. Bioelectromagnetics (e.g. magnetic therapy).

This list was developed in the United States by the National Center for Complementary and Alternative Medicine (1999b). Some of the therapies listed are an important part of conventional healthcare for pain, as well as alternative/complementary interventions. Therapies such as acupuncture, spinal manipulation, massage, hypnosis, imagery and relaxation are more widely accepted in conventional healthcare (Ernst et al 1995) particularly for pain, than homeopathy, chelation, energy fields, therapeutic touch, or bee stings. The mind–body approaches are used by occupational therapists, psychologists, and by many physiotherapists. TENS and several other interventions are commonly used by many physiotherapists (discussed in Chapter 11).

Some ACTs are accessible to a client primarily through a practitioner who is knowledgeable about their use. In some cases, specialized training and certification specific to the intervention is required (e.g. chiropractic, acupuncture and hypnosis). Other therapies are easily available to a client without the use of either a conventional health practitioner or an alternative/complementary specialist (e.g. herbs, diet supplements). These differences may affect how widely they are used and the potential benefit or harm.

Usage of ACTs

Alternative/complementary therapies are widely used. Conventional healthcare can relieve some problems but at times it causes others, resulting in a person's frustration and disillusionment with conventional healthcare (Berman et al 1998). The likelihood that a person will seek help from an ACT is particularly increased in the presence of chronic or progressive health problems, especially if they involve pain or mood disturbances (Eisenberg et al 1993). For example, Krauss et al (1998) found that 57% of adults with physical disabilities used ACTs compared to 34% of the national general population. In this population, the primary reason for use of these therapies was to obtain pain relief and secondarily to relieve depression or anxiety.

Approximately 31–94% of adults with arthritis also use some form of ACT (Southwood et al 1990). Rao et al (1999) found that two-thirds of patients at six rheumatology clinics used these therapies. Use of ACTs is also associated with higher education (Eisenberg et al 1993, Warrick et al 1999). Possibly, clients with more education may have more access to sources of healthcare information, particularly the Internet, where considerable information about ACTs is readily available, although the completeness and accuracy can be extremely variable.

People with cancer are also frequent consumers of ACTs with 7–64% reporting use of one or more ACTs

(Cassileth 1999). Thirty-seven percent of cancer outpatients attending a pain and symptom clinic (Oneschuk et al 1998), and 22% of patients with head and neck cancer use ACTs (Warrick et al 1999). Nam et al (1999) reported that 25–80% of patients with prostate cancer used ACTs. For people with cancer who are in pain and faced with a threat to their mortality, the possibility of relief or possible cure through ACTs may be especially compelling.

It is important to note that while the major group of ACT consumers are adults, ACTs are frequently used by adults for children. Sixty-nine percent of parents who use ACTs for their own healthcare, also use them for their children's health problems (Spigelblatt et al 1994). The number of different ACTs used for children by their parents increases with the child's age (Southwood et al 1990). A Canadian survey of 2055 children attending a general paediatric clinic found that 34% of the children had used an ACT in the previous year and one-third had been seen by an alternative therapist (Spigelblatt et al 1994). 39–86% of children with arthritis from Sweden, Australia, New Zealand or Canada have used an ACT for the management of this condition (Hoyeraal et al 1984, Southwood et al 1990).

Why are ACTs popular?

Many clients that we meet in our professional practice will be faced with situations similar to the one that is described in the Reflective exercise 12.1.

Often, clients will find that conventional healthcare is unable to effectively treat all of the problems that are associated with having a persistent pain or a progressive health problem. For example, rheumatoid arthritis frequently has a fulminating course, with periods of improvement followed by regression. There are times when the disease is responsive to medication and other times when medications do not slow disease progression and may even cause serious health side-effects. This irregular and often unpredictable progress might be interpreted as ineffective medical care and the client may seek out an ACT to achieve more control and relief over symptoms. Frustration with conventional care, progressive illness and easy access to ACTs provide some of the initial impetus for their use.

Another attraction of ACTs is that they appear to be more natural and therefore safer, particularly if the person has experienced negative side-effects from conventional healthcare. For example, a troublesome side-effect frequently seen with opioid medication is constipation. Many people also worry about addiction to pain medication. A person with cancer may have concerns about the side-effects of chemotherapy or radiation. Such experiences increase the appeal of ACTs.

Most, if not all ACTs, promote a holistic view of health, active involvement in health and wellness, and an enhancement of the mind–body connection. Promotion of the mind–body connection may enable a person to regain a new perspective over her or his health problem, less helplessness, more control and more relief. Although conventional health professionals such as occupational therapists and physiotherapists also promote active involvement and often a holistic orientation, practitioners of ACTs may achieve this perspective more easily because they are situated outside of the conventional health framework.

Many ACTs emphasize the importance of the interpersonal relationship between the client and the practitioner. As a result, the client may feel better understood and may perceive that his or her health and overall quality of life matter to the ACT therapist. This point is particularly important for people with persistent pain. Often, in conventional healthcare, a person with pain will have encountered considerable doubt about the legitimacy of the pain. Consequently, more energy may be expended on trying to prove the existence of the pain than on recovering from the pain. A practitioner of ACT typically begins where the client is at, believes that the pain is legitimate, and allows the client to get on with getting better (Kenny & Guy 2000).

People who use ACTs and feel that they have been helped often advocate the use of ACTs to others with similar problems. Hearing that someone else with a similar problem managed to overcome or eliminate it by use of a particular ACT can be very persuasive, particularly since research findings typically contain considerable technical literature related to methodology

---

Reflective exercise 12.1

Imagine for a moment that you have had abdominal pain quite frequently. You've seen your family physician about it. You were given some advice about stress and diet. Still, the pain is bothersome and it doesn't seem to be getting any better. You wonder if the doctor just thought you were a bit of a complainer.

A good friend mentions that she has been using an alternative/complementary product that is supposed to relieve a variety of pains. Would you give it a try? Think about what information you might want to know about the product.

and statistics that may be bewildering. The persuasiveness of testimonials is borne out in a survey about the use of alternative treatments by parents (Spigelblatt 1995). Hearing about ACTs by word of mouth was the most common reason given by these parents for using an ACT for their children.

Lastly, some people use ACTs not to relieve pain, depression, anxiety or treat illness, but as an adjunct to other health behaviours. Vitamins and other herbal remedies are sometimes used in this way to promote health. In these instances, it may seem natural to turn to other ACTs if health problems do develop. Using ACTs may be more consistent with the individual's personal belief systems and past behaviours.

Clearly, there are many reasons for the appeal of ACTs. It is human nature to consider all options to find relief from persistent pain. ACTs provide this opportunity generally at a low cost and with seemingly fewer risks of harm (Boisset & Fitzcharles 1994, Eisenberg et al 1993). In a later section of this chapter, we will be examining what is known about the benefits and potential harm of some of the more common ACTs used for pain.

Acceptance of ACTs by conventional health professionals

Physiotherapy and occupational therapy are two professions which developed from innovative approaches to complex health problems that were not easily managed by conventional medical care. Many accepted techniques employed in rehabilitation were at one point considered 'alternative'.

An example from physiotherapy comes from Elizabeth Dicke, a German physiotherapist, who developed circulatory complications after a leg infection. In bed, with back pain and one leg at risk of gangrene and probable amputation, Ms Dicke discovered that deep massage to her back resulted in improved circulation to her leg. Amputation was avoided and connective-tissue massage was born (Gifford & Gifford 1994).

Sensory integration was developed by Jean Ayres, an American occupational therapist, as an approach for treating children with learning disabilities (Spitzer et al 1996). Sensory integration is widely used for learning disabilities and a variety of other problems.

Often, health professionals have had to come up with innovative approaches to enable their clients to live better with their health problems. Their perspective is quite different from medicine where the primary goal is to cure disease and provide relief of symptoms. Possibly for these reasons, professionals

such as physiotherapists, occupational therapists and nurses have been more accepting of ACTs, in some cases even including some of them as a legitimate aspect of conventional practice.

Some ACTs are gaining acceptance by conventional health professionals. For example, when health professionals with expertise in low back pain were surveyed about ACTs, they rated osteopathy and chiropractic as effective for acute uncomplicated low back pain, and acupuncture as effective for chronic, uncomplicated, low back pain, but neither homeopathy or herbalism was considered effective (Ernst & Pittler 1999).

In a Canadian survey, general practitioners perceived that alternative therapies were useful for musculoskeletal problems, chronic pain and chronic illness (Verhoef & Sutherland, 1995). In the same survey, chiropractic, hypnosis and acupuncture were thought to be effective for chronic pain. Using a meta-analysis examination of physicians' attitudes, Ernst et al (1995) found that the majority of physicians believed that manipulation and acupuncture were moderately useful or effective.

As noted previously, the ACTs that are most readily accepted in conventional healthcare are those therapies that 'fit' most easily into conventional frameworks. For example, cognitive–behavioural therapies, relaxation and hypnosis fit comfortably into conventional pain management programmes and generally would not be considered as ACTs. However, prior to Melzack and Wall's (1965) formulation of the Gate Control theory of pain, these therapies were not so well accepted. The Gate Control theory provided an explanation of how these therapies might have a positive benefit on pain.

Other therapies, such as massage, may be accepted intuitively because many health professionals have experienced personal benefit from a relaxing massage. Vertebral manipulation and acupuncture are not always accepted by conventional health professionals but they have a long history and there is growing evidence of their benefit. When the ACT is relatively new, or the theory underlying it is foreign to conventional healthcare, then the ACT is treated with more skepticism. For example, interventions based on shifts in the circulation of an undetectable energy in invisible conduits (i.e. vibrational medicine) will not readily gain acceptance.

Accessing information about ACTs

Obtaining accurate information about any ACT is challenging. Many of these therapies have long been regarded as incompatible with conventional medicine. Until recently, they have not been well researched or published in peer-reviewed healthcare journals. Discussions are mostly found in books concerned with health and wellness, in health-related magazines, and through organizations or businesses concerned with alternative/complementary healthcare.

In the last decade, two very powerful and efficient ways of information-gathering have become available for anyone with access to a computer. One approach is to gather information via a computerized search of electronic databases (e.g. Cochrane Library, Medline, CINAHL). Such searches can be done at university or hospital libraries. The second approach is to use a search engine on the Internet to find information about a particular strategy. It is important to recognize that the way in which one searches for information, and the reason for conducting the search, will determine the kind of information that is retrieved.

Searching an electronic database such as Medline or the Cochrane Library will retrieve papers and peer-reviewed studies published in the conventional health literature. The Cochrane Library database is focused on empirical research. Medline will identify research as well as clinical discussions.

Searching the Internet opens up many possibilities. Research sites, advertisements, email lists, centres, practitioners and fraudulent individuals or companies may all be located in this way. Accurate information about ACTs may exist both in electronic databases of traditional medical and health-related journals, and on the Internet. However, potential bias exists in both locations. Conventional literature sources may give greater attention to the publication of identified risks than to the benefits associated with ACTs. Conversely, literature emanating from ACT practitioners or producers may be biased towards publication of benefits with minimization of risks. The reason for the search also influences the type of information that the searcher may be looking for and the way in which the information will be appraised. A client's need for information is often more pressing and has more personal consequences than the search conducted by a health professional. A therapist may search for information to be helpful or to broaden his or her understanding of an ACT.

The Reflective exercises 12.2 and 12.3 present two scenarios about an ACT that illustrate how questions about an ACT might emerge for a client or a therapist. Exercise 12.2 describes a therapist scenario. Exercise 12.3 presents the scenario from the client's perspective.

Bee-sting therapy is the focus of Reflective exercises 12.2 and 12.3. One of the authors (A.U.) first became aware of bee-sting therapy for pain in the process of conducting a large community survey of the way people appraise and cope with a recent pain event. Several respondents spontaneously commented that they were using bee stings to relieve chronic pain. There is no known prevalence data about how widespread the use of bee-sting therapy for pain might be. Bee-sting therapy is a good illustration of an ACT that is not well-known among conventional health professionals, but may be known to people who experience chronic pain.

Let's consider the information that might be retrieved on bee-sting therapy for pain. We conducted a search via CINAHL, Medline, and the Internet. A search of CINAHL and Medline identified two papers related to bee-sting therapy. A search of the references of these two papers identified one additional publica-

---

Reflective exercise 12.2

Joan Smith is one of your clients. She was diagnosed with multiple sclerosis 2 years ago. She is well motivated in her therapy but unpredictable bouts of pain and fatigue have interfered with her progress and involvement with therapy despite her best intentions.

In her self-help support group, she heard that some members were using bee stings to treat their pain and fatigue. Joan asked you about this treatment. Is it just some crazy scheme or is there some evidence of effectiveness? You have never heard of using bee stings to relieve pain.

- How would you find more information? Conduct a search.
- What advice would you give Joan?

Reflective exercise 12.3

Two years ago, you were diagnosed with multiple sclerosis. The diagnosis was a relief because it explained your symptoms, but it was very upsetting. You have been particularly troubled by unpredictable but frequent pain and fatigue.

Recently, you joined a self-help support group. Several people mentioned that they were using bee stings to relieve pain and found it to be very helpful. The idea of bee stings is not appealing but you are feeling desperate about having more control over this disease. You have access to the Internet at the local library and decided to find out more about this therapy. Conduct the Internet search. Does the information you obtain convince you to try bee-sting therapy for your pain?

tion. The first paper was a letter to the editor expressing concern about the increasing usage of this ACT in the writers' own country (Italy) because of the risks of granulomata due to retention of stinger fragments, and the possibility of anaphylactic shock (Altomare & Capella 1994). The second paper presented a case of painful nodular lesions in a 65-year-old man (Veraldi et al 1995). He had used bee-sting therapy for 1 month for pain due to arthrosis of the spinal column. Conventional treatment was used to treat the lesions, but at 1-year follow-up, there was only partial regression of the lesions. The third paper described the following types of reactions associated with bee stings: urticaria and generalized oedema, local swelling, shock and collapse, laryngeal oedema, bronchospasm, angioneurotic oedema, partial or complete coma, tachycardia, itching, rash, faintness, face swelling, vomiting and cyanosis (Ordman 1968).

These reactions may occur with a bee sting or with injection of the bee venom. In addition, Ordman (1968) discussed the way in which increased exposure to bee venom can increase sensitivity and increase the probability of adverse reactions and their severity. These papers gave the impression that bee-sting therapy, or apitherapy as it is also termed, is dangerous, and that it was once a common therapy for arthrosis, rheumatic diseases and sciatica, but has now fallen into disuse (except perhaps in Italy).

In contrast, a 10-minute search of the Internet located two apitherapists, five books directly concerned with bee-venom therapy, two electronic discussion lists, an American Apitherapy Society, and four testimonials about the effectiveness of apitherapy. These sources did emphasize the need for allergy-testing in advance of using apitherapy, but there was no discussion about other possible side-effects or the risk of sensitivity with increased use. Evidence of effectiveness was presented in an anecdotal format. There were no testimonials from anyone for whom the therapy was ineffective or harmful. The apitherapists presented themselves as nurturing individuals concerned about the welfare of others and convinced that bee-venom therapy was an effective remedy for many problems.

An occupational therapist or physiotherapist who conducted these two searches might conclude that bee-sting therapy is uncommon, has a number of serious risks, and is without any scientific evidence of effectiveness. In contrast, a client who is suffering from pain due to arthritis, multiple sclerosis or sciatica might conclude that conventional medicine knows little about this therapy, the risks were possibly overstated and rare, and that the therapy was helpful for people with similar problems.

For the therapist and the client, it is instructive to search both the conventional and the alternative health literature to obtain the most balanced and comprehensive understanding of the benefits, limitations and possible risks of any health intervention (Newall et al 1996).

Very often, an ACT is based on a theoretical foundation by the originator or a master teacher, and the founding publication may be a helpful source of information. It should contain clear statements that the approach is not intended to replace conventional medicine or healthcare. It should provide discussion about possible harm and how to monitor for side-effects. Claims about research-evidence of effectiveness should be treated cautiously. Case stories and correlational research is not convincing evidence. We discuss these issues in the next section.

BENEFITS AND LIMITATIONS OF ACTs

Alternative/complementary interventions may be beneficial, ineffective or harmful, in the same way as interventions that are used in conventional healthcare. In this section, we will examine the potential benefits and harm of alternative/complementary approaches, and then, in the following section, we will review the data on some of the more common ACTs used for pain.

Benefits

There are a number of potential benefits of ACTs. Some of these benefits are psychological and others are physiological. In large part, the psychological benefit can be attributed to the emphasis on the interaction between the mind and the body. The mind–body medicine approaches are more likely to decrease feelings of helplessness and to promote feelings of hopefulness and optimism about recovering from pain. By emphasizing the client–therapist relationship, the client feels that she or he is treated with more compassion and understanding. The client may also have more perception of being in control over his or her healthcare. The perception that many of these therapies are more natural than those associated with conventional healthcare leads to the conviction that they can be trusted at least to cause no harm. Both directly and indirectly, these three factors likely promote placebo effects as were discussed in detail in Chapter 5.

Some ACTs have a physiological benefit in reducing pain. Some of this benefit may be due to reduced stress, improved muscle relaxation and attention to environmental or lifestyle factors that exacerbate pain. Other therapies have a more direct physiological benefit on reduction of pain. For example, there is sufficient research to demonstrate that acupuncture is effective in reducing some types of pain (Alltree 1994, Baldry 1989, Gadsby & Flowerdew 1997, 1999, Patel et al 1989, Pomeranz 1995, Ter Reit et al 1990, Winlentz 1998).

Unfortunately, for other ACTs, there is insufficient research to demonstrate whether or not the therapy is beneficial. Much of the evidence is only at the level of case stories. Often the stories are biased because they are used to sell the product or the approach. Some therapies will have evidence of correlational relationships between the product or therapy and beneficial outcomes, such as reduction of pain. However, correlational studies do not provide evidence that the reduction in pain is caused by the use of the ACT. The beneficial effect may be due to something else that the person was doing in addition to using the ACT, or some other factor. With the growing emphasis on evidence-based practice, in the next few years there will likely be a significant increase in the number of studies assessing the efficacy of ACTs.

Aside from any direct therapeutic (psychologic or physiologic) effect on pain, the holistic approach of ACT encourages the reduction of unhealthy habits such as a sedentary lifestyle, smoking and consumption of high-fat foods, with a simultaneous improvement of health through a nutritionally balanced diet and participation in an active lifestyle. These changes will likely result in a general improvement in health. Although this positive change in health may be the only benefit conferred by the therapy, this effect may enable the consumer to cope more effectively with pain. Improved coping is an important positive benefit.

Harm

There are a number of ways in which ACTs can be harmful. Some harm is caused directly by the use of an ACT, particularly if it is used as an alternative rather than as a complementary therapy. Harm may also result from problems in the regulation of products, belief that apparently natural products are inherently safe, financial costs and possible exploitation by unskilled practitioners.

ACTs that are used as alternative strategies may exacerbate the underlying cause of the pain, even if the ACT is effective in providing some pain relief or relief from other symptoms. This can be a significant problem for diseases such as arthritis, cystic fibrosis, diabetes, cancer and others. Of course, this difficulty may also occur in conventional healthcare, but ACT practitioners may not be trained to identify malignancy or other underlying problems. The client may also be harmed if the conventional therapies are not used. With some chronic or life-threatening conditions (e.g. rheumatoid arthritis, morbid obesity, cancer), the timing of effective intervention may be critical to prevent the development of side-effects or further complications of the disease.

Unfortunately, a client who chooses the alternative therapy route (i.e. conventional medicine is rejected) may find that his or her condition deteriorates. In some instances, the disease may progress sufficiently that the impact of conventional treatment (if the client chooses to switch back) is less effective due to physiological changes associated with the disease.

The potential for physiological harm is of particular concern for children, whose developing nervous system may be at greater risk. The most common pain problem in children that parents treat with ACT (reports as high as 70% of patients) is juvenile arthritis (Hoyeraal et al 1984, Southwood et al 1990). Deterioration in management and control of arthritic disease, growth retardation, very early onset of puberty and life-threatening starvation have been reported as consequences of alternative/complementary diet manipulations and medicines (Southwood et al 1990, Spigelblatt 1995). Chiropractic manipulation for congenital torticollis in a 4-month-old child resulted in quadriplegia (Shafrir & Kaufman 1992). Mercury poisoning, hyponatremia, oedema, severe pruritis and urticaria have been reported in children treated with homeopathy (Spigelblatt 1995). Careful monitoring of benefits and possible side-effects will assure the parent that the benefits of therapy are maximized, particularly if conventional health professionals remain involved with the child's care.

Some ACTs are not well-regulated. Most biologically-based therapies are not systematically tested before they are released to the public, so there is no formal mechanism to monitor benefits or harmful effects. There are no controls to ensure that the product on a shelf, or that is bought through the Internet or mail-order sources, actually contains sufficient active ingredient to achieve a positive effect. Since there are no regulations to control the shelf-life of the product, even a product whose efficacy is known may no longer be effective by the time it is purchased. There are no requirements to alert the consumer on the product labels about possible side-effects. The current interest in ACTs may result in significant changes to the control of these therapies and may provide better consumer protection.

Many alternative therapies (e.g. herbal remedies, diet supplements, ointments and homeopathic remedies) can be administered independently by a client without the guidance of an alternative or a conventional health practitioner. An individual who uses these strategies in this way is typically more attentive to noting positive effects, in part because the strategy is considered natural and therefore safe. Negative consequences may take some days to emerge. An individual may not make the connection between the intervention and any negative health effects.

Some therapies have the potential to become more personal and intimate. Relaxation, hypnosis, or therapies which involve physical contact (e.g. massage) may cause significant emotional release on the part of the client. Anyone providing such strategies should be aware of this possibility and should be prepared to respond appropriately to such occurrences. Clients who have a history of abuse require sensitivity and considerable professional skill before such therapies are attempted.

Most ACTs are not covered by governmental or private insurance programmes. If the therapy has a known benefit, then the cost may be reasonable, but it may still be beyond what is manageable as a personal expense for many people. For ACTs with unknown or questionable benefits, the additional cost can be an unnecessary burden.

Unfortunately, the lack of regulation of many ACTs enables people whose primary intention is to exploit people for their own profitable gain to enter this area of practice. There is often little recourse for consumers to seek disciplinary action in the event of malpractice. The potential for exploitation is also increased by the easy access to the Internet for clients and charlatans. It is often difficult to discern useful information from fraudulent material.

In summary, ACTs can be beneficial and harmful to the client. This caution is also true for many interventions offered in conventional healthcare for pain. For example, surgery for back pain often causes more pain, indeed one study found that 15% of patients were worse after spinal surgery (Waddell et al 1979). Accessing multiple sources of information, attending to positive and potentially harmful effects, consultation with conventional health professionals and ACT practioners, and exercising reasonable caution to avoid exploitation, will enable a client to make informed choices.

EVIDENCE FOR EFFECTIVENESS OR HARM FOR COMMON ACTs FOR PAIN

In this section, we refer to Cochrane reviews, meta-analyses or systematic reviews where they exist, and other sources of evidence, to examine the benefits or harm for some of the more well-known ACTs used for pain.

Mind–body approaches

The two mind–body strategies most commonly used for pain are hypnosis and cognitive–behavioural therapy. Hypnosis, the attempt to influence the mind–body interaction through suggestion, has a lengthy history. There is good evidence of the effectiveness of hypnosis over pain perception (Hilgard & Hilgard 1983, Hilgard & LeBaron 1984, Nickelson et al 1999, Simon & Dahl 1999). Experimental studies have demonstrated decreased pain perception when hypnotized subjects are compared with non-hypnotized subjects (Hilgaard & Hilgaard 1983).

Recently, Rainville et al (1999) demonstrated that hypnosis was successful in modulating pain perception. Hypnotherapy out-performs physical therapy in clients with fibromyalgia who do not respond well to most other forms of treatment (Haanen et al 1991).

Cognitive–behavioural therapy is based on the premise that behavioural responses to illness are influenced by both positive and negative reinforcement, and treatment is aimed at improving management and coping strategies. Cognitive–behavioural therapy and hypnosis are effective in decreasing pain and pain-related anxiety in children undergoing bone-marrow aspiration (Liossi & Hatira 1999). A meta-analysis of 51 studies revealed that cognitive coping strategies were effective at reducing the perception of chronic pain (Fernandez & Turk 1989).

Another ACT, imagery, uses all of the senses to evoke images that will have a positive effect on clients' interpretation of symptoms. Imagery is thought to affect the autonomic nervous system (Hawk 2000). Imagery is used to modify or relieve pain (Roberto 1994) and is not usually used alone but in combination with relaxation strategies. Relaxation therapies are broadly employed by healthcare practitioners. In a critical review of relaxation techniques, Kerr (2000) concluded that relaxation strategies (including physical and non-physical approaches) had a positive effect on physiologic indicators of stress (as shown by heart-rate electromyography and blood pressure) and psychological markers.

Mind–body therapies influence the way people think, feel and behave. When a person is willingly placed under the influence of suggestion, he or she is in a vulnerable state, therefore appropriate training and ethical practice are necessary and essential.

Alternative medical systems

Acupuncture has been known in China for more than 3000 years, first reaching the Western world about 300 years ago (Baldry 1989). Acupuncture is a component of traditional Chinese medicine which is based on the theory that two opposing forces, yin and yang, must be balanced in order to keep an optimal flow of energy to maintain a healthy mind and body. Traditional Chinese medicine uses a complex assessment including many systems (hearing, skin, pulse, the external ear and the tongue) to diagnose where there is an imbalance. Treatment involves acupuncture and herbal remedies with the objective of establishing homeostasis, improving the immune response and often calming or sedating the person.

Although traditional Chinese medicine requires extensive training and a completely different interpretation of how the human body functions, the treatment modality, acupuncture, can be selectively and successfully learned and incorporated into Western health practice without the necessary shift to occidental belief systems.

The majority of Westerners who use acupuncture for pain treatment use the musculoskeletal approach, stimulating acupuncture points which are tender (ah-shi points), and are highly correlated with myofascial trigger points (Chaitow 2000, Melzack et al 1977). Acupuncture points can be located by skin-conductance devices, because they are associated with superficial nerve endings, musculotendinous junctions, intramuscular and visceral nerve endings, where there is increased sweating and vasomotor activity (Gunn et al 1976, Liu et al 1975, Wu 1988).

Dry-needling of trigger points has become widely used by acupuncturists and others (mostly physiotherapists, physicians and dentists). Trigger points are identified by symptom patterns and palpation, not through traditional Chinese diagnostic practice, and are therefore straightforward for a conventional healthcare professional to learn. Needles are widely available and weekend courses will instruct practitioners in how to insert them. Acupuncture points can also be stimulated using non-invasive techniques such as massage (shiatsu massage), TENS, laser and ultrasound.

A consensus panel of the National Institutes of Health in the US concluded that there was strong evidence to support the use of acupuncture by itself or in combination with conventional medicine for postoperative dental pain and several other problems unrelated to pain (Wilentz 1998). The panel also concluded that acupuncture may be effective for headache, menstrual cramps, fibromyalgia, tennis elbow, carpal tun-

nel syndrome and low back pain. However, for these types of pain the data was less convincing.

Acupuncture provides relief from acute and chronic pain in some studies but in other studies there is no evidence of positive effect (Ter Reit et al 1990). A Cochrane review found that there was no evidence at this time that acupuncture was effective for low back pain (van Tulder et al 1999). However, only two high-quality studies of acupuncture for chronic low back pain were found. Ezzo et al (2000) reviewed 51 randomized controlled trials of acupuncture for a variety of chronic pains representing 2423 clients. The researchers concluded that there is:

Limited evidence that acupuncture is more effective than no treatment for chronic pain; and inconclusive evidence that acupuncture is more effective than placebo, sham acupuncture or standard care. (Ezzo et al 2000 p 217)

Of the studies reviewed, six were considered to have high methodological quality, but of these studies only one reported positive benefit. Deluze et al (1992) found that acupuncture was beneficial for the treatment of fibromyalgia. Two other studies were rated as high in methodological quality (though not as highly scored as Deluze et al), and these studies reported a benefit of acupuncture for headache (Hansen & Hansen 1985), and face pain (Hansen & Hansen 1983).

It is important to note that Ezzo et al (2000) concurred with van Tulder et al (1999) that, 'low-quality scores were significantly associated with positive findings' (Ezzo et al 2000 p 222), concluding that weaker studies may bias outcomes and overestimate positive effects.

The experience and the training of the acupuncturist, years of experience, and the type and duration of acupuncture treatment delivered have a strong impact on whether a study might determine that acupuncture is effective or not effective. Until the recent development of a placebo acupuncture needle (Streitberg & Kleinhertz 1998), blinding of the subject in a controlled study has not been possible. Although sham acupuncture points have been determined and used in an attempt to blind subjects, studies using that approach cannot account for the stimulatory effect of the insertion of acupuncture needles, which may also have a positive benefit (Ezzo et al 2000). These problems reduce the comparability of studies and potentially obscure beneficial outcomes.

There are some risks associated with acupuncture. Inadequate sterilization of needles can cause infection and the spread of disease. HIV infections, hepatitis and subacute bacterial endocarditis have been caused by the use of non-sterile needles (van Tulder et al 1999). The easy availability of disposable needles has reduced this risk in many countries. If needles are not inserted correctly then insertion may cause soreness and pain, and in some cases may cause damage to underlying structures, perforation of internal organs (such as lungs, intestines or the bladder), or epileptic seizure. Needles that are not inserted correctly may break. People who have needle phobia are poor candidates for acupuncture unless they receive prior therapy for fear of needles. These negative effects are uncommon and are considerably reduced if the individual is properly qualified and licensed as an acupuncture practitioner.

The World Health Organization has taken the position that practitioners who use acupuncture must be properly trained in diagnosis and treatment 'to ensure safety and competence' (Alltree 1994 p 100). Anyone planning to incorporate acupuncture into her or his practice should consult the local regulatory body to obtain information about licensure. There is considerable variation between jurisdictions about who is permitted to perform acupuncture and under what conditions.

Biologically-based therapies

Increasing awareness about herbal remedies, also known as nutraceuticals, combined with an abundance of choice, has lead to the proliferation of anecdotal reports regarding the benefits of such products for pain. Unfortunately, as Towheed and Anastassiades (2000) have written, these remedies are often less beneficial than what the labels proclaim:

As with many nutraceuticals that currently are widely touted as beneficial for common but difficult-to-treat disorders, the promotional enthusiasm often far surpasses the scientific evidence supporting clinical use. (Towheed & Anastassiades 2000 p 1470)

Pharmacists may also not be sufficiently knowledgeable about ACT products.

Chrubasik and Roufogalis (1999) listed the following biologically-based products for pain: devil's claw, stinging nettle, willow bark, blackcurrant leaf, blackcurrant seed, evening primrose seed, borage seed, goldenrod herb, aspen bark with ash bark, capsicum, arnica flower, comfrey herb and root, white mustard seed, sweet clover herb, tea tree oil, feverfew, butterbur, peppermint oil, St John's Wort, and Kava-Kava. Chrubasik and Roufogalis (1999) argued that in a number of clinical studies, herbal products have demonstrated greater effectiveness than a placebo with a lower incidence of side-effects than conventional medications used for pain.

Currently, of these herbal products, only St John's Wort has been examined in a Cochrane review. This herb does have a positive impact on depression. It may also have a direct benefit on pain-relief but this outcome has not been well researched. There are also some side-effects.

There are a few compounds that merit special mention. Selenium deficiency may contribute to the muscle pain of fibromyalgia (van Rij 1979). A study using selenium supplements resulted in improvement after 12 weeks in nearly 60% of the subjects in a double-blind study (Robinson et al 1981).

Caffeine is an additive in many over-the-counter analgesic preparations and is easily accessed through many popular drinks and foods. Many clinical trials have investigated the effectiveness of caffeine for pain, and benefit has been noted with does above 65 mg (Wallenstein 1975). It is recommended that caffeine doses should not exceed 200 mg and should not be taken more frequently than every 3–4 hours (Food and Drug Administration 1975).

Glucosamine sulfate and chondroitin sulfate have received public and research attention. The pain of osteoarthritis is partly due to loss of cartilage and studies of these compounds have led to the conclusion that they may aid in cartilage production and repair (Burkhardt & Ghosh 1987, Leffler et al 1999). They may also have anti-inflammatory effects (Ronca et al 1998, Towheed & Anastassiades 2000). McAlindon and colleagues (2000) recently completed a comprehensive meta-analysis of glucosamine and chondroitin for the treatment of osteoarthritis and concluded that symptoms improved to a moderate extent, but not to the degree that would be expected based upon advertisement and publicity.

Many chronic pain patients report that marijuana is an effective intervention for pain and useful as a sleep aid. Clinical trials have demonstrated the value of cannabinoids for their analgesic effect, however there is a high incidence of side-effects (drowsiness, hypotension and bradycardia) (Herzberg et al 1997). These substances are not available in most countries by prescription, but patients gain access through illegal 'street' markets (determination of dose is even more uncertain in the illegal market than with unregulated herbal remedies). Currently, pharmaceutical research is developing analgesic compounds with cannabinoid content (Howlett et al 1990).

Aromatherapy uses essential oils from herbs, plants and flowers to relieve pain (Urba 1996). The oil can be applied directly to the skin or the aroma of the oil can be inhaled. It is often used in combination with massage to treat pain due to arthritis (Brownfield 1998), cancer pain (Urba 1996) and chronic pain (Buckle 1999). It has also been used to treat nausea, vomiting and pain due to labour in childbirth, and improve mood during labour (Burns & Blamey 1994). There is little evidence that aromatherapy has a positive benefit on pain or sleep, but aromatherapy in combination with massage may improve subjective perceptions of wellbeing (Brownfield 1998).

Manipulative and body-based systems

Touch plays a powerful role in human health and wellbeing (Montague 1971). The term 'body-works' refers to therapies that hypothesize that combined emotional and physical stressors cause long-standing alterations in neuromusculoskeletal structures. These changes in alignment and posture result in further stress, pain, joint restriction, discomfort and fatigue, which trigger more changes. The body-works approach uses external manual techniques, along with increased self-awareness, to achieve a posturally balanced, flexible and strong body alignment (McPartland & Miller 1999).

The number of forms of body works is rapidly increasing, with 197 named techniques thus far in the USA (McPartland 1992). There is no common nomenclature for these therapies. For example, Reiki may be considered as a 'body-work', but it is also a 'biofield' approach. The goals of the therapy and the amount of physical force that is used in treatment are important considerations to determine if there are any contraindications (e.g. someone with osteoporosis should not undergo therapies that involve significant forces, particularly through bones or joints).

The target of body-work techniques can be quite diverse. Balanced energy flow is a common objective to these therapies and is generally achieved through gentle techniques. Some techniques target the circulation of fluids such as cerebrospinal fluids (CSF), as in craniosacral therapy. Other techniques focus on muscles, tendons and fascia. These techniques closely overlap with physiotherapy. Many types of massage fall into this category, along with techniques such as shiatsu, myofascial release and rolfing. These latter techniques involve direct movement and manipulation of bones and joints. Nevertheless, none of these therapies, with the exception of massage, have been sufficiently examined in empirical research to provide convincing evidence of effectiveness.

The amount of force applied by the practitioner varies with the technique. Generally, lighter forces are used when influencing energy or CSF flow, and

increasing forces when the target is connective tissues. Joint manipulation requires significant force, but delivered under controlled conditions limiting the force transmission to specific joint structures (there is more detailed discussion of these techniques in Chapter 10 on physical therapies).

Craniosacral therapy is based upon the undemonstrated belief that a practitioner can feel the pulsations of CSF and through subtle cranial bone movement can influence its circulation. There are some reports of attempts to measure a practitioner's ability to sense CSF movements and craniosacral rhythm, without success (Hanten et al 1998, Rogers et al 1998). Measurement can be difficult as the targets of the craniosacral therapy become less and less tangible, therefore reports of effectiveness must be examined carefully.

Myofascial release uses sustained postures, stretching and deep massage, targeting fascia that has shortened due to injury and faulty posture. Hanten and Chandler (1994) compared an isometric contract–relax manual technique to myofascial release (leg pull technique) for increasing hip range of motion (ROM). Both techniques were effective but the isometric technique achieved greater increased ROM than the myofascial release technique. Nevertheless, the outcome measure, hip ROM, was more likely to demonstrate an effect for the physiotherapy technique than for the application of myofascial release. Myofascial release techniques target the entire body fascia; typically one area is not treated in isolation. A physiotherapy technique might single out a shortened hip extensor muscle and target it specifically. ROM is more likely to improve when the affected muscle group is targeted specifically.

Massage is frequently used to relieve stress and ease musculoskeletal pain, back pain, and headaches. Although there are currently no Cochrane reviews of massage for pain, there are some studies of importance. A systematic review was conducted on massage for low back pain and found that although massage seemed to have some potential as a therapy for low back pain, the existing research had too many major methodologic flaws to provide evidence for or against its efficacy (Ernst 1999).

In a different review, Ernst (1998) found that massage had some potential to relieve pain associated with muscle soreness following exercise. Unfortunately, the studies included in this review suffered from many methodologic problems. Massage was also included in a review of non-pharmacological therapies for cancer pain, but in this review massage did not appear to have a beneficial effect on pain relief (Sellick & Zaza 1998).

Back massage was included with bath and mobilization for low back pain associated with labour, but this intervention was not as effective as intracutaneous sterile water injections (Labrecque et al 1999) in relieving pain intensity or unpleasantness of the pain. Interestingly, although water injections provided significantly more pain relief, fewer women in this group indicated that they would choose this treatment again if they experienced back pain in another delivery.

A randomized controlled trial compared a 15-minute workplace massage to brief seated rest, for staff in a hospital setting (Katz et al 1999). The Swedish massage technique was used and carried out by registered massage therapists. The groups were not different in any variable measured before intervention or in their attendance. Participants who received massage reported significantly lower pain (pain in the head, neck or shoulders) and decreased tension. They also reported feeling more relaxed and in a more positive mood. For 70% of the participants, pain relief, tension reduction and relaxation persisted for up to a day or longer. This study demonstrated that massage may have an impact on pain relief for common pains that are experienced in the workplace and that massage can decrease tension and improve mood.

Research about massage thus far has only provided limited evidence regarding the benefits of massage for pain. However, other studies have shown a positive effect of massage on depression, anxiety, fatigue and confusion (Field 1998 Field et al 1996, 1997). Improvement of mood may be very important to enable clients with chronic pain to readjust to daily life and maintain a better quality of life while managing persistent pain. These studies do not report negative effects associated with massage, but massage may be contraindicated for clients with a history of physical or sexual abuse, or who are otherwise uncomfortable with this degree of physical contact.

Biofield therapies

This category includes the field of vibrational medicine; it encompasses many types of therapy. The notions of energy balance clearly echo traditional Chinese medicine. In addition, there is an intersection between spirituality and this unique belief of how the human body functions. The foundation of the field of study is the Einsteinian paradigm, which sees 'human beings as networks of complex energy fields that interface with physical/cellular systems' (Gerber 1988 p 39). The flow of this energy is considered central to wellness. Its interruption or change heralds illness, and its correction, a return to balance and health.

Therapeutic touch is a well-known biofield approach that has gained some acceptance among some health professions, particularly nursing (Gordon et al 1998). The technique attempts to achieve a balance by manipulating a person's energy field using specific hand placements and strokes, without actually making any physical contact with the client. It is unknown how therapeutic touch has its effect on clients, however, people often report feeling more relaxed. Preliminary research suggests that therapeutic touch may decrease anxiety in hospitalized patients (Quinn & Strelkauskas 1993) and may have some effect on improving pain and function in clients with osteoarthritis of the knee (Gordon et al 1998), however, thus far there is no clearly convincing evidence of a positive benefit.

There are also several other therapies based on energy flow. Reiki is believed to be a 2500-year-old therapy originally developed in Tibet. Reiki means 'boundless and universal' (Japanese, *rei*) and 'life force, vital energy' (*ki*). With this technique, the practitioner lightly places his or her hands on a client's body, directing healing energy in 12 places.

Polarity therapy uses massage to seek balance in the circulation of *prana* or energy through channels similar to the meridians of traditional Chinese medicine (McPartland & Miller 1999).

None of the interventions mentioned in this section have been examined in randomized controlled trials. Their effectiveness or risk for harm similarly remains unknown.

Bioelectromagnetics

The use of magnetic therapy dates to Paracelsus in the fifteenth century (Livingston 1998). Paracelsus argued that magnets could attract disease out of the body, in much the same way that they attracted iron. Franz Anton Mesmer (1734–1815) is famous for his work which laid the foundation for modern-day hypnosis. In his sessions, patients sat around a tub filled with water and iron filings, and held iron rods through which his magnetic influence might reach their bodies. Mesmer would then transfer his animal magnetism to the clients (Hilgard & Hilgard 1983). Magnets have been used in various fashions to draw disease and illness out of the body, although their popularity has also come and gone through the centuries.

At present, magnets for therapeutic purposes are sold in band-aid-like patches, as belts, wraps, insoles, headbands, earrings, necklaces, bracelets, cushions, pillows and mattresses (Livingston 1998). Some products are multipolar (i.e. they have alternating north- and south-pole magnets), whereas other products are unipolar. For the most part, there is no research demonstrating the effectiveness of magnetic therapy for pain. However, a recent randomized, double-blind study comparing magnetic therapy with sham magnets to relieve post-polio pain did find a substantial and significant pain reduction for magnetic therapy as compared to controls (Vallbona et al 1997). Nevertheless, there were some important limitations to this study and much more research is needed to determine whether magnetic therapy is indeed beneficial for post-polio pain or for any other type of pain.

IMPLICATIONS FOR PHYSIOTHERAPISTS AND OCCUPATIONAL THERAPISTS

There are two important considerations concerning ACTs for physiotherapists and occupational therapists.

First, therapists may have an interest in providing ACTs as part of their own practice for clients with pain. Whether the intervention is considered conventional practice or ACT, a therapist should be cognizant of the degree of evidence of benefit that exists for any intervention that is offered to a client, and any associated harm. As noted, some ACTs, such as cognitive–behavioural therapies, chiropractic and acupuncture, do have some degree of evidence for positive benefit and minimal side-effects when provided by qualified practioners: and they are generally well-accepted in conventional healthcare. However, the evidence for other therapies such as biofield strategies or bioelectromagnetic interventions is weak.

Secondly, occupational therapists and physiotherapists will likely have clients with pain who are using ACTs. In most cases, when this information becomes known to the therapist, these therapies will be used as complementary to the interventions used by the therapist and other conventional treatments. However, occasionally the client may indicate his or her intention to terminate conventional care for alternative therapies. Often when the client is sharing this information with the therapist, he or she is directly looking for the therapist's opinion or perspective about such a decision. The client has the right to determine what care is in his or her best interests. Nevertheless, it is important that the therapist avoid endorsing a therapy about which he or she may have insufficient knowledge or expertise. The therapist should ensure that the client has access to accurate information.

Box 12.2 Tips for the consumer of ACTs (adapted from the National Center for Complementary & Alternative Medicine, National Institutes of Health 2001)

Assessing the usefulness, the safety and the effectiveness of the therapy
- Search the Internet for information. Search electronic databases such as Medline, Cinahl and the Cochrane Library for evidence about whether or not the therapy is effective.
- Ask a librarian for assistance.
- Determine advantages, disadvantages, risks, side-effects and expected results. What is the expected length of treatment?
- Is the therapy applicable for one of your health problems but not others?
- Do the claims for the therapy seem reasonable or are promises of cures made that seem too good to be true?
- Do the benefits outweigh the risks?
- Are there research findings to support claims?
- Ask the advice of a conventional healthcare practitioner.
- Ask the advice of an alternative/complementary therapist.
- Be an informed consumer and continue to gather information.

Determining the practitioner's expertise if you decide to try the alternative therapy
- Find out the qualifications, competence, training and licensure of the practitioner you intend to consult.
- Talk with those who have had experience with this practitioner.
- Talk with the practitioner. The practitioner should be open and receptive to questions.
- You should feel comfortable with him or her.

Consider the service delivery
- How is the therapy given? Under what conditions?
- Visit the practitioner's office and ask how many clients they see in a day.
- Is the environment clean and safe?

Consider the costs
- Alternative therapies are not usually reimbursed by health insurance. Are the costs reasonable and affordable?
- Find out what several practitioners charge for the same treatment.

Using an alternative/complementary therapy
- If you are receiving conventional treatment for an underlying illness, disease or disability, advise these health professionals of your intention.
- Determine whether there may be harmful interactions between the ACT under consideration and conventional treatments that are being used.
- Be extremely cautious about rejecting conventional healthcare interventions in preference for an ACT to manage an underlying illness or disease.
- Monitor health over the period during which the alternative therapy is being used, paying attention to positive and negative aspects of health.
- Report any troubling symptoms to your conventional health practioner and your alternative health therapist.

The National Center for Complementary and Alternative Medicine in the USA is a good resource for information about ACTs for clients and professionals (http://nccam.nih.gov). This field is changing rapidly; interested clients and therapists should periodically search databases such as Medline, CINAHL, or the Cochrane Library for recent research about the effectiveness of a therapy. A client may also appreciate assistance with identifying credible ACT practitioners and obtaining information about ACTs. Box 12.2 lists some suggestions for consumers that we have adapted from the National Center for Complementary and Alternative Medicine (1999, 2001).

Health professionals may not always agree with a client's decisions, particularly if the client chooses to use an alternative rather than a complementary approach. As long as the client is considered to be capable of making an informed decision, a client has the right and responsibility to decide what is in his or her best interests. However, the situation can be more problematic if the client is a child. Decisions about a child's healthcare are usually made by a caregiver on behalf of the child. Sometimes, a child may also indicate his or her own preferences, thereby raising questions about when a child is able to truly provide informed consent about his or her healthcare. Conflict about interventions between children, parents and health professionals can involve institutional ethical committees, children's protection services and legal action. These issues will be less conflictual if the child, the parents, and the health professionals are able to consider all possibilities and work out a mutually agreed-upon solution that accepts some compromise.

CONCLUSION

Alternative/complementary therapies have become increasingly popular. Pain relief is one of the most common reasons people give for the use of these therapies. The distinction between ACTs and conventional therapies is sometimes unclear, since some therapies are used both by conventional health professionals and by alternative/complementary specialists.

One of the appeals of ACTs is the perception that they are natural and unlikely to cause harm. Because ACTs are less carefully monitored and not rigourously studied, little is known about their benefits and potential harm. There is emerging evidence that therapies such as acupuncture, chiropractic and massage have beneficial outcomes for some types of pain. However, the strength of the evidence for many other ACTs is weak or non-existent.

Increased interest in these therapies by consumers will improve the quality of the research about ACTs for pain and will improve our knowledge about their associated benefits and harms. Ultimately, it is the client who must decide what is in his or her best interest.

Study questions/questions for revision

1. What is the difference between an alternative and a complementary therapy?
2. Name five reasons why a client might want to try an ACT for persistent pain?
3. What are the risks associated specifically with alternative therapy?
4. What biases might be inherent in the publications about ACTs?

REFERENCES

Alltree J 1994 Acupuncture. In: Wells P, Frampton V, Bowsher D (eds) Pain Management by Physical Therapy, 2nd Edn. Butterworth-Heinemann Ltd, Oxford

Altomare G F, Capella G L 1994 'Bee sting therapy': the revival of a dangerous practice. Acta Dermato Venereologica 74: 409

Baldry P 1989 Acupuncture, Trigger Points and Musculoskeletal pain. Churchill Livingstone, New York

Berman B M, Jonas W, Swyers J P 1998 Issues in the use of complementary/alternative medical therapies for low back pain. Physical Medicine and Rehabilitation Clinics of North America 9: 497–513

Boisset M, Fitzcharles M A 1994 Alternative medicine use by rheumatology patients in a universal health care setting. Journal of Rheumatology 21: 148–152

Brownfield A 1998 Aromatherapy in arthritis: a study. Nursing Standard 13(5): 34–35

Buckle J 1999 Use of aromatherapy as a complementary treatment for chronic pain. Alternative Therapies in Health and Medicine 5(5): 42–46, 48–51

Burkhardt D, Ghosh P 1987 Laboratory evaluation of antiarthritic drugs as potential chrondroprotective agents. Seminars in Arthritis and Rheumatism 17 (2 Suppl 1): 3–34

Burns E, Blamey C 1994 Using aromatherapy in childbirth. Nursing Times 90(9): 54–58

Cassileth B 1999 Complementary therapies: overview and state of the art. Cancer Nursing 22: 85–90

Chaitow L 2000 Fibromyalgia Syndrome: a Practitioner's Guide to Treatment. Churchill Livingstone, New York

Chrubasik S, Roufogalis B 1999 Herbal medicinal products for the treatment of pain. Rheumatic Pain, Newsletter of the IASP Special Interest Group on Rheumatic Pain, November: 1–4

Deluze C, Bosia L, Zirbs A, Chantraine A, Vischer T L 1992 Electroacupuncture in fibromyalgia: results of a controlled trial. British Medical Journal 305: 1249–1252

Eisenberg D, Kessler R, Foster C, Norlock F, Calkins D, Delbanco T 1993 Unconventional medicine in the United States. New England Journal of Medicine 328: 246–252

Ernst E 1998 Does post-exercise massage treatment reduce delayed onset muscle soreness? A systematic review. British Journal of Sports Medicine 32: 212–214

Ernst E 1999 Massage therapy for low back pain: a systematic review. Journal of Pain and Symptom Management 17: 65–69

Ernst E, Pittler M H 1999 Experts' opinion on complementary/alternative therapies for low back pain. Journal of Manipulative Physiological Therapy 22(2): 87–90

Ernst E, Resch K-L, White A R 1995 Complementary medicine – What physicians think of it: a meta-analysis. Archives of Internal Medicine 155: 2405–2408

Ezzo J, Berman B, Hadhazy V A, Jadad A R, Lao L, Singh B B 2000 Is acupuncture effective for the treatment of chronic pain? Pain 86: 217–225

Fernandez E, Turk D 1989 The utility of cognitive coping strategies for altering pain perception: a meta-analysis. Pain 38: 123–135

Field T M 1998 Massage therapy effects. American Psychologist 53: 1270–1281

Field T, Grizzle N, Scafidi F, Schanberg S 1996 Massage and relaxation therapies' effects on depressed mothers. Adolescence 31: 903–911

Field T, Quintino O, Henteleff T, Wells-Keife L, Delvecchio-Feinberg G 1997 Job stress reduction techniques. Alternative Therapies and Health Medicine 3: 54–56

Food and Drug Administration 1975 Advisory Review Panel on OTC Sedative, Tranquilizer, and Sleep-Aid Drug Products (40FR57292). Fed Reg 42: 35482–85

Gadsby G, Flowerdew M 1997 Nerve stimulation for low back pain – a review. Nursing Standard 16: 11(43): 32–33

Gadsby J G, Flowerdew M W 1999 Transcutaneous electrical nerve stimulation and acupuncture-like transcutaneous electrical nerve stimulation for chronic low back pain. Cochrane Library, Issue 4: 33 pages

Gerber R 1988 Vibrational Medicine: New Choices for Healing Ourselves. Bear & Company, Santa Fe

Gifford J, Gifford L 1994 Connective tissue massage. In: Wells P, Frampton V, Bowsher D (eds) Pain Management by Physical Therapy, 2nd Edn. Butterworth, Oxford

Gordon A, Merentstin J, D'Amico F 1998 The effects of therapeutic touch on patients with osteoarthritis of the knee. Journal of Family Practice 47: 271–277

Gunn C, Ditchburn F, King M, Renwick G 1976 Acupuncture loci: a proposal for their classification according to their relationship to known neural structures. American Journal of Chinese Medicine 4: 183–195

Haanen H, Hoendrerdos H, van Romunde L, Hop W, Mallee C, Terwiel J, Hekster G 1991 Controlled trial of hypnotherapy in the treatment of refractory fibromyalgia. Journal of Rheumatology 18: 72–75

Hansen P E, Hansen J H 1983 Acupuncture treatment of chronic facial pain – a controlled cross-over trial. Headache 23: 66–69

Hansen P E, Hansen J H 1985 Acupuncture treatment of chronic tension headache – a controlled crossover trial. Cephalgia 1985: 137–142

Hanten W, Chandler S 1994 Effects of myofascial release leg pull and sagittal plane isometric contract-relax techniques on passive straight-leg raise angle. Journal of Orthopedic Sports Physical Therapy 20: 138–144

Hanten W, Dawson D, Iwata M, Seiden M, Whitten F, Zink T 1998 Craniosacral rhythm: reliability and relationships with cardiac and respiratory rates. Journal of Orthopaedic and Sports Physical Therapy 27: 213–218

Hawk C 2000 (personal communication) http://www.therapeutictouch.com/crystal.html

Herzberg U, Eliav E, Bennett G, Kopin I 1997 The analgesic effects of R(+)-WIN 55,212-2 mesylate, a high affinity cannabinoid agonist, in a rat model of neuropathic pain. Neuroscience Letters 221(2–3): 157–160

Hilgard E, Hilgard J 1983 Hypnosis in the Relief of Pain, 2nd Edn. William Kaufmann, Los Altos

Hilgard J, LeBaron S 1984 Hypnotherapy of Pain in Children with Cancer. William Kaufmann, Los Altos

Howlett A, Johnson M, Melvin L 1990 Classical and nonclassical cannabinoids: mechanism of action–brain binding. In: Drugs of Abuse: chemistry, pharmacology, immunology and AIDS, NIDA Research Monograph 96. US Department of Health and Human Services, Rockville

Hoyeraal H M, Brewer E J, Giannini E H, et al 1984 Unconventional therapies in pediatric rheumatology (abstract). Scandinavian Journal of Rheumatology Supplement 53: 113

Katz J, Wowk A, Culp D, Wakeling H 1999 A randomized, controlled study of the pain- and tension-reducing effects of 15 min workplace massage treatments versus seated rest for nurses in a large teaching hospital. Pain Research and Management 4: 81–88

Kenny D T, Guy L 2000 Pain-making: ritual dances between chronic pain patients and their doctors. The Progress of Pain: Before, Betwixt, & Beyond. Australian Pain Society 21st Annual Scientific Meeting, March 2000, p 36

Kerr, K 2000 Relaxation techniques: a critical review. Critical Reviews in Physical and Rehabilitation Medicine 12: 51–89

Krauss H H, Godfrey C, Kirk J, Eisenberg D M 1998 Alternative health care: its use by individuals with physical disabilities. Archives of Physical Medicine and Rehabilitation 79: 1440–1447

Labrecque M, Nouwen A, Bergeron M, Rancourt J F 1999 A randomized controlled trial of nonpharmacological approaches for relief of low back pain during labor. Journal of Family Practice 48: 259–263

Leffler C T, Philippi A F, Leffler S G, Mosure J C, Kim P D 1999 Glucosamine, chondroitin, and manganese ascorbate for degenerative joint disease of the knee or low back: a randomized, double-blind, placebo-controlled pilot study. Military Medicine 164: 85–91

Liossi C, Hatira P 1999 Clinical hypnosis versus cognitive behavioural training for pain management with pediatric cancer patients undergoing bone marrow aspirations. International Journal of Clinical and Experimental Hypnosis 47: 104–116

Liu Y, Varela M, Oswald R 1975 The correspondence between some motor points and acupuncture loci. American Journal of Chinese Medicine 3: 347–358

Livingston J D 1998 Magnetic therapy: plausible attraction? Committee for the Scientific Investigation of Claims of the Paranormal, Skeptical Inquirer, http://www.csicop.org/si/9807/magnet.html

McAlindon T, LaValley M, Gulin J, Felson D 2000 Glucosamine and chondroitin for treatment of osteoarthritis: a systematic quality assessment and meta-analysis. Journal of the American Medical Association 283: 1469–1472

McPartland J 1992 Alternative schools of manual medicine practicing in the United States. American Academy Osteopathy Journal 2: 23–24

McPartland J, Miller B 1999 Bodywork therapy systems. Physical Medicine and Rehabilitation Clinics of North America 10: 583–602

Melzack R, Wall P 1965 Pain mechanisms: a new theory. Science 150: 971–979

Melzack R, Stillwell D, Fox J 1977 Trigger points and acupuncture points for pain: correlations and implications. Pain 3: 3–23

Montague A 1971 Touching: the Human Significance of the Skin, 2nd Edn. Harper & Row New York

Nam R, Fleshner N, Rakovitch E, et al 1999 Prevalence and patterns of the use of complementary therapies among prostate cancer patients: an epidemiological analysis. Journal of Urology 161: 1521–1524

National Center for Complementary and Alternative Medicine 1999a, Frequently asked questions. http://www.nccam.nih.gov/nccam/what-is-cam/faq.shtml

National Center for Complementary and Alternative Medicine 1999b Considering alternative therapies? http://nccam.nih.gov/nccam/what-is-cam/classify.shtml

National Center for Complementary and Alternative Medicine 2001 Considering alternative therapies? http://nccam.nih.gov/nccam/what-is-cam/consider.html

Newall C, Anderson L, Phillipson J 1996 Herbal medicines: a guide for health-care professionals. Pharmaceutical Press, London

Nickelson C, Brende J O, Gonzalez J 1999 What if your patient prefers an alternative pain control method? Self-hypnosis in the control of pain. South Medical Journal 92: 521–523

Oneschuk D, Fennell L, Hanson J, Bruera E 1998 The use of complementary medications by cancer patients attending an outpatient pain and symptom clinic. Journal of Palliative Care 14(4): 21–26

Ordman D 1968 Bee stings in South Africa. South Africa Medical Journal 42: 1194–1198

Patel M, Gutzwiller F, Paccaud F, Marazzi A 1989 A meta-analysis of acupuncture for chronic pain. International Journal of Epidemiology 18: 900–906

Pomeranz B 1995 Scientific basis of acupuncture. In: Stux G, Pomeranz B (eds) Basics of Acupuncture. Springer-Verlag, Berlin, pp 1–36

Portenoy R K, Lesage P 1999 Management of cancer pain. Lancet 353: 1695–1700

Quinn J, Strelkauskas A 1993 Psychoimmunologic effects of therapeutic touch on practitioner and recently bereaved recipients: a pilot study. Advances in Nursing Science 15: 13

Rainville P, Carrier B, Hofbauer R, Bushnell M, Duncan G 1999 Dissociation of sensory and affective dimensions of pain using hypnotic modulation. Pain 82: 159–171

Rao J K, Mihaliak K, Kroenke K, Bradley J, Tierney W M, Weinberger M 1999 Use of complementary therapies for arthritis among patients of rheumatologists. Annals of Internal Medicine 131: 409–416

Roberto K 1994 Older Women with Chronic Pain. Harrington Park Press, New York

Robinson M, Campbell D, Stewart R, Rea H, Thomson C, Snow P, Squires I 1981 Effect of daily supplements of selenium on patients with muscular complaints in Otago and Canterbury. New Zealand Medical Journal 93: 289–292

Rogers J, Witt P, Gross M, Hacke J, Genova P 1998 Simultaneous palpation of the craniosacral rate at the head and feet: intrarater and interrater reliability and rate comparisons. Physical Therapy 78: 1175–1185

Ronca F, Palmieri L, Panicucci P, Ronca G 1998 Anti-inflammatory activity of chondroitin sulfate. Osteoarthritis and Cartilage 6 Suppl A: 14–21

Sellick S M, Zaza C 1998 Critical review of five nonpharmacological strategies for managing cancer pain. Cancer Prevention and Control 2: 7–14

Shafrir Y, Kaufman B A 1992 Quadriplegia after chiropractic manipulation in an infant with congenital torticollis caused by a spinal astrocytoma. Journal of Pediatrics 120: 266–269

Simon E P, Dahl L F 1999 The sodium pentothal hypnosis interview with follow-up treatment for complex regional pain syndrome. Journal of Pain and Symptom Management 18: 132–136

Southwood T R, Malleson P N, Roberts-Thomson P J, Mahy M 1990 Unconventional remedies used for patients with juvenile arthritis. Pediatrics 85: 150–153

Spigelblatt L S 1995 Alternative medicine: should it be used by children? Current Problems in Pediatrics 25: 180–188

Spigelblatt L, Laine-Ammara G, Pless B, Guyer A 1994 The use of alternative medicine by children. Pediatrics 94: 811–814

Spitzer S, Roley S S, Clark F, Parham D 1996 Sensory integration: current trends in the United States. Scandinavian Journal of Occupational Therapy 3: 123–138

Streitberg K, Kleinhertz J 1998 Introducing a placebo needle into acupuncture research. The Lancet 352: 364–365

Ter Reit G, Kleijnen J, Knipschild P 1990 Acupuncture and chronic pain: a criteria-based meta-analysis. Clinical Epidemiology 43: 1191–1199

Towheed T, Anastassiades T 2000 Glucosamine and chondroitin for treating symptoms of osteoarthritis. Journal of the American Medical Association 283: 1469–1475

Urba S G 1996 Nonpharmacological pain management in terminal care. Clinics in Geriatric Medicine 12: 301–311

Vallbona C, Hazelwood C F, Jurida G 1997 Response of pain to static magnetic fields in postpolio patients: a double-blind pilot study. Archives of Physical and Rehabilitation Medicine 78: 1200–1203

van Rij A 1979 Selenium deficiency in total parenteral nutrition. American Journal of Clinical Clinical Nutrition 32: 2076–2085

van Tulder M W, Cherkin D C, Berman B, Lao L, Koes B W 1999 Acupuncture for low back pain. Cochrane Library, Issue 4: 15 pages

Veraldi S, Raiteri F, Caputo R, Alessi E 1995 Persistent nodular lesions caused by 'bee sting therapy'. Acta Dermato Venereologica 75: 161–162

Verhoef M J, Sutherland L R 1995 General practitioners' assessment of and interest in alternative medicine in Canada. Social Science and Medicine 41: 511–515

Waddell G, Kummel E, Lotto W, Graham J, Hall H, McCulloch J 1979 Failed lumbar disc surgery and repeat surgery following industrial injuries. Journal of Bone and Joint Surgery 61A: 201–207

Wallenstein S 1975 Analgesic studies of aspirin in cancer patients. In: Dale T (ed) Proceedings of the Aspirin Symposium. The Aspirin Foundation, London, pp 5–10

Warrick P, Irish J, Morningstart M 1999 Use of alternative medicine among patients with head and neck cancer. Archives of Otoloaryngology Head and Neck Surgery 125(5): 573–579

Wilentz J 1998 NIH Consensus Development Conference on acupuncture. APS Bulletin 8(2): 1, 21 (http://consensus.nih.gov)

Wu D Z 1988. Traditional Chinese rehabilitative therapy in the process of modernization. International Disability Studies 10: 140–142

13

Exercise and pain

Julie Hides   Carolyn Richardson

OVERVIEW

Providing patients with effective and efficient pain relief, as well as preventing pain re-occurring is a high-priority health issue. Treating pain, especially chronic pain associated with injury to the musculoskeletal system, is now recognized as a complex management issue.

There are many conservative methods available to the allied health professionals to achieve pain relief. These range from manual techniques such as massage and joint mobilizations to electrophysical modalities such as interferential or TENS applications (see Chapter 11) and other approaches such as relaxation training. This chapter explains an exercise approach, which has been shown to affect pain relief, as well as decreasing recurrences of injury and pain.

Low-level, specific isometric exercises aim to re-activate and train the muscles closely linked to joint stabilization (see Box 13.1). Muscles such as the lumbar multifidus, in the case of low back pain, and vastus medialis oblique, in the case of patellofemoral joint pain, can be specifically exercised, independently of

---

Box 13.1   Key terms defined

Joint stabilization – The mechanical control of the joint, preventing injuries to ligaments and capsules.

Reflex inhibition – The situation that occurs when sensory stimuli impede the voluntary activation of a muscle.

Arthrogenous muscle weakness – Weakness of muscles acting about an injured or inflamed joint.

Specific stabilization training – Training the isolated or independent control of specific muscles directly linked to joint stabilization. This term is also referred to as 'segmental stabilization training' when the training is related to muscles concerned with spinal stability.

adjacent muscles, to re-establish their important function of joint stabilization. This chapter describes the type of exercise, giving the probable mechanisms by which these exercises affect pain. Two main clinical models are used in the chapter as examples, but the principles can be applied to other musculoskeletal conditions, e.g. exercising the rotator cuff muscles for pain relief for shoulder impingement syndrome.

Learning objectives

On completing the chapter, readers will have an understanding of:

1. Joint stabilization and the muscles designed primarily for such stabilization.
2. The muscle problems associated with joint pain and injury.
3. The link between muscle dysfunction, poor joint stabilization and implications for the development of acute and chronic musculoskeletal pain.
4. The concepts and principles involved in specific (segmental) stabilization exercise

MUSCULOSKELETAL PAIN

Formal exercise programmes (used in conjunction with other methods of treatment) are one of the main forms of conservative treatments used to treat painful musculoskeletal conditions.

Due to the high cost and morbidity of chronic musculoskeletal conditions, it is important that the most efficient and effective pain management treatments are given to patients with these conditions. One of the most common musculoskeletal pain problems is low back pain, encompassing acute as well as recurrent episodic and chronic low back pain. Low back pain (LBP) and knee pain will be the two main clinical models used in this chapter to illustrate general principles of exercise therapy for musculoskeletal disorders.

Chronic low back pain is acknowledged to be a complex problem, which may be associated with various psychological, behavioural and environmental changes. Chronic pain has been described (Chapter 1) as the maintenance of pain long after the expected period of healing. This was explained as the inability of the body to restore its physiological functions to normal, e.g. the nervous system may be altered following the original injury, in such a way that it is unable to restore itself to normal functioning.

For mechanical LBP, our contention is that the physiological function of deep muscles close to the spine, such as the lumbar multifidus, is impaired following the original injury. These muscles, and the central nervous system pathways responsible for their control, are unable to return to their normal function of stabilization and protection of the spine and specific exercise techniques are required to reverse and correct this situation. Similarly, in peripheral joints such as the knee, the function of the quadriceps muscle group (particularly vastus medialis oblique) is likely to be impaired after joint injury or disease and so it becomes important to use specific exercise principles to re-educate the function of this muscle.

Therefore this chapter deals with only one aspect of the treatment of chronic pain, i.e. how specific exercise techniques can help in the management of the painful symptoms of musculoskeletal diseases such as mechanical low back pain or patello-femoral joint dysfunction. Exercise should be seen as one method of self-help management used in the conservative care of such painful musculoskeletal disorders.

In order to gain an understanding of how exercise can help a painful musculoskeletal condition such as low back pain or knee pain, it is essential to have an understanding of active support and stabilization of the spine and peripheral joints, the link between acute pain and muscle dysfunction, the pathophysiological consequences of painful joint injury, specific muscle problems and the development of persistent pain, and the role of specific (segmental) stabilization exercise.

ACTIVE SUPPORT AND STABILIZATION OF JOINTS

Lumbopelvic region

There are many muscles that have been associated with the maintenance of lumbopelvic stabilization. Our research group has focused on the stabilization role of transversus abdominis and multifidus (for review see Richardson et al 1999). While both muscles contract together to protect the spine, we will focus in this chapter on the segmental multifidus (Fig. 13.1). This muscle surrounds the zygapophyseal joints and provides a good illustration of the relationship between joint injury, pain and the effect of pain and injury on muscles closely associated with that joint.

The multifidus muscle plays an important part in lumbopelvic stability in the non-pathological situation. There is considerable evidence to support this claim. Evidence is found in four main areas of

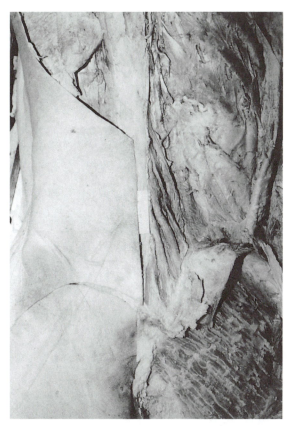

Figure 13.1 Anatomical dissection of the five fascicles of the lumbar multifidus (with kind permission from Richardson et al 1999 p 22).

investigation: morphological, muscle composition, biomechanical and activation studies.

On the basis of morphological evidence, the factors that are most important in providing lumbar stability are the segmental arrangement of multifidus fascicles (Macintosh et al 1986), the large size of the muscle at the lumbosacral junction (Amonoo-Kuofi 1983, Macintosh et al 1986) and the close relationship between the multifidus and the zygapophyseal joints (Lewin et al 1962, Macintosh et al 1986). Muscle composition studies provide further evidence of this important stability role in terms of the predominance of type I fibres in the multifidus, in line with its tonic stabilizing role (Jorgensen et al 1993, Sirca & Kostevc 1985, Verbout et al 1989).

Evidence of the stability role of the multifidus has been provided in the area of biomechanical research. These studies have linked the stability role of the multifidus with control of neutral zone motion (Crisco & Panjabi 1991, Panjabi et al 1989, Wilke et al 1995), maintenance of the lumbar lordosis (Aspden 1992,

Bergmark 1989), control of shear forces, and enhancement of lumbar spine stiffness (Wilke et al 1995). Finally, muscle activation studies have made an important contribution to our knowledge of the stability function of multifidus by demonstrating that it is often active in situations where activity is unexpected (Donisch & Basmajian 1972, Pauly 1966).

With its important role in providing lumbar stability, any dysfunction in the multifidus of low back pain patients must have a significant effect on the protection and support of the lumbar vertebral segments.

Muscular control of the patellofemoral joint of the knee

The vasti, the muscles that control the knee, have a common insertion, and the question of whether each has an individual action has been a subject of much research and scientific debate. As early as 1968, the vastus medialis oblique was recognized as a key muscle for the stabilization and control of the patella, rather than an extensor of the knee joint. The classical anatomical studies of Lieb and Perry (1968, 1971) confirmed that the oblique fibres of the muscle function to keep the patella controlled and centred in the femoral groove, rather than functioning with the other heads of the quadriceps to extend the knee.

The individual stabilizing function of vastus medialis oblique was also investigated during rapid (ballistic) movement of the knee. Electromyography (EMG) was used to observe the pattern of muscle activity in vastus medialis oblique, rectus femoris and vastus lateralis during three speeds of rapid flexion–exension movements of the knee (Richardson & Bullock 1986). Two aspects of this study are relevant to the argument for a stability role of vastus medialis oblique.

All muscles (except vastus medialis oblique), increased their levels of EMG activity (measured over three movement cycles) with progressive increases in speed (Fig. 13.2A). This result is to be expected as more muscle activation is required with faster alternating movements. However, the levels of EMG activity of vastus medialis oblique remained unchanged over three cycles, in line with its patella-supporting role rather than contributing to knee movement as the other components of the quadriceps do.

In addition, while the other quadricep muscles demonstrated phasic activity during the rapid, phasic alternating movements (as expected from biomechanics), the vastus medialis oblique demonstrated a tonic, continuous EMG pattern (Fig. 13.3). Such a pattern, during alternating phasic knee movement would be in line with a stabilization role of the muscle.

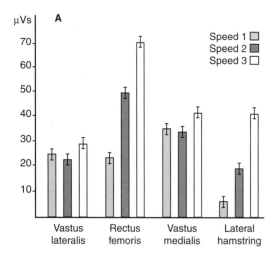

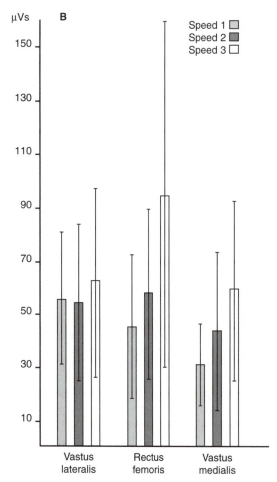

Figure 13.2 Comparison of changes in muscle activity with increases in speed for (**A**) normal subjects and (**B**) patellofemoral pain subjects (with kind permission from Richardson 1987b).

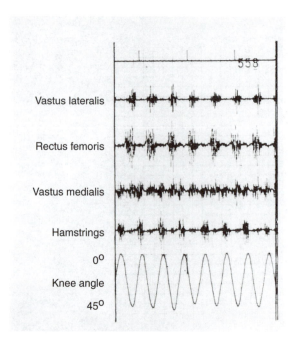

Figure 13.3 EMG of the quadricep and hamstring muscles during rapid repetitive knee flexion–extension movements, performed in a prone-lying position. Note the tonic pattern of activity for vastus medialis (oblique) in normal subjects (with kind permission from Richardson et al 1999).

Interestingly, a similar tonic pattern had been seen in transversus abdominis by Cresswell et al (1992) during alternating trunk movements. This and other studies (Hodges & Richardson 1996, 1997) have established transversus abdominis as a muscle with similar EMG characteristics to vastus medialis oblique, that is, designed for the function of joint stabilization rather than initiating or controlling joint movement.

PAIN AND MUSCLE DYSFUNCTION

Multifidus and low back pain

Increased fatigability (or decreased endurance) of the multifidus muscle has been demonstrated in low back pain (LBP) patients in several research studies (Biedermann et al 1991, Roy et al 1989). These findings are also in line with studies on the fibre-type composition of multifidus in the low back pain population who had undergone surgery. Poor functional recovery after surgery was linked with increased abnormalities of the type I fibres (Rantanen et al 1993). These are the fibres linked to the endurance capacity of the muscle.

Additional important evidence of dysfunction at localized segmental levels of multifidus in patients with acute LBP has been provided in the form of studies demonstrating a segmental decrease in multifidus cross-sectional area, using real-time ultrasound imaging (Hides et al 1994) (Fig. 13.4). This decrease in size occurs rapidly (within days), and was found to be significantly greater in subjects with a duration of symptoms of less than 2 weeks than in those with a duration of symptoms greater than 2 weeks. The decreased multifidus size was localized to the side of painful symptoms in patients with unilateral LBP. Examination of the possible mechanisms associated with this local decrease in multifidus cross-sectional area provides valuable information to guide appropriate rehabilitation of the segmental multifidus, based on the cause of the dysfunction.

Possible causes of decreased multifidus size include reflex inhibition and disuse atrophy. The rapidity of onset and localized distribution of the decrease in muscle size, suggest that disuse atrophy was not the cause and that a selective mechanism (reflex inhibition) was in operation (Hides et al 1994).

Quadriceps (vastus medialis oblique) dysfunction and knee pain

Evidence of dysfunction of vastus medialis oblique has been demonstrated in patients with patellofemoral pain syndromes. The individual function of vastus medialis oblique was investigated in patients with patellofemoral pain syndromes during rapid (ballistic) movement of the knee in a study similar to that described by Richardson and Bullock (1986). There was some evidence that the stability role of vastus medialis oblique had been lost in patients with patella pain (Richardson 1987a, 1987b). The EMG patterns recorded from vastus medialis oblique were phasic during the alternating knee movements, similar to the other quadriceps. The distinctive, continuous holding role of the vastus medialis oblique was not present in patients with patellofemoral pain. In addition, this muscle increased its EMG activity with the increasing speeds of alternating knee movement, in a similar way to the rest of the quadriceps (Fig. 13.2B). Thus, some evidence exists for muscle dysfunction in patients with patella pain. There is a loss of control in one of the quadriceps, vastus medialis oblique, the individual muscle of the quadriceps responsible for stabilization of the patella.

In addition, Voight and Weider (1991) have demonstrated, through measuring reflex response times, another change in the vastus medialis oblique in patients with patellofemoral pain. While vastus medialis oblique fired significantly faster than vastus lateralis in normal subjects, the reverse was true in the patients with patellofemoral pain, i.e. vastus lateralis was activated earlier than the vastus medialis. This change in muscle timing of vastus medialis oblique is interesting, considering that inhibition of the vastus medialis oblique is known to be associated with patellofemoral pain syndrome.

The neurophysiological basis of reflex inhibition, which is related to the muscle dysfunction found in both multifidus in LBP and vastus medialis oblique in patellofemoral pain problems, will be discussed further below.

REFLEX INHIBITION AND MUSCLE FUNCTION

Reflex inhibition of a muscle has been defined as the situation that occurs when sensory stimuli impede the voluntary activation of a muscle. To understand the phenomenon of reflex inhibition and how it could influence exercise design, it is necessary to review briefly the possible neurophysiological pathways involved, the patterns of muscle wasting and possible explanations of the rapid muscle response.

Neurophysiological pathways involved in reflex inhibition

The specific sensory pathway involved in reflex inhibition is not known. It involves joint afferents and articular nerves, terminating in the spinal cord. The main sensation attributed to the joint is pain (Schaible & Grubb 1993). Joints are supplied by articular branches descending from main nerve trunks or their muscular, cutaneous and periosteal branches (for review of joint innervation, morphology, types and location of joint receptors, see Freeman & Wyke 1967 and Schaible & Grubb 1993). The mechanosensitivity of articular afferents is increased when joints are inflamed. Recordings from afferent fibres innervating joints have shown that sensory units are sensitized during inflammation (Schaible & Grubb 1993). Mechanosensitivity is altered by both physical changes that occur during inflammation (e.g. synovial effusion) and chemical changes.

The pathways from joint afferents have extensive projections in the spinal cord (Craig et al 1988). Animal research has shown that sensory input from the knee joint is conveyed to interneurones, motor neurones and supraspinal structures, including the cerebral cortex and the cerebellum (see Chapter 2). Information

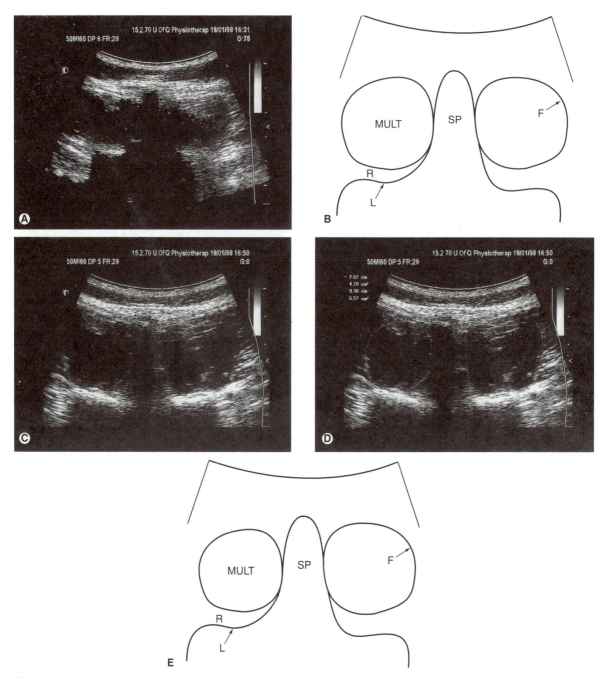

Figure 13.4 (**A**) Sonographic appearance of the multifidus (axial image) at the level of the fifth vertebra in a normal subject. (**B**) The multifidus muscle (MULT) is bordered by the vertebral lamina/zygapophyseal joint (L) inferiorly, the spinous process (SP) medially, fascia, fat and skin superiorly, and the fascia between the multifidus and the lumbar longissimus and iliocostalis (F) laterally. The brightness seen at the interior border of the multifidus is reflection (R) of sound waves from the vertebral lamina and zygapophyseal joints. Acoustic shadowing is seen inferior to this landmark, as the ultrasound waves are unable to penetrate the bone. (**C**) Sonographic appearance of the multifidus (axial image) at the level of the fifth vertebra in a patient with unilateral left-sided low back pain. (**D**) In this image the borders of the multifidus have been traced to demonstrate the asymmetry. The multifidus on the left (symptomatic) side is 4.78 cm², while the larger multifidus on the right side is 6.57 cm². This represents a decrease on the left side of 27%. (**E**) Note the decreased size of the left multifidus in comparison with the right side. Labels are as in (**B**) (with kind permission from Richardson et al 1999 p 72).

from joint afferents ascends in the dorsal columns and in the spinothalamic, spinoreticular and spinocerebellar pathways (Johansson et al 1991). Electrical stimulation of the posterior articular nerve of the cat knee joint has been shown to excite interneurones (Gardner et al 1949), motor neurones (Eccles & Lundberg 1959a, 1959b) and neurones of the spinocerebellar (Haddad 1953) and spinocervical tract (Harrison & Jankowska 1985) in the lumbar spinal cord. A number of transmitters, neuromodulators and receptors are involved in spinal cord activity when nociceptive input from joints is processed (Schaible & Grubb 1993) (see Chapter 3). Variables such as joint inflammation affect the levels of transmitters and neuromodulators present in the dorsal root ganglion and the spinal cord and alters the sensitivity of spinal cord neurons.

The sensory pathways involved in reflex inhibition are complex. Research has been conducted on animals (mainly cats) to investigate the motor reflexes. Reflexes in limb muscles and reflex discharges in motor neurones can be elicited by either electrical stimulation of articular nerves or activation of receptors in the joint capsule or the joint ligaments (either directly or by pressure applied by inflation of the joint). Electrical stimulation of articular nerves provided the first evidence that reflex motor pathways actually exist (Eccles & Lundberg 1959a, Gardner 1950, Hongo et al 1969, Lundberg et al 1978). Activation of receptors in the joint capsule and the joint ligaments confirmed this motor response (Baxendale et al 1987, Ekholm et al 1960, Grigg et al 1978). Motor reflexes may be considered as a feedback mechanism, from the joint back to the joint, since sensory information arising in the joint may influence the motor output to the muscles that move and stabilize the joint (Schaible & Grubb 1993). It is interesting to examine the pattern of muscle wasting found in studies of reflex inhibition, as this may help to guide specific rehabilitation approaches.

Patterns of muscle wasting in reflex inhibition

Most research concerning patterns of muscle wasting in reflex inhibition has been conducted at the knee joint. Initial evidence of patterns of motor responses was provided by the classic study of Ekholm et al (1960), which involved stimulation of joint receptors by pinching of the joint capsule. This led to inhibition of the knee extensors and facilitation of the knee flexors. This pattern of response is similar to that proposed by the pain adaption model described in Chapter 3.

These results have been used to explain the common finding of isolated wasting of the quadriceps with hamstring sparing in knee joint injuries. Furthermore, it has been demonstrated in several studies that the pattern of reflex responses in the spinal cord can be changed by the induction of joint inflammation by chemical stimulants which activate fine afferent fibres (nociceptors) (Ferrell et al 1988, He et al 1988, Woolf & Wall 1986). The response to inflammation was a pronounced and prolonged increase in alpha motor neurone excitability in the flexor muscles. The prolonged facilitation of the flexor reflex did not require any ongoing input, i.e. peripheral activation of the afferent fibres (C fibres) modified the functional response of the spinal cord. This shows that sensory and motor alterations are found after peripheral tissue injury. Ferrell et al (1988) proposed that these findings provide a possible mechanism for the development of flexion contractures, as seen in arthritic patients. These findings also relate directly to joint resting positions in acute joint injury.

In summary, these studies have demonstrated that sensory stimuli can exert potent effects on motor neurone excitability. Preferential inhibition of extensor motor neurones and facilitation of flexor motor neurones has been demonstrated when receptors in the joint capsule have been activated (Ekholm et al 1960). Evidence of flexor motor neurone facilitation has been provided by joint inflammation studies.

Even more specific changes than inhibition of extensor muscles and facilitation of flexor muscles have been found to exist. There is evidence that the inhibition response may be focused on individual muscles within the functional muscle group. This has been demonstrated predominantly in the quadriceps muscles. Studies conducted on human knee joints using experimentally induced effusions to stimulate joint receptors, have shown preferential inhibition of the vastus medialis muscle (Kennedy et al 1982, Spencer et al 1984). These studies used the Hoffman reflex (H reflex) to measure inhibition. The H reflex was elicited by selective recruitment of 1a spindle afferents in the femoral nerve with a consistent low-voltage stimulus. This generated a reproducible quadriceps contraction. Within the spinal cord, this transmission comes under the influence of modulating sensory inputs, acting through the internuncial pool. Inputs arriving from the articular receptors can facilitate or inhibit the reflex.

By maintaining a constant stimulus, Kennedy et al (1982) and Spencer et al (1984) were provided with an indirect assessment of the activity of articular afferents by measuring the degree of the quadriceps contraction, using EMG, as they increased the volume of intra-articular fluid in the subjects' knees. Similar findings of selective vastus medialis muscle inhibition measured using EMG have been reported by Wise et al (1984) in patients with patellofemoral pain syndromes. It has been reported that the rectus femoris muscle is the component of the quadriceps muscle group least affected by inhibition following injury (Stener 1969, Wolf et al 1971). These findings are in line with the findings of a dysfunction of vastus medialis oblique (rather than the other quadriceps) in patients with patella pain described by Richardson (1987a) and described in detail earlier in his chapter. However, in contrast to these findings, Wild et al (1982) found that the quadriceps muscles were all equally inhibited in patients with patellofemoral disorders.

Imaging techniques have also been used to provide information on selective atrophy of parts of muscle groups. Results using imaging techniques are conflicting. Gerber et al (1985) reported selective atrophy of the vastus medialis muscle, while other results suggested a more uniform atrophy (Halkjaer-Kristensen et al 1980, Young et al 1982). Although some of the findings in this area are contradictory, the weight of the evidence suggests that parts of muscles can be selectively inhibited. Further evidence of this phenomenon has been provided by the findings of localized inhibition of the multifidus in acute LBP patients (Hides et al 1994). It appears that muscles, or components of muscle groups that perform specific synergistic functions, to limit or control unwanted movement, may be particularly susceptible to inhibition.

Examination of the possible mechanism of selective inhibition of part of a muscle group is intriguing. In the case of knee joint injuries, explanation on a neurophysiological basis for the common clinical finding of isolated wasting of the quadriceps with hamstring sparing is not forthcoming. It is the sensory innervation of the injured joint or structure which is the crucial element in reflex inhibition. From definitions of reflex inhibition, sensory stimuli impede the voluntary activation of a muscle. The afferent stimuli arise from injury to a joint at which the muscle functions. However, in the case of the knee joint, the nerves which supply the joint are derived from the obturator, femoral, tibial and common peroneal nerves (Kennedy et al 1982). The segmental supply of the knee joint and capsule is therefore widespread (from L2–S3). On the basis of the sensory innervation of the knee joint, almost any muscle in the lower limb could potentially be inhibited. Yet, the actual response in clinical practice is isolated to the quadriceps group, which is innervated by the femoral nerve (L2–4), and an even more specific effect has been observed in part of the quadriceps (the vastus medialis). This finding implies that input from the joint is processed and modulated in the spinal cord to produce a specific effect in specific muscles and even parts of muscles. However, the actual mechanism is not understood at this time.

A similar argument applies in the case of localized segmental inhibition of the lumbar multifidus in acute LBP patients. The innervation of the zygapophyseal joints is derived from branches of the dorsal rami (Bradley 1974). The capsule receives a number of branches from either two nerves (the medial branch of the dorsal ramus at that level and the level above (Bogduk & Twomey 1987, Bradley 1974) or three nerves (one spinal nerve higher, one lower and the spinal nerve of the level in question (Paris 1983, Wyke 1981).

Lumbar discs are supplied by the sinuvertebral nerves, which are recurrent branches of the ventral rami that re-enter the intervertebral foramen to be distributed within the intervertebral canal (Bogduk & Twomey 1987). Each lumbar sinuvertebral nerve supplies the disc at its level of entry into the vertebral canal and the disc above, i.e. the L3–4 disc is supplied by the L3 and L4 sinuvertebral nerves. There are countless other vertebral structures which are innervated and could be injured in acute LBP. Yet the response to injury in the case of the multifidus, as with the knee joint, is specific and localized to the part of the multifidus muscle that crosses the affected vertebral segment (Hides et al 1994).

Another interesting phenomenon is the speed of muscle atrophy after any joint injury, for example the multifidus in the case of patients with acute LBP and vastus medialis oblique in the case of patients with knee or patellofemoral pain. An explanation for this requires review of other causes of muscle atrophy.

Possible explanations for the rapid muscle response to reflex inhibition

Muscle atrophy is known to occur very rapidly in the case of reflex inhibition (Stener 1969). In the clinical situation, rapid atrophy of muscle is also a commonly observed phenomenon. Yet, the actual mechanism of rapid muscle atrophy in reflex inhibition is not yet fully understood.

The size of muscle fibres is determined multifactorially, with influences exerted by various factors including activity and innervation, hormones, growth, stretch and nutrition (Jennekens 1982). Muscle atrophy is one of the most common responses of a muscle fibre to a loss of neural influences, to processes that prevent normal contractile activity, and to various pathological stimuli (Cullen & Mastaglia 1982). It involves a phase of negative growth and a regression in volume. The mechanisms underlying myofibre atrophy are not fully understood.

Shrinkage of a cell or tissue may be brought about either by an increase in the normal rate of protein degradation, or by a reduction in protein synthesis, or by the occurrence of both processes together (Goldberg 1975). The enzymes involved in the degradation of muscle protein have not been identified. Proteinases, which are present in muscle and capable of breaking down myofibrillar proteins have been examined in animal studies. In rats, myofibrillar protein breakdown can be rapid during myofibre atrophy, with a potential for total myosin degradation within 6–9 days (Schwartz & Bird 1977). However, the intracellular control mechanisms of protein degradation are not understood (Cullen & Mastaglia 1982).

Denervation atrophy

In order to understand the mechanism of rapid muscle atrophy in reflex inhibition, it is useful to review explanations of decrease in muscle size in conditions such as denervation atrophy and disuse atrophy. Reports of the time taken for a decrease in muscle-fibre size as a result of denervation vary. It is common to find reports of atrophy of human muscles taking a few weeks to become evident following denervation (Jennekens 1982).

Animal research models have commonly been adopted for atrophy studies, due to ethical restrictions. Muscle fibres of the Australian opossum atrophy rapidly in the initial weeks following denervation. Atrophy becomes evident in cats after a month, and rats show evidence of decreases of approximately 20% within 3 weeks (Jennekens 1982). A more rapid rate of muscle atrophy in humans has been documented in immobilization studies. Muscle weight, fibre size and muscle strength decrease most dramatically during the first week of immobilization (Appell 1990). In the rat gastrocnemius muscle, a weight loss of 30% was already present within 3 days of immobilization (Max et al 1971). Similar findings have been reported for muscle fibre size, with little further reduction in fibre diameter after 1 week (Appell 1986a, 1986b). It would seem that the rapid atrophy described in immobilization studies provides a basis for understanding some of the possible mechanisms involved in the case of reflex inhibition.

Rapid muscle atrophy is a commonly observed clinical phenomenon in various conditions. Following spinal cord injury, a decrease in quadriceps depth of 16% within days of injury has been reported using ultrasound imaging (Taylor et al 1993). Up to 50% of quadriceps depth was lost in the first 3 weeks following injury. Clinical observations would suggest that rapid atrophy is more evident in certain muscles following injury, e.g. the quadriceps and especially the vastus medialis muscle in knee joint injuries or the multifidus in lower back injuries. This observation may be explained on the basis of the susceptibility of different fibre types.

It has been suggested that extensor (i.e. antigravity) muscles undergo more severe atrophy than flexors in studies of reflex inhibition. This has also been demonstrated in immobilization studies, and the explanation for this finding has been based on the fact that the extensor muscles contain more type I fibres than the flexor muscles. Interestingly, the vastus medialis contains more type I fibres than other components of the quadriceps, potentially making it the most vulnerable to immobilization-induced atrophy (Appell 1990). Furthermore, Appell (1990) suggested that muscles that function as antigravity muscles, cross a single joint and contain a relatively large proportion of slow fibres are most vulnerable to atrophy due to immobilization. This may well be similar in the case of reflex inhibition, and may help to explain the finding of rapid atrophy of the multifidus, which has similar muscular characteristics.

Dysfunction of the multifidus has also been found to particularly involve the deep ventromedial corner of the muscle. Interestingly, the known anatomical distribution of type I and type II fibres may provide an explanation for this finding. The numerical proportions of the fibre types are not constant throughout the cross-sectional area of the muscle, with type I fibres tending to predominate in a deeper plane, near to the trunk (Jennekens et al 1971, Johnson et al 1973, Pullen 1977). If these deep type I fibres are more susceptible to atrophy, this could explain the location of the changes found in the multifidus. Furthermore, type I muscle fibres are innervated by beta motoneurones (Landon 1982) which are frequently activated, and receive a more continuous impulse flow than the type II fibres, which receive stimulation in the form of bursts of impulses (Burke 1980, Burke & Edgerton 1975).

The greater susceptibility of slow fibres may relate to their dependence on tonic and ongoing neural input, and may also depend on their more rapid rates of turnover and thus a higher rate constant for protein degradation (Goldberg 1967).

Biochemical changes

At a biochemical level, Appell (1990) explained rapid muscle atrophy in terms of increased protein degradation, the autophagic response and decreased succinate dehydrogenase activity. Increased protein degradation results in a net loss of muscle protein during atrophy. Evidence of autophagic activity has been demonstrated in atrophic muscle. It was found that lysosomal enzymes may be important in the initiation of muscle atrophy. A decrease in succinate dehydrogenase activity occurs as a consequence of muscular disuse in animals (Booth 1978) and humans (Häggmark et al 1981). These changes further highlight the susceptibility of type I fibres, as they are dependent on oxidative metabolism.

In conclusion, rapid muscle atrophy is known to occur in cases of reflex inhibition. The mechanisms involved at a muscular level may be similar to those described for disuse atrophy, which also leads to rapid muscle atrophy. Disuse atrophy presents a similar pattern of muscle dysfunction as demonstrated in the multifidus, with type I muscle fibres being predominantly affected, parts of muscles more affected than others and deep portions of the muscle specifically affected.

THE DEVELOPMENT OF CHRONIC MUSCULOSKELETAL PAIN

While the study of reflex and pain inhibition does give some insight into what needs to be achieved in rehabilitation, it is also the relationship between inhibition and the eventual development of chronic musculoskeletal pain that is of some additional practical value to the clinician.

The muscle system has been considered previously with respect to control of joints and a role in preventing re-injury. Stokes and Young (1984a, 1984b) presented a 'vicious circle' model of arthrogenous muscle weakness which was based on the knee model. 'Arthrogenous muscle weakness' was defined as weakness of muscles acting about an injured or inflamed joint. It is very apparent that there is a strong link between injury, pain, muscle inhibition and disuse and that inhibition and disuse must be specifically reversed by exercise and activity.

It was considered in this model (that refers to quadriceps inhibition and knee injury) that joint damage leads to reflex inhibition and muscle weakness and wasting, which in turn leaves the joint unprotected and vulnerable to further joint damage, which in turn leads to further reflex inhibition and the cycle is perpetuated. The cycle of increasing pain can be broken by activation and exercise of the affected muscles, in this case the quadriceps. In addition, many interventions which help to relieve pain, i.e. manual therapy and electrotherapy, should be used in conjunction with exercise to promote healing and to modulate pain.

Imaging studies have shown evidence of fatty infiltration of the muscles of the erector spinae group including multifidus, in older patients with chronic LBP (Hultman et al 1993). These fatty changes in the deep multifidus are commonly observed on the MRI images of chronic LBP patients (Vert Mooney, personal communication). Laasonen et al (1984) showed both unilateral and bilateral atrophy of the multifidus in postoperative patients. When atrophy was partial, it always included the medial multifidus. Unilateral atrophy on the affected side ranged from 10–30% of the unaffected side, and fatty degeneration of the muscles was evident.

Replacement of contractile tissue by scar tissue can also occur after spinal surgery. In these situations where non-contractile tissue replaces some of the contractile elements of the muscle, it will be more difficult to activate the muscle and restore its normal function. For these reasons, it would be more challenging for the therapist to break the vicious circle of arthrogenous muscle weakness.

Our research on the multifidus has been conducted using real-time ultrasound imaging (Hides et al 1995a). Hides et al (1994) found that the lumbar multifidus muscle is impaired in the acute LBP patient. Following pain or injury, our research has shown rapid pathological changes and decrease of muscle size at the painful segmental level, which is likely to be due to reflex inhibition (Hides et al 1996). Pain resolved in 90% of the patients within 4 weeks, but multifidus muscle size did not return to normal spontaneously. Furthermore, this decrease in multifidus muscle size did not return to normal spontaneously. Furthermore, this decrease in multifidus muscle size did not resolve with 6 weeks of normal pain-free work, sport and leisure activities.

From the model above, it could be hypothesized that persistent muscle weakness (or loss of control of the segmental multifidus) could leave the patient vulnerable to re-injury and recurrent episodes of pain. A long-term follow-up of these patients was conducted to evaluate this hypothesis (Hides et al 2001). The results demonstrated high recurrence rates at 3 years following the initial episode. These results could be extrapolated to patients with persistent chronic LBP of mechanical origin, where the muscles are unable to return to normal and require exercise techniques to reverse and correct this situation.

THE SPECIFIC STABILIZATION EXERCISE APPROACH

While it cannot be disputed that general strength and endurance work is necessary for deconditioned and atrophied muscles of patients with an overall lack of strength and endurance, more specific training of the deep muscles of the local system in their stabilizing role is not included in the more traditional exercises approaches. This chapter describes a new approach to exercise, specific stabilization training, specially designed to take into account the dysfunction of individual muscles or parts of a muscle. This type of exercise is directed to re-activating inhibited muscles and necessarily occurs early in rehabilitation, prior to proceeding to traditional strength and endurance programmes.

Principles for rehabilitation are, to a large extent, based on reflex inhibition investigations and the related specific and localized muscle dysfunction. The principles for the specific stabilization exercises are summarized in Box 13.2 and include:

1. Excite the motor neurone pool at a local level (including the use of facilitation and feedback techniques)
2. Commence rehabilitation early following injury
3. Regular performance of the exercise
4. Decrease stress on joint structures and avoid pain
5. Include some features of general stability programmes (e.g. muscle co-contraction).

Low-load isometric exercise techniques of a continuous or semicontinuous nature, based on these principles of rehabilitation, are also known as 'segmental stabilization training' (Richardson et al 1999) in the case of rehabilitation of spinal muscle dysfunction. This type of training, based on reversing reflex inhibition, has been shown in clinical research trials to be effective in the treatment of both acute (Hides et al 1996, 2001) and chronic (O'Sullivan et al 1997) LBP.

For the rehabilitation of patellofemoral pain, the isometric techniques are those based on the research and clinical innovations of McConnell (1993). More recently these techniques have been detailed by McConnell and Fulkerson (1996). These two treatment methods, concerning the specific rehabilitation of the stabilizing musculature of the spine and the patellofemoral joint, have been more rigorously studied than the stabilizing muscles of other joints but the same principles can be applied in other body regions. For example, re-education of the rotator cuff (especially subscapularis) is important for the rehabilitation of shoulder impingement syndrome and gluteus medius (especially gluteus medius posterior) is essential for the rehabilitation of painful hip conditions which are related to inadequate stabilization of the femoral head (e.g. osteoarthritis).

Principles for rehabilitation

The exercise technique involves teaching the patient to perform voluntary (cognitive) isometric contractions of the specific stabilizing muscle. This is best performed in a neutral joint position. As this type of isometric contraction is not familiar to the patient, it does require some form of facilitation to achieve such a contraction, e.g. deep manual pressure in the case of multifidus, taping the patella in the case of vastus medialis oblique (to lengthen the soft tissues attached to the lateral side of the patella), to assist contraction of vastus medialis oblique.

Excite the motor neuron pool

The spinal cord is an integrative site for sensory and motor functions. It shows plasticity during inflammatory and other types of lesions. This leads to modification of spinal processing of afferent input and thus to changes in spinal cord output (see Chapter 3). The functional status of the spinal cord is dependent on afferent, spinal and supraspinal influences. This means that the spinal cord actively contributes to nociceptive processing and that it changes as a consequence of nociceptive (Schaible & Grubb 1993).

Retraining must therefore focus on exciting the inhibited motor neuronal pool. Stener and Petersen (1962) stated that retraining was very important after injury, as the muscles that are inhibited will not be retrained automatically. Various strategies exist to enhance muscle retraining. The possibilities are to actively decrease inhibition and/or facilitate the inhibited muscles. Decreasing muscle inhibition involves decreasing stress on joints (this may include decreasing oedema) and avoidance of pain. Facilitation will be more successful if factors actively causing or perpetuating reflex inhibition can be minimized. Facilitation may actually work in two ways in the case of inhibition; it is known that sensory stimuli can block other afferent sensory stimuli in the spinal cord (Wolf 1978) and cutaneous sensory nerve stimulation can also increase motor neuron excitability in humans. Facilitation techniques may reduce inhibition of motor neurons by either preventing activation of inhibitory synapses (disinhibition) or by increasing the excitability of anterior horn cells (Stokes & Young 1984a).

Techniques of facilitation have been described in the propriceptive neuromuscular facilitation literature (Knott & Voss 1968). Techniques include manual contact, verbal commands, stretch facilitation, traction and approximation and resistance. Manual contacts use pressure as a facilitating mechanism. Manual feedback, via gentle pressure on the muscle, is very effective in facilitation of the multifidus. Communication with the patient may include manual contact, use of visual cues and verbal cues, and timing of verbal commands. Preparatory commands can be made more meaningful by demonstration of the desired movement and by providing a visual cue. A photograph of the muscle and its location is useful. Patient motivation may be positively influenced by verbal cues.

Muscle stretch may be used to facilitate muscle contraction due to the physiology of the stretch reflex. The stretch reflex can be used to initiate voluntary motion, as well as to increase strength and enhance the response in weak muscles. Vibration may also be used to stimulate muscle via the stretch reflex. Traction (separation of joint surfaces) and approximation (compressing the joint surfaces) affect the joint receptors, which are receptive to alterations in joint position and intra-articular pressure. Traction and approximation are used to stimulate the proprioceptive centres supplying the joint structures themselves.

EMG biofeedback has been used successfully to retrain inhibited quadriceps muscles (Krebs 1981, LeVeau & Rogers 1980, Wise et al 1984). Biofeedback techniques provide auditory and visual feedback, which are important for re-education of muscle function, especially in the cognitive phase of motor relearning (Martenuik 1979). In isometric strengthening programs, the addition of EMG biofeedback has been shown to lead to greater strength gains than isometric exercise alone (Lucca & Recchuiti 1983). Increases in quadriceps strength, associated with biofeedback, could be the result of both motor unit firing rate and recruitment patterns (Asfour et al 1990).

While EMG biofeedback is useful to help activate the superficial vastus medialis oblique muscle (McConnell & Fulkerson 1996), this technique is not useful to activate a muscle such as multifidus, which lies deep, close to the underlying joints. Real-time ultrasound has recently been introduced as a biofeedback modality (Hides et al 1995b, 1998, Stokes et al 1997) and has proved to be a potent addition to assist in the efficiency and effectiveness of the specific segmental training of multifidus (Fig. 13.5).

Early commencement of rehabilitation

In the case of inhibited muscles, the exercise programme should be instituted early after injury, and the frequency, intensity and duration tailored to the individual (Morrissey 1989). The programme should be of an intensity, frequency and duration that results in a training effect but does not result in increased inflammation (and increased muscle inhibition) of the injured joint. It is important to commence rehabilitation of inhibited muscles early following injury, as the effects of reflex inhibition are so rapid.

Severe muscle inhibition, demonstrated by a decrease in the maximal voluntary activation of the

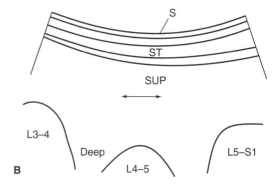

Figure 13.5 (A) Ultrasound image of the multifidus in longitudinal section. (B) Superiorly are the skin (S) and subcutaneous tissue (ST). The multifidus fibres run in the direction of the arrow (↔). Inferiorly are the zygapophyseal joints L3-L4, L4-L5 and L5-S1. The deep fibres of the multifidus are seen surrounding the zygapophyseal joints. Deep, deep multifidus fibres; SUP, superficial. (with kind permission from Richardson et al 1999 pp 137)

quadriceps of 50–70%, has been demonstrated within hours in humans undergoing open meniscectomy (Stokes & Young 1984a). Furthermore, the magnitude and duration of reflex inhibition following injury is unexpectedly high. In the study of Stokes and Young (1984a), quadriceps inhibition became more pronounced over the first 24 hours (80%) and by 3–4 days post-operation was still very severe (70–80%). Even 10–15 days postoperatively there was still 35–40% inhibition. This occurred despite the fact that patients were discharged from hospital, were experiencing minimal or no pain and were fully weight-bearing. Other quadriceps muscle EMG studies have supported the findings of Stokes and Young (1984a) with regard to the persistence of reflex inhibition. Krebs et al (1983) found decreased quadriceps activity 3 or more weeks post-meniscectomy, and Santavirta (1979) found EMG changes up to at least 12 weeks after surgery. The fact that reflex inhibition lasts for such a long period of time following injury supports the concept that facilitation of the motor neuronal pool should be commenced as early as possible in an attempt to curtail these prolonged effects.

Other evidence comes from biopsy studies. Biopsy analysis has been used in an attempt to determine the relative effects of reflex inhibition on different muscle fibre types. Häggmark et al (1981) showed that type I atrophy occurred very rapidly (within the first week) following knee joint injury. In a cross-country skier who was treated operatively, a drop from 81% to 57% in slow twitch fibres was noted. The patient was given very early active rehabilitation, and after some months returned to his pre-injury fibre distribution. It was concluded that very early onset of rehabilitation following injury is important for the restoration of type I fibre function. Because it has been shown that the multifidus muscle contains a higher proportion of type I fibres than type II fibres, early commencement of rehabilitation to maintain type I fibres would seem appropriate, considering that dysfunction of type I fibres has been seen in LBP patients.

Regular performance of rehabilitation

It can be argued, from the nature of reflex inhibition, that the rehabilitation exercises chosen would need to be repeated regularly and often. The long duration and large magnitude of the reflex inhibition response in itself suggests that rehabilitation exercises must be performed very regularly to affect this phenomenon. As the goal of treatment is to increase the excitability of anterior horn cells, while the injury is still acute, it can be argued that bombardment of the inhibited motor neuronal pool, through regular performance of exercises, would be necessary to promote over-riding of the inhibitory sensory stimuli.

The greater sensitivity of type I muscle fibres to disuse, pain and reflex inhibition compared to type II fibres also has implications for the frequency of rehabilitation required. It has been demonstrated that the type I fibres (which are connected to low-threshold motor neurons) receive a more continuous impulse flow from the motor neurons in the spinal cord than type II fibres, which receive stimulation in the form of bursts of impulses (Burke & Edgerton 1975). Häggmark and Eriksson (1979) proposed that occasional exercise sessions would maintain type II fibres, but that type I fibres require a more constant nervous-system activation. A more constant nervous-system activation would require frequent and regular rehabilitation sessions with a strong emphasis on increased holding time in order to restore the oxidative potential of the type I fibres.

Decrease stress on joint structures

The importance of decreasing stress on joint structures for rehabilitation relates to preventing or minimizing the effects of reflex inhibition. A considerable amount of information pertaining to this area has been derived from both animal and human studies of inflammation and joint distension (effusion).

Models of experimentally induced joint inflammation have been used to investigate the position in which animals hold their injured limbs. This position has been described as a semiflexed or 'resting position'. Induction of joint inflammation by chemical stimulants which activate joint afferents is known to alter the pattern of neuronal function in the spinal cord (Ferrell et al 1988, He et al 1988, Woolf & Wall 1986). He et al (1988) showed that inflammation of the cat knee produced significant and often large increases in the response of flexor motor neurons to local pressure and movement of the leg. However, some flexor motor neurons were inhibited by the inflammation. The inhibitory reflex response modified the stereotypical flexion response, to allow the joint to be kept at a midrange position, or 'resting position'. This position is one where afferent feedback from the joint receptors is at a minimum.

These findings have important clinical implications for the treatment of inflamed joints. If the aim of the treatment is to facilitate muscle activity, this should be performed with the joint in a midrange position where the nociceptive joint afferents are least activated (Schaible & Grubb 1993).

The potent effect of reflex inhibition on muscles has also been clearly displayed in studies that have involved joint effusion. These studies have been conducted on both animal and human subjects, and the effects of both experimentally and non-experimentally induced effusions have been investigated.

In human subjects, knee joint effusion is known to produce quadriceps inhibition (DeAndrade et al 1965, Jayson & Dixon 1970, Kennedy et al 1982, Spencer et al 1984, Stratford 1981). One classic study that investigated this phenomenon was performed by Jayson and Dixon (1970). The effects of human knee joint effusion and increased articular pressure were investigated in normal subjects and patients with rheumatoid arthritis. The position in which the intra-articular pressure and the quadriceps inhibition was least was in 30° of knee flexion. The proposed mechanism of the reflex was that joint distension stimulated the type I corpuscles and produced afferent impulses leading to quadriceps inhibition (Jayson & Dixon 1970). Joint distension will also stimulate type IV afferents.

Similar findings with respect to joint position were found when EMG was used to assess the electrical activity of the quadriceps, in a group of patients with painless acute knee effusions (Stratford 1981). Decreased activation was demonstrated at full knee extension but not at 30° flexion. This difference was also attributed to the decreased intra-articular pressure (and therefore decreased inhibition) at 30° of flexion.

Further evidence of the importance of joint position in effused joints has been provided by animal studies. When cat knee joints were inflated, changes in discharge patterns were observed. The lowest discharge rates were observed when the joint was in midposition. Synovial pressure was normally lowest when joints were positioned in a resting position, but rose and often became positive during knee flexion (Ferrell et al 1986).

In summary, evidence of the importance of a neutral or midrange position has been provided through investigations of inflamed and effused joints. To minimize the effects of inhibition, the joint should be positioned in a neutral position (Krebs et al 1983). This is especially relevant in the acute pain situation, where both inflammation and effusion may be present. Effused and inflamed joints should be exercised only within a range of motion that does not stimulate afferent inhibitory impulses (DeAndrade et al 1965).

Exercise under painless conditions

Various investigators have studied the relationship between pain and muscle inhibition (Arvidsson & Eriksson 1986, Arvidsson et al 1986, Mariani & Caruso 1979, Stener & Petersen 1962, Stokes & Young 1984a, Wild et al 1982, Young et al 1983).

In an attempt to clarify the relationship between pain and muscle inhibition. Arvidsson et al (1986) recorded integrated EMG (IEMG), during maximal voluntary contraction of the quadriceps muscle in 10 patients on day 1 post-operation (anterior cruciate ligament repair). Recordings were taken before and after epidural injection of 20 ml of 0.25% lignocaine with adrenalin 2.5 ug ml^{-1}. As pain subsided, the IEMG increased by a mean of 27–28% in the 20–25 minutes following injection. The authors therefore concluded that the quadriceps inhibition was due to pain inhibition of normal muscle activation. Available evidence therefore suggests that it is important to decrease or minimize pain to minimize muscle inhibition.

With respect to pain inhibition and its possible effects on fibre type, Gydikov (1976) demonstrated that painful stimulation of the sural nerve caused selective inhibition of type I muscle fibres, whereas 'tactile' stimulation caused facilitation. If pain directly affects type I fibres, this must also direct the rehabilitation program towards specific exercises that stimulate these fibres. This relates to the frequency of exercise, the amount of load applied during exercise and the type of contraction. It has been proposed that isometric exercises are more appropriate, especially when pain is an inhibitory factor, as isometric exercises involve less joint movement and therefore, in general, less pain production (Bower 1986).

Segmental stabilization training (Richardson et al 1999) and the segmental alignment rehabilitation approach of McConnell (McConnell & Fulkerson 1996), which focuses on the retraining of vastus medialis oblique, are based on low-load isometric exercise in the early stages of rehabilitation.

Use of low-load exercise

One of the strongest arguments for implementation of low-load exercises in the acute situation relates to the response of inhibited muscles to resistance. Resistance to muscle contraction is generally considered to be one of the most effective muscle facilitation techniques, as the number of activated motor units increases approximately in proportion to the magnitude of the resistance (Knott & Voss 1968). However, muscle activity can be inhibited by resistance to contraction in the pathological situation (Janda 1986). Janda (1986) proposed that increased loading in this case would cause a decrease of activity in the muscle being loaded. To continue the exercise against the applied resistance, the inhibited muscle will be eliminated from the movement pattern and replaced by non-inhibited and sufficiently strong muscles.

In the case of the multifidus, possibilities include other muscles of the general extensor group, the lumbar and thoracic components of the erector spinae muscles. Repetition of exercises in this case could further intensify muscle inhibition, and under these circumstances, exercise against resistance may harm the patient.

Similar patterns can be seen at the knee joint, where there may be an increased activation of rectus femoris at the expense of the vasti. This situation may even occur during high-resistance quadriceps exercises, in the non-pathological situation. For example, exercise in sitting and completing knee extension with resistance produces high quadriceps motor unit activity, especially in inner range (Duarte Cintra & Furlani 1981). It is of interest that Andres (1979) found that as the load was increased during the knee extension exercise (i.e. from 50–100% maximum), rectus femoris increased its level of activity in comparison with the vasti. This dominance of rectus femoris activity during high-resistance exercise could produce further problems for the patient with patellofemoral pain.

Further evidence for low-load exercise relates to fibre type. To stimulate type I fibres, which are affected by reflex inhibition, requires low-intensity holding contractions suitable for type I oxidative fibres (Richardson & Jull 1994). It has been shown that repeated isometric training increased the oxidative potential of the quadriceps muscle (Grimby et al 1973), suggesting that frequent low-load exercises of this type may be of benefit in rehabilitation of patients with inhibition.

Precise control of the neutral joint position

Exercise which incorporates re-education of the precise control of the neutral joint position should be included in the specific stabilization exercise programme. The reasons for this have been earlier explained and relate to decreasing stress on joints, especially the joints of the spine. One of the mechanisms which allows control of stresses applied to the lumbar intervertebral segments is control of the lumbar lordosis in flexion and extension (Saal 1990). Furthermore, attainment of adequate musculoligamentous control of lumbar spine forces may also prevent further injury to damaged lumbar structures.

The control of the neutral joint position with an emphasis on rehabilitation of kinaesthetic awareness has always been an important part of general stabilization programmes. These exercise programmes have mainly evolved for the treatment of LBP. Proponents of stabilization training include Harvey and Tanner (1991), Irion (1992), Kennedy (1980), Leimohn (1990), Morgan (1988), Richardson et al (1992), Robison (1992), Saal (1990) and Saal and Saal (1989).

In these programmes it is considered that co-contraction muscle patterns should be used to stabilize the lumbar spine in its 'neutral spine' position. However, definitions of neutral spine position vary. One classic definition of neutral spine is, 'the position in which the overall stresses in the spinal column and the muscular effort to hold that posture are minimal' (Panjabi 1992 p 391). Although the muscles are described by Panjabi (1992) as being minimally active, Damiano (1993) considers that in this position, the muscles are in a state of maximal preparedness. This description would apply to the concepts of stabilization training, where patients are required to hold this position for progressively longer periods of time (Morgan 1988). Robison (1992) defines neutral spine position clinically as the position or range of motion where patients are pain-free. Robison (1992) calls this 'the functional range'.

Developing control of the functional range relates to the basic underlying goal of stabilization training, which is pain control via muscle control. Control of neutral spine is usually conducted in a position of low spinal load initially, e.g. supine crook-lying (Harvey & Tanner 1991). Progressions are then made to the quadruped position, sitting, standing and movements in different positions.

Training patients to be aware of positions such as neutral spine and functional range require development of kinaesthetic awareness (Morgan 1988, Robison 1992, Saal 1990). Yet, the measurement of proprioception of the low back is difficult. Recently, position–reposition tasks have been used for evaluating the position sense of the spine, and it has been shown that young healthy individuals are capable of repositioning the pelvis and back (absolute error of approximately 2°) during both standing and sitting (Brumagne et al 1999a, 1999b). Both exercise-induced fatigue and mechanical LBP have a deleterious effect on lumbosacral positioning accuracy (Brumagne et al 1999c, 2000). It is thought that the degraded position sense is due to altered multifidus muscle spindle afferent input and central processing of this sensory input, and that deficits in the spinal reflex system might also contribute.

This means that specific exercises to enhance lumbosacral proprioceptive acuity are important in the management of LBP and prevention of recurrences. To facilitate this, meticulous technique and precision of

---

Box 13.2 Summary of the features of specific stabilization training

1. Teach patient to perform a voluntary (cognitive) isometric contraction of the specific stabilizing muscle.
2. Low load exercise.
3. Emphasis on neutral joint position and improving kinaesthetic awareness.
4. Use a variety of feedback techniques to facilitate the inhibited muscle (EMG and real-time ultrasound).
5. Decrease inhibition on the muscle (decrease stress on joints, avoidance of pain, decrease joint effusion).
6. Early commencement of rehabilitation (immediately after injury if possible).
7. Repeat isometric stability exercises regularly and often.
8. Gradually increase holding time.

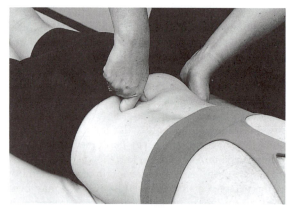

Figure 13.6 Therapist hand position to provide deep segmental pressure for multifidus facilitation (with kind permission from Richardson et al 1999 p 130).

performance is required (Morgan 1988, Robison 1992, Saal 1990). Achieving quality of movement and developing kinaesthetic awareness to control spinal posture automatically also requires exhaustive practice (Robison 1992). Careful repetition is required to allow engram motor programming to occur. Once this has occurred, the routine is patterned in the motor cortex (Saal 1990), and conscious effort is not required.

Specific stabilization programme for the multifidus for acute and chronic LBP

An optimal rehabilitation programme for the locally inhibited multifidus in LBP patients requires assimilation of the basic principles (summarized in Box 13.2) with clinically based techniques which are currently known to be effective.

The prone-lying or side-lying positions are suitable for commencement of exercises in acute LBP patients; as these are positions of low load on the spine, the spine can be placed in a neutral position and it allows access to the multifidus muscle. The type of contraction used should be a cognitive, slowly developing isometric contraction, which is localized and low-load. Deep manual pressure by the therapist is placed each side of the spine at the affected segmental level (Fig. 13.6). The usual instructions are to 'gently swell your muscles out against my fingers'.

It is important that no cheating or substitution occurs. This can be usually be detected by a lack of multifidus contraction, sometimes combined with lumbar flexion and posterior tilt or contraction of multifidus as a result of lumbar spine extension combined with anterior pelvic tilt.

The multifidus can be activated using techniques of facilitation, including instruction, demonstration, touch and pressure, in a co-contraction pattern with the deep abdominal muscles. Recent studies have also implicated transversus abdominis in the muscle dysfunction associated with chronic LBP (Hodges & Richardson 1996). The relationship between transversus and multifidus is important and is described in detail elsewhere (Richardson et al 1999). Based on this relationship with other supporting muscles, facilitation techniques for multifidus include contraction of transversus abdominis and/or the pelvic floor muscles.

Once activation has been achieved, patients should be encouraged to hold the specific multifidus contraction for longer periods of time, within pain limits, and repeat regularly.

Apart from progressing the multifidus programme in terms of holding capacity, another method of progression would be to change the exercise position. The basic principles described relating to position restrictions for acute LBP patients should still be maintained, i.e. the lumbar spine should be positioned in a neutral position, exercise should be isometric, low-load and painless. A suitable progression would be the standing position. This is a functional position, and one in which patients spend a considerable amount of time. The principle of increasing the muscle's holding capacity would also be followed in this position.

The patients should be given a formal home programme to ensure that multifidus exercises are performed frequently. The exercises should be performed as often as possible, as long as they are performed accurately and precisely with no signs of fatigue or substitution. In addition, this exercise programme should be structured into the patient's daily functional activities to improve compliance.

Real-time ultrasound imaging has been used to provide confirmation of multifidus activation (Hides et al 1995b, 1998). This technique can be used to ensure that the activation of the multifidus occurs at the affected vertebral segment. It provides a potent form of visual feedback to enhance local and specific multifidus re-education, which in turn helps to efficiently train the muscle for its functional role of joint stabilization and protection.

Hides et al (1996) have conducted a randomized clinical trial which supports the use of this approach. Two groups of acute LBP patients with a unilateral decrease in cross-sectional area of multifidus (at a segmental level) participated in the study. One group were trained in the specific exercise approach for multifidus while the other group acted as controls. Manual palpation as well as ultrasound biofeedback were used to facilitate the affected level of multifidus in the specific exercise group. In the control group, the decrease in multifidus muscle size did not resolve with 6 weeks of normal pain-free work, sport and leisure activities. For the specific exercise group, the cross-sectional area of multifidus had returned to normal within the 4-week exercise period.

A long-term follow-up was conducted to evaluate the recurrence rate in both the control and exercise group. The results demonstrated significantly higher recurrence rates at 3 years (following the initial episode) in the control group compared with the specific exercise group (Hides et al 2001). These results could be extrapolated to patients with persistent chronic LBP of mechanical origin who demonstrate decreases in the cross-sectional area of multifidus, where the muscles are unable to return to normal and require exercise techniques to reverse and correct this situation.

Specific stabilization programme for the vastus medialis oblique

An optimal rehabilitation programme for the locally inhibited vastus medialis oblique in knee problems requires adherence to the same basic principles (summarized in Box 13.2). Some innovative clinical techniques such as EMG biofeedback and taping have added to the effectiveness of the method. Details of the programme are described elsewhere (McConnell & Fulkerson 1996, McConnell 1986, 1993).

To rehabilitate vastus medialis oblique, the patient is usually in the walk/standing position with the affect-

ed knee in flexion (Fig. 13.7). The patient is asked to perform a cognitive, slowly developing isometric contraction, which is localized and low-load. EMG biofeedback, with electrodes placed directly on the oblique fibres of vastus medialis oblique, is an important tool to help develop an independent action of the muscle. Taping of the patella to ensure correct patella alignment is often used during the exercise. Once the contraction of vastus medialis oblique is achieved, the patient learns to hold the contraction during slow and controlled ranges of knee movement in this position.

Additional techniques of facilitation include using different types of instruction, demonstration, touch and pressure, and activating in co-activation patterns with the hip musculature. Hodges and Richardson (1993) found that the activation of vastus medialis oblique compared to the other quadriceps increased when a relatively low-level hip adduction contraction (15% of maximum voluntary contraction) was performed in a weight-bearing position. Based on this relationship with other supporting muscles, facilitation techniques for vastus medialis oblique include contraction of some hip muscles, e.g. adductor magnus and gluteus medius (McConnell & Fulkerson 1996).

Once activation has been achieved, patients should be encouraged to hold the specific vastus medialis oblique contraction for longer periods of time, within pain limits, and repeat regularly. Progression would be achieved through isometric holding contractions

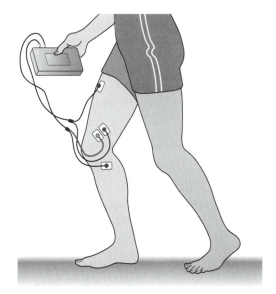

Figure 13.7 Patient developing an isometric contraction of vastus medialis oblique with the aid of EMG biofeedback and taping of the patella (with kind permission from McConnell & Fulkerson, 1996 p 718).

maintained during more functional joint movement tasks. An example of a useful exercise involving a functional activity is the controlled lowering of the body-weight down stairs.

A formal home programme is also required to ensure that exercises are performed frequently. The exercises should be performed as often as possible, as long as they are performed accurately and precisely with no signs of fatigue, substitution or loss of control of the more proximal joints (i.e. hip and trunk). The patient needs to learn how to recognize if these situations have occurred. Observation in mirrors, self-palpation of vastus medialis oblique and EMG biofeedback are all techniques which are suitable for home-use. While it would be hoped that the contraction of vastus medialis oblique would eventually become automatic, it is usually recommended that the patient remain on a maintenance programme.

CONCLUSION

For musculoskeletal pain associated with joints, our contention is that the physiological function of specific muscles closely associated with the stability of the joint are damaged from an original injury to the joints (or associated joint structures) and, without treatment, are unable to return to their normal function of stabilization and protection of that joint. If not treated, a cycle of recurrent pain and injury can result. It has been argued that specific activation of the inhibited muscles in their supportive role is required to alleviate the problem. For this reason, formal exercise pro-

grammes known as segmental stabilization training have become one of the main forms of conservative treatments used by physiotherapists to treat LBP.

The principles of this type of exercise treatment are also used in the treatment of other painful musculoskeletal conditions such as anterior knee pain, neck pain, osteoarthritis of the hip and shoulder impingement syndrome. This new approach to exercise will need to be compared to other methods of conservative care in future research studies, to ensure the most effective and efficient treatments are offered to the LBP patient and other patients suffering from painful musculoskeletal conditions.

Study questions/questions for revision

1. What are the physical changes found in the multifidus muscle of LBP patients?
2. What do you understand by the term 'reflex inhibition'?
3. Describe the vicious circle of arthrogenous muscle weakness which is proposed to occur as a result of knee injury.
4. Why should the rehabilitative exercise for the multifidus muscle be given at a low load i.e. without external resistance?
5. What is the significance of exercising in a neutral position of the spine?
6. Briefly describe the randomized clinical trial which demonstrated that segmental stabilization training was effective in decreasing recurrence rate after acute LBP.

REFERENCES

Amonoo-Kuofi H S 1983 The density of muscle spindles in the medial, intermediate and lateral columns of human intrinsic post-vertebral muscles. Journal of Anatomy 136: 509–519

Andres T L 1979 Involvement of selected quadricep muscles during a knee extension exercise. American Corrective Therapy Journal 33(4): 111–114

Appell H J 1986a Skeletal muscle atrophy during immobilisation. International Journal of Sports Medicine 7: 1–5

Appell H J 1986b Morphology of immobilised skeletal muscle and the effects of a pre- and post-immobilisation training program. International Journal of Sports Medicine 7: 6–12

Appell H J 1990 Muscular atrophy following immobilisation: A review. Sports Medicine 10(1): 42–57

Arvidsson I, Eriksson E 1986 Post-operative TENS pain relief after knee surgery: objective evaluation.

Orthopedics 9: 1346–1351

Arvidsson I, Eriksson E, Knutsson E, Arner S 1986 Reduction of pain inhibition in voluntary muscle activation by epidural analgesia. Orthopedics 9: 1415–1419

Asfour S S, Khalil T M, Waly S M, Goldberg M L, Rosomoff R S, Rosomoff H L 1990 Biofeedback in back muscle strengthening. Spine 15: 510–513

Aspden R M 1992 Review of the functional anatomy of the spinal ligaments and the lumbar erector spinae. Clinical Anatomy 5: 372–387

Baxendale R H, Ferrell W R, Wood L 1987 The effect of mechanical stimulation of knee joint afferents on quadriceps motor unit activity in the decerebrate cat. Brain Research 415: 353–356

Bergmark A 1989 Stability of the lumbar spine. Acta Orthopaedica Scandinavica 60: 1–54

Biedelmann H J, Shanks G L, Forrest W J, Inglis J 1991 Power spectral analyses of electromyographic activity.

Discriminators in the differential assessment of patients with chronic LBP. Spine 16: 1179–1185

Bogduk N, Twomey L T 1987 Clinical Anatomy of the Lumbar Spine. Churchill Livingstone, Melbourne

Booth F W 1978 Regrowth of atrophied skeletal muscle in adult rats after ending immobilisation. Journal of Applied Physiology 44: 225–230

Bower K D 1986 The role of exercises in low back pain. In: Greive G (ed) Modern Manual Therapy of the Vertebral Column. Churchill Livingstone, Edinburgh

Bradley K C 1974 The anatomy of backache. Australia and New Zealand Journal of Surgery 44: 227–232

Brumagne S, Lysens R, Spaepen A 1999a Lumbosacral repositioning accuracy in standing posture: A combined electrogoniometric and videographic evaluation. Clinical Biomechanics 14: 361–363

Brumagne S, Lysens R, Spaepen A 1999b Lumbo-pelvic position sense during pelvic tilting in men and women without low back pain: Test development and reliability assessment. Journal of Orthopedic and Sports Physical Therapy 29: 30–36

Brumagne S, Lysens R, Swinnen S 1999c Effect of exercise-induced fatigue on lumbopelvic position sense. Physical Therapy, submitted

Brumagne S, Cordo P, Lysens R, Verschueren S, Swinnen S 2000 The role of paraspinal muscle spindles in lumbo-pelvic position sense in individuals with and without low back pain. Spine 25: 989–994

Burke R E 1980 Motor units in mammalian muscle. In: Summer A J (ed) The Physiology of Peripheral Nerve Disease. W B Saunders, Philadelphia p 133

Burke R E, Edgerton V R 1975 Motor unit properties and selective involvement in movement. In: Exercise and Sports Science Reviews. Academic Press, New York, pp 31–81

Craig A D, Heppelmann B, Schaible H G 1988 The projection of the medial and posterior articular nerves of the cat's knee to the spinal cord. Journal of Comparative Neurology 276: 279–288

Cresswell A G, Grundstrom A, Thorstensson A 1992 Observations on intra-abdominal pressure and patterns of abdominal intra-muscular activity in man. Acta Physiologica Scandinavica 144: 409–418

Crisco J J, Panjabi M M 1991 The intersegmental and multisegmental muscles of the lumbar spine. A biomechanical model comparing lateral stabilising potential. Spine 16: 793–799

Cullen M J, Mastaglia F L 1982 Pathological reactions of skeletal muscle. In: Skeletal Muscle Pathology. Churchill Livingstone, Edinburgh, pp 88–139

Damiano D L 1993 Reviewing muscle co-contraction: Is it a developmental, pathological or motor control issue. Physical and Occupational Therapy in Paediatrics 12: 3–20

DeAndrade J R, Grant C, Dixon A J 1965 Joint distension and reflex muscle inhibition in the knee. Journal of Bone and Joint Surgery 47A: 313–322

Donisch E W, Basmajian J V 1972 Electromyography of deep back muscles in man. American Journal of Anatomy 133: 25–36

Duarte Cintra A I and Furlani J A 1981 Electromyographic study of quadriceps femoris in man. Journal of Electromyography and Clinical Neurophysiology 21: 539–554

Eccles R M, Lundberg A 1959a Synaptic actions in motoneurones by afferents, which may evoke the flexion reflex. Archives Italiennes de Biologie 97: 199–221

Eccles R M, Lundberg A 1959b Supraspinal control of interneurones mediating spinal reflexes. Journal of Physiology 147: 565–584

Ekholm J, Eklund G, Skoglund S 1960 On the reflex effects from the knee joint of the cat. Acta Physiologica Scandinavica 50: 167–174

Ferrell W R, Nade S, Newbold P J 1986 The interrelation of neural discharge, intra-articular pressure and joint angle in the knee of the dog. Journal of Neurophysiology 373: 353–365

Ferrell W R, Wood L, Baxendale R H 1988 The effect of acute joint inflammation on flexion reflex excitability in the decerebrate low spinal cat. Quarterly Journal of Experimental Neurophysiology 73: 95–102

Freeman M A R, Wyke B 1967 The innervation of the knee joint. An anatomical and histological study in the cat. Journal of Anatomy 101: 505–532

Gardner E 1950 Reflex muscular responses to stimulation of articular nerves in the cat. American Journal of Physiology 161: 133–141

Gardner E, Latimer F, Stilwell D 1949 Central connections for afferent fibres from the knee joint of the cat. American Journal of Physiology 159: 195–198

Gerber C, Hoppeler H, Claasen H, Robotti G, Zehndu R 1985 The lower extremity musculature in chronic symptomatic instability of the anterior cruciate ligament. Journal of Bone and Joint Surgery 67: 1034–1043

Goldberg A L 1967 Protein synthesis in tonic and phasic skeletal muscle. Nature 216: 1219–1220

Goldberg A L 1975 Mechanisms of growth and atrophy of skeletal muscle. In: Carcina R G, Institute of Muscular Biology (eds) Muscle Biopsy, Vol. 1. Marcel Dekker, New York, pp 89–115

Grigg P, Harrigan E P, Fogarty K E 1978 Segmental reflexes mediated by joint afferent neurons in cat knee. Journal of Neurophysiology 41(1): 9–14

Grimby G, Björntorp P, Fahlén M, Hoskins T, Höök O, Oxhöj H, Saltin B 1973 Metabolic effects of isometric training. Scandanavian Journal of Clinical and Laboratory Investigation 31: 301–305

Gydikov A A 1976 Pattern of discharge of different types of alpha motor units during voluntary and reflex activities under normal physiological conditions. In: Komi P V (ed) Biomechanics. University Park Press, Baltimore, pp 45–57

Haddad B 1953 Projection of afferent fibres from the knee joint to the cerebellum of the cat. American Journal of Physiology 172: 511–514

Häggmark T, Eriksson E 1979 Hypotrophy of the soleus muscle in man after achilles tendon rupture: Discussion of findings obtained by computed tomography and morphologic studies. American Journal of Sports Medicine 7: 121–126

Häggmark T, Jansson E, Eriksson E 1981 Fibre type area and metabolic potential of the thigh muscle in man after knee surgery and immobilisation. International Journal of Sports Medicine 2: 12–17

Halkjaer-Kristenen J, Ingemann-Hansen T, Saltin B 1980 Cross-sectional and fibre size changes in the quadriceps muscle of man with immobilisation and physical training. Muscle and Nerve 3: 275

Harrison P J, Jankowska E 1985 An intracellular study of descending and non-cutaneous afferent input to spinocervical tract neurones in the cat. Journal of Physiology 356: 245–261

Harvey J, Tanner S 1991 Low back pain in young athletes. A practical approach. Sports Medicine 12(6): 394–406

He X, Proske V, Schaible H G, Schmidt R F 1988 Acute inflammation of the knee joint in the cat alters responses of flexor motoneurones to leg movements. Journal of Neurophysiology 59(2): 326–340

Hides J A, Stokes M J, Saide M, Jull G A, Cooper D H 1994 Evidence of lumbar multifidus muscle wasting ipsilateral to symptoms in patients with acute/subacute low back pain. Spine 19(2): 165–172

Hides J A, Richardson C A, Jull G A 1995a Magnetic resonance imaging and ultrasonography of the lumbar multifidus muscle: Comparison of two different modalities. Spine 20: 54–58

Hides J A, Richardson C A, Jull G A, Davies S E 1995b Ultrasound imaging in rehabilitation. Australian Journal of Physiotherapy 41: 187–193

Hides J A, Richardson C A, Jull G A 1996 Multifidus muscle recovery is not automatic following resolution of acute first episode low back pain. Spine 21(23): 2763–2769

Hides J A, Richardson C A, Jull G A 1998 Use of real-time ultrasound imaging for feedback in rehabilitation. Manual Therapy 3(3): 125–131

Hides J A, Jull G A, Richardson C A 2001 Long-term effects of specific stabilizing exercises for first episode low back pain. Spine, in press

Hodges P W, Richardson C A 1993 An investigation into the effectiveness of hip adduction in the optimisation of the vastus medialis oblique contraction. Scandinavian Journal of Rehabilitation Medicine 25: 57–62

Hodges P W, Richardson C A 1996 Inefficient muscular stabilisation of the lumbar spine associated with low back pain: a motor control evaluation of transversus abdominis. Spine 21: 2640–2650

Hodges P W, Richardson C A 1997 Feedforward contraction of transversus abdominis is not influenced by the direction of arm movement. Experimental Brain Research 114: 362–370

Hongo T, Jankowska E, Lundberg A 1969 The rubrospinal tract II. Facilitation of interneuronal transmission in reflex paths to motoneurones. Experimental Brain Research 7: 365–391

Hultman G, Nordin M, Saraste H, Ohlsen H 1993 Body composition, endurance, strength, cross-sectional area and density of mm erector spinae in men with and without low back pain. Journal of Spinal Disorders 6(2): 114–123

Irion J M 1992 Use of the gym ball in rehabilitation of spinal dysfunction. Orthopaedic Physical Therapy Clinics of North America 1(2): 375–399

Janda V 1986 Muscle weakness and inhibition (pseudoparesis) in back pain syndromes. In: Grieve G (ed) Modern Manual Therapy of the Vertebral Column. Churchill Livingstone, Edinburgh

Jayson M, Dixon A 1970 Intra-articular pressure in rheumatoid arthritis of the knee. III Pressure changes during joint use. Annals of the Rheumatic Diseases 29: 401–408

Jennekens F G I 1982 Neurogenic disorders of muscle. In: Mastaglia F L, Walton J (eds) Skeletal Muscle Pathology. Churchill Livingstone, Edinburgh, pp 204–234

Jennekens F G I, Tomlinson B E, Walto J N 1971 The sizes of the two main histochemical fibre types in five limb muscles in man. An autopsy study. Journal of the Neurological Sciences 14: 245

Johansson H, Sjölander P, Sojka P 1991 Receptors in the knee joint ligaments and their role in the biomechanics of the joint. CRC Critical Reviews in Biomedical Engineering 18: 341–368

Johnson M A, Polgar J, Weightman D, Appleton D 1973 Data on the distribution of fibre types in thirty-six human muscles: an autopsy study. Journal of the Neurological Sciences 18: 111–129

Jorgensen K, Mag C, Nicholaisen T, Kato M 1993 Muscle fibre distribution, capillary density and enzymatic activities in the lumbar paravertebral muscles of young men. Significance for isometric endurance. Spine 18: 1439–1450

Kennedy B 1980 An Australian programme for measurement of back problems. Physiotherapy 66: 108–111

Kennedy J C, Alexander I J, Hayes K C 1982 Nerve supply to the knee and its functional significance. American Journal of Sports Medicine 10(6): 329–335

Knott M, Voss D E 1968 Proprioceptive Neuromuscular Facilitation, 2nd Edn. Harper and Row, New York

Krebs D E 1981 Clinical E M G biofeedback following menisectomy. Physical Therapy 61: 1017–1021

Krebs D E, Staples W H, Cuttita D, Zickel R E 1983 Knee joint angle: its relationship to quadriceps femoris in normal and post arthrotomy limbs. Archives of Physical Medicine and Rehabilitation 64: 441–447

Laasonen E M 1984 Atrophy of sacrospinal muscle groups in patients with chronic diffusely radiating lumbar back pain. Neuroradiology 26: 9–13

Landon D N 1982 Skeletal muscle – normal morphology, development and innervation. In: Mastaglia F L, Walton J (eds) Skeletal Muscle Pathology. Churchill Livingstone, New York, pp 1–88

Leimohn W 1990 Exercise and arthritis; Exercise and the back. Rheumatic Diseases Clinics of North America 16(4): 945–970

LeVeau B F, Rogers C 1980 Selective training of the vastus medialis muscle using EMG biofeedback. Physical Therapy 60: 1410–1415

Lewin T, Moffett B, Viidik A 1962 The morphology of the lumbar synovial joints. Acta Morphologica Neerlando Scandinavica 4: 299–319

Lieb F J, Perry J 1968 An anatomical and mechanical study using amputated limbs. Journal of Bone and Joint Surgery 50A: 1535–1548

Lieb F J, Perry J 1971 Quadriceps function. Journal of Bone and Joint Surgery 53A(4): 749–758

Lucca J A, Recchuiti S J 1983 Effect of electromyographic biofeedback on an isometric strengthening program. Physical Therapy 83: 200–203

Lundberg A, Malmgren K, Schomburg E D 1978 Role of joint afferents in motor control exemplified by effects on reflex pathways from lb afferents. Journal of Physiology 284: 327–343

Macintosh J E, Valencia F, Bogduk N, Munro R R 1986 The morphology of the human lumbar multifidus. Clinical Biomechanics 1: 196–204

Mariani P P, Caruso I 1979 An electromyographic investigation of subluxation of the patella. Journal of Bone and Joint Surgery 16B: 169–171

Martenuik R E 1979 Motor skill performance and learning: Considerations for rehabilitation. Physiotherapy Canada 31: 187–202

Max S R, Maier R F, Vogelsang L 1971 Lysosomes and disuse atrophy of skeletal muscle. Archives of Biochemistry and Biophysics 146: 227–232

McConnell J 1986 The management of chondromalacia patellae: A long term solution. Australian Journal of Physiotherapy 32(4): 215–223

McConnell J 1993 Promoting effective segmental alignment. In: Crosbie J, McConnell J (eds) Key Issues in Musculoskeletal Physiotherapy. Butterworths, London, pp 172–194

McConnell J, Fulkerson J 1996 The knee: patellofemoral and soft tissue injuries. In: Zachazewski J E, Magee D J, Quillen W S (eds) Athletic Injuries and Rehabilitation. W B Saunders and Co, Philadelphia, pp 693–728

Morgan D 1988 Concepts in functional training and postural stabilisation for the low back injured. Top Acute Care Trauma Rehabilitation 2(4): 8–17

Morrissey M C 1989 Reflex inhibition of thigh muscles in knee injury: Causes and treatment. Sports Medicine 7(4): 263–276

O'Sullivan P B, Twomey L T, Allison G T 1997 Evaluation of specific stabilizing exercise in the treatment of chronic low back pain with radiologic diagnosis of spondylolysis or spondylolisthesis. Spine 22: 2959–2967

Panjabi M 1992 The stabilising sysem of the spine. Part I. Function, dysfunction, adaptation and enhancement. Journal of Spinal Disorders 5: 383–389

Panjabi M, Abumi K, Duranceau J, Oxland T 1989 Spinal stability and intersegmental muscle forces. A biomechanical model. Spine 14: 194–200

Paris S V 1983 Anatomy as related to function and pain. Orthopaedic Clinics of North America 14: 475–489

Pauly J E 1966 An electromyographic analysis of certain movements and exercises: Some deep muscles of the back. Anatomical Record 155: 223–234

Pullen A H 1977 The distribution and relative sizes of three histochemical fibre types in the rat tibialis anterior muscle. Journal of Anatomy 123: 1

Rantanen J, Hurme M, Falck B, Alaranta H, Nykvist F, Lehto M, Einola S, Kalimo H 1993 The lumbar multifidus muscle five years after surgery for a lumbar intervertebral disc herniation. Spine 18: 568–574

Richardson C 1987a Atrophy of vastus medialis in patello-femoral pain syndrome. In: Proceedings Tenth International Congress World Confederation of Physical Therapy, Sydney, pp 400–403

Richardson C A 1987b Investigations into the optimal approach to exercise for the knee musculature. PhD Thesis, Department of Physiotherapy, The University of Queensland

Richardson C, Bullock M 1986 Changes in muscle activity during fast alternating flexion-extension movements of the knee. Scandinavian Journal of Rehabilitation Medicine 18(2): 51–58

Richardson C A, Jull G A 1994 Concepts of assessment and rehabilitation for active lumbar stability. In: Boyling and Palastanga N (eds) Grieve's Modern Manual Therapy, 2nd Edn. Churchill Livingstone, Edinburgh, pp 705–720

Richardson C A, Jull G A, Toppenberg R, Comerford M 1992 Techniques for active stabilisation for spinal protection: A pilot study. Australian Journal of Physiotherapy 38(2): 105–112

Richardson C, Jull G, Hodges P, Hides J 1999 Therapeutic Exercise for Spinal Segmental Stabilization in Low Back Pain – Scientific Basis and Clinical Approach. Churchill Livingstone, Edinburgh

Robison R 1992 The new back school prescription: Stabilisation training part 1. Occupational Medicine 7(1): 17–31

Roy S H, DeLuca C J, Snyder-Hackler L, Emley M S, Crenshaw R L, Lyons J P 1990 Fatigue, recovery and low back pain in vaisity rowers. Medicine and Science in Sports and Medicine 22: 463–469

Saal J A 1990 Dynamic muscular stabilization in the nonoperative treatment of lumbar syndromes. Orthopaedic Review 19(8): 691–700

Saal J A, Saal J S 1989 Nonoperative treatment of herniated lumbar intervertebral disc with radiculopathy. An outcome study. Spine 14: 431–437

Santavirta S 1979 Integrated electromyography of the vastus medialis muscle after meniscectomy. American Journal of Sports Medicine 7: 40–42

Schaible H G, Grubb B D 1993 Afferent and spinal mechanisms of joint pain. Pain 55: 5–54

Schwartz W N, Bird J W C 1977 Degradation of myofibrillar proteins by cathepsins B and D. Biochemical Journal 167: 811

Sirca A, Kostevc V 1985 The fibre type composition of thoracic and lumbar paravertebral muscles in man. Journal of Anatomy 141: 131–137

Spencer J D, Hayes K C, Alexander I J 1984 Knee joint effusion and quadriceps reflex inhibition in man. Archives of Physical Medicine and Rehabilitation 65: 171–177

Stener B 1969 Reflex inhibition of the quadriceps elicited from a subperiosteal tumour of the femur. Acta Orthopaedica Scandinavica 40: 86–91

Stener B, Petersen I 1962 Electromyographic investigation of reflex effects upon stretching the partially ruptured medical collateral ligament of the knee joint. Acta Chirurgica Scandinavica 124: 396–415

Stokes M, Young A 1984a The contribution of reflex inhibition to arthrogenous muscle weakness. Clinical Science 67: 7–14

Stokes M, Young A 1984b Investigations of quadriceps inhibition: Implications for clinical practice. Physiotherapy 70(11): 425–428

Stokes M, Hides J, Nassiri K 1997 Musculoskeletal ultrasound imaging: Diagnostic and treatment aid in rehabilitation. Physical Therapy Reviews 2: 73–92

Stratford P 1981 EMG of the quadriceps femoris muscles in subjects with normal knees and acutely effused knees. Physical Therapy 62: 279–283

Taylor P N, Ewins D J, Fox B, Grundy D, Swain I D 1993 Limb blood flow, cardiac output and quadriceps muscle bulk following spinal cord injury and the effect of training for the Odstock functional electrical stimulation standing system. Paraplegia 31: 303–310

Verbout A J, Wintzen A R, Linthorst P 1989 The distribution of slow and fast twitch fibres in the intrinsic back muscles. Clinical Anatomy 2: 120–121

Voight M, Wieder D 1991 Comparative reflex response times of the vastus medialis and the vastus lateralis in normal subjects and subjects with extensor mechanism dysfunction. American Journal of Sports Medicine 10: 131–137

Wild J J, Franklin T D, Woods G W 1982 Patellar pain and quadriceps rehabilitation: An EMG study. American Journal of Sports Medicine 10(1): 12–15

Wilke H J, Wolf S, Claes L E, Arand M, Wiesend A 1995 Stability increase of the lumbar spine with different muscles groups. A biomechanical in vitro study. Spine 20: 192–198

Wise H H, Fiebert I M, Kates J L 1984 EMG biofeedback as treatment for patellofemoral pain syndrome. Journal of Orthopaedic and Sports Physical Therapy 6: 95–103

Wolf S L 1978 Perspectives on central nervous system responsiveness to transcutaneous electrical nerve stimulation. Physical Therapy 58: 1443–1449

Wolf E, Magora A, Gonen B 1971 Disuse atrophy of the quadriceps muscle. Electromyography 11: 479–490

Woolf C J, Wall P D 1986 Relative effectiveness of C primary afferent fibres of different origins in evoking a prolonged facilitation of the flexor reflex in the rat. Journal of Neuroscience 6(5): 1433–1442

Wyke B D 1981 The neurology of joints: A review of general principles. Clinics of the Rheumatic Diseases 7: 223–239

Young A, Hughes I, Round J M, Edwards R H T 1982 The effect of knee injury on the number of muscle fibres in the human quadriceps femoris. Clinical Science 62: 227–234

Young A, Stokes M, Shakespeare D T, Sherman K P 1983 The effect of intra-articular bipuvicaine on quadriceps inhibition after menisectomy. Medicine and Science in Sports and Exercise 15: 154

14

Re-integration into work

*Libby Gibson   Shelley Allen
Jenny Strong*

OVERVIEW

Return to work is often a highly valued goal for the individual with chronic pain. However, work is often an area of functioning that is very difficult for the person with chronic pain (Strong 1996). Because chronic pain from work disability causes high personal and economic costs, many countries around the world support early intervention to return the injured worker to work.

Occupational therapists and physiotherapists play a major role in the work rehabilitation process. These professionals contribute to a multidisciplinary approach for the person with pain through assessments, interventions and case management of work rehabilitation programmes. With appropriate assessment and intervention, both with the individual and the workplace, it is possible for a person with chronic pain to return to productive employment (Johns & Bloswick 1994, Schmidt et al 1995).

This chapter provides an overview of the process of re-integrating the individual with pain into work. We outline the different work rehabilitation roles of the occupational therapist and physiotherapist. We explain the steps of a comprehensive evaluation of the worker with pain. Next, we provide an overview of the strategies that can be used to assist the individual with pain achieve the goal of return-to-work. Finally, we explore some of the issues that can influence the work rehabilitation process for the individual with pain.

Smith (1989) suggested that the overall goal of the work rehabilitation process is to rehabilitate the client to meet the job demands upon return to work. However, with the advent of early intervention, rehabilitation often occurs with the worker at the workplace. Such early intervention rehabilitation is called occupational rehabilitation. Box 14.1 gives definitions

> **Box 14.1** Key terms defined
>
> **Work rehabilitation** – This is the generic term for both occupational and vocational rehabilitation. It applies to rehabilitation of clients who have retained their employment, lost their employment, or never been employed due to impairment or disability. Interventions include medication, surgery, work conditioning, retraining, graded return to work, counselling and workplace modifications (Allen 1999).
>
> **Occupational rehabilitation** – This is a managed process involving early intervention with appropriate, adequate and timely services based on assessed needs, which is aimed at maintaining injured or ill employees in, or returning them to, suitable employment' (National Occupational Health
>
> & Safety Commission 1995 p 2). Occupational rehabilitation typically takes place at the workplace.
>
> **Vocational rehabilitation** – This is the comprehensive process of assessments and interventions designed to enable clients with a disability to obtain and retain alternative employment after loss of functional ability for their former work. Vocational rehabilitation commonly involves vocational assessment, counselling and training (Schmidt et al 1995). Characteristics of vocational rehabilitation include longer programmes, more professions involved and increased costs. It may result in a change in job title, duties and tasks for the worker.

of work rehabilitation, occupational rehabilitation and vocational rehabilitation to explain the differences between these terms.

A tabular representation of the relationship between occupational and vocational rehabilitation process is shown in Table 14.1. It includes the assessments and interventions to be provided by the occupational therapist and physiotherapist at each stage, and the most frequent site for each rehabilitation type.

Learning objectives

At the end of this chapter students will have an understanding of the following:

1. Some roles of the occupational therapist and physiotherapist in re-integration of the person with pain into work.
2. The work rehabilitation process for the person with pain.
3. The return-to-work evaluation process.
4. Some return-to-work strategies.
5. Some of the issues that can affect performance in return-to-work and maintenance of the worker role.

The trend to workplace-based rehabilitation

Some countries, such as Australia, have advocated workplace-based rehabilitation since the 1980s (Innes

Table 14.1 Stages of work rehabilitation, therapy services and sites (from Allen, unpublished work, 2000)

Injury or disability event	Occupational rehabilitation or workplace-disability management	Vocational rehabilitation
Self-treatment or attendance at acute medical treatment facility, first-aid station, or physiotherapy practice	1. Return to work (RTW) without time off • Functional capacity evaluation (FCE), job analysis and RTW interventions are not required • Occurs at workplace 2. RTW to same job or employer after time off work • May receive restorative rehabilitation • Work-site FCE, job analysis and graded RTW; job / work modifications may be required • Occurs concurrently at workplace and in community 3. RTW to same job or employer but unable to maintain employment • FCE, job analysis, RTW interventions may assist the person maintain employment • Occurs concurrently in workplace and in community • Referral for vocational rehabilitation is required	Unable to return to same employer or enter workforce due to pain • FCE, job analysis and RTW Interventions required • Community-based

1997a). This is reflected in Australian workers' compensation systems that advocate occupational rehabilitation as means of reducing the personal and financial cost of work injury (Innes 1997a). The importance of workplace-based interventions has been increasingly advocated in other countries, including the USA (Jundt & King 1999) and Canada (Shrey & Hursh 1999). The term 'workplace disability management' is often used, particularly in North America, to refer to return-to-work programmes for workers with disabilities (Shrey & Hursh 1999). Recognition of the importance of workplace-based services is reflected by the recently published results of a survey of occupational therapists involved in work programmes in the USA by Jundt & King (1999). This survey found that there is an emphasis on provision of services in the workplace with fewer programmes focusing only on the individual's condition.

An emphasis on workplace-based interventions has also been endorsed for the person with pain. Among the major recommendations of the Task Force on Pain in the Workplace by the International Association for the Study of Pain (Fordyce 1995) was the need for an emphasis on 'worksite-based interventions as a method for minimising and limiting disability' (p xiii). The report of the taskforce called for a proactive approach to workplace injury management, aimed at prevention of injuries in the first instance, and early intervention when injuries occur. As noted by Mital and Pennathur (1999), years of ergonomic interventions have not prevented workplace injuries. These authors reported that ergonomists concede that only two-thirds of workplace injuries can be prevented by improved design of jobs through ergonomic interventions. They presented an integrated model of injury management that incorporates ergonomics as a method of intervention within a comprehensive disability management programme.

One of the primary workplace-based approaches in reintegrating the person with pain into work is through a 'modified' or 'suitable duties programme'. There are many benefits for the worker with pain from such programmes. An important benefit is that it helps the worker to keep a link with the workplace and his or her role as a worker, thereby helping to mitigate the secondary physical and psychosocial problems that a long time off work can cause. There are also the physical benefits of keeping active and maintaining work-specific fitness. For the worker with more chronic pain who has been off work for an extended period, a valuable strategy for return to work is by a graded return-to-work programme that helps minimize the potential aggravation of his or her pain, and to build up work-specific fitness.

Modified return to work or suitable duties programmes may also be referred to as 'transitional work'. Shrey and Hursh (1999) defined transitional work as:

Any combination of tasks, functions, or jobs that a worker who has functional restrictions, can perform safely, for pay, and without the risk of injury to self or other workers (Shrey & Hursh 1999 p 58).

This definition highlights the value of return-to-work programmes in that they can allow a safe return to work based on an evaluation of the person's functional restrictions. This approach is preferable to the alternatives of either staying off work with long periods of inactivity or going back to work and risking aggravation or re-injury without any consideration of the specific needs of the individual, such as the nature of the injury, job demands and workplace organizational factors. As noted by Innes (1997a), providing suitable duties for a worker with an injury as part of a rehabilitation programme aims to 'enable a safe and speedy return to work' (p 18). The suitable duties 'should avoid risk of further injury' while allowing ongoing recovery (p 18).

Waddell (1998) noted that there is conflicting evidence about the effectiveness of recommending a return to modified work duties for the worker with back pain. However, he also noted that all the current guidelines for management of back pain recommend a return to work as soon as possible and that, 'all the evidence . . . shows that early return to work does not increase the chance of recurrence of back pain' (Waddell 1998 p 249).

In a review of the research on modified return-to-work programmes, Krause et al (1998) found overall support for their effectiveness. From their review of studies that met high standards for their soundness of methodology, these investigators found that workers with injuries who had access to programmes for modified return to work were twice as successful in return to work than workers who did not have access to such programmes. A study on the impact of vocational rehabilitation and working on a trial basis had a similar finding (Schmidt et al 1995). This study looked at the value of vocational rehabilitation for patients with a variety of conditions including back pain. It found that, 'the probability of obtaining work was 2 times higher for people who participated in vocational rehabilitation than for those who did not' (Schmidt et al 1995 p 953). Matheson et al (1995) and Matheson and Brophy (1997) reported success in a workplace-based early intervention programme providing modified duties to workers with work-related back injury. This study reported high return-to-work rates from a managed care approach that focused on early identification of injury and provision of short-term lighter work duties. We will discuss modified return-to-work or suitable duties programmes again in this chapter in the section on interventions for re-integration into work.

The trend to workplace-based rehabilitation has meant less emphasis is being placed on centre-based, tertiary multidisciplinary programmes, such as the functional restoration approach. This approach, described by Mayer and Gatchel (1988), is a multidisciplinary approach to rehabilitation for spinal disorders. The aim of functional restoration is to, 'focus on function in spite of disability and pain' (Bendix et al 1998 p 718) rather than diagnosis and elimination of pain. Mayer et al (1995) described how functional restoration programmes use principles of physical sports medicine, 'combined with psychologic and disability management education' (Mayer et al 1995 p 2061).

Some research has been reported that supports the effectiveness of this combination in improving functional capacity and return to work (Bendix et al 1998, Burke et al 1994, Haider et al 1998, Mayer et al 1998). Bendix et al (1998) reported reasonable results for a modified functional restoration programme with patients with chronic back pain. They described their 3-week programme which had three main components including:

1. Intensive physical training for 5 hours per day led by physical and occupational therapists.
2. Psychological pain management 2 hours per day, guided by clinical psychologists.
3. Education for 1 hour per day with topics by medical practitioners, therapists, psychologists, a social worker and a nutritionist.

As seen by this programme outline, such programmes are resource-intensive. Mayer et al (1995) explained that functional restoration programmes are high-intensity programmes for the 5–8% of individuals with chronic disability that require tertiary care. According to Mayer et al (1995), such high-intensity tertiary care programmes require medical direction and all the disciplines involved (medical, psychologic, vocational, physical and occupational therapy) to be located on-site. The more common scenario that is available to the person with pain, is secondary level care. Mayer et al (1995) described this care as involving, 'the skills of a qualified allied health practitioner (usually a physical or occupational therapist) providing cost-effective care by use of limited space and equipment, mainly with consultative medical, psychologic, and vocational adjuncts' (Mayer et al p 2065).

Feuerstein et al (1994) described a multidisciplinary approach to return to work for clients with occupational back pain that has a workplace emphasis. This approach includes medical, physical, psychoeducational/psychosocial, ergonomic and vocational components. Services in the physical component include provision of 'therapeutic exercise/physical conditioning, work conditioning/simulation and physical therapy modalities' (Feuerstein et al 1994 p 232). In the ergonomic component services include, 'worksite ergonomic job analysis' and 'redesign of work-station/work method to reduce risk' (p 232). Other components of this approach relevant to occupational therapists and physiotherapists are the psychoeducational/psychosocial components of pain management, back school and stress management. Some of these occupational therapy or physiotherapy services will be discussed later in this chapter in the section on interventions. Another multidisciplinary approach, work-hardening, will also be discussed later in the chapter.

This chapter will not deal with broader multidisciplinary approaches to work rehabilitation. Rather it will address the specific role of the occupational therapist and physiotherapist in the work rehabilitation process whether it is in a multidisciplinary centre or as a sole practitioner. The roles of the occupational therapist or physiotherapist in this process will not necessarily be delineated. Rather the services and strategies common to both disciplines will be described.

ROLES OF THE OCCUPATIONAL THERAPIST AND PHYSIOTHERAPIST

Occupational therapists and physiotherapists can play major roles at various stages of the work rehabilitation process for workers with pain. They can obviously be involved at the traditional intervention or treatment phase, aimed at facilitating recovery from the injury by treatment and injury management. These interventions are covered in other chapters in this book. The main role in work rehabilitation is in direct provision of services aimed at addressing any mismatch between the person's residual capacities and the demands of the job. This role is the primary focus of this chapter and will be reviewed in depth. Another increasingly important role is in coordination or management of the overall work rehabilitation process.

High levels of coordination and communication are required for return-to-work (RTW) programmes to succeed (Shrey & Hursh 1999). Coordination and communication are required both within the workplace and with external providers. The coordination role may be managed within the workplace by a rehabilitation coordinator (National Occupational Health & Safety Commission 1995) or disability management coordinator

(Shrey & Hursh 1999). Occupational therapists and physiotherapists often fill this role either within or external to the organization where the worker is employed.

The coordination role is often called case management or disability management. There is potential for confusion about these terms as case management is sometimes used as an umbrella term for early-intervention rehabilitation (for example Shrey & Hursh 1999), which in other systems is called occupational rehabilitation. Case-management services are being increasingly used in North America as a strategy to reduce occupational disability from low back pain (Frank et al 1996) and work injury in general (Jundt & King 1999). Management of RTW programmes is a major role for therapists working in work rehabilitation. In a survey of occupational therapy work programmes in the USA, 45% of participating occupational therapists reported that they offered case-management services (Jundt & King 1999).

An important part of managing the overall RTW process is developing the plan, in conjunction with the worker, employer, treating medical practitioner and other key parties. As a case manager, the occupational therapist or physiotherapist needs to be able to select and consult appropriate members of a multidisciplinary team, including the person's medical practitioners, in order to propose and then monitor and review the RTW programme. Referral may come from several sources. These include medical practitioners, insurers, employers, health and welfare professionals, solicitors/attorneys, the injured worker or client, or their family. Regardless of the referral source, the programme needs to be funded. It is in the interests of all stakeholders to resolve the issue of payment early and to have the client return to productive work as quickly and safely as possible.

In cases where the person with chronic pain cannot return to work, the occupational therapist and physiotherapist play an important role. The physiotherapist aims to help the person with chronic pain to optimize his or her physical activity level and pain management, while the occupational therapist aims to optimize the person's participation in other life roles. Other avenues for productive participation can be explored with the person, such as voluntary work or hobbies.

In all the above roles, knowledge in a number of important areas is required. These include the relevant legislation, such as workers' compensation and occupational health and safety legislation, the nature, prognosis and functional impact of the injury, risk management and ergonomic principles, measurement principles and programme evaluation (Gibson, unpublished work, 1999).

As mentioned previously, the emphasis in this chapter will be on the role of the occupational therapist or physiotherapist in the process of returning the person with pain to work using a RTW programme. The occupational therapist or physiotherapist can assist at various stages throughout the programme. They can initially be involved in assessing the individual needs of the person in relation to work. Later they can assist in the upgrading of duties or hours (if indicated). Later still, upon successful return to work, they can assist in the maintenance of work status.

THE WORK REHABILITATION PROCESS
Goal-setting

Any RTW programme must be based on an individualized assessment of the person's functional capacities, in conjunction with a through assessment of the demands of the job (Innes 1997a, Shrey & Hursh 1999). Such assessment is needed to determine the most appropriate RTW goal. The work rehabilitation process has a preferred hierarchy of goals for return to work (National Occupational Health & Safety Commission 1995). The hierarchy, outlined in Figure 14.1, encompasses all work rehabilitation types outlined in the definitions earlier in this chapter.

A framework for the process

A framework for the work rehabilitation process is presented in this chapter. In Figure 14.2 are the basic

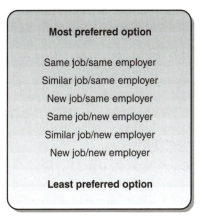

Most preferred option

Same job/same employer

Similar job/same employer

New job/same employer

Same job/new employer

Similar job/new employer

New job/new employer

Least preferred option

Figure 14.1 Hierarchy of preferred return-to-work outcomes. (Adapted from National Occupational Health & Safety Commission 1995.)

Assessment phase

1. Assess the demands of the job/workplace

↓

2. Assess the capacity of the worker with injury/disability

↓

Intervention phase

3. Improve the match between the demands of the job/workplace and the functional capacity of the worker

↓

4. Facilitate a return to work (or maximal independence in community if unable to return to work)

Figure 14.2 The work rehabilitation process.

steps of the occupational therapist or physiotherapist's involvement in the work rehabilitation process. The steps may not necessarily occur in the order in which they are presented in each phase. Steps 1 and 2 may in fact occur concurrently, especially if the person can be assessed on the job in the workplace. Steps 3 and 4 may also occur concurrently. Although the worker with pain needs to be medically stable enough to safely return to work, he or she may not necessarily be at 100% of his or her potential functional capacity before returning to some form of productive work duties.

The first two steps of the work rehabilitation process involve the assessment of the match between the demands of the person's job and his or her capacity to perform these demands. Innes (1997b) referred to the assessment of this match as identification of the 'person–activity–environment fit', that is the 'match and/or mismatch which exists between the person, the job performed and environment or context in which it is performed' (Innes 1997b p 227). We will now provide an overview of how to assess the workplace–worker match.

First, we will look at assessing the demands of the job, which is broadly called workplace assessment. The workplace includes both the job tasks and the environment in which they are undertaken. Next, we will look at how to assess the person with pain for return to work, broadly called work assessment. In practice, the order these steps in the assessment process occur can vary, depending on many factors such as the purpose of the referral and whether assessment at the workplace provides sufficient information to determine readiness for return to work.

If the person does not have an identified job to which to return, an assessment of work capacity will take precedence over the analysis of any potential job.

Evaluating the demands of the job and workplace

Where possible, the demands of the person's job should be assessed, or at least considered, before assessment of the person's capacities for return to work. Such assessment of the demands of the job allows criteria to be set against which the person's capacity can be measured (Gibson & Strong 1997). A workplace assessment involves assessment of the demands of the person's job and the workplace environment.

The job needs to examined and sub-divided into the major tasks. The tasks are then assessed for the demands they place on the person with pain. A detailed job analysis involving observation of the job is often required to establish the demands of the job that will be critical for return to work. Various formats, guidelines and tools are available to assist the job analysis process. In practice, the primary methods of job analysis for an individual client are interview and observation, using checklists. More specialized analysis can be conducted using more sophisticated methods if indicated. Texts such as Chaffin et al (1999) and Jacobs (1999) are valuable resources for occupational therapists and physiotherapists in the field of ergonomics.

There are many job demands that can impact on the person with pain for return to work. These include physical or sensorimotor, psychological, psychosocial, cognitive, perceptual and environmental demands (Jacobs 1999). For people with physical injury or disability, the physical and environmental demands of work need to be assessed routinely. For the person with pain, it is important to also assess the psychosocial demands of the work to determine the impact for the person. For example, work that requires high levels of contact with a demanding public may place additional demands on a person with pain. Alternatively, the contact with people may distract the person from focusing on pain.

Similarly, it may also be important to assess the cognitive demands of work. Chronic pain and medication may impact on cognitive capacities. The therapist needs to determine when the safety of the person, co-workers, plant and equipment are dependent on those cognitive capacities. The psychosocial and cognitive demands are not discussed in depth in this chapter. They are, however, acknowledged as important components of a job analysis and may be the critical factors in any reintegration into work.

Factors in the workplace that can contribute to musculoskeletal disorders are also the factors that are potentially aggravating for the worker with pain from such disorders. Factors such as handling of loads, static working positions and whole-body vibrations such as when driving, can all contribute to back injury (Department of Employment, Training and Industrial Relations (DETIR) 2000). Such factors can also be major aggravators of pain for a worker with back pain. The therapist needs to observe the tasks of the job to look out for any such factors. Rodgers (1984) provided a practical guide to potential aggravating factors in the workplace for workers with back pain and strategies to overcome them. Box 14.2 lists examples of these factors that are potential aggravators of back pain.

Factors that contribute to upper limb musculoskeletal disorders include the following:

- 'Repeated or sustained exertions, including gripping with or without high force
- Static postures involving the neck, shoulders and arms, such as while using tools or computers or when lifting or carrying loads
- Repeated use of vibrating tools and equipment, especially while working in cold conditions' (DETIR 2000 p 5).

Such factors are also potentially aggravating factors for the worker with upper limb pain.

Box 14.2 Low back pain aggravators (Rodgers 1984)

Standing postures
- Stooping
- Hyperextending back
- Extended forward reaches
- Crouching/awkward postures
- Constant standing

Sitting postures
- Lack of foot support
- Twisting of trunk
- Extended forward reaches
- Constant sitting, inadequate support

Manual handling
- Heavy lifting
- Twisting while lifting/pushing/pulling
- Uneven lifting/carrying
- Over-sized loads
- Sustained heavy handling/awkward postures

Each of the following elements of a job need to be considered in assessing the workplace for potentially aggravating factors for pain:

- Forceful exertions
- Working postures
- Repetition and duration
- Vibration
- Work area design
- Hand-tool use
- Load handling
- Individual factors
- Work organization
- Work environment.

These elements are based on the areas of risk in the Manual Tasks Advisory Standards 2000 (DETIR 2000). This wide range of factors may exacerbate pain for the worker after injury. However, occupational therapists and physiotherapists are often required to concentrate on assessment of the load-handling demands of the job and abilities of their clients with pain. The therapist needs to identify any combination of lifting, bending and twisting, as these combinations are likely to cause and exacerbate injury (Aja & Laflin 1999).

There are a number of guides available to assist the therapist to assess the demands of jobs that require lifting of loads (Aja & Laflin 1999). Well known guides are the 1981 and 1991 formulas or equations developed by the National Institute of Occupational Safety and Health (NIOSH) in the USA. The 1981 formula (NIOSH 1981) and the revised NIOSH formula (1991) provide a method for calculating the recommended weight for two-handed lifting tasks (Aja & Laflin 1999). Both equations are based on four aspects of lifting derived from the scientific literature and the judgement of experts. The aspects are:

- Biomechanical (specifically disc compression force)
- Physiological (specifically energy expended)
- Psychophysical (specifically maximum acceptable weight)
- Epidemiological (specifically population data about injuries by occupational tasks, body location and severity).

The NIOSH (1981) version identified several factors as influencing the loads that may be lifted safely. Factors included the weight of the load, the horizontal distance of the load, the vertical distance of travel, and the frequency of the lift. Two additional factors were included in the revised NIOSH (1991) version as impacting on a safe lift. They were the coupling between hands and the object, and the asymmetry of the lift. Aja and Laflin (1999) found the revised NIOSH (1991) lift formula more useful than the NIOSH (1981) version to therapists in industrial settings, but recommended that it be used in conjunction with therapist observation of postures and positions.

Other elements of the job and tasks within the job need to be considered. DETIR (2000) identified that the total time spent doing particular tasks, the tools and equipment used, organizational factors such as job rotation, timing of tasks, rest breaks and the use of personal protective equipment, may all contribute to or reduce the risk of injury.

When assessing the work demands the therapist needs to select equipment that will provide the best information for the client within time-limitations of an individual programme. In addition to the checklist referred to previously, therapists can use a range of recommended equipment to assist them to quantify and record the demands of the job. These include a stills camera or video camera, tape measure, scales, push/pull gauge, and stopwatch. Permission should be sought from the workplace before photographing employees and the workplace. Therapists need to ensure their own safety and demonstrate their awareness of the workplace through wearing appropriate personal protective equipment such as hard-hat and steel-toecap boots.

Assessment when there is no job to return to

It is often the case for the individual with chronic pain that they do not have a job to which they can return. The longer a person is off work, the less likely it is that they will return to work (Waddell 1998). This is why it is essential that efforts aimed at returning the worker with chronic pain to productive employment be commenced as soon as possible.

The process of exploring potential alternatives to employment and implementing strategies for this to happen is usually termed vocational rehabilitation (see definitions in Box 14.1). Occupational therapists and physiotherapists also play a vital role in this process. They are required to help establish the residual functional capacity of the person with chronic pain and assess the suitability of the alternative occupation or position. Vocational counselling may be needed to identify and locate work that is different to the person's pre-injury position or occupation and which is suitable for the person's condition (National Occupational Health & Safety Commission 1995).

Evaluating the capacity of the worker for work

Once the demands of the person's job or potential job are known, the person's capacity to meet these demands must be established. This process is broadly termed work assessment. Work assessment can occur by a number of methods. It can be workplace-based, where the person is observed performing the duties of the job. It can be centre-based, where the person performs a range of tasks that attempt to simulate the demands of the job or work in general. Sometimes, both approaches are needed to accurately establish the person's potential for return to work.

Work assessment, in the broadest use of the term, can evaluate a range of factors. In addition to assessment of physical and psychomotor capacities, Jacobs (1991) also noted that work assessment could include assessment of variables such as intellectual capacities, vocational interests and achievements, work skills and tolerances, work habits such as punctuality and job-seeking skills. The usual role for occupational therapists and physiotherapists in work assessment of the person with chronic pain is primarily to assess the person's physical capacities for return to work. The main means by which this is achieved in practice, apart from workplace-based assessment and self-report, is by use of functional capacity evaluation. Assessments of the non-physical components of a work assessment may be required but are not addressed in this chapter.

Functional capacity evaluation (FCE) evaluates the person's performance of the physical demands of the job, or when there is no job available to which the person can return, the person's performance of the physical demands of work in general. The trained therapist observes the person performing physical tasks, such as sitting, standing, lifting and carrying, and notes the person's abilities and limitations. The physical tasks observed in FCE are usually based on the physical demands defined in 'The Revised Handbook of Analyzing Jobs' (United States Department of Labor 1991b). This book is a companion publication of the 'Dictionary of Occupational Titles' (DOT) (United States Department of Labor 1991a). The DOT system is widely used to evaluate the match between the person's functional capacity and the physical demands of the job (King et al 1998, Lechner et al 1994, Randolph 1996, Spektor 1990, Wickstrom 1996). Table 14.2 lists the physical demands of work defined in 'The Revised Handbook of Analyzing Jobs' (United States Department of Labor 1991b) arranged to demonstrate potential areas of difficulty for the person with back pain, with the first column showing those items most

Table 14.2 The physical demands of the job for the person with pain (adapted from United States Department of Labor 1991b)

Strength demands	Other physical demands	Sensory and communication demands
Position: standing, walking, sitting Weight/force: lifting, carrying, pushing, pulling, Use of hand–arm and foot–leg controls	Climbing Balancing Stooping Kneeling Crouching Crawling Reaching Handling Fingering	Feeling Talking Hearing Tasting/smelling Vision: near acuity, far acuity, depth perception, accommodation, colour vision, field of vision

likely, and the third column those items least likely to pose barriers to work participation.

Before the FCE is undertaken, the therapist needs to determine which of the physical demands the person needs to be observed performing. The physical demands of the job that are evaluated can be dependent on the demands of the job or the diagnosis of the person being assessed. For example, crawling may not be one of the job demands of a warehouse attendant. For the worker with back pain, it is often unnecessary to observe the physical demand of fingering or fine manipulation.

When using the system of job analysis outlined by The Revised Handbook of Analyzing Jobs (United States Department of Labor 1991b), the occurrence, frequency and importance of these physical demands of a job are noted. This information is used to make a comparison of the requirements of the job with the capacities of the person to perform these requirements, as assessed in the FCE. Based on the person's performance of the demands in the FCE, the therapist extrapolates whether the person could perform these demands in the workplace at the frequency required by the job. The therapist also comments on any limitations in the performance and restrictions that may be required for safe performance of the demands in the workplace. It is important to note whether the demands of the job are critical to the performance of the job. For example, in some jobs lifting may constitute less than 15% of the job and be considered less critical than good teamwork and safe use of manual handling devices.

Based on the performance of the physical demands, the therapist may also extrapolate the physical level of

work the person can perform. This is especially relevant if the person has no job to which they can return and the FCE needs to determine the level of physical work the person can perform that would be suitable to their condition. Again, FCE systems borrow definitions from the DOT job analysis system in categorizing the different levels of work the person can perform. These levels include sedentary, light, medium, heavy and very heavy.

There are many different approaches to FCE, both commercial, standardized approaches and non-standardized. Research to date on these approaches has been limited. Innes and Straker (1999a, 1999b) provided reviews of the reliability and validity of the many different commercial approaches available. These reviews and the same authors' three-part series of a clinician's guide to work-related assessments (Innes & Straker 1998a, 1998b, 1998c) are valuable resources for occupational therapists and physiotherapists working in this area. Innes and Straker (1999a, 1999b) called for more research into the psychometric properties of these assessments, which has been commonly recognized as a major limitation.

As well as the limited research on FCE, particularly its reliability and validity, and the many competing commercial interests of the different approaches, FCE has other limitations. It can only give an indication of function on a particular day at a particular time (Vasudevan 1996). Furthermore, FCE is influenced by motivation, cognitive, behavioural and environmental factors (Rudy et al 1996, Vasudevan 1996), and it may not necessarily reflect actual job-specific demands (Sen et al 1991).

Despite these limitations, FCE has many benefits. According to Waddell (1998), one of the values of FCE is that it is a more objective measure of the person's functional capacity for return to work than only self-report from interview and questionnaires. Furthermore, Waddell noted, it is standardized and is 'much better than "clinical impression" ' (Waddell 1998 p 41). FCE can be of great value in ensuring a *safe* return to work program. It is also a valuable baseline, review and outcome performance measure. FCE can help to clarify any uncertainties about a person's capacities for return to work and can be of much assistance in determining the match between the demands of the job and the person's ability to perform these demands.

Another benefit of FCE is its focus on function. For the person with pain wanting to return to work, evaluation of impairment may provide a distorted understanding of functional abilities. The person's diagnosis may be a poor indication of their actual function

(World Health Organization 1998). Similarly, impairment is poorly correlated with function during work activities. Impairment refers to the loss or abnormality of body structure or of physiological or psychological function (WHO 1998). The therapist is most interested in function during the activities the person would normally perform at work, rather than the level of impairment. Impairment measures, such as range-of-motion or muscle-strength testing, will provide important information about the potential impact of the injury or condition on functional activities. However, they will not show what the therapist needs to know, that is, what the person with pain can or cannot do in the workplace. The therapist may need to evaluate the person's impairment level before an FCE as a means of screening for potential underlying problems, precautions or contraindications for testing. However, the focus should be on the functional performance of the physical demands of work and potential function for return to work.

The process of FCE usually involves several steps (Gibson, unpublished work, 1999), outlined in Box 14.3. We will now briefly explain each of the steps in this process.

Referral/collection of background information

Before the FCE is undertaken it is important to establish that the person is medically stable and physically ready to undergo the FCE. Apart from needing advice from the treating medical practitioner that the person's pain-related condition is stable, the therapist also needs to know that there are no other medical precautions or contraindications for testing that need to be considered, such as cardiovascular or pulmonary disease. Hart et al (1993) provided some guidelines for conducting FCE of people with medical conditions. Other important information to collect is:

- Medical history and treatments to date
- Information about the original injury

> **Box 14.3** The steps of the FCE process (Gibson, unpublished work, 1999)
>
> 1. Referral/collection of background information
> 2. Screening
> 3. Measurement of the person's perceived functional capacity
> 4. Observation of performance of the physical demands
> 5. Follow-up after the FCE
> 6. Interpretation and reporting of the results

- Compensation or litigation status
- Job or vocational situation
- Job description in cases where a job analysis has not been conducted
- Possible job options if no job is available
- Employment history
- Perceived capacity for activities of daily living (ADL)
- Leisure and community participation.

Screening

As mentioned previously, it is important to conduct a screening before observation of the physical demands, to check for any underlying impairments or precautions or contraindications. As well as confirming medical stability and the absence of contraindications, quantifying the level of impairment, such as range of motion, can be useful for comparison with the functional limitations found in the subsequent performance of physical demands (Hart et al 1993).

Screening can consist of measurement of any or all of the following, depending on the purpose of the FCE and the nature of the condition: resting heart rate and blood pressure, height, weight, range of motion, muscle strength, posture, gait and neurological status.

Measurement of perceived functional capacity

The extent of measurement of the person's perceived functional capacity also depends on the purpose of the evaluation and the nature of the person's condition. For the person with chronic pain, this can be an important component of the FCE process, as perceived capacity can be highly influential on performance of the physical demands and function, such as return to work (Gibson & Strong 1998).

Important aspects to assess by interview include the person's symptoms and signs, and their current participation in work, activities of daily living and leisure. If not already completed, the therapist needs to conduct some level of pain assessment as discussed in Chapter 7. This should include at least some measurement of the intensity, location and quality of the person's pain. Other variables worth including in a comprehensive FCE are the person's perceived capacity for performance of the physical demands, perceived disability, expectation of return to work and self-efficacy, especially for work. Strong (1996) and Gibson and Strong (1998) provide a review of these variables and corresponding tools that can be used by therapists to conduct comprehensive FCE and work assessment of individuals with chronic pain.

Observation of performance of the physical demands

Observation of the person's performance of the physical demands is the primary component of the FCE. Important aspects of this component in either standardized or non-standardized FCE's include:

- Which physical demands are observed and in what order
- How the physical demands are performed
- Equipment used to perform the demands
- Positioning of the person and the equipment to perform the demand
- Procedure used to perform the physical demand
- Instructions used with the person to evaluate the physical demand
- Technique the person uses to perform the physical demand
- Cues the therapist uses during the performance of the physical demands to facilitate the evaluation
- Method used by the therapist to determine the end-points of the person's performance of the physical demands (Gibson, unpublished work, 1999).

The method for determining the end-points of performance is usually referred to as the model of the evaluation. There are three main possible models to use in FCE. Gibson and Strong (1997) described these three models and 'how each model relates to how the individual works within the constraints of a particular body system' (p 4). The three models, as described by Matheson (1988), are:

- The biomechanical model, 'the ability of the individual to perform work with his/her musculoskeletal and neuromuscular systems'
- The physiological, cardiovascular or metabolic model, 'the ability of the individual to perform work with his/her cardiovascular, pulmonary and metabolic systems'
- The psychophysical model, 'the ability of the individual to perform work within his/her self-perception, beliefs and expectations' (Matheson 1988 p 3).

In the application of these models, there can be two extremes. At one extreme, the therapist determines the person's performance by only heeding observed signs of increased demands on the body. At the other extreme, the therapist is guided by feedback from the client, such as reports of pain.

Gibson and Strong (1997) supported use of the three models in combination. For the person with chronic pain, this requires a balance between acknowledgement and consideration of the person's reported pain, while maintaining an emphasis on function and observed indicators of performance. Rudy et al (1996) cautioned against regular rating of pain during FCE, as this may have a negative influence on the person's performance and focus the person on the pain. Other authors (Innes & Straker 1998c) have also supported the use of a combination of the three models as a means of considering all the realms of the person's performance during the FCE (Gibson & Strong 1997).

Follow-up 1–2 days after the FCE

An important, and sometimes neglected component of the FCE process, is follow-up of the client 1–2 days after the evaluation to determine the effects of the performance of the physical demands. The person with chronic pain may experience more difficulty in the days after the evaluation than during it. The therapist needs to ascertain the nature and severity of any symptoms and signs.

The person who has been physically inactive is likely to experience a level of delayed-onset muscle soreness that can be expected to subside. Any after-effects need to be taken into account in any decisions or recommendations made from the FCE. Such after-effects can provide an indication of the person's endurance for physical tasks, which the performance of the physical demands during a 2–3 hour assessment cannot necessarily provide.

Interpretation and reporting of the results

The last components of the FCE are interpretation and reporting of the results. There are many issues involved with interpretation of the results from FCE. It may be difficult to extrapolate the performance in the FCE to performance in the workplace, however, the performance in the FCE can provide an indication of many aspects of the person's functional capacity for work. The FCE provides specific indications of the person's abilities and limitations to perform the physical demands of work, and an understanding for the reasons for any limitations in performance. Biomechanical factors (e.g. limited strength or range of motion), physiological factors (e.g. reduced cardiovascular fitness), or psychophysical factors (e.g. symptomatic responses to activity or fear of pain or movement) may limit performance. Such reasons for limited performance can point the therapist to interventions that may improve performance and function in the workplace (Gibson, unpublished work, 1999).

In order to increase proficiency in extrapolating from the FCE data, the novice FCE practitioner can confer with and read reports of more experienced colleagues. The therapist can also follow an action learning cycle for each client. In an action learning cycle the therapist might follow the return-to-work outcomes for the client at 3-monthly intervals for a period of up to 1 year. During this time the therapist would make notes about the accuracy of his/her predictions, reflecting on and planning how to improve recommendations in the future. Such follow-up would only be done with the client's consent.

The FCE can also help make specific recommendations for any restrictions in performance of the physical demands of the job, such as no lifting of items at certain heights, or limiting the amount of low-level work. In this way, the FCE assists the process of planning a safe return to work with a minimized chance of aggravation of the person's pain. However, therapists must be cautious about not being over-restrictive in their recommendations for return to work. One study found that some work restrictions by therapists had no sound basis and that provision of restrictions for the return-to-work process were associated with less likelihood of a successful return to work than if no restrictions were recommended (Hall et al 1994). When the person has no job to which he or she can return, the FCE provides an indication of the level of work the person may be able to perform, thus assisting the vocational redirection process.

The written report of the results from an FCE will vary depending on the purpose of the evaluation and the type of approach used. However, there are elements that are common to many reports. Box 14.4 shows some of the topics that are covered in FCE reports in practice (Gibson & Strong 1997).

For the person who is changing employment, recommendations may include information about the person's work interests, values and expectations. Job satisfaction has been found to be not only related to the person's capacity to physically perform a different job with a different employer, but also to gaining employment consistent with the person's interests and values (Allen 1999).

After assessing the work demands and the person's capacity (Steps 1 and 2) the occupational therapist or physiotherapist needs to compare the results and identify the areas of mismatch. For example, a person may be required to lift 10 kg frequently during the working day, but only have demonstrated the capacity to lift up to 5 kg on an occasional basis during the FCE.

It is important to note not only the job demands that the person is unable to perform but also the person's capacities that exceed job demands, as these may have potential for future employment directions. The therapist then needs to decide which areas of mismatch are the most critical barriers to return to work. For example, the person may be able to return to work in an office if lifting can be avoided because another worker gives assistance with this minor component of the job. Box 14.5 lists some of the common problems for workers with pain identified during assessment.

We have looked at how to assess the match between the worker and the job. Now, we will look at strategies to improve any mismatch found by such an assessment.

IMPROVING MATCH BETWEEN DEMANDS OF JOB/WORKPLACE AND FUNCTIONAL CAPACITY OF WORKER

The therapist needs to determine whether any improvements made to the work tasks, the work

---

Box 14.4 Common topics in FCE reports (based on Gibson & Strong 1997 with kind permission)

- Purpose of the FCE
- Injury information
- Self-report of capacity
- Work history/job description
- Consistency of performance
- Pain behaviour
- Safety of body mechanics used
- Abilities, limitations and restrictions
- Recommended level of physical work
- Recommendations for return to work
- Recommendations for rehabilitation

Box 14.5 Common problems for worker with pain identified during assessment

- Reduced fitness
- Symptomatic responses to activity (pain)
- Fear of pain and/or fear of movement/re-injury
- Limited static positional tolerances (e.g. sitting, standing)
- Limited mobility (e.g. walking, crouching)
- Limited manual handling ability

environment or the worker's function, would decrease or eliminate the areas of mismatch to enable the person to return to work. The resources such as time, money and personnel required to make the changes may affect the options for interventions. There are a number of strategies available to the therapist that will improve the match between the demands of the workplace and the capacities of the worker with pain. Figure 14.3 provides a framework for the intervention phase. The work reintegration or rehabilitation plan may incorporate all three areas of intervention.

We will discuss some of the strategies aimed at improving either the ergonomics of the workplace or the worker's function, that is, the match between the work demands and the worker. Some of these strategies may be necessary before the person returns to work, or can occur in conjunction with a return-to-work programme either within or outside the workplace, or both. The strategies are discussed assuming that they are occurring within the context of a planned return-to-work programme, as discussed earlier in the chapter.

Maintaining our focus on the importance of the workplace, we will discuss strategies to improve the demands of the workplace first. Then we will outline some of the strategies that can be used to improve the function of the worker. We will then cover the important aspects of planning and monitoring return to work programmes. In practice, a combination of strategies is usually required to improve the match between the demands of the workplace and worker's capacities. Box 14.6 has a hierarchy of strategies for the occupational therapist or physiotherapist to use to consider the options for either improving the workplace or the worker's function or both.

Box 14.6 Hierarchy of strategies for improving the match between the demands of the job/workplace and the functional capacity of the worker with pain

1. Eliminate/avoid
   - unnecessary and/or aggravating tasks

2. Re-design
   - workstation
   - environment
   - tasks

3. Adapt by
   - improving general and work-specific fitness
   - using adaptive equipment
   - using modified or graded return to work

4. Train/educate
   - anatomy and physiology relating to injury and recovery
   - manual handling techniques
   - pain management

Improving the workplace

The therapist can use interventions in the workplace to reduce the potential aggravators in the job's tasks or the work environment. Apart from assisting the person with pain to return to work after injury or chronic pain, such reduction of aggravating factors will also increase the chances of the worker with pain being able to maintain his or her job. Rodgers (1984) provided suggestions for how job tasks and the work environment can be improved for a worker with back pain. These guidelines can also be applied to workers with pain from conditions other than back pain. Rodgers suggests the following areas that need to be considered to improve the work tasks or environment:

- Provide appropriate heights and distances of the location of tasks
- Provide adequate seating
- Improve the design of manual handling tasks
- Improve the size and design of objects to be handled
- Provide adequate recovery time for workers' muscles
- Improve work patterns to accommodate pacing.

The therapist needs to consider and apply basic ergonomic principles in modifying the work tasks and environment to improve the match between the worker's functional capacity and the demands of the job and to minimize the potential effects of any aggravating factors.

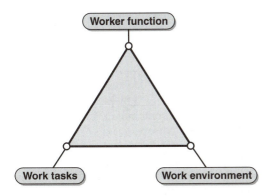

Figure 14.3 Framework of interventions for the person with pain.

One of the first considerations about any potentially aggravating factor in the workplace is whether it can be eliminated altogether by redesign or adaptive equipment, or at least be avoided by the worker with pain. Where this cannot occur, the next strategy is to minimize its effects. The worker with pain may still be able to perform the task through use of adaptive equipment. Provision of workplace aids and equipment will usually only be funded for workers receiving workers' compensation support if the aids and equipment are directly related to the specific functional limitations of the worker with pain (National Occupational Health & Safety Commission 1995). The aids and equipment must be essential for restoring or maintaining a person at work and cannot be provided only to improve the general ergonomics of a workplace.

Rodgers (1984) discussed a range of special workplace aids for people with low back pain to help avoid the common back-pain aggravators (Box 14.7).

Box 14.7 List of back pain aggravators and aids to mitigate their effects (based on Rodgers 1984)

- Stooping
  — adjustable-height table/bench
  — platforms
- Hyperextending back
  — step stools or platforms
- Extended forward reaches
  — tool or control extenders
  — reach extenders
- Twisting of trunk
  — roller conveyors
  — swivel chairs
- Constant standing
  — appropriate seating
  — sit/stand seating
  — foot-rail
  — foot-rest
  — shoes with cushioned inserts or soles
  — shock-absorbent floor covering
- Sitting postures
  — appropriate seating with adjustable seat height, appropriate seat width and depth, and adequate lumbar support
  — adjustable footrest
  — document holders
  — forearm supports
- Manual handling
  — straps with a D-handle for sheet handling
  — carts/trolley/forklifts
  — overhead hoists
  — levelators, lowerators and scissor lifts
  — conveyors
  — sliding aids
  — pallets/platforms

When the task or the environment cannot be redesigned, or there is no suitable workplace aid or equipment to minimize the aggravating effects of a particular task, the only remaining strategy may be education or training of the worker. This can be aimed at educating the worker on the risks associated with the task and training him or her in the most appropriate technique to minimize aggravation of pain. We will discuss some principles of such functional education later in the chapter, and it is also addressed in Chapter 15 on Lifestyle management.

Another major strategy for returning the worker with chronic pain to work is to use a graded return-to-work (RTW) or a modified-duties programme. For the worker with pain, a graded return to work can be the main way they can return to productive work duties with minimal aggravation. There may be little or no risk of re-injury for someone with pain returning to work. However, without some modification to the work tasks, there is often a risk of aggravation of the pain, such that the person cannot stay at work and requires further time off. We will now discuss some of the practical issues in planning and monitoring modified or suitable duties programmes to make them a successful strategy in re-integrating the worker with pain back to work.

Modified RTW or suitable-duties programmes have to be based on a thorough assessment of the match between the demands of the job and the person's functional capacities (Shrey & Hursh 1999, Innes 1997c). They also need to be planned in conjunction with the recommendations of the treating medical practitioner and in close liaison with the workplace. The first step is to consider the hierarchy of RTW goals, which we discussed earlier. The therapist determines the most appropriate RTW goal in conjunction with the worker, employer, treating medical practitioner and other key parties.

It is important to involve all such key parties in the planning and monitoring of RTW programmes. Other key people are the person's family, the insurer, and in the workplace his or her direct supervisor and co-workers and any union representative. Any medical restrictions imposed by the treating medical practitioner(s) need to be adhered to in planning the duties for a RTW programme. The selected duties need to match the person's functional abilities. They also need to be safe, meaningful, productive and compatible with the person's age, education, skills and experience (Innes 1997a). The hours and duties to be performed depend upon the nature of the condition and the stage of recovery (National Occupational Health & Safety Commission 1995).

Various options for grading duties and tasks can be used. Duties can be graded in terms of heaviness (from light to heavy), frequency (occasional to frequent), pace (slow to fast) or structure (from structured to unstructured). Hours can be graded from part-time to full-time and days can be graded, from a few days per week to 5 days per week. In upgrading the graduated RTW programme, it is important that only a limited number of options are changed at any one time. This allows the therapist to know what may be the cause of any possible aggravation of the person's pain. It is also important to monitor the programme regularly, both formally and informally.

The therapist can use a variety of tools to assist this monitoring process. Pain scales, pain location drawings and pain diaries, reviewed in Chapter 7, can be valuable aids in the monitoring process. The worker can complete these during the week, then the therapist can review them to look for any patterns in activities and corresponding aggravation of pain. The therapist plays an important role in supporting the client in minimizing any such aggravation.

One of the difficulties in planning RTW programmes is determining what the person should and should not do in the workplace, to prevent aggravation of their condition or re-injury or both. An individualized evaluation of the person's capacities for the physical demands of work through thorough workplace assessment or FCE or both will assist in determining what the person can and cannot do in the workplace. However, there often remains concern that there are tasks a person should not do because of the risk of recurrence or re-injury.

Current guidelines for management of back pain agree that the person with back pain should be encouraged to avoid bed-rest and be as active as possible, including early RTW activities, if possible (Waddell 1998). However, there are few specific guidelines for activities that are suitable for the person with back injury to do in the workplace. The US Clinical Practice Guidelines for acute low back problems in adults provide some guidelines for sitting and unassisted lifting, according to the severity of the person's symptoms (Waddell 1998). These may assist the therapist in planning RTW programmes for people with back pain.

The therapist should always be cautious in using any single-load limits in all situations, as individual factors such as the nature of the load, environmental factors and personal characteristics are important considerations in recommendations for manual handling in the workplace. The US guidelines urge clinicians to:

Make it clear to patients and employers that: even moderately heavy unassisted lifting may aggravate back

symptoms; any restrictions are intended to allow for spontaneous recovery or time to build activity tolerance through exercise (Waddell 1998 p 286).

The US guidelines also caution that any restrictions on work activities should only be short-term, suggesting that there are no benefits to restrictions 'beyond 3 months' (p 288). Obviously, the therapist needs to be cautious about the RTW recommendations he/she makes, that they do not cause re-injury and that they provide a high chance of a successful return to work. However, the therapist also needs to be careful to not be too restrictive in the recommendations he/she makes (Hall et al 1994) and should plan to gradually reduce the restrictions over a suitable period wherever possible.

Mazanec (1996) noted that return to work restrictions are often based on pain report and 'unfounded fears of further injury' (p 169). He too argued the need for RTW restrictions to be temporary and to be based on individual assessment of the match between the demands of the job and the person's functional capacities. He commented that, 'patients with back pain usually do not need restrictions on sedentary or light work, particularly if they have some freedom of movement during the workday' (Mazanec 1996 p 169).

Johns (1996) and Johns and Bloswick (1994) provided some specific guidelines for workers at risk of recurrent low back pain, including guidelines for lifting, stooping or bending and pushing and pulling. These may assist the therapist in making recommendations for the worker with chronic back pain to return to work, in conjunction with individualized assessment of the specific demands of the job and the person's functional capacities.

One of the main challenges for therapists in devising a modified or suitable duties programme is determining duties that are suitable within those offered by the employer. In a survey of employers in one Australian state, Kenny (1999) found that more than half of employers found it difficult to find suitable duties for their injured workers, especially employers with less than 20 employees. Such difficulties can mean that the person is not recommended to return to work unless fully fit (Kenny 1999). Therapists need to think broadly and creatively in devising RTW programmes and may be able to assist the employer in examining potential suitable duties for different injury types.

Improving the functional capacity of the worker with pain

There are a number of strategies the occupational therapist or physiotherapist may use with the person with pain to improve their functional capacity for re-integration into work. The therapist may provide conventional treatment strategies and other interventions for the person with pain that have been reviewed elsewhere in this book. In this chapter, we will deal with strategies that have a work focus. In practice, a combination of strategies may be used concurrently or progressively to improve the person's functional capacity for re-integration into work. Strategies include improving fitness for work and functional education or training for work duties. We discussed the use of workplace assistive devices in the section on improving the workplace. We will also discuss the approach of work-hardening and discuss the differences between this and work-conditioning. Finally we review some group strategies for improving worker capacity for return to work.

Improving fitness for work

Innes (1997b) provided an overview of different approaches to improving work fitness, with an emphasis on improving the neuromusculoskeletal and motor components of work fitness. She differentiated between the terms work fitness and physical fitness. Work fitness was described as the 'capacity to meet successfully the present and potential challenges of work requirements with vigour, and to demonstrate the traits and capacities associated with low risk of premature development of occupational injuries and diseases' (Innes 1997b p 228). Physical fitness refers to components such as 'cardiorespiratory endurance, muscle strength and endurance, flexibility and body composition' (p 228). Occupational therapists and physiotherapists may be concerned with improving both of these types of fitness in assisting the worker with pain to return to work.

After time off work and recovering from injury, the worker with pain can be de-conditioned. An important role of the occupational therapist and physiotherapist in rehabilitation is to encourage a return to physical activity, including fitness activities and meaningful productive activities. Rodgers (1984) provided the following simple guidelines for the worker to minimize aggravation of pain in the workplace: avoid factors in the workplace that aggravate pain (see the earlier section on back-pain aggravators), keep muscles fit, and lift safely. These strategies require the therapist to help the worker to improve their fitness for work and to understand the ways they can minimize aggravation of their pain or re-injury.

There are a number of different strategies for improving the fitness of the worker with pain for work.

These can include home or gym-based exercise programmes, individually prescribed for the person by a physiotherapist. Exercise programmes are discussed in Chapter 13. Such exercise programmes are aimed at improving aspects of physical fitness such as cardiorespiratory endurance, strength and flexibility. Modified or suitable duties programmes can also allow the development of work-specific fitness. More formal strategies for improving the worker's fitness for return to work include work-hardening and work-conditioning.

Work-hardening is a multi- or interdisciplinary approach to improving the worker's function. According to King (1998), the Commission on Accreditation of Rehabilitation Facilities in the US officially defined work-hardening as, 'a highly structured, goal-oriented, individualized treatment programme designed to maximize the individual's ability to return to work' (King 1998 p 258). It has been described as a comprehensive interdisciplinary approach to work rehabilitation that 'addresses biomedical and psychosocial problems' (Niemeyer et al 1994 p 328), and an approach to 'fill the gap between medical intervention and return to work' (King 1998 p 258). The primary means by which the aims of work-hardening are achieved are by use of 'real or simulated work activities in conjunction with conditioning tasks' (Wyrick et al 1991 p 109).

The physical demands that form the basis of the FCE, as described earlier in this chapter, also often provide the framework for the activities that a person performs on a work-hardening programme. These include activities of lifting, carrying, walking and reaching. The person often performs a circuit of activities aimed at improving his or her tolerance for the different physical demands of work. As well as aiming at improving 'the injured worker's biomechanical, neuromuscular, cardiovascular-metabolic, and psychosocial functioning', work-hardening should also address 'issues of productivity, safety, physical tolerances and work behaviours' (Wyrick et al 1994 p 109).

While work-hardening has broad multi-faceted aims, work-conditioning programmes have an emphasis on the physical conditioning of the worker using exercise equipment and aerobic conditioning, with less use of work-related tasks than work-hardening (King 1998). Work-conditioning requires less professionals, space and time commitment on behalf of the client (King 1998) and has less of a behavioural component than work-hardening.

Historically, large centre-based work-hardening programmes have been used in North America to provide intensive rehabilitation of the injured worker for return to work. In Australia, the trend has been to use the workplace in graded RTW programmes to improve worker fitness. In the USA, the cost-effectiveness of multidisciplinary centre-based programmes has been questioned and the trend is to workplace-based programmes and managed care (Niemeyer et al 1994).

Functional education

Functional education should be directed at assisting the person to understand and manage pain associated with work tasks. This may include anatomy and physiology related to mechanisms of injury and repair of soft tissue, an understanding of pacing and fatigue, and the physical and physiological demands of work, domestic and leisure tasks. The therapist may need to facilitate decisions about the best use of low-pain or pain-free periods, and about how to avoid individual lifestyle factors that exacerbate pain. In order to perform critical work tasks the person may need to delegate domestic tasks such as cleaning floors or food preparation, or forego leisure activities such as sports or handcrafts that may increase pain. The person with pain may need to be prepared to work with a certain level of pain if re-integration into work is an important goal.

A major role for occupational therapists and physiotherapists in rehabilitation of the person with chronic pain for return to work is in back education. As principles of back care are covered in Chapter 15 we will consider education that is specific to workers with pain.

Innes (1997c) reviewed some of the issues concerned with the effectiveness of this education for prevention of back injuries. She also reviewed guidelines for the content that should be included in such education. These guidelines are relevant for educating the worker with pain for return to work:

- Anatomy of the spine and posture
- Resting positions, correct sitting, standing, lifting
- Practice of these static and dynamic postures
- Job-specific activities and situations and practice of these
- Physical fitness
- Impact of psychological aspects.

All workers should use sound manual handling techniques. However, it is even more important for the worker with pain to use these techniques to avoid further injury and to minimize potential aggravation of pain. There are various theories about manual handling techniques. Current practice advocates the use of general principles rather than a specific technique (Department of Employment, Training and Industrial Relations 2000). The therapist needs to consider the demands of the workplace before recommending an appropriate manual handling technique. Some of the current basic principles of manual handling are outlined in the next chapter.

It is important in all education or workplace-based training programmes that adult learning principles are used. This means that the occupational therapist or physiotherapist needs to be conversant with the person's workplace and workplace demands, to demonstrate preferred behaviours, to provide opportunities for practice of new skills and to provide feedback to the worker during the learning process (King 1995).

One of the main ways of improving worker function is through interventions to improve self-management of the pain. The person needs to be informed of his/her abilities and limitations as assessed by the FCE and other evaluations. In addition, the person may avoid re-injury if he/she knows and understands the implications of any restrictions imposed by medical practitioners and therapists.

Group strategies to improve worker function

A number of these strategies may be undertaken in group settings. The opportunity to listen and contribute to problem-solving sessions may be beneficial to the person with pain. Main and Watson (1995) reported reasonable results for a group programme for a group of unemployed people with back pain. This programme included:

Active physical rehabilitation, individual and group psychological intervention, education in basic anatomy and function of the spine, simple ergonomic advice, interviewing and job-seeking skills, advice on appropriate employment, and information on how to cope with the changes in benefits and finances that occur on re-entering employment (Main & Watson p 213).

Ekberg (1995) described an innovative approach to work rehabilitation using a problem-based rehabilitation (PBR) strategy. This PBR strategy was aimed at improving participants' intrinsic motivation and coping abilities for rehabilitation and return to work. This approach was integrated into a model of rehabilitation that also addressed workplace and individual injury factors.

Effective combinations of interventions

In this chapter we have outlined a number of interventions and intervention frameworks for the occupational therapist and physiotherapist to use when assisting the person with pain to return to work. A number of

Table 14.3 Example of combined strategies for workers with back pain under the proposed frameworks

Problem area	Strategy	Type of strategy	Action
Reduced fitness	Specific strengthening programme	Worker function	Adapt
	Work-hardening	Worker function	Adapt
	Graded return to work	Work task	Adapt
	Education about fitness	Worker function	Train/educate
Limited static positional tolerances (e.g. sitting and standing)	Avoid prolonged standing with sit/stand stool	Work environment	Eliminate/adapt
	Modify height of standing workstation to appropriate height	Work environment	Redesign
	Graded RTW to build up standing and sitting tolerances	Work task	Adapt
	Alternate sitting and standing	Work task	Adapt
	Supportive shoes	Worker function	Adapt
	Mat to prolong standing tolerance	Work environment	Adapt
	Alternate sitting, standing, walking	Work task	Adapt
Limited mobility	Re-organise work layout and locations to reduce prolonged walking and need for crouching	Work environment	Redesign
	Fitness program	Worker function	Adapt
	Work conditioning	Worker function	Adapt
Limited manual handling ability	Eliminate by use of mechanical devices	Work environment	Eliminate
	Work conditioning/work hardening	Worker function	Adapt
	Re-organize layout so loads are handled between shoulder and mid-thigh height or at waist height where possible	Work environment	Redesign
	Break-up loads into smaller loads	Work task	Redesign
	Manual handling training	Worker function	Train/educate

strategies may be used concurrently in an effective return to work programme. To assist the therapist devise a return to work programme Table 14.3 illustrates how strategies may address particular problem areas. These strategies are categorized according to the framework of interventions for the person with pain (see Figure 14.3) and represent a range from the hierarchy of strategies for improving the match between the demands of the job/workplace and the functional capacity of the worker with pain (see Box 14.6).

ISSUES IN RE-INTEGRATION OF THE PERSON WITH CHRONIC PAIN INTO WORK

Research into RTW of individuals with pain, especially chronic back pain, highlights the complexity of the many factors involved. There are many variables that affect RTW of the individual with chronic back pain and these variables interact in a complex interplay that varies across individuals and situations.

It is increasingly acknowledged that psychosocial variables, including job-related psychosocial variables, play a major role in influencing RTW of the person with back pain (Waddell 1998). Aspects of the job such as the amount of autonomy and support are examples of these important workplace-based psychosocial variables (Waddell 1998).

Other, more personal, psychosocial variables that are associated with RTW include self-efficacy for work and RTW (Gibson & Strong 1998) and fear of pain and of movement/re-injury (Gibson & Strong 1999, Vlaeyen & Linton 2000, Vlaeyen et al 1995). These variables need to be evaluated or at least considered by the therapist to improve chances of a successful outcome. There are many tools available to the occupational therapist or physiotherapist to evaluate these important variables (Gibson & Strong 1998, 1999).

A relatively new tool designed for evaluating the psychosocial and environmental aspects of work and to be used in conjunction with FCE is the Worker Role Interview (WRI) (Velozo et al 1998). The WRI aims to aid the therapist to consider the influential psychosocial and environmental aspects of the person's job and potential for RTW. This semi-structured interview based on the Model of Human Occupation is 'designed to be used as the psychosocial/environmental component of the initial rehabilitation assessment process for the injured worker' (Velozo et al 1998 p 1). There has been some research conducted on the WRI (Fisher 1999, Velozo et al 1999).

One of the most controversial issues in RTW of people with chronic pain is the influence of litigation or compensation (Waddell 1998). Contrary to popular belief, there is conflicting evidence for the influence of litigation and compensation on outcome from chronic pain including RTW (Fields 1995). There has been a suggestion that the person with chronic pain makes 'secondary gain' in economic, physical or emotional terms from their condition (Waddell 1998). Based on the evidence, Waddell commented that the 'secondary losses' from back pain 'usually outweigh secondary gains' (Waddell 1998 p 219). As noted by Teasell and Merskey (1997), 'the notion that patients' pains improve and they return to work shortly after the final settlement of compensation claims remains unfounded' (Teasell & Merskey p 232).

In fact, in a recent review of the research on disability exaggeration or malingering in patients with chronic pain, Fishbain et al (1999) found that no conclusions can be drawn from the research to date on the prevalence of malingering in this population. The questionable quality of the studies led the authors to only a guarded conclusion that malingering does occur and it may be present in 1.25–10.4% of chronic pain patients. The authors called for research into the prevalence of malingering and development of reliable and valid methods for identifying malingering. The authors also cautioned pain practitioners against 'believing that malingering can be conclusively identified in some way' (Fishbain et al p 271) and against believing that existing methods for such identification are valid. They provide a review of the very limited evidence for current methods in malingering identification, that is useful for occupational therapists and physiotherapists working in the rehabilitation of clients with chronic pain.

Indeed, the experience of the authors suggests that therapists need to be alert for the over-eager worker with pain who may ignore the advice of health professionals and risk aggravation of pain and of re-injury. Examples include the manual labourer with arthritis who is unwilling or unable to retrain for a less physically demanding job, or the person with family and financial commitments who is reluctant to take time off work.

The report of the Task Force on Professional Education of the International Association for the Study of Pain (Fields 1995) provides a summary of the evidence on compensation, disability assessment and pain in the workplace that provides a valuable resource for occupational therapists and physiotherapists working in this area. The reader is also referred to the work of Mendelson and Mendelson (1997) for a review of the medicolegal aspects of pain management.

A final word of caution is needed for therapists to not allow the person's compensation or litigation status to influence judgements or recommendations for return to work. A study of the influence of knowledge of patient's workers compensation status by physiotherapists on their clinical judgements, showed that it did not affect assessment results (Simmonds & Kumar 1996). However, it did affect predictive judgements of outcome.

CONCLUSION

This chapter has presented an overview of the process used by the occupational therapist or physiotherapist to evaluate and improve the match between the worker's capacities and the demands of the job in the work rehabilitation of the person with chronic pain. Despite the best efforts at interventions with the individual and the workplace, societal change such as social legislation and labour market policy (Alaranta & Rytokoski 1994) is required to fully achieve the goal of integration of individuals with pain into the workforce.

Study questions/questions for revision

1. What are the three significant roles of occupational therapists and physiotherapists that are referred to in this chapter? How does each role contribute to the re-integration into work of the person with pain?
2. List the phases of the work rehabilitation process and two components of each phase.
3. What are the steps in a Functional Capacity Evaluation?
4. Identify four physical demands of the job that need to be assessed for the person with pain.
5. Provide one strategy for each of the following limitations: reduced fitness, limited static positional tolerances, limited mobility, and limited manual handling ability.
6. What are some of the issues for the person with pain who is attempting to return to work?

REFERENCES

Aja D, Laflin K 1999 Lifting analysis. In: Jacobs K (ed) Ergonomics for Therapists, 2nd Edn. Butterworth-Heinemann, Boston, pp 179–218

Alaranta H, Rytokoski U 1994 Intensive physical and psychosocial training program for patients with chronic low back pain: a controlled clinical trial. Spine 19(12): 1339–1349

Allen M M 1999 Successful Employment Change: the experiences of people who changed employment due to disability. The University of Queensland, Brisbane

Bendix A F, Bendix T Labriola M, Boekgaard P 1998 Functional restoration for chronic low back pain: two-year follow-up of two randomized clinical trials. Spine 23(6): 717–725

Burke S A, Harms-Constas C K, Aden P 1994 Return to work/work retention outcomes of a functional restoration program. Spine 19(17): 1880–1886

Chaffin D B, Andersson G B J, Martin B J 1999 Occupational Biomechanics. John Wiley, New York

Department of Employment, Training and Industrial Relations 2000 Manual Tasks Advisory Standard 2000. Goprint, Brisbane

Ekberg K 1995 Workplace changes in successful rehabilitation. Journal of Occupational Rehabilitation 5(4): 253–269

Feuerstein M, Menz L, Zastowny T, Barron B A 1994 Chronic back pain and work disability: vocational outcomes following multidisciplinary rehabilitation. Journal of Occupational Rehabilitation 4: 229–251

Fields H L (ed) 1995 Core Curriculum for Professional Education in Pain. IASP Press, Seattle

Fishbain D A, Cutler R, Steele-Rosomoff R 1999 Chronic pain disability exaggeration/malingering and submaximal effort research. Clinical Journal of Pain 15(4): 244–274

Fisher G S 1999 Administration and application of the worker role interview: looking beyond functional capacity. Work 12: 25–36

Fordyce W E (ed) 1995 Back Pain in the Workplace: management of disability in nonspecific conditions. IASP Press, Seattle

Frank J W, Brooker A S, DeMaio S E, Kerr M S, Maetzel A, Sharnon H S, Sullivan T J, Norman R W, Wells R P 1996 Disability resulting for occupational low back pain. Part II: What do we know about secondary prevention? A review of the scientific evidence on prevention after disability begins. Spine 21(25): 2918–2929

Gibson L, Strong J 1997 A review of functional capacity evaluation practice. Work 9: 3–11

Gibson L, Strong J 1998 Assessment of psychosocial factors in functional capacity evaluation of clients with chronic back pain. British Journal of Occupational Therapy 61: 399–404

Gibson L, Strong J 1999 Work Rehabilitation: the role of fear-avoidance. Proceedings, OT Australia 20th National Conference, Canberra

Haider T T, Kishino N D, Gray T P, Tomlin M A, Daubert H B 1998 Functional restoration: comparison of surgical and nonsurgical spine patients. Journal of Occupational Rehabilitation 8(4): 247–253

Hall H, McIntosh G, Melles T, Holowachuk B, Wai E 1994 Effect of discharge recommendations on outcome. Spine 19(18): 2033–2037

Hart D L, Isernhagen S J, Matheson L N 1993 Guidelines for functional capacity evaluation of people with medical conditions. Journal of Orthopaedic and Sports Physical Therapy 18: 682–686

Innes E 1997a Work assessment options and the selection of suitable duties: an Australian perspective. New Zealand Journal of Occupational Therapy 48(1): 14–20

Innes E 1997b Work programmes to enhance motor and neuromuscuoloskeletal performance components. In: Pratt J, Jacobs K (eds) Work Practice: international perspectives. Butterworth-Heinemann, Oxford, pp 224–244

Innes E 1997c Back injury prevention programs: do they make a difference? Proceedings OT Australia 19th National Conference, Perth, pp 215–219

Innes E, Straker L 1998a A clinician's guide to work-related assessments: 1 – purposes and problems. Work 11: 183–189

Innes E, Straker L 1998b A clinician's guide to work-related assessments: 2 – design problems. Work 11: 191–206

Innes E, Straker L 1998c A clinician's guide to work-related assessments: 3 – administration and interpretation problems. Work 11: 207–219

Innes E, Straker L 1999a Reliability of work-related assessments. Work 13(2): 107–124

Innes E, Straker L 1999b Validity of work-related assessments. Work 13(2): 125–152

Jacobs K 1993 Occupational Therapy: work-related programs and assessments, 2nd Edn. Little, Brown & Co, Boston

Jacobs K (ed) 1999 Ergonomics for Therapists, 2nd Edn. Butterworth-Heinemann, Boston

Johns R E 1996 Fitness for duty considerations in disabling occupational low-back pain. Journal of Back and Musculoskeletal Rehabilitation 7: 151–166

Johns R E, Bloswick D S 1994 Chronic recurrent low-back pain – a methodology for analyzing fitness for duty and managing risk under the Americans with Disabilities Act. Journal of Occupational and Environmental Medicine 36: 537–547

Jundt J, King P M 1999 Work rehabilitation programs: a 1997 survey. Work 12: 139–144

Kenny D T 1999 Employers' perspectives on the provision of suitable duties in occupational rehabilitation. Journal of Occupational Rehabilitation 9(4): 267–276

King P M 1995 Employee ergonomics training: current limitations and suggestions for improvement. Journal of Occupational Rehabilitation 5(2): 115–123

King P M 1998 Work hardening and work conditioning. Sourcebook of Occupational Rehabilitation. Plenum, New York, pp 257–275

King P M, Tuckwell N, Barrett T 1998 A critical review of functional capacity evaluations. Physical Therapy 78(8): 852–866

Krause N, Dasinger L K, Neuhauser F 1998 Modified work and return to work: a review of the literature. Journal of Occupational Rehabilitation 8(2): 113–139

Lechner D E, Jackson J R, Roth D L, Straaton M D 1994 Reliability and validity of a newly developed test of physical work performance. Journal of Occupational Medicine 36: 997–1004

Main C J, Watson P J 1995 Screening for patients at risk of developing chronic incapacity. Journal of Occupational Rehabilitation 5(4): 207–217

Matheson L N, Brophy R G 1997 Aggressive early intervention after occupational back injury: some preliminary observations. Journal of Occupational Rehabilitation 7(2): 107–117

Matheson L N, Brophy R G, Vaugh K D, Nunez C, Saccoman K A 1995 Workers' compensation managed care: preliminary findings. Journal of Occupational Rehabilitation 5(1): 27–36

Matheson L N 1988 Integrated work hardening in vocational rehabilitation: an emerging model. Vocational Evaluation and Work Adjustment Bulletin 22(2): 1–9

Mayer T G, Gatchel R J 1988 Functional Restoration for Spinal Disorders: the sports medicine approach. Lea & Febiger, Philadelphia

Mayer T G, Polatin P, Smith B et al 1995 Contemporary concepts in spine care: spine rehabilitation secondary and tertiary nonoperative care. Spine 20: 2060–2066

Mayer T, McMahon M, Gatchel R, Sparks B, Wright A, Pegues P 1998 Socioeconomic outcomes of combined spine surgery and functional restoration in worker's compensation spinal disorders with matched controls. Spine 23: 598–606

Mazanec D J 1996 The injured worker: assessing 'return-to-work' status. Cleveland Clinic Journal of Medicine 63: 166–171

Mendelson G, Mendelson D 1997 Medicolegal aspects of pain management. Pain Reviews 4: 244–274

Mital A, Pennathur A 1999 Musculoskeletal overexertion injuries in the United States; mitigating the problem through ergonomics and engineering interventions. Journal of Occupational Rehabilitation 9(2): 115–149

National Occupational Health & Safety Commission 1995 Guidance note for best practice rehabilitation management of occupational injuries and disease. National Occupational Health & Safety Commission, Sydney, pp 2–3

National Institute of Occupational Safety & Health 1981 Work practices guide for manual lifting. US Department of Health and Human Services, technical report no 81122. National Institute of Occupational Safety & Health, Cincinnati

National Institute of Occupational Safety & Health 1991 Scientific support documentation for the revised NIOSH lifting equation: technical contract report. US Department of Commerce, Technical Information Service. National Institute of Occupational Safety & Health, Cincinnati

Niemeyer L O, Jacobs K, Reynolds-Lynch K, Bettencourt C, Lang S 1994 Work hardening: past, present, and future – the work programs special interest section national work-hardening outcome study. American Journal of Occupational Therapy 48(4): 327–339

Randolph D C 1996 Functional capacity evaluation and disability management. Journal of Back and Musculoskeletal Rehabilitation 7: 181–186

Rodgers S H 1984 Working with backache. Perinton, Fairport

Rudy T E, Lieber S J, Boston J R 1996 Functional capacity assessment: influence of behavioural and environmental factors. Journal of Back and Musculoskeletal Rehabilitation 6: 277–288

Schmidt S H, Oort-Marburger D, Meijman T F 1995 Employment after rehabilitation for musculoskeletal

impairments: the impact of vocational rehabilitation and working on a trial basis. Archives of Physical Medicine and Rehabilitation 76: 950–954

Sen S, Fraser K, Evans O M, Stuckey R 1991 A comparison of the physical demands of a specific job and those measured by standard functional capacity assessment tools. Proceedings of the 27th Annual Conference of the Ergonomic Society of Australia, Coolum, pp 263–268

Shrey D E, Hursh N C 1999 Workplace disability management: international trends and perspectives. Journal of Occupational Rehabilitation 9(1): 45–59

Simmonds M, Kumar S 1996 Does knowledge of a patient's workers' compensation status influence clinical judgements? Journal of Occupational Rehabilitation 6(2): 93–107

Smith E R 1989 Ergonomics and the occupational therapist. In: Hertfelder S, Gwin C (eds) Work in Progress. American Occupational Therapy Association, Rockville, pp 127–156

Spektor S 1990 Chronic pain and pain-related disabilities. Journal of Disability 1: 98–102

Strong J 1996 Chronic Pain: the occupational therapist's perspective. Churchill Livingstone, Edinburgh

Teasell R W, Merskey H 1997 Chronic pain disability in the workplace. Pain Forum 6(4): 228–238

United States Department of Labor 1991a Dictionary of Occupational Titles, 4th Edn. Government Printing Office, Washington DC

United States Department of Labor 1991b Revised Handbook for Analyzing Jobs. US Department of Labor, Employment and Training Administration, Washington DC

Vasudevan S V 1996 Role of functional capacity assessment in disability evaluation. Journal of Back and Musculoskeletal Rehabilitation 6: 237–248

Velozo C, Kielhofner G, Fisher G 1998 A user's guide to worker role interview (WRI). Model of Human Occupational Clearinghouse. Department of Occupational Therapy, College of Health and Human Development Sciences, University of Illinois, Chicago

Velozo C, Kielhofner G, Gern A, Fang-Ling L, Azhar F, Lai J S, Fisher G 1999 Worker role interview: toward validation of a psychosocial work-related measure. Journal of Occupational Rehabilitation 9(3): 153–168

Vlaeyen J W S, Linton S J 2000 Fear avoidance and its consequences in chronic musculoskeletal pain: a state of the art. Pain 85: 317–332

Vlaeyen J W S, Kole-Snijders A M J, Rotteveel A N, Ruesink R, Heuts P H T G 1995 The role of fear of movement/(re)injury in pain disability. Journal of Occupational Rehabilitation 5: 235–252

Waddell G 1998 The Back Pain Revolution. Churchill Livingstone, Edinburgh

Wickstrom R J 1996 Evaluating physical qualifications of workers and jobs. In: Bhattacharya A, McGlothin J D (eds) Occupational Ergonomics: theory and application. Marcel Dekker, New York, pp 367–386

World Health Organization 1998 Towards a common language for functioning and disablement. ICIDH-2: the International Classification of Impairments, Activities and Participation. World Health Organization, Geneva

Wyrick J M, Niemeyer L O, Ellexson M, Jacobs K, Taylor S 1991 Occupational therapy work-hardening programs: a demographic study. American Journal of Occupational Therapy 45(2): 109–112

15

Lifestyle management

Jenny Strong

OVERVIEW

In addition to work, individuals occupy a number of life roles, such as homemaker, parent, student, employee, sportsperson, spouse, etc. Many people with chronic pain have disruptions to several of these occupational roles, and hence to aspects of their lifestyle which are important to them. This chapter will focus on strategies to assist the patient to regain desired lifestyle goals or attain new ones. Such an approach is integral to the practice of occupational therapists, who consider clients as occupational beings embedded within particular environmental systems.

When working with clients with pain, an emphasis will be placed on assisting the client in selecting realistic lifestyle goals, and on fostering a philosophical approach to living well, despite pain. Strategies to use in attaining these goals will be considered. These strategies will include adaptive equipment use, good body mechanics, back care, pacing, and relaxation and biofeedback. Particular problems experienced by clients in the areas of intimacy, sexuality and sleeping are included in this chapter.

Learning objectives

At the end of this chapter students will have an understanding of:

1. Lifestyle factors which impinge on pain management.
2. Principles of lifestyle management which have been shown to be effective.
3. Some particular techniques which may be of use.

This chapter should be read in conjunction with Chapter 9, which explained a number of strategies therapists can use with clients, including client education, goal setting, self-efficacy enhancement, self-esteem development and coping-skills enhancement.

BACKGROUND ISSUES IN MANAGING A LIFESTYLE WITH PAIN

At the current stage of our knowledge and skill in assessing and treating chronic pain, there are many people for whom a 'cure' is not readily available. The reality for such individuals is that they must *learn to live with pain*; they must learn to adjust their patterns of living, their dreams and aspirations, and their expectations, to accommodate a chronic pain problem, in much the same way as someone newly diagnosed with multiple sclerosis or someone with a spinal injury must learn to accommodate and adjust. For people with chronic pain conditions, this may seem particularly vexatious for a number of reasons:

- The pain is not an obvious tangible thing to others around the person. Many clients comment that this makes their adjustment a much harder process, because people don't believe they have a problem.
- Secondly, while health professionals such as occupational therapists may be saying 'we can help you learn to live with your pain', there will be others who are promoting the latest panacea, be it a new wonder drug or particular machine or surgical technique. Very often those around a client will be offering help and support, but without a uniformity of approach.
- Thirdly, many clients have a perception when they are advised to learn to live with their pain that health professionals believe they are putting it on. With little objectivity to their condition, there is often difficulty establishing and/or maintaining credibility.

For such clients, the input of the occupational therapist in helping the client with lifestyle management and adjustment can be invaluable.

Those seeking help are not representative of those experiencing pain in the general population. Many will be capable of working out individual and highly effective ways to manage their pain and maintain the most satisfying lifestyle possible, while others will require considerable help and still manage only a minimally rewarding lifestyle. For each of these two ends of the spectrum the therapist will take a different approach. Those who are active in working out solutions will need less support but may profit most from technical advice and information. Clients who are less able to see solutions will require considerable support and encouragement and possibly cognitive restructuring, as well as information and technical advice.

Henriksson (1995) interviewed 40 women with pain from fibromyalgia in two countries and found some were able to actively accept their limitations in a way which allowed them to plan their lives and introduce effective changes. However, some women were resistant to change. They continued to work at the same rate, to hide their problems, and had little leisure. During their 'time for themselves' they were in a state of collapse, or they were unable to change their practices, spending the majority of their time in rest. While many clients are able to think of and to utilize effective lifestyle changes, some are less resourceful in this area. Therapists then:

1. Help the person with pain to analyse their lifestyle
2. Help the person to prioritize activities and roles that are important to maintain
3. Provide information about and training in alternative strategies to improve the quality of lifestyle
4. Support the person during changes to their lifestyle.

There are several personal concepts that may need to be modified to produce a rewarding lifestyle. These include: reviewing expectations of life and pain, setting goals, pacing, and active involvement in decision-making. Techniques to use include cognitive restructuring, education in such things as back care and good body mechanics, relaxation training, exercise for conditioning, use of adaptive equipment and daily activity scheduling.

As has been already mentioned in Chapter 9, cognitive–behavioural approaches to pain management are very successful. In managing alterations to lifestyle, a cognitive–behavioural approach is likely to be most useful for several reasons. Firstly, changing well established aspects of a person's lifestyle requires the active, thoughtful (well considered) involvement of that person. Active involvement in decision-making has been said to be essential to a positive outcome in many pain management programmes, and this involvement is most likely to be achieved using the cognitive approach. Secondly, if a client is to feel capable of involvement in decision-making, then she or he must have a personal sense of agency, or of self-efficacy.

Learning to live with pain is primarily a cognitive and behavioural process. Without at least some understanding that waiting for a 'cure' and return to a previous lifestyle is not useful (i.e. an understanding of the need to 'get on with' life even if pain still exists), any attempts to devise a more manageable lifestyle will be doomed to limited success at best, if not failure. But there is also an emotional component. The client may need to grieve for those parts of a familiar lifestyle that must be discarded temporarily or permanently to ensure a quality of life despite pain.

An aspect of psychological adjustment to living with chronic pain is fear-avoidance beliefs, which were previously mentioned in Chapter 9. Clients' own beliefs of how physical activity might affect their pain can lead them to avoid activities. Fear of pain, and what to do about it, may be more disabling than pain itself.

Waddell et al (1993) found that there was little direct relationship between pain and disability, but a strong relationship between fear-avoidance beliefs about work and both work loss and disability in activities of daily living. This has obvious implications for achieving a lifestyle with independent and rewarding features. Clients may need reassurance that in contrast to acute pain, chronic pain is not necessarily a signal of continuing underlying tissue damage that requires active medical treatment. Hurting is not synonymous with harming. Fear that the presence of pain is a signal that continued activity will result in more tissue damage will inhibit clients from further activity. Lifestyle changes may be needed long-term or permanently, such as those reported by Henriksson (1995) from her interviews with clients affected by fibromyalgia, or those adopted by the people with low back pain included in our study of coping with back pain (Strong & Large 1995).

STRATEGIES FOR LIFESTYLE MANAGEMENT

Exercise and conditioning

There have been a number of studies which suggest that a more functional and enjoyable lifestyle is possible if the person with chronic pain is able to resist or counteract body deconditioning. In our study of successful copers who had chronic low back pain, regular exercise was a recurring theme (Strong & Large 1995, Large & Strong 1997).

Participants in our study had weighed up the costs and benefits of exercise, and chosen to exercise in a variety of ways ranging from bellydancing, or jogging to work each day, to more simple exercises. To this end, exercise programmes are often included as a component of a multidisciplinary pain-management programme.

Protas (1996) reviewed the evidence from published papers for the usefulness of aerobic exercise in the rehabilitation of clients with chronic low back pain. Aerobic exercise is commonly suggested for this condition. There were imperfections in the studies found

and reviewed, but most had found improved endurance, even if back pain or functional capacity didn't alter. There was evidence from one study of improvement in return to work and reduced sick days, and in another of less physical dysfunction and depression with the aerobic exercise programme. Overall, the aerobic exercise was responsible for some positive effects, and no negative effects were isolated. With fibromyalgia, clients have found that even if overall they can do less in their life than previously, regular physical activity has a beneficial effect on their lifestyle (Henriksson 1995).

Physiotherapists also provide specific rehabilitation exercises to clients with chronic pain (see Chapter 13) When prescribing exercises, a physiotherapist needs to consider variables such as history of previous injuries, mechanism of current injury, training goals and other factors specific to the individual (McGill 1998). Physiotherapists may recommend a combination of stretching and strengthening exercises to the client. While exercise has consistently been demonstrated to have positive outcomes for individuals with chronic pain, a major difficulty encountered with recommending exercise therapy in clinical practice is non-compliance (Jensen & Lorish 1994). Thus, physiotherapists need to be aware of strategies to enhance clients' adherence to exercise programmes.

Techniques which may improve compliance with exercise programmes include strategies which enhance the client's level of internal control, such as increasing the patient's understanding of the problem, involving the client in the design and implementation of treatment (Friedrich et al 1998, Jensen & Lorish 1994). A recent study, which compared two exercise programmes for clients with chronic pain, found that the one which addressed motivational factors was more effective in reducing disability and pain in the participants (Friedrich et al 1998).

Chapter 13 provides further information on the role of exercise in the management of clients with chronic musculoskeletal pain. In addition, there are a number of self-help books available, which have useful sections on developing fitness and exercise tolerance, for example the book by Parker and Main (1995) has a chapter on increasing fitness and activity levels. A more recent book on managing pain is the one by Nicholas et al (2000).

Back care and body mechanics

As there are a large number of people with low back pain, it follows that back care strategies need to be taught. Many comprehensive rehabilitation programmes include 'back schools' for clients with chronic low back pain. The effectiveness of back schools in reducing work-related injuries has been demonstrated in the rehabilitation literature (Bettencourt 1995). Back schools provide information on basic anatomy and function of the spine, posture re-education, and training in manual handling techniques. Therapists also use these strategies to assist clients with chronic back pain who they see in other settings. Strategies explored in greater detail in this chapter include manual handling techniques, posture re-education and physical conditioning.

Education in the use of safe lifting and handling can help prevent further pain and improve the quality of life for clients with chronic low back pain. Therefore, therapists must be aware of methods of moving, lifting and handling objects, which are bio-mechanically safe and energy-efficient. Despite extensive research in this area there is controversy regarding which lifting techniques should be recommended to clients with low back pain. For example the popular 'back straight, knees bent' approach has received mixed support throughout the literature (Bettencourt 1995). A number of different styles have been advocated, depending on factors relating to the person performing the lift, the load to be lifted, and the environment in which the lifting will occur. A critique of the different approaches is beyond the scope of this book, however further information on the advantages and disadvantages of various lifting styles may be obtained from ergonomic publications referred to in Chapter 14.

While there is a lack of consensus in the literature regarding specific lifting techniques, there are numerous publications outlining the basic principles of safe manual handling. These core principles may be applied to most lifting situations, and are outlined in Box 15.1. Guidelines for manual handling have been published for a variety of industries. Therapists can obtain such guidelines, and Manual Handling Advisory Standards from the relevant occupational health and safety authority in their state or country (e.g. http://www.detir.qld.gov.au/hs/advisory).

When educating clients in lifting and handling techniques, therapists must ensure that the programme is suited to the client's lifestyle. This may involve the client learning more than one lifting technique if different lifting situations occur routinely in the client's life (lifting a small child from the floor at home is associated with different demands than lifting boxes from the back of a van at work).

It is important that the client is given the opportunity to practice the lifting techniques in the situations in which they will occur, and provided with feedback if an adjustment to the technique is necessary. Sometimes

---

Box 15.1 Basic principles of lifting/carrying
1. Plan the move. Consider safe work methods, eliminate obstacles and obtain assistance if required.
2. Reduce manual handling. Lighten the load.
3. Test the load: ensure there is adequate grip on the load.
4. Avoid lifing with a fully bent back.
5. Keep the load as close to the body as possible.
6. Reduce bending, twisting and reaching movements.
7. Perform the lift in a smooth, even motion.
8. Move feet if a change in direction is necessary.
9. Avoid muscle fatigue – warm up first and take frequent rest breaks.
Source: Employment, Training and Industrial Relations Workplace Health and Safety 2000

---

the therapist will need to compromise so that the most appropriate lifting style that the client will use is selected. The use of video feedback can be helpful to clients. It is also useful for therapists to give the client 'permission' to avoid doing certain lifts that are unsafe. Clients need to be able to judge what is a safe lift within their capabilities, and to ask for help or an alternative technique when the lift is unsafe. It has been observed that the least effective way of reducing risk of injury is to rely on 'safe' behaviour by the worker (DETIR 2000). Hence, therapists need to be pro-active in examining the client in context with their environment.

Another important component of back care involves posture re-education. Back, neck and shoulder pain can result from adopting poor posture in daily activities. Physiotherapists and occupational therapists can provide the client with advice regarding the most efficient postures for a number of activities such as driving, sitting, standing, sleeping, resting and leisure activities. There is evidence that sustained postures are important risk factors in the development of a variety of musculoskeletal disorders (Wallace & Buchle 1987).

Postures that constantly compress the intervertebral disc (such as prolonged sitting) upset the normal metabolic processes of the disc, leading to back pain and disc deterioration (Kramer 1981). Changes in posture encourage bloodflow to the muscles, which is important for adequate oxygen delivery and the removal of toxins. Therapists need to educate clients with back pain about the importance of taking rest breaks and changing positions to prevent problems associated with prolonged postures.

In addition to sustained postures, poor body alignment may exacerbate chronic pain. Enwemeka and colleagues (1986) noted that people with neck pain and upper thoracic back pain often worked in a protruded head position. Habitual asymmetry of posture (such as leaning on one arm while sitting) has also been identified as a risk factor in the development of certain musculoskeletal problems. Therapists will find the general postural recommendations provided by Pheasant (1986) to be useful ones. Encourage the client to:

1. Make frequent changes to posture
2. Avoid forward leaning of the head and trunk
3. Avoid using the upper limbs in a static elevated position
4. Avoid positions which make the body twisted or asymmetrical
5. Avoid postures which require a joint to be used constantly at the limits of its range of motion (Pheasant 1986).

When applying these recommendations to a clinical setting, therapists need to keep in mind that individuals vary greatly in their tolerance of postural stresses. Some individuals may require frequent rest breaks, while others may find visual cues to remind them to take rest breaks beneficial. Still and videotape photography of a client's usual working posture are useful tools to assist therapists in posture re-education.

Physiotherapists and occupational therapists may be required to provide advice regarding lumbar lordosis to an individual with back pain who experiences pain while sitting. While there are contrasting views about what constitutes correct sitting posture, it is important to avoid slumping, which places joints at end-range. Ensuring there is adequate support for the back, and encouraging regular rest breaks may help to minimize slumping.

Aids and equipment may be of help to some individuals to enhance posture. A lumbar roll, for instance, may be used to provide an individual with support for the lower back while sitting. Williams et al (1991) demonstrated the use of the lumbar roll to reduce lumbar and referred pain in the sitting position. Modification to the individual's environment may also promote better posture. Therapists can provide advice regarding rearrangement of the home or work space in order to minimize bending, twisting and reaching movements.

Physical conditioning exercises are important for the mobility and strength of the spine. Physiotherapists advise on specific muscle-strengthening exercises, which help protect the spinal ligaments, joints and discs, and stretching exercises to overcome the stiffness associated with prolonged postures or tense mus-

cles. Such exercises are based on a thorough physical examination of the client (see Chapter 13).

Common strengthening exercises for individuals with chronic low back pain include abdominal, gluteal and quadriceps strengthening (Oliver 1994). Stretching exercises generally involve the iliopsoas, hamstring, erector spinae, upper trapezious and suboccipital muscles (Oliver 1994). Exercises should be simple to perform and the patient can be provided with written instructions to enhance compliance. Physiotherapists may also educate the client on a variety of pain-relieving postures, depending upon the nature of the individual's back pain.

Goal-setting and pacing

Clients with chronic pain can find it immensely useful to engage in goal-setting activities with their occupational therapist or physiotherapist. Rather than an umbrella (and possibly unachievable) goal of 'getting rid of the pain', the person can be assisted to identify and focus on other life goals involving useful functioning, such as travelling to visit family or friends or starting a vocational course to learn new skills.

The practical implications of an approach to lifestyle management based on a 'living despite' pain philosophy are the need to gradually introduce more activities into the client's lifestyle, and the need to ensure that managing these activities is both rewarding and enjoyable for the client.

Clients with chronic pain often experience a change in their usual activity pattern, in addition to changes in expectations about what they can achieve while they have pain. Many clients with chronic pain (and 'well' people!) underestimate their functional abilities. Often this results in a reduction in activity level, although some clients may increase their level of activity in an attempt to 'cope' with their pain. Too much inactivity can lead to physical deconditioning which may contribute to muscle pain and stiffness. Alternatively, overdoing oneself can exacerbate symptoms and cause setbacks for several days.

Therapists encourage clients with chronic pain to re-establish more normal levels of activity (Moran & Strong 1995). Clients are encouraged to change daily activity patterns so that they may function successfully in spite of symptoms. This may involve challenging beliefs that activity is 'bad' for pain, and providing clients with education regarding work-simplification techniques and good body mechanics. Therapists may also encourage family members to shift their responses from concerns about the patient's pain to interest in activity performance.

An important consideration in improving the activity levels of clients with chronic pain involves the setting of sequential, achievable goals. Both short-term and long-term goals need to be considered. Goal setting involves a collaborative process between the patient and the therapist, and therapy is more efficacious when there is a collaborative approach to goal setting (Law et al 1995, Neistadt 1995). Clients are more likely to be satisfied with the service if they have been able to participate in decision-making.

The goal-setting process may include both formal and informal methods to set goals. Formal methods of setting goals usually involve the use of a questionnaire or scale, such as the Occupational Performance History Questionnaire (Kielhofner & Henry 1988) or the Neuropsychiatric Institute (NPI) Interest Checklist (Matsutsuyu 1969). These assessments assist therapists in identifying activities which are important to the client, which can be used to determine goals. The Canadian Occupational Performance Measure (COPM) (Law et al 1991) is a useful tool for goal setting. The COPM utilizes a client-centred philosophy in assisting clients to identify their priorities for therapy (Law et al 1994, Lidstone 1996, Toomey et al 1995), and addresses the client's functioning in the areas of self-care, productivity and leisure (Pollock 1993).

Setting goals can also occur informally during an interview with the client. Key questions to consider when setting goals include:

- The client's daily living routines
- The client's life roles
- The client's interests, values and goals
- The client's perception of ability and assumption of responsibility
- Human and non-human components of the client's environment (Kielhofner & Henry 1988).

It is essential that the goals are realistic and meaningful to the client, and that the client gradually introduces them to their lifestyle. Once goals have been established the client may need to adjust the activity level in order to achieve them. This involves an approach referred to as 'pacing'. Pacing involves introducing tasks in a graded manner, in order for the client to build skills, confidence and tolerance for the activity, so that activity level may be increased. Gradual increases in activity are expected (Harding & Williams 1995). This is particularly important in clients with chronic pain who may be physically deconditioned as a result of reduced activity. In Henriksson's (1995) study, women with fibromyalgia discussed pacing techniques which they found helpful in managing everyday activities. Common techniques included:

- Organizing – the majority of women learned to organize their daily schedule to allow more time to complete tasks and to include necessary rest breaks. Many required several hours to get ready in the morning, due to morning stiffness. Activities were often spaced out to ensure adequate 'downtime'.
- Prioritizing – Many women would complete the most important tasks first, while pain levels were relatively low. Tasks which were deemed most important, varied between the women, reflecting differences in the women's roles and values.
- Flexibility – Many women found that they developed more flexibility in the way they approached tasks. For example, they were able to alternate between light and heavy tasks, change work positions frequently, and adjust their level of activity according to fluctuating pain levels.

Therapists need both to monitor clients' progress in achieving their goals and to help the clients develop the skills to do this themselves, for future use. Barriers to achieving goals will need to be identified and clients should be encouraged to develop problem-solving skills to overcome these barriers. It is also important that the client and therapist re-evaluate their goals to determine whether they are still relevant to the patient's lifestyle.

An important aspect of pacing is taking an overall approach to an activity, to a single day, a week and indeed, to life activities in the long-term. People without their full fitness, agility and freedom of movement may have to accept a reduction in the ability to be as spontaneous, and to act when the desire tempts them, and learn to organize their whole lives in a much more predictable and regular manner. This recommended reduced spontaneity, and freedom, is a significant loss and intrusion upon quality of life for many people. Clients may need guidance to gain confidence in adjusting to a way of thinking which considers the long-term, delayed, benefits of more successful functioning. This requires a shift from a short-term perspective and measure to a long-term view, something that is challenging for people whose confidence and trust may be rather battered by their current and past life experiences.

Box 15.2 provides an example of the integration of goal setting and pacing strategies in the rehabilitation

---

Box 15.2 Case example

Name: Mr S
Age: 53 years
Marital status: Married
Employment: Senior Public Servant, Administrative
History – presenting illness: Low back pain and headache

These complaints related to degenerative vertebral changes for which no curative surgical or medical option was available.

He was supported by his wife who tolerated, but did not support, his obsessional attitudes to almost all activities.

He previously prided himself on putting '110%' into all endeavours, including his job, football coaching and gardening. This approach had been instrumental to his considerable early career advancement, with early promotions, great responsibility, commendations and great expectations. He had similarly been given great recognition and responsibility with football coaching.

He routinely worked very long hours, after hours at home, and on weekends. Holidays, when they were taken, were usually focused on catching up even further on these tasks, leaving little time for rest and recovery, which was increasingly required because of both his condition and the loss of the reserves of youth.

He was a friendly, gregarious but busy gentleman, very generous and well liked, but with little insight regarding the contribution of his approach to his difficulties, especially about how he could aggravate his physical condition by his excessive expectations and habits.

In his usual tendency to extremes, he completely ceased working, coaching and mowing the lawn, berating himself for his inadequacies.

He did, however, have a very good set of standards when advising others, particularly those close to him, and for whom he believed he had a duty of care. He accepted the wisdom of other employees not routinely arriving early, not leaving late, not taking work home and not having holidays, and saw that this provided them with an opportunity for recovery, and to enjoy their lives.

Using his very overgrown lawn as an easily available and controllable project, he gradually accepted the proposition that doing the overall task in steps was a better option than doing nothing, and without the necessity to achieve the level of perfection he had previously demanded. In the past, he did not stop until he had mown all of the considerable lawn, cut and trimmed the edges, and weeded all the garden beds, all in one effort. Following his injury, he needed several days of bed-rest to recover from this task.

Accepting that it would be useful for him to use his considerable skills in good management and coaching, with a graduated programme, with built-in review and encouragement on a 'current personal best' basis, he was eventually able to start the mower and complete a square yard only, as a planned first step.

He learned how to stop the task when it was useful for him, without a period of extended recovery required, rather than being 'externally' dictated to in his activity by the amount of work available.

Again, using his skills of perseverance and self-discipline, he mapped out a plan of graduated increase, based upon his demonstrated recovery time, to do the lawn, edges, and garden in sections, as well as to deal with the considerable emotional turmoil this programme precipitated within him as he battled against his own obsessional impulses. To accomplish this, he had to confront and control emotional pressures based on a personal value system that was no longer useful.

Having achieved control of his 'lawn project' he was then able to generalize, and to apply the new conceptual approach to coaching, accepting new limitations, developing new techniques, and being mindful to develop a balance of his activities such that he no longer worked to exhaustion before he allowed himself to stop.

Replenishment of his reserves had particularly been a more recent issue because of his age, and because of the development of employment and business practices which placed less value on the encouragement from senior management, but which relied on individually competitive outputs. Being somewhat dependent, he was not adept at encouraging himself but excessively reliant upon the praise of others.

Returning to work was more difficult. Initially, he experienced considerable nausea approaching his workplace. The nausea itself was disabling and required a behavioural desensitization programme to eliminate this problem. This program used initially very small goals with a very high probability of achievement, in his own estimation, then increasingly more complicated steps as he became more comfortable.

He initially drove past his building, then walked, then entered it after hours, and later visited during hours, before he recommenced work. He returned to work in a different capacity, with the support of his superior who was also informed about the usefulness of a step-wise approach for returning to work. It is worthwhile remembering that Mr S had been a very successful worker prior to being overcome by his chronic pain condition. He had been consumed by his work, and derived great benefits from it, both economic and personal. And yet the anxiety he felt about returning to his work was a big issue for him, one that needed a sensitive and supportive approach from his therapist (who in this case was a consultant psychiatrist).

Graduated duties recommenced, with an emphasis on having precisely formulated the details of the project before he left home, based upon the degree of confidence (not desire) he had developed from his recent level of functions, with many small increments planned. The finishing point had to be defined before he started each step, not continuing on the basis of how he felt at the time but on the basis of the track record he had recently established. He had to guard against continuing, while he felt good, to the point of failure again.

Relapses occurred, giving an opportunity for review, further learning and a re-commitment to a disciplined approach to resist the temptation to yield to previously well established old desires, which were once cued by the old environment, and which arose again to challenge the new order. Implementing life-long changes is often a challenge, especially for a person with chronic pain.

of a 53-year-old man with low back pain and headache.

Relaxation and biofeedback

Relaxation strategies can be used by clients with chronic and acute pain conditions (e.g. pain of childbirth, dental pain or procedural pain, postoperative pain and chronic back pain). By relaxation we mean 'active relaxation', or the experience of a positive, restful, nonstressful amount of time. It has both a physical and a mental dimension. The main aims of relaxation are:

1. To reduce unnecessary strain on the body
2. To treat stress-related disorders which have already developed
3. As a skill for everyday use for better coping (Payne 1995).

All of these aims can be relevant for the patient with a pain problem. McCaffery and Beebe (1989) suggested that people with pain might benefit from relaxation, due to the influence of pain, muscle tension and anxiety. A study by Strong (1990a) suggested that relaxation for patients with back pain helped in reducing the sensory and affective components of the back pain experience.

Biofeedback is a process whereby the client is provided with relatively immediate information about one of his covert bodily functions (such as muscle tension or skin temperature) via some biophysiological instruments (Blanchard & Young 1974). The client is then encouraged to make voluntary efforts to alter that bodily function.

Relaxation methods can be categorized as primarily physical or mental techniques (Payne 1995). Chronic pain may precipitate tension and spasm in the musculoskeletal system, and around the injury site, which can be reduced by relaxation procedures that are predominantly physical. Chronic pain may also precipitate anxiety, depression and stress-related symptoms which can be positively influenced by both physical and mental techniques. Often the cognitive–behavioural approaches to pain management will include elements of relaxation, particularly goal-directed mental types, as an aid in cognitive restructuring.

The types of physical relaxation techniques which are commonly used, and are suitable for most clinical settings are Mitchell's (1987) physiological relaxation, progressive muscular relaxation, the Alexander technique, stretching and exercise, and breathing methods. Common mental techniques include imagery, goal-directed visualization, mediation and Benson's relaxation response (Benson 1976). These and others are described in various books about relaxation. The book by

Payne (1995) is a particularly useful resource for therapists. Methods which require considerable training (such as meditation) are rarely used by therapists in everyday practices. There are some very useful books with instructions for relaxation (e.g. Bernstein & Borkovec 1973)

Relaxation methods need to be individually tailored. It may take several attempts before the 'best fit' relaxation method is chosen for a particular patient. Aspects to be considered in selecting a relaxation method include:

1. Time available for learning and using it
2. Method of learning most preferred by client
3. Environment to be used
4. Prior experience with types of relaxation
5. The nature of the client's pain condition.

Because relaxation is learned, the client must practice relaxation techniques on a daily basis (Nicholas et al 2000). The individual should begin with short periods of practice, for example 10 minutes, which can be gradually increased over time. Between 20 minutes and an hour is the recommended time-period for daily practice. Clients also need to learn how to integrate relaxation techniques into their daily life. This may involve, for example, assisting clients to identify cues for muscle tension at work. Reminders, such as post-it notes stuck to the computer, can be useful so clients become more aware of muscle tension throughout the day, and can implement relaxation techniques as required.

There will be many pain situations in which some type of relaxation will need to be part of the management regime. Concomitantly, there are almost no pain situations in which relaxation should not at least be considered. Relaxation is not indicated for clients who refuse to participate, clients with a history of psychotic hallucinations or delusions, clients with cardiac problems, or clients who are severely depressed (McCaffery & Beebe 1989).

While relaxation may seem like the most inoffensive technique that could be taught by anyone, therapists need to be aware of the possible powerful effects of relaxation. It is recommended that therapists trial techniques with the clients rather than putting on a relaxation tape and leaving the room. Clients may become very distressed during relaxation sessions, when their defences are lowered. Being there with the client enables the therapist to support the client and help them work through issues. It may be necessary to refer a client on for further assistance, depending upon the problems being faced by the client.

Always try to individualize the relaxation methods used with clients. This is, of course, easier to do in one-to-one sessions with clients, than in group sessions. One of us still remembers running a group relaxation class with a group of nurses in the middle of winter. In keeping with the weather, images of warmth were developed. One participant become more and more tense. In debriefing after the session, it was discovered that the participant lived in the tropics and disliked the heat. Always check out clients' preferences and styles when using imagery in relaxation.

An example of a relaxation script which incorporates Mitchell's physiological relaxation and mental imagery is contained in Box 15.3.

Box 15.3 Relaxation script

Relaxation can be used by an individual to help ease pain, lessen tension in your body, and help you to cope better with stressful situations. Relaxation is a method which has been used extensively with people with pain problems. Relaxation is a method for lessening tension in body and mind. It is a behaviour that can be learned. Learning relaxation is an active process: it requires some time and patience, some self-discipline to practice, and a desire to help better manage with your pain. You should try and practise using relaxation for at least 10 minutes, twice per day. Over a period, you will find that you can more easily develop a relaxed feeling.

A source of considerable stress to a lot of people is the presence of chronic pain. Pain which remains day in and day out can really tire people, and wear them out, wear them down. Relaxation can help the individual to better deal with the stress of living with a chronic pain problem.

There are many techniques that you can use to relax. This tape utilizes a technique where you move different parts of your body to achieve relaxation in the muscles. For example, when you bend your wrist forwards, one set of muscles (your extensors) relax, while the other set of muscles (the flexors) contract.

There are a few pointers which can assist in doing relaxation. First, try and chose a quiet room in which to practice relaxation. Make sure that you are comfortable and warm. Rest on a comfortable bed. Try and avoid interruptions during the session. If there is any part of your body that is feeling particularly painful, don't feel you need to move that part, just concentrate on your normal steady breathing, and join in again after we have passed the painful body part. Let's begin the session now . . .

Just settle yourself comfortably back on the bed or carpet. Loosen any tight clothing, make sure your whole body is supported. Arms resting by your side, your legs straight, feet comfortably resting. Let your eyes gently close, and concentrate on my voice and the instructions I give. Try and block all other thoughts out of your mind and concentrate on my words. Block out all background noises, let them fade from your mind, and begin to focus on your normal steady breathing. As you breathe in, feel your chest wall expand, then as you breathe out, feel the sense of ease that comes into your muscles. Breathe in . . . and out . . . In . . . and out . . . In . . . and out . . . . Just continue to breathe at your own steady pace, and begin to feel the calmness entering your body, feel the tension begin to leave your body . . . breathe in . . . and out.

I want you now to concentrate your thoughts onto your shoulders. Put all other thoughts out of your mind. Now 'pull your shoulders towards your feet'. Now, stop pulling. Notice the feeling. Notice the lengthening and stretching out of your trapezius muscles.

Now, concentrate on your elbows. Move 'your elbows out and open' then, stop moving, and notice the sensations and feelings of this position. Enjoy this new position of ease. Move your thoughts to your hands and move your fingers so they are long and lean instead of curled up and tight. Stretch out your fingers and become aware of the barely perceptible change in your muscles; the elimination of muscle tightness. Concentrate on this new position, and how it feels.

Move your thoughts onto your breathing, your steady normal breathing, breathing in . . . and out . . . In . . . and out. Just keep breathing at this normal steady pace.

Move your thoughts to your lower limbs. Roll your hips outwards, then stop. Notice the ease that comes from moving your hips into this position. Move your thoughts down to your knees and move them so they become comfortable. Move your thoughts down to your feet, and 'push your feet away from your face and then stop'. Note the feeling in your feet. Feel your legs and feet stretched out, relaxed, lengthened. Now push your body back against the surface you are lying on. Then stop pushing. Push your head back into the surface you are lying on, and then stop. Notice how your head and body are being supported. Think of your jaw now, letting your jaw open comfortably. Enjoy this relaxed position for a few moments. Now move your thoughts to your tongue and push it down against your bottom jaw, and then stop and notice how it feels, with your tongue relaxed. Smoothing out the muscles around your eyes and forehead. Feel a sense of ease coming into your face, relaxing, heavy, comfortable. Letting the smile lines around your eyes and the furrows on your brow smooth out and relax. Your whole body now should be feeling really comfortable, very relaxed.

I want you now to enjoy the relaxed feeling of body and mind. Notice how nice it feels, how calm and restful your body feels. Spend a few moments feeling relaxed, comfortable, heavy, too heavy to even move . . . Picture yourself in your favourite place. Imagine this place in your mind's eye. Picture yourself there now. Imagine the colours around you, the noises you can hear in this place. Let yourself enjoy being relaxed in body and mind, in this favourite place . . .

Now, I want you to become aware of where you are, the noises around you, the room in which you are, become aware of your body and how it is feeling. Gently begin to move again, wriggle your toes and fingers. As you do so, remember that this is a relaxation method you can use to help manage better with daily living and to help cope with ongoing pain. Open your eyes, and when you feel ready, you can sit up.

of relaxation training and biofeedback with ...s with various types of pain problems has been well studied (e.g. Linton et al 1985, Strong et al 1989, Strong 1990a, Turner & Chapman 1982). Relaxation has been found to be useful in reducing pain intensity (Level II evidence) (Linton 1986, NIH 1996).

Use of assistive devices

Clients with chronic pain commonly experience limitations in strength, endurance, coordination and range of motion. These limitations can affect the client's ability to perform self-care, household, leisure and vocational tasks. A study by Verbrugge and colleagues (1991) found that elderly clients with chronic pain (arthritis) had more difficulty in physical functions, personal care and household activities than their peers who did not experience chronic pain. Individuals with chronic low back pain experience significant impairment in physical, psychosocial, work and recreational activities (Strong 1996). Such activities may aggravate pain to the extent that the individual is unable to perform them.

Limitations in functional capacities can result in loss of self-esteem and an increased sense of dependence for clients with chronic pain (Strong 1996). A comprehensive evaluation of the client's abilities and limitations in self-care, work and leisure activities is therefore warranted. The occupational therapist assesses the client's occupational performance skills, and works with the client to identify problems that interfere with functional performance. Depending upon limitations identified in the assessment, the occupational therapist may recommend an assistive device to help the client achieve a higher level of functioning.

An assistive device refers to equipment that is purchased 'off-the-shelf' or is modified for a particular purpose (Schemm & Gitlin 1998). The purpose of an assistive device for a client with chronic pain is to improve the client's ability to perform tasks independently and to assist with reducing discomfort and pain (Strong 1996). Assistive devices commonly used by clients with chronic pain include lumbar support cushions, dressing sticks, shoehorns, etc.

There is some controversy in the literature regarding the use of assistive devices for clients with chronic pain (Engel 1990, Strong 1990b, Tyson & Strong 1990). Assistive devices may reinforce a client's pain behaviour, encourage dependency and reduce self-confidence (Dear & Steuart-Corry 1997). However, the use of a simple assistive device may mean the difference between enabling a person with chronic pain to perform an activity which others take for granted, or not performing the activity at all (Strong 1996).

Furthermore, a study examining the use and perceived benefit of assistive devices among 40 clients with chronic low back pain, found that 85% of participants perceived the device to be of some benefit (Tyson & Strong 1990). Nonetheless, a proper evaluation of the patient's need for the assistive device is important to ensure that the device is appropriate for the individual in question. The client's values, roles, interests and motivation for acquiring and using the device need to be considered, in addition to the patient's functional limitations.

Another important consideration in providing a client with an assistive device, involves education and training in the use of the device (Weilandt & Strong 2000). Research has shown that instruction and training in the use of equipment for clients and the family is a major factor in the acceptance and subsequent use of a device (Tyson & Strong 1990). Furthermore, *adequacy* of instruction influences assistive device use (Schemm & Gitlin 1998). Clients need to be able to practice using the devices during treatment sessions, and be given opportunities to integrate the device into their daily life.

Other methods used to facilitate the functional performance of individuals with chronic pain include: education in work-simplification techniques, advice regarding environmental modification and exercises for physical conditioning. These techniques are discussed elsewhere in this chapter.

PERSONAL ISSUES OF A LIFESTYLE WITH PAIN

Managing sexuality with pain

Sexuality, and other aspects of intimate relationships, can be considerably affected by the presence of pain. While acute pain may briefly impair this area of life, it is in the chronic pain conditions that the therapist needs to consider assessment and intervention.

Clients with rheumatoid arthritis and those with chronic low back pain often experience difficulties with sexual activity, and there is some likelihood that depression associated with pain may play a part. Kraaimaat et al (1996) reported other studies that found that sexual activity and pleasure are reduced in clients with rheumatoid arthritis. In their study, they also found that clients who report higher levels of impact of their rheumatoid arthritis on their sexuality differed on self-report of mobility, self-care, pain and depression from those who reported low levels of impact. The study also examined gender differences, but found that being male or female did not influence intrusiveness of rheumatoid arthritis on sexuality.

While the relief provided by analgesic medication can help, other side-effects such as reduced libido from narcotics and antidepressant medication, and sedation from benzodiazepines, may need to be assessed.

Fear of pain and fatigue may also impact on sexual activity in individuals with chronic pain. Methods commonly employed to reduce pain and prevent fatigue are: using supportive positions such as lying in the most comfortable positions and using pillows, selecting suitable times of day or night when medications are most effective, and resting prior to and after sexual activities (Kennedy 1987). There are a number of books and a video (Hunter Region Rehabilitation Services 1985) available which discuss positions for sexual activity and the issue of sex for individuals with chronic pain (e.g. Nicholas et al 2000, Parker & Main 1995, Strong 1996).

The implications of these findings for therapists are that they need to deal with mobility, self-care and pain as much as possible in treatment, with the aim of improving capacity for a pleasurable sexual lifestyle. Some clients should be referred for sexual counselling. Kraaimaat et al (1996) indicated that clients might benefit from help to focus on pleasurable sensations or fantasies instead of on pain. A cognitive–behavioural approach may be very useful, because it involves a restructuring of focus for the client.

Issues of sexuality may not be easy to introduce, because reserve and embarrassment may be felt by both the patient and the therapist. On the therapist's part, he or she must understand that sexuality is an essential part of lifestyle, and needs to be considered if the whole person is to be treated. Usually the reserve felt by the therapist in raising and discussing the issue will diminish over time and experience. It is useful to have read some of the studies which give information about problems pain clients have with sexuality and the methods which have been used successfully. Being sure of your information can provide confidence in a difficult discussion. Additionally, practising talking about sexuality – perhaps with other therapists or colleagues – may increase confidence.

Therapists should remember that if the therapist declines to address the issue of sex and pain, it might not be discussed with the patient by anyone. People often assume they need permission from others before they can discuss such intimate personal issues, and the therapist has an important role in normalizing and modelling by providing an example as to how such a discussion can be reasonably conducted while still respecting proper interpersonal boundaries. Alter-

natively, if therapists do no raise the issue of sexuality, clients who do have sexual difficulties may assume that the problems are untreatable, adding considerably to relationship stress.

Often it may be tactful to introduce the topic to the client by providing some background information – either written or verbal – about problems with sexuality that clients with pain experience, and later exploring if this is an area of concern to the client. A direct question about the client's sexuality may be a little too blunt for both parties. However, some persistence may be required to explore the area. It is then possible to refer the person to an appropriate therapist, if there are indications that a problem exists.

Managing sleep with pain

Many individuals with chronic pain report difficulties with sleeping. Problems may include: an inability to fall asleep, an inability to maintain sleep and early awakening. Several laboratory-based studies indicate that clients with chronic pain have more light sleep, less deep sleep and more waking than clients without pain (Lamberg 1999, Wittig 1982).

In describing their sleeping problems, clients with chronic pain may report that they have difficulty obtaining and maintaining a comfortable position in which to go to sleep – they 'roll over' onto the painful part and wake up. Others may state that they are frequently wakened due to pain from a sustained position or a change in position while in bed. There are also clients who report problems with sleeping, who do not cite pain as a specific cause. In these cases, characteristics of the chronic pain syndrome such as anxiety and depression may be a contributing factor.

Specific enquiry is normally needed to obtain a history about snoring with this being important because of the association with sleep apnoea, and subsequent serious health problems.

Difficulties with sleeping may pose serious implications for clients with chronic pain. A study which examined the sleeping habits of 100 out-clients with chronic pain, found clients with sleep difficulties were more likely to report greater degrees of pain and physical disability (Pilowsky et al 1985). Poor sleep has also been associated with increased daytime fatigue, irritability and somatic complaints (Lamberg 1999). Research has found that clients complaining of chronic pain and poor sleep show significantly more affective disturbance, particularly depression, than clients reporting good sleep (Pilowsky et al 1985, Wittig et al 1982). It is unclear whether clients experience disturbed sleep as a result of depression or whether poor sleep leads to depression. Regardless of the cause, therapists need to be aware of the relationship between poor sleep and depression, when treating clients with chronic pain. The patient's underlying depression needs to be addressed before improvement in sleep can be expected.

Considering the impact poor sleep may have on an individual's lifestyle it is important that therapists are aware of strategies which may alleviate sleep disturbance in clients with chronic pain. Successful management of sleep difficulties generally involves both behavioural and psychological strategies (Lamberg 1999, Rogers 1997). A simple behavioural strategy involves the patient keeping a sleep-diary, in which the quantity and quality of his or her sleep is recorded. Important observations and concerns may be revealed by discussion with an observant partner who may be harbouring significant concerns about this aspect. Clients keep an account of behaviour and mood prior to going to bed, which may be used to identify particular behaviours or attitudes which interfere with sleep. Additionally, it may reveal to the patient that his or her sleeping pattern is within a healthy, average range. This knowledge may serve to improve sleep by reducing anxiety.

Using information obtained from the sleep-diary or by interview with the patient the therapist can educate clients about behaviours that are inconsistent with good sleep. This process is referred to as 'sleep hygiene'. Practices which interfere with good sleep include: excessive intake of caffeine, vigorous exercise near bedtime and sleeping in an uncomfortable environment (Rogers 1997). Sleeping late in the mornings, taking naps whenever tired and having an irregular schedule for activities can make falling asleep difficult, as this interferes with the self-sustaining properties of a regular sleep–wake pattern (Lamberg 1999, Rogers 1997).

The therapist's role is to assist the patient in recognizing the impact of their behaviour on sleep and in making the necessary modifications in behaviours or sleep environments. This may involve strategies such as reducing caffeine and alcohol intake, smoking cessation, reducing noise in the sleeping environment and establishing a regular time for going to bed at night and getting out of bed in the morning.

Another practice which contributes to sleep difficulties is the habit of staying in bed for activities other than sleep (Rogers 1997). Individuals with chronic pain may spend a considerable amount of time resting in bed, in an attempt to relieve pain or because of fatigue. Clients are encouraged to reserve the bed for night-time sleeping and to rest elsewhere, to minimize the association between the patient's bed and being awake. This technique is referred to as stimulus control, and attempts to re-associate the bed with sleep. The aim is to develop an appropriate conditioned response of bed and sleep instead of bed and work or worry or pain.

Exercise has a positive effect on sleep, however many individuals with chronic pain decrease their level of activity as a result of their pain. It is important to encourage the individual to increase his or her activity, while pacing the activity within pain levels. Guidelines for exercise for individuals with chronic pain are discussed in Chapter 13.

Moderate exercise should be avoided several hours before going to bed, as exercise late during the day raises the level of autonomic arousal which can create problems falling asleep. Additionally, engaging in frustrating activities or excessive anxiety close to bedtime may result in arousal and prevent sleep. Clients are therefore encouraged to establish a relaxing routine in preparation for sleep. Reading and listening to music are often chosen as sedentary activities for this, as long as they do not involve a lot of problem-solving or excitement.

Pain is a major factor which may disrupt sleep in individuals with chronic pain. Therapists may provide clients with education about postures likely to aggravate pain and advice regarding sleeping postures to relieve pain. For example, sleeping on the stomach as been associated with neck pain, because the individual must sustain their head in rotation in order to breathe. Pain-relieving postures may involve the positioning of pillows for support and comfort. A client's pain medication may also interfere with sleeping. For instance non-steroidal anti-inflammatory drugs may increase waking and delay deep sleep (Lamberg 1999). Clients may benefit from discussing their pain medication regime with their doctor. If possible, the clients' medication timing may be altered to match the periods when the patient is awake and asleep. If pain medication is needed during the night, then it should be kept close beside the bed with anything else that is required for taking the medication. Use of sedative medication during the day can encourage an unwise reverse sleep–wake cycle.

Some clients may find it helpful to train and habituate their body to a longer sleep cycle. To use this strategy, clients record the time when they fell asleep and the time at which they awoke for 4–5 days. An alarm is then set for approximately half an hour before the patient's earliest recorded wake period for the next few days. For example, if the patient woke up at 5.30, 6.00, 6.15 and 6.00, then the alarm is set for 5.00. The patient must get up at 5.00 am. The alarm is set for 5.00 until the patient is reliably sleeping until 5.00, waking when the alarm rings. Then the alarm is readjusted to 5.15 or 5.30. The intervals of increase should be small if the patient has had difficulty sleeping until the ringing of the alarm. This programme can be continued until the client has achieved a more restful sleep. Unfortunately, although this strategy has been used successfully in some clinics, there is no published data to show whether this approach is better than any other.

Psychological techniques are often used to assist clients with sleeping difficulties. Useful techniques for clients with chronic pain include cognitive–behavioural techniques and relaxation training. Cognitive–behavioural techniques have been described more fully in Chapter 9. Cognitive–behavioural therapy can help alter negative thoughts and attitudes about sleep, and promote clients' perception of control of the sleeping process. For example, clients may be encouraged to alter their thoughts from, 'it is impossible to sleep when I am in pain', to 'it is sometimes difficult to sleep when I am in pain, but I have managed to sleep in the past'.

Cognitive–behavioural techniques often include relaxation training. The goal of relaxation is to reduce the patient's level of cognitive and physiological arousal, thereby assisting with the induction of sleep. Studies have demonstrated that relaxation reduces the level of sympathetic activity and increases parasympathetic activity, which promotes the onset of sleep (NIH Technology Assessment 1996).

There are a number of approaches to help clients with chronic pain to obtain a restful night's sleep. It is important to encourage the client to try a number of strategies, in order to discover those most effective for the patient. However it is important that sleep is not treated in an isolated manner. Aspects of the patient's daily life, ranging from spousal relationships to work demands, also impact on sleep. A holistic framework when working with clients with chronic pain is therefore recommended.

Active involvement of the client in decision-making

Increasingly, health services are moving away from the traditional medical model in which health professionals define problems and make decisions for their clients, to an enablement model that aims to shift autonomy, control and responsibility back to the client. Pollock (1993) argues that if the client is not the problem-definer then it will be unlikely that she or he will

be the problem-solver either. The concept of client involvement in decision-making reflects a core philosophy of occupational therapy and physiotherapy, and is a recurring theme throughout this book.

An approach in which clients become active participants in their healthcare acknowledges aspects of the patient's lifestyle which are unique to the individual. One person's occupational needs and abilities will not be the same as any other persons. When clients are actively involved in decision-making, treatment is likely to be more meaningful for the patient, as it reflects the importance of their roles, environments and culture. This is important when working with clients with chronic pain, as chronic pain is a multidimensional phenomenon, involving physical, psychological and social domains.

The role of the occupational therapist and physiotherapist, in the client-centred approach, is to provide information and guided experience to enable the client to make appropriate decisions regarding therapy. While clients are considered to be experts about their occupational function, the occupational therapist possesses the expertise to facilitate solutions to a broad range of occupational performance issues associated with chronic pain. For example, occupational therapists may provide advice on body mechanics, environmental modification, relaxation techniques or assistive devices. Information should be provided in a format that is understandable and that will enable clients to make decisions about their needs.

It is important that clients recognize that all activities, and avoidance of activities, have both a possibility of benefit and a risk of failure of varying degree (Law et al 1995). Practice can be used as a valuable learning experience, provided that the client is able to understand the risks associated with the decision (Law et al 1995). However, therapists need to be able to openly discuss such issues with clients. Obviously therapists cannot support actions which are unethical, could involve excessive risk of harm or are considered malpractice. In such instances therapists must firmly state that they cannot support the client's plan. On the other hand, some clients may be reluctant to assume responsibility for their care.

It is important to explore reasons why clients are reluctant to accept responsibility in their treatment. Lack of confidence, anger, excessive reliance on others, fear of pain, depression, lack of knowledge regarding pain or belief in a medical 'cure' are just some of the reasons which may affect a client's willingness to accept responsibility in their treatment. Occupational therapists and physiotherapists must discuss these issues with the client, and work together towards potential solutions. An important role of the occupational therapist and physiotherapist is to help the client develop a judgement which is useful and appropriate to their changed situation. The judgements and practices of the past, or of others, are no longer necessarily applicable.

Client involvement in decision-making during therapy has been shown to facilitate the development of rapport, promote treatment participation and satisfaction, and empower the patient by encouraging independence, personal control, self-determination and self-esteem (Mew & Fossey 1996). Studies have demonstrated that active involvement of clients in decision-making can result in shorter hospital stays (Shendell-Falik 1990), and better goal attainment and outcomes for the patient (Czar 1987) than a traditional medical model approach. Considering the escalating costs associated with treatment of clients with chronic pain, approaches which enhance the effectiveness of therapy are of great importance. Involving the patient in decision-making is a relatively simple, yet effective, means of achieving more effective outcomes

The role of social support

The type and degree of social support available to an individual with chronic pain will have some influence on their lifestyle. In most chronic conditions the presence of social support is a positive factor. Linton (1994) suggested that the family might provide a source of social support that provides a buffer to the problems associated with chronic pain. For example, family members are able to offer encouragement, distraction, praise and compassionate listening. In addition to support, family members can also provide tangible assistance to an individual with chronic pain.

On the other hand, support from family members may sometimes serve as positive reinforcement of pain behaviours. An individual with chronic pain may learn that displays of pain behaviour lead to positive social consequences such as attention, sympathy, and avoidance of unwanted marital or family responsibilities (Gil et al 1987). Consequently, family support may actually sustain pain behaviours and encourage disability in individuals with chronic pain. A study by Latham and Davis (1994) found that higher levels of pain and lower levels of activity are reported by clients with low back pain who are married to spouses who were viewed as being solicitous.

An important role of the therapist is to educate the patient's family about the chronic pain cycle. This should include the role of social learning in the maintenance of pain behaviours and advice on appropriate responses to pain behaviours. An example of an appropriate response may be for family members to allow clients with chronic pain more time to complete an activity, rather than completing the activity on the patient's behalf. Families need to appreciate the importance of focusing on an individual's achievements and adaptive behaviours. This strategy fits in well with the operant–behavioural model, and has an overall goal of reducing pain behaviours and increasing activity levels in clients with chronic pain (further discussion of the operant–behavioural approach can be found in Chapter 9).

Individuals with chronic pain may find some support from those in a similar situation. Support or self-help groups for people with chronic pain may provide fertile ground for the exchange of ideas and information regarding techniques for lifestyle management (Baptiste & Herman 1982, Herman & Baptiste 1981). Shared problem-solving and positive role modelling are other potential benefits. Not all clients, however, would be suited to support groups, and it is recommended that people with chronic pain maintain contact with non-pain-related social outlets. Some caution is needed to ensure that the well-intended supporters are not encouraging inappropriate and unhelpful approaches.

There is considerable evidence in the literature regarding the buffering effect of social support gained from outside family networks. Social support has been found to buffer against adverse effects of life stress on physical and mental health (Iso-Ahola & Park 1996). This is particularly important for clients with chronic pain as, for many, ongoing pain is seen as a source of considerable stress (Turner et al 1987). Individuals with chronic pain, however, often experience a limited social network as a result of withdrawing from activities due to pain or depression. Clients who can maintain membership of, and active involvement in, such groups as sporting clubs, church, volunteer work, hobby groups and so on, will often fare better in maintaining a positive focus. Consequently, the maintenance of social contacts and involvement in leisure activities is an important component of a pain management programme, assisting towards the balanced lifestyle that most people aspire to.

Leisure and the individual with chronic pain

A major problem faced by individuals with chronic pain is an increase in discretionary time. This particularly applies to individuals who no longer work, or who have experienced limitations in other roles due to pain. Lyons (1987) considered that discretionary time may provide the opportunity for self-fulfillment through activity or it may lead to boredom, loneliness and depression. Despite recognition of the problems associated with increased discretionary time, leisure receives little attention in chronic pain practice. In clinical settings the focus is generally on essential functions such as activities of daily living and work, rather than leisure (Strong 1996). Strong (1996) observed that this neglect is reflected in the lack of attention leisure receives in the chronic pain literature.

Leisure is a difficult concept to define. Generally a leisure activity contains components of enjoyment, lack of evaluation, relaxation, freedom of choice and intrinsic motivation (Shaw 1985), although there is no universally accepted definition of leisure in the literature. The meaning of leisure varies between individuals, yet it is frequently cited as a problem among clients with chronic pain (Follick et al 1985). Lack of recreation, isolation and loneliness can be most *distressing* problems encountered by people with physical disabilities, although issues such as work, money and daily living feature as the most prominent problems (Blaxter 1976). A person who has been particularly preoccupied and dependent upon work before illness/injury may have few skills, and at times significant personal issues (e.g. guilt) regarding use of leisure time.

Leisure-generated social support has been consistently related to positive adjustment to stress. Companionship in shared leisure activities has been shown to buffer life stress and enhance psychological wellbeing of those who are exposed to varying levels of stress. The buffering effect is related to the individual's belief that friends or family would provide assistance should a crisis arise. Perceived support has been shown to be more important than received support in predicting adjustment to stressful life events (Coleman & Iso-Ahola 1993).

While leisure-generated support has been identified as an important tool for stress management, it can also enhance stress, especially if it undermines an individual's sense of freedom and control (Coleman & Iso-Ahola 1993). A client may experience obligatory and unwanted social contacts through leisure, or a number of well meaning friends may provide the individual with conflicting advice. It is important, therefore, that the client is able to be assertive. Occupational therapists can offer training in communication skills, if clients experience stress when dealing with their existing social support structure.

Leisure is also a buffer against stress because it can foster a sense of control and mastery, and can be considered a coping strategy in itself (Coleman 1993). A qualitative study by Reynolds (1997) looked at the impact of leisure participation in 35 women with chronic pain. Leisure participation was associated with a number of positive effects relating to increased sense of achievement and personal worth, relief from anxiety and depression, and distraction from other negative feelings (such as pain). Some women described leisure participation as a means of providing structure to their day, which helped to overcome feelings of boredom. Many people may benefit from leisure because it brings opportunities for enjoyment and happiness into daily life, for alternative outlets, roles, achievement and skills.

Leisure activities need to be appropriate for the individual in question. Interest checklists and activity configurations may be used by the occupational therapist to identify suitable leisure activities for clients with chronic pain. Individuals with chronic pain may find it difficult to engage in physically orientated pursuits (Strong 1996). Activities which can help with the physical aspects of pain, for example yoga or a tai-chi group, can be encouraged. Similarly sedentary activities may increase pain in individuals with chronic pain. Techniques to facilitate leisure participation include social skills training, environmental adaptation, rest breaks, and advice on body mechanics.

It is common for people not to have considered or explored their full potential in alternative activities, often enjoying a preoccupation with one or two. The forced need to change is again a significant loss, often associated with grief, despair and irritation, but the task of assisting a person in the gentle art of having fun, often in an area of activity not previously contemplated, is a most important and enjoyable aspect of helping them towards an improved quality of life.

CONCLUSION

In this chapter, an examination has been made of a number of lifestyle issues which therapists would do well to consider when working with clients with chronic pain problems. Given the chronicity of many pain problems, it is important that therapists broaden their focus beyond the mere elimination of the person's pain. This is, of course, not to deny the value of a focus upon pain relief. However, for many of the clients therapists see with chronic pain, a more fruitful focus may be upon living despite the pain. Attention to lifestyle issues can help clients to live better with chronic pain.

Study questions/questions for revision

1. Identify why it is important for therapists to consider lifestyle issues with clients with chronic pain.

2. How can you go about goal-setting with a patient?
3. What types of relaxation techniques can you use with clients with chronic pain?
4. What are the essential principles of good manual handling techniques?

ACKNOWLEDGEMENTS

I would like to thank Dr Frank New, for his expert comments on this chapter and for the case reported in Box 15.1, Mrs Thea New, for reviewing the chapter from the physiotherapy perspective, and Ms Jennifer Sturgess and Ms Michele Adams, for their help in the preparation of this chapter.

REFERENCES

Baptiste S, Herman E 1982 Group therapy: A specific model. In Roy D, Tunks E (eds) Chronic Pain – Psychosocial Factors in Rehabilitation. Williams & Wilkins, Baltimore, pp 166–177

Benson H 1976 The Relaxation Response. Collins, London

Bernstein D A, Borkovec T D 1973 Progressive Relaxation Training: a manual for the helping professions. Research Press, Champaign, Illinois

Bettencourt C M 1995 Ergonomics and injury prevention programs. In: Jacobs K, Bettencourt CM (eds) Ergonomics for Therapists. Butterworth-Heinemann, Boston pp 185–203

Blanchard E B, Young L D 1974 Clinical applications of biofeedback training, a review of evidence. Archives of General Psychiatry 30: 573–589

Blaxter M 1976 The Meaning of Disability. Heineman Educational Books Ltd, London

Coleman D 1993 Leisure based social support, leisure dispositions and health. Journal of Leisure Research 25: 350–361

Coleman D, Iso-Ahola S E 1993 Leisure and health: the role of social support and self-determination. Journal of Leisure Research 25: 111–128

Czar M 1987 Two methods of goal setting in middle-aged adults facing critical life changes. Clinical Nurse Specialist 1: 171–177

Dear J, Steuart-Corry L 1997 Provide skills, not equipment. Therapy Weekly 23: 7

Engel J 1990 Commentary on 'adaptive equipment: its effectiveness for people with chronic lower back pain'. Occupational Therapy Journal of Research 10: 122–130

Enwemeka C S, Bonet I M, Ingle J A 1986 Postural correction in persons with neck pain. Journal of Orthopaedic and Sports Physical Therapy 8: 240–242

Follick M J, Smith T W, Ahern D K 1985 The sickness impact profile: a global measure of disability in chronic low back pain. Pain 21: 67–76

Friedrich M, Gittler G, Halberstadt Y, Cermak T, Heiller I 1998 Combined exercise and motivation program: Effect on the compliance and level of disability of patients with chronic low back pain: A randomized controlled trial. Archives of Physical Medicine Rehabilitation 79: 475–487

Gil K M, Keefe F J, Crisson J E, Van Dalfsen P J 1987 Social support and pain behaviour. Pain 29: 209–217

Harding V, Williams A C de C 1995 Extending physiotherapy skills using a psychological approach: cognitive–behavioral management of chronic pain. Physiotherapy 81: 681–687

Henriksson C M 1995 Living with continuous muscular pain – patient perspectives. Part II: Strategies for daily life. Scandinavian Journal of Caring Sciences 9: 77–86

Herman E, Baptiste S 1981 Pain control: Mastery through group experience. Pain, 10, 79–86

Hunter Region Rehabilitation Services 1985 Back to sex: lower back pain and sexuality (video). Medical Communications Unit, Royal Newcastle Hospital in association with the Hunter Region Rehabilitation Services, Newcastle, Australia

Iso-Ahola S E, Park C J 1996 Leisure-related social support and self-determination as buffers of stress–illness relationship. Journal of Leisure Research 28: 169–187

Jensen G M, Lorish C D 1994 Promoting patient cooperation with exercise programs. Arthritis Care and Research 7: 181–189

Kennedy M 1987 Occupational therapists as sexual rehabilitation professionals using the rehabilitative frame of reference. Canadian Journal of Occupational Therapy 54: 189–193

Kielhofner G, Henry A 1988 Development and investigation of the occupational performance history interview. American Journal of Occupational Therapy 42: 489–498

Kraaimaat F W, Bakker A H, Janssen E, Bijlsma J W 1996 Intrusiveness of rheumatoid arthritis on sexuality in male and female patients living with a spouse. Arthritis Care and Research 9(2): 120–125

Kramer J 1981 Intervertebral disc disease. Year Book Publishers, Chicago

Labbe E E 1988 Sexual dysfunction in chronic back pain patients. Clinical Journal of Pain 4: 143–149

Lamberg L 1999 Chronic pain linked with poor sleep; exploration of causes and treatment. Journal of the American Medical Association 281: 691–692

Large R G, Strong J 1997 The personal constructs of coping with chronic low back pain. Pain 73: 245–252

Latham J, Davis B D 1994 The socioeconomic impact of chronic pain. Disability and Rehabilitation 16: 39–44

Law M, Baptiste S, Carswell-Opzoomer A, McColl M A, Polatajko H, Pollock N 1991 Canadian Occupational Performance Measure. Canadian Association of Occupational Therapists, Toronto

Law M, Baptiste S, Mills J 1995 Client-centered practice: What does it mean and does it make a difference? Canadian Journal of Occupational Therapy 62: 250–257

Law M, Polatajko H, Pollock N, McColl M A, Carswell A, Baptiste S 1994 Pilot testing of the Canadian Occupational Therapy Performance measure: clinical and measurement issues. Canadian Journal of Occupational Therapy 61: 191–197

Lidstone P J 1996 Family-centred assessment and goal-setting for occupational therapy in early education. Honours Thesis, Department of Occupational Therapy, University of Queensland

Linton S J 1982 A critical review of behavioural treatments for chronic benign pain other than headache. British Journal of Clinical Psychology 21: 321–337

Linton S J 1986 Behavioural remediation of chronic pain: a status report. Pain 24: 125–141

Linton S J 1994 The role of psychological factors in back pain and its remediation. Pain Reviews 1: 231–243

Linton S J, Melin L, Stjernlof K 1985 The effects of applied relaxation on chronic pain. Behavioural Psychotherapy 13: 87–100

Lyons R F 1987 Leisure adjustment to chronic illness and disability. Journal of Leisurability 14: 4–10

Matsutsuyu J 1969 The Interest Checklist. American Journal of Occupational Therapy 23: 368–373

McCaffery M, Beebe A 1989 Pain: Clinical manual for nursing practice. C V Mosby, St Louis

McGill S M 1998 Low back exercises: Evidence for improving exercise regimens. Physical Therapy 78: 754–763

Melvin J L 1986 Fibromyalgia syndrome: getting healthy. American Occupational Therapy Association, Bethesda

Mew M M, Fossey E 1996 Client-centered aspects of clinical reasoning during an initial assessment using the Canadian Occupational Performance Measure. Australian Journal of Occupational Therapy 43: 155–166

Mitchell L 1987. Simple relaxation. The Mitchell method for easing tension, 2nd Edn. John Murray, London

Moran M, Strong J 1995. Outcomes of a rehabilitation program for patients with chronic back pain. British Journal of Occupational Therapy 58: 55–60

Neistadt M E 1995 Methods of assessing clients' priorities: A survey of adult physical dysfunction settings. American Journal of Occupational Therapy 49: 428–436

Nicholas M, Molloy A, Tonkin L, Beeston L 2000 Practical and positive ways of adapting to chronic pain. Manage your pain. Australian Broadcasting Corporation, Sydney

NIH Technology Assessment Panel 1996 Integration of behavioral and relaxation approaches into the treatment of chronic pain and insomnia. Journal of the American Medical Association 276: 313–318

Oliver J 1994 Back Care. An illustrated guide. Butterworth Heinemann, Oxford

Parker H, Main C J 1995 Living with Back Pain. Manchester University Press, Manchester

Payne R A 1995 Relaxation Techniques: A practical handbook for the health care professional. Churchill Livingstone, Edinburgh

Pheasant S 1986 Bodyspace. Anthropometry, Ergonomics and Design. Taylor & Francis, London

Pilowsky I, Crettenden I, Townley M 1985 Sleep disturbance in pain clinic patients. Pain 23: 27–33

Pollock N 1993 Client-centered assessment. American Journal of Occupational Therapy 47: 298–301

Protas E J 1996 Aerobic exercise in the rehabilitation of individuals with chronic low back pain: a review. Clinical Reviews in Physical and Rehabilitation Medicine 8: 283–295

Reynolds F 1997 Coping with chronic illness and disability through creative needlecraft. British Journal of Occupational Therapy 60: 352–358

Rogers A E 1997 Nursing management of sleep disorders Part 2: Behavioural interventions. American Nephrology Nurses' Association 24: 672–680

Schemm R L, Gitlin L N 1998 How occupational therapists teach older patients to use bathing and dressing devices in rehabilitation. American Journal of Occupational Therapy 52: 276–282

Shaw S M 1985 The meaning of leisure in everyday life. Leisure Sciences 7: 1–24

Shendell-Falik N 1990 Creating self-care units in the acute care setting: A case study. Patient Education and Counselling 15: 39–45

Sjogren K, Fugl-Meyer A R 1981 Chronic back pain and sexuality. International Journal of Rehabilitation Medicine 3: 19–2

Strong J 1990a Relaxation and chronic pain. British Journal of Occupational Therapy 54: 216–218

Strong J 1990b Commentary response on 'adaptive equipment: its effectiveness for people with chronic lower back pain'. Occupational Therapy Journal of Research 10, 131–133

Strong J 1996 Chronic Pain: The occupational therapist's perspective. Churchill Livingstone, Edinburgh

Strong J, Cramond T, Maas F 1989 The effectiveness of relaxation techniques with patients who have chronic low back pain. Occupational Therapy Journal of Research 9: 184–192

Strong J, Large R G 1995 Coping with chronic pain: an idiographic exploration through focus groups. International Journal of Psychiatry in Medicine 25: 361–377

Toomey M, Nicholson D, Carswell A 1995 The clinical utility of the Canadian Occupational Performance Measure. Canadian Journal of Occupational Therapy 62: 242–249

Turner J A, Chapman C R 1982 Psychological interventions for chronic pain: a critical review. I. Relaxation training and biofeedback. Pain 12: 1–21

Turner J A, Clarcy S, Vitaliano P P 1987 Relationships of stress, appraisal and coping to chronic low back pain. Behaviour Research Therapy 25: 281–288

Tyson R, Strong J 1990 Adaptive equipment: its effectiveness for people with chronic lower back pain. Occupational Therapy Journal of Research 10: 111–121

Verbrugge L M, Lepkowski J M, Konkol L L 1991 Levels of disability among U S adults with arthritis. Journal of Gerontology 46: s71–83

Waddell G, Newton M, Henderson I, Somerville D, Main C J 1993 A Fear–Avoidance Beliefs Questionnaire (FABQ) and the role of fear-avoidance in chronic low back pain and disability. Pain 52: 157–168

Wallace M, Buchle P 1987 Ergonomic aspects of neck and upper limb disorders. International Review of Ergonomics 1: 173–198

Wielandt T, Strong J 2000 Compliance with prescribed

adaptive equipment: a literature review. British Journal of Occupational Therapy 63: 65–75

Williams M M, Hawley J A, McKenzie R A, van Wijmen P M 1991 A comparison of the effects of two sitting postures on back and referred pain. Spine 16: 1185–1191

Wittig R M, Zorick F J, Blumer D, Heilbronn M, Roth T 1982 Disturbed sleep in patients complaining of chronic pain. Journal of Nervous and Mental Disease 170: 429–431

16

Pharmacology of pain management

Anthony Wright
Heather A. E. Benson
James O'Callaghan

OVERVIEW

Drug therapies provide an important means of managing pain, both in the acute and chronic situations. A number of different groups of drugs are available that produce analgesia through a variety of mechanisms and with varying degrees of effectiveness (see Box 16.1). These drugs may also be administered in a variety of ways to provide effective treatment in different situations. This chapter highlights distinctions between inflammatory pain and neuropathic pain and outlines a range of drug therapies for each type of pain. Distinctions are made between the various

---

Box 16.1   Key terms defined

Analgesic drug – A drug that relieves pain due to multiple causes.

Adjuvant drugs – Drugs used in combination with analgesic drugs in the management of pain.

Endogenous opioids – A generic term referring to three groups of endogenous opioid peptides: the enkephalins, the endorphins and the dynorphins.

Non-steroidal anti-inflammatory drugs (NSAIDs) – Drugs with an anti-inflammatory action that are not classified as steroids.

Opioids – Exogenous and endogenous chemicals acting on opioid receptors.

Tolerance – The reduction in physiological response to a drug after repeated administration.

Physical dependence – This is a physiological problem in which a withdrawal syndrome will develop if the drug is suddenly withdrawn or if an antagonist drug is administered.

Psychological dependence/addiction – A behavioural problem involving the compulsive search for and use of the drug for reasons other than the intended medical indication. It involves a 'craving' for the drug.

categories of drugs and information is provided about the mechanisms of action of different drugs, their routes of administration, their effects and effectiveness and any side-effects that they might cause. Some examples are given of clinical situations in which particular drugs or methods of administration might be used and some examples of effective combinations of pharmacological therapies and physical therapies are suggested.

Melzack and Wall's (1965) 'Gate Control Theory' provides an important explanation of the body's ability to modulate nociceptive signals passing through the dorsal horn of the spinal cord (Melzack & Wall 1965). This gating mechanism opens at times, resulting in significant pain being experienced, while at other times, central inhibitory mechanisms are active, markedly reducing the nociceptive signal travelling to the brain. An explanation of these processes is provided in Chapter 3. Following damage to the nervous system itself, either peripherally or centrally, these pain inhibitory systems may become less effective. Further information on this topic is provided in Chapter 18.

There is now evidence showing that, with chronic pain, changes occur in both the peripheral and central nervous systems, leading to increased sensitivity of the nociceptive system (see Chapter 3 for a detailed explanation of these processes).

A clear understanding of the neurophysiology of pain perception and pain modulation provides an important basis for understanding the actions of various classes of analgesic drugs. In this chapter, different classes of analgesic drugs will be discussed in terms of their mechanisms of action, their site of action, their effects and side-effects, and the clinical situations in which they could be used.

Learning objectives

Having studied this chapter, students will:

1. Be able to identify different classes of analgesic drugs.
2. Be able to identify different routes of administration of analgesic drugs.
3. Understand distinctions between inflammatory and neuropathic pain.
4. Understand the concepts of tolerance and dependence.
5. Be able to describe the likely sites of action and mechanism of action for drugs used in pain management.
6. Understand the side-effect profiles of commonly used analgesic drugs.

INFLAMMATORY PAIN AND NEUROPATHIC PAIN

Pain is often classified as either inflammatory pain, where the peripheral nociceptors are being activated by chemical mediators of inflammation, or as neuropathic pain, where the cause of the pain is damage to the nervous system or disease processes affecting the nervous system (Woolf 1995). Inflammatory pain may arise from somatic structures such as muscles and joints, or from visceral structures such as the liver or gut (Fig. 16.1).

Inflammatory pain involves activation of nociceptors, which are the free nerve endings of C fibres and A delta fibres (see Chapter 2). Activation of nociceptors involves the release of a variety of chemical mediators, as well as direct physical stimulation (see Chapter 3 for a detailed explanation). The 'inflammatory soup' of sensitizing chemicals and associated changes in the function of molecular receptors provide targets for peripherally acting drugs (Dray 1995). Changes related to the process of central sensitization also provide potential mechanisms for pharmacological interventions to control inflammatory pain using a variety of drugs (Yaksh 1988).

When damage to the nervous system occurs, pain is generated within the nervous system, rather than at the nociceptor. This results in a very distinctive pattern of pain that is not easily modified by endogenous pain inhibitory systems, as these systems may also have been damaged as a result of the injury or disease process. The hypersensitive state that develops in peripheral and central nervous system neurons appears to be greater than that which occurs with inflammatory pain. Chapter 18 provides a more in-depth discussion of the pathophysiology of neuropathic pain.

Clinically, neuropathic pain can present in at least two ways: either as a constant pain, often burning in nature, or as a lancinating pain, also referred to as neuralgia (Woolf & Mannion 1999). A subgroup of neuropathic pain states, termed sympathetically maintained pain states (SMP) has been identified in which the sympathetic nervous system is thought to contribute to the pain experienced (see Fig. 16.2); it has been hypothesized that these disorders may be linked to an

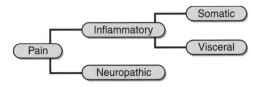

Figure 16.1 Classification of pain.

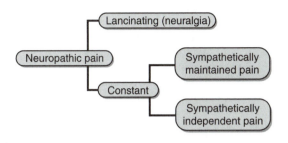

Figure 16.2 Classification of neuropathic pain.

acquired sensitivity to circulating noradrenaline in peripheral nociceptors (Devor 1995, Perl 1999).

DRUG THERAPY OF INFLAMMATORY PAIN

As discussed previously, inflammatory pain involves the activation of peripheral nociceptors by chemical mediators of inflammation, and transmission of the nociceptive signal along the peripheral nerve, through the dorsal horn of the spinal cord, and up to the brain (Fig. 16.3). Chapter 2 provides a detailed explanation of the neuroanatomical pathways involved in transmitting nociceptive information.

Current drug therapy modulates the nociceptive stimulus at four major sites (as shown in Fig. 16.4 and Figs 16.6–16.8):

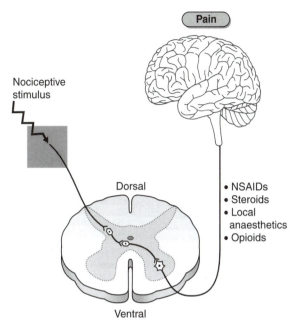

Figure 16.4 Drugs acting on the peripheral inflammatory response. Shaded area denotes site of drug action.

1. Peripheral tissues
2. Peripheral nerve fibres
3. Dorsal horn of spinal cord
4. Supraspinal sites

Drugs acting on the peripheral inflammatory response

Orally administered non-steroidal anti-inflammatory drugs (NSAIDs)

Non-steroidal anti-inflammatory drugs (NSAIDs) have analgesic, anti-inflammatory and antipyretic effects (Insel 1996). While all NSAIDs are analgesic, anti-inflammatory and antipyretic, considerable variability exists in the relative degree to which various drugs exert each of these actions (reviewed in Insel 1996). For example, paracetamol/acetaminophen has a weak anti-inflammatory action but is an effective analgesic and antipyretic. Their effects have been attributed primarily to their ability to reduce the biosynthesis of prostaglandins by inhibition of cyclo-oxygenase (COX) enzymes (Vane 1971) (Fig. 16.5), however, they do not inhibit the formation of other important inflammatory mediators such as leukotrienes.

Other mechanisms that have been postulated for the anti-inflammatory action of NSAIDs include inhibition of leucocyte adherence and function, reduction of

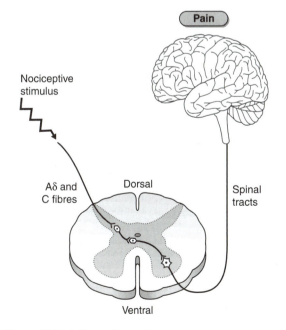

Figure 16.3 Inflammatory pain.

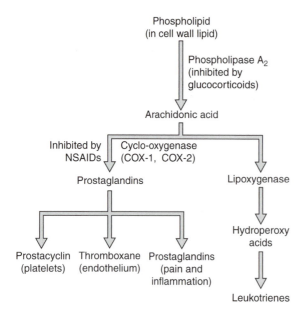

Figure 16.5 Inflammatory biochemistry.

One of the primary actions of NSAIDs is to inhibit cyclooxygenase activity. This enzyme catalyses the conversion of aracidonic acid into PGH_2. PGH_2 is then rapidly converted to prostaglandins (PGD_2, PGE_2, $PGF_{2\alpha}$), prostacyclin (PGI_2 or thromboxane A_2 (TxA_2)) (O'Banion 1999). Research over the last decade has identified two different forms of the cyclooxygenase enzyme, described as cyclooxygenase-1 (COX-1) and cyclooxygenase-2 (COX-2). COX-1 is present in many tissues and is constitutively expressed; COX-2 on the other hand is only induced in response to a variety of stimuli including the presence of inflammation (O'Banion 1999).

It is thought that inhibition of COX-1 is responsible for many of the side-effects seen with administration of NSAIDs. Consequently, there has been an intensive effort to develop drugs that specifically inhibit COX-2, in the belief that these drugs will be more effective in limiting pain and inflammation, and that they will exhibit fewer side-effects. Although COX-2-specific NSAIDs have been developed (e.g. celecoxib, rofecoxib, nimesulide), it remains to be seen if they will have better side-effect profiles in practice (O'Banion 1999, Rainsford 1999).

Side-effects of NSAIDs include gastrointestinal ulceration, increased bleeding times and reduced renal function (Jones & Tait 1995, Rainsford 1999). Hypersensitivity reactions may also occur, particularly with aspirin. Differences exist in the severity of side-effects among different NSAIDs depending on the physicochemical properties of the drugs (Insel 1996, Jones & Tait 1995, Rainsford 1999). However, due to these side-effects, caution is required in chronic administration, particularly in the elderly patient.

Some drugs may be better tolerated than others and considerable inter-patient variability in response and side-effect profiles exists, so that patients may switch from one NSAID to another to find the drug with the best efficacy/side-effect profile for their individual needs. Paracetamol/acetaminophen does not cause gastrointestinal or renal side-effects, but should be restricted to not more than 4 g per day to avoid liver toxicity. In general, long-term regular use of oral NSAIDs for pain relief is not recommended due to their toxic effects on the gastrointestinal tract and kidneys.

platelet aggregation, modulation of lymphocyte responsiveness, inhibition of cytokine production, suppression of proteoglycan production in cartilage, amelioration of complement-mediated cell-lysis and inhibition of free radical formation (Insel 1996). Their mechanism of analgesic action is not clearly understood and may involve both peripheral and central effects (Gebhart & McCormack 1994).

Drugs classed as NSAIDs include aspirin, paracetamol (acetaminophen in the USA), ibuprofen, indometacin, piroxicam, diclofenac, ketoprofen, ketorolac and naproxen. NSAIDs are usually effective against pain of low to moderate intensity for which there is a clearly discernable inflammatory cause. Their primary clinical applications are as antiinflammatory/analgesic agents in the management of rheumatoid arthritis, osteoarthritis, ankylosing spondylitis and soft-tissue disorders. It is important to note that, in general, NSAIDs provide only symptomatic relief of these conditions and are not diseasemodifying.

Other drugs, known as second-line or diseasemodifying antirheumatic drugs (DMARDs), such as azathioprine, cyclosporine, methotrexate, glucocorticoids, penicillamine, hydroxychloroquine, sulfasalazine and gold are required to modify the progression of pathological processes in affected tissues. Unlike the NSAIDs, they do not produce an immediate alleviation of symptoms, but require 4–6 months of treatment for a full therapeutic response.

Topically applied NSAIDs

NSAID creams, gels and sprays applied topically to the skin at the site of pain can provide local pain relief. A number of these preparations, containing NSAIDs, such as benzydamine, ibuprofen, diclofenac, ketoprofen, piroxicam and salicylates, are available for sale at pharmacies. The rationale for topical application of NSAIDs to the skin surface over the target site is that local tissue levels of drug will be achieved with minimal systemic absorption. If drug delivery can be targeted to the site of action in this way, the dosage required can be reduced, thereby minimizing side-effects while achieving a therapeutic outcome.

To exert a therapeutic action, a sufficient quantity of the applied NSAID must reach the site of action. This may occur due to direct penetration across the skin, via the systemic circulation or by a combination of these routes. The NSAID must diffuse across the stratum corneum (the outermost layers of dead epidermal cells, that present the major barrier to the penetration of NSAIDs), the viable epidermis and dermis. In the dermis, systemic absorption of the NSAID may occur via the blood vessels of the dermis, or penetration into deeper tissues can result. In their recent review, Vaile and Davis (1998) concluded that there have been a sufficient number of studies of soft-tissue conditions to demonstrate the superiority of topical NSAIDs over placebo, and equivalent efficacy compared with oral administration. Direct penetration of topically applied NSAIDs to underlying soft tissues has been demonstrated; tissue levels achieved are clinically relevant and plasma levels are relatively low compared with oral administration (Vaile & Davis 1998). Systematic studies comparing the relative efficacy of different topically applied NSAIDs are not available, though it is likely that both the properties of the NSAID and the formulation in which it is applied will influence the rate and extent of penetration across the stratum corneum barrier.

There is less evidence to support topical application of NSAIDs in the treatment of arthropathies, as direct penetration to the synovial fluid has not been demonstrated. The adverse-effect profile of topical applications appears to be favourable compared to oral administration, due to the lower plasma concentrations following topical application. Cutaneous adverse reactions such as erythema, pruritis and irritation are the most common effects reported, typically occurring in 1–2% of patients (De Beneditis & Lorenzetti 1996).

It has been suggested that a synergistic treatment effect may be achieved by combining the application of a topical NSAID and therapeutic ultrasound. A NSAID gel could be used as a suitable ultrasound couplant during therapy (Benson & McElnay 1994). The ultrasound could potentially increase penetration of the NSAID to the site of action and at the same time provide the therapeutic advantages of the ultrasound therapy itself. However, evidence to support this treatment protocol has not been demonstrated

(Meidan et al 1995) and it would probably be of more benefit to have the patient apply the NSAID preparation some time in advance of their scheduled ultrasound treatment. This would allow a great deal more time for penetration of the NSAID into the skin than that offered during a typical ultrasound treatment. The subsequent ultrasound treatment, together with the presence of the NSAID in the tissues, could be beneficial.

Steroids (corticosteroids or glucocorticoids)

Although symptom relief can be dramatic, steroids are of limited value in the management of chronic pain, due to their severe side-effects. However, they are extremely potent anti-inflammatory agents, and a short course of high-dose oral steroids for a few days is sometimes indicated for certain painful conditions, such as polymyalgia rheumatica. In these cases a high initial dose of corticosteroid is given to induce remission, and the dose is then gradually reduced and discontinued. In some cases, pulse doses of corticosteroid (e.g. up to 1 g methyl prednisolone intravenously on 3 consecutive days) may be used to suppress highly active inflammatory disease, while longer-term and slower-acting medication is commenced (British National Formulary 1999, p 435).

Steroids act to depress inflammation by suppressing neutrophil and macrophage function, including the release of inflammatory mediators and the effects of these mediators on blood capillaries. They also have effects on many other body organs and functions. In chronic pharmacotherapy with steroids, the over-intensive production of these physiological or pharmacological actions results in adverse side-effects such as iatrogenic Cushing's syndrome (Orth 1995), insomnia and mental disturbances, muscle wasting, peptic ulceration, cataracts and glaucoma, osteoporosis, diabetes mellitus and growth retardation in children (British National Formulary 1999).

Patients who have symptoms confined to a few joints may benefit from intra-articular steroid injections (the three drugs most commonly injected into joints are triamcinolone, methylprednisolone and betamethasone); these are used to relieve pain, increase mobility and reduce deformity in the affected joint. Full aseptic procedure is required to avoid infection in the joint. Triamcinolone acetonide is the steroid of choice for intra-articular injection, as the drug is relatively insoluble and therefore provides a long-acting effect. Local steroid injections into soft tissues may also be used in the treatment of tendonitis (British National Formulary 1999, p 436). Following an initial rest period, patients who receive an intra-articular steroid injection will require graduated restoration of range of movement and muscle function.

Topically applied local anaesthetics

Local anaesthetic drugs act by causing a reversible block to conduction of impulses along nerve fibres. There are a number of local anaesthetic drugs available that vary in their potency, toxicity and duration of action. They are administered by various routes, such as topical to skin and mucous membranes, infiltration, injection into tissues, regional nerve block, epidural or spinal block. Local anaesthetic preparations for topical application to the skin include EMLA cream and patch (containing a eutectic mixture of lignocaine (lidocaine in USA) and prilocaine) and Ametop gel (amethocaine). EMLA can produce a small area of cutaneous anesthesia, but long-term use is limited due to the frequent development of skin reactions with repeated use. EMLA and Ametop are indicated for reducing pain at the site of venepuncture or venous cannulation. In both cases the product is applied to the site under an occlusive dressing to speed-up skin penetration. A minimum of 30-minutes or 1-hour application time is recommended prior to venepuncture for EMLA and Ametop, respectively. EMLA is also used during harvesting and placement of split skin grafts (British National Formulary 1999, p 551).

Orally administered opioid analgesics

The term opium is derived from the Greek term for juice, the drug being derived from the juice of the poppy, *Papaver somniferum*. Drugs such as morphine mimic endogenous opioid chemicals known as the enkephalins, endorphins and dynorphins. Enkephalin in the dorsal horn of the spinal cord and β-endorphin in the periaquaductal grey (PAG) region of the brain are neurotransmitters involved in 'closing the pain gate', thereby inhibiting the transmission of nociceptive information.

Until recently it was believed that this opioid inhibitory system existed only in the central nervous system (CNS). Over the past few years however, researchers (Coggeshall et al 1997, Stein et al 1995) have shown that the inflammatory response leads to activation of opioid receptors in the peripheral nervous system and increased production of opioid receptors in dorsal root ganglion cells, thereby allowing endogenous opioids to exert an important peripheral effect. Opioids act by binding at specific receptor sites in body tissues.

To date, three main classes of receptor have been identified, namely Mu (μ), Kappa (κ) and Delta (δ) receptors (Pleuvry 1983). Subgroups within these major divisions have been identified and there has been debate as to the existence of other forms of opioid receptors (Pleuvry 1983). Although both μ and δ receptors are present in the periphery, the μ receptor seems to be of most relevance to the production of peripheral analgesic effects (Coggeshall et al 1997). Opioid drugs are therefore likely to have a peripheral analgesic action in the presence of inflammation.

Within each of the three classes of opioid receptor there are a number of subtypes, for example morphine analgesia can be elicited supraspinally via μ_1 or spinally via μ_2 receptors. Binding of opioids at these receptors, when they are present on neurons within the nociceptive system, elicits analgesia, which is the pharmacological response desired in pain therapy. Binding to these and related receptors at other sites in the body elicits side-effects such as gastrointestinal tract effects including reduced motility, constipation and emesis, central nervous system effects including euphoria and tranquility, respiratory depression, peripheral vasodilation and inhibition of baroreceptor reflexes leading to orthostatic hypotension and fainting.

Drugs in this class are sub-divided into weak and strong opioids. Weak opioids are codeine, dihydrocodeine and dextropopoxyphene, which are available as single-agent oral preparations or more frequently in combination with paracetamol/acetaminophen. These preparations are sometimes used as an alternative to NSAID therapy, but are not an alternative to strong opioid analgesics when such therapy for inflammatory pain is indicated.

Strong opioid analgesics include morphine, dihydromorphone, methadone, buprenorphine and pethidine (meperidine in USA). Morphine is the most frequently used opioid analgesic. It has a duration of effect of about 4 hours from standard formulations. Sustained-release capsule, tablet and liquid formulations are available which provide the patient with longer dosing intervals (Reisine & Pastarnak 1996). Methadone is available for oral administration; it is an effective analgesic that is used primarily in the treatment of withdrawal symptoms in physically dependent individuals. Because the drug is heavily protein-bound, withdrawal from methadone produces less severe symptoms than withdrawal from some other opioids (Reisine & Pastarnak 1996). Buprenorphine is available as a sublingual tablet, which is placed under the tongue and allowed to dissolve. The drug is absorbed directly across the oral mucosa to the circulation to provide its analgesic effect. It therefore produces a more rapid onset of analgesia than oral morphine. Buprenorphine also has a longer duration of effect than morphine (6 hours) and a dosing interval of 8 hours (Reisine & Pastarnak 1996).

Intravenous administration of opioids

Morphine may be administered by continuous infusion or intermittent intravenous dosing. Patient-controlled analgesia (PCA), a special kind of drug administration system in which the patient has some measure of control over their dosing amount and/or interval, has been used with opioids with considerable success (Barkas & Duafala 1988). PCA is generally accomplished with a portable device consisting of a pump that infuses the drug from a reservoir, at a rate that can be controlled by the patient. PCA is used most commonly in the management of postoperative pain or chronic cancer pain (Barkas and Duafala 1988).

Common side-effects of morphine therapy include nausea, vomiting, constipation and drowsiness. Euphoria may be seen with acute use of opioids, but does not commonly occur in chronic use. Larger doses produce respiratory depression and hypotension. A number of other opioids including pethidine/meperidine are also available for intravenous administration.

Topical administration of opioids

Fentanyl is available as a sustained-release transdermal patch for application to the skin. In this case the intention is not simply to topically administer the drug to a specific site, but to provide systemic delivery of the drug over a sustained period. The patch releases a constant level of drug continuously for 72 hours, hence providing a steady blood concentration. The patch is replaced every 3 days, and the patient often has a short-acting opioid preparation available in case of breakthrough pain, and to provide coverage until steady-state plasma concentrations are established following the initiation of therapy. The fentanyl transdermal therapeutic system is not recommended in the management of acute postoperative pain, however it does appear to be an effective alternative to morphine administration in chronic cancer pain and in chronic pain of non-malignant origin (Jeal & Benfield 1997). Data suggest that patients prefer the convenience of the transdermal application system to other forms of administration (Jeal & Benfield 1997).

Disadvantages of opioid analgesics

Chronic administration of opioids in pain management may result in the development of physical dependence, but rarely results in psychological dependence (Porter & Jick 1980). Repeated administration may also result in the development of tolerance, which means that there is a reduced effect of the drug (Reisine & Pastarnak 1996). If tolerance occurs, the dosage should be increased, the method of administration changed, or another opioid substituted to ensure continued control of pain symptoms. Opioids can be discontinued in dependent patients without subjecting them to withdrawal symptoms by gradual dose-reduction over several days. Specific dose-reduction schedules have been devised and the provision of alternative medications such as methadone and other supplementary medications can provide effective treatment for physical dependence (O'Brien 1996).

Side-effects following the administration of these drugs are relatively common and can be significant. The range of possible side-effects includes respiratory depression, nausea, vomiting, dizziness, drowsiness, dysphoria, pruritis, constipation, urinary retention and hypotension (Reisine & Pastarnak 1996).

Drugs acting on peripheral nerve fibres

Local anaesthetics

Local anaesthetic blockade of a peripheral nerve (see Fig. 16.6) can be a useful technique in treating many conditions involving inflammatory pain. A wide range of techniques is available to produce regional analgesia and a number of different drugs are used depending on the extent and duration of analgesia required. Some of the more commonly used drugs include procaine, lignocaine (lidocaine in USA), prilocaine, mepivacaine, bupivacaine, etidocaine and ropivacaine (Veering 1996). Procaine, a derivative of ρ-aminobenzoic acid, is a weak local anaesthetic with a slow onset and short duration of action. It is used primarily for skin infiltration and for diagnostic purposes. Lignocaine/lidocaine is the most versatile and commonly used local anaesthetic with good potency, rapid onset and moderate duration of action (Veering 1996). There is some potential for systemic toxicity with repeated administration. Prilocaine is another amino-amide local anaesthetic that has a similar profile to lignocaine/lidocaine. It produces a good anaesthetic effect with relatively rapid onset and a moderate duration of effect. It is the least toxic of the amino-amide group of local anaesthetics.

Mepivacaine has a longer duration of effect than lignocaine/lidocaine, however it is not as potent as lignocaine/lidocaine. Bupivacaine has a relatively long duration of action and it can be used effectively to produce a differential block of sensory and motor fibres.

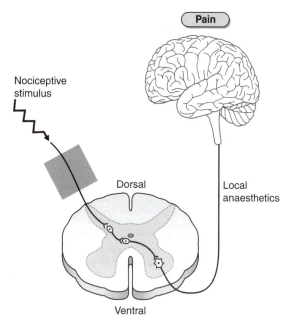

Figure 16.6 Drugs acting on the peripheral nerves. Shaded area denotes site of drug action.

This makes it particularly useful for several applications in postoperative and out-patient pain management. Etidocaine is similar to lignocaine/lidocaine, however it has a rapid onset of effect and a prolonged duration of effect with its most profound influence being on motor fibres. Ropivacaine is similar to bupivicaine in that its effect is relatively long-lasting. It also produces a differential sensory and motor block. Different agents or combinations of agents may be selected for specific purposes (Veering 1996).

A host of different techniques are available for regional anaesthesia/analgesia in relation to surgical procedures, and in relation to pain management, in both the postoperative and out-patient settings (Lubenow 1996). Some of the more commonly used techniques for pain management include brachial plexus, intercostal, ilioinguinal, sciatic and tibial nerve blocks (Lubenow 1996, Rogers & Ramamurthy 1996). When used appropriately, regional anaesthetic blocks are relatively safe, however some of the potential complications and technical errors include systemic cardiovascular and central nervous system toxic responses, hypotension, neurological complications, intravascular injection and neuropathy (Concepcion 1996).

The analgesia provided by regional blocks is often sufficient to allow physical therapy to a body area previously too painful to touch or move. A painful joint

for instance, can be mobilized using a continuous passive mobilization device under the analgesic cover of a regional infusion of local anaesthetic (Urmey 1996). Similarly, daily brachial plexus blocks (interscalene approach) can provide analgesia to allow mobilization of a painful, stiff shoulder joint. Thoracic nerve blocks can provide pain relief and facilitate respiratory therapy in patients with multiple rib fractures (Kopacz 1996).

Drugs acting on the dorsal horn of the spinal cord

Opioid analgesics

In selected situations, morphine may be administered epidurally or intrathecally (Foley 1985, Gustafsson & Wiesenfeld-Hallin 1988). Morphine is by far the most commonly used opioid for spinal administration, however a number of other opioids can be delivered by this method (Carr & Cousins 1998, Rawal 1996). Other opioids such as fentanyl, sufentanil, buprenorphine and pethidine/meperidine are also administered via the epidural or intrathecal routes but there is little evidence to suggest that this route of administration has clear-cut advantages over parenteral administration for these more lipophilic drugs (Rawal 1996). The relatively hydrophilic nature of morphine helps to ensure that it is more potent when administered spinally (Rawal 1996). The mechanism of action of morphine has been outlined above and appears to be associated with binding to receptors in the dorsal horn of the spinal cord (Fig. 16.7), although spread to higher centres may also occur. Direct administration of morphine to the CNS can be used in postoperative pain management where meta-analysis of randomized clinical trials has demonstrated clear benefits (Carr & Cousins 1998).

Typically, opioids are administered in combination with local anaesthetics. Effective postoperative analgesia with minimal motor block facilitates early mobilization and return to function; this is particularly important for mobilization of patients after major surgery.

Epidural or intrathecal opioid administration can also be used for the long-term management of cancer pain or for the management of chronic pain of benign origin. In these cases, an implanted infusion pump is often used to control drug delivery. These devices are normally implanted under the skin of the chest wall and include a reservoir that can be topped up from time to time (Carr & Cousins 1998). Beneficial outcomes of this treatment approach have been demonstrated in clinical trials (Carr & Cousins 1998).

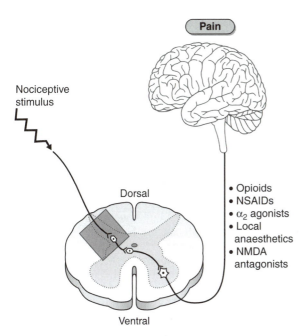

Figure 16.7 Drugs acting on the dorsal horn. Shaded area denotes site of drug action.

Combination approaches

The spinal route of administration has become a popular approach for the management of both postoperative and chronic pain states. Limitations and side-effects associated with particular drugs have prompted consideration of various combination therapies for epidural or intrathecal administration in the management of pain. Combinations of local anaesthetics, opioids, ketamine, clonidine and NSAIDs have all been utilized to varying degrees. The objective in general is to provide effective treatment at relatively low dosage, minimize side-effects and promote synergistic effects.

A variety of local anaesthetic agents can be used in varying combinations depending on the objectives of a particular epidural block. As indicated above, different anaesthetics produce motor and sensory blockade to varying degrees and their duration of action may vary. Different combinations of bupivacaine, lignocaine/lidocaine, ropivacaine and etidocaine can be used to produce blocks that have a greater or lesser degree of sensory and motor blockade (Cousins & Veering 1998). Local anaesthetics are also regularly used in combination with opioids such as morphine, pethidine/meperidine and fentanyl to manage postoperative pain (Carr & Cousins 1998).

The α_2-agonist clonidine is also frequently used for spinal analgesia, either in combination with local anaesthetics or in combination with opioids (Brownridge et al 1998, Carr & Cousins 1998). It appears to enhance and prolong the effects of the other agents, resulting in a synergistic effect. The action of clonidine is thought to involve an interaction with the descending noradrenergic pain-modulation system.

Ketamine is an NMDA antagonist that can be used in combination with other agents to produce spinal analgesia. By blocking activation of the NMDA receptor it is thought to have an important influence on the central sensitization process (see Chapter 3 for further information). Combination of ketamine and morphine provides a greater duration of analgesia and reduces the requirements for postoperative analgesia (Carr & Cousins 1998). On the other hand, administration of ketamine alone does not produce satisfactory analgesia (Carr & Cousins 1998). Combination of opioids with ketamine may also be useful in the management of neuropathic pain (see below) (Wiesenfeld-Hallin 1998).

Combination of epidural local anaesthetics or opioids with systemic NSAIDs has also been considered as a potential therapeutic approach influencing a number of different spinal mechanisms (Gordh et al 1995, Kehlet 1995). It is apparent that increasingly more complex combinations of drugs may be considered as the complexity of spinal pain transmission and modulation becomes better understood.

NSAIDs

As outlined in Chapter 3, up-regulation of the nociceptive system involves the release of prostanoids within the CNS. Sensitization of the nociceptive system resulting in increased intracellular $[Ca^{2+}]$ will lead to activation of phospholipase and increased production of aracidonic acid (Malmberg & Yaksh 1992). Cyclooxygenase can then convert this substrate to the various elements of the prostaglandin cascade outlined above; prostaglandins are then released to diffuse through the spinal cord and alter the sensitivity of adjacent neurons (Malmberg & Yaksh 1992, Yaksh 1999).

There is now increasing evidence that NSAIDs exert an important action on the CNS to block or reverse a component of the increased sensitivity that develops in the nociceptive system following a peripheral nociceptive input. Studies using the formalin test in rats have shown that a range of NSAIDs block the second-stage pain response in the test, without demonstrating any significant influence on the first-stage response (Dirig et al 1997, Malmberg & Yaksh 1992, Willingale et al 1997). The second-stage response is thought to be related to altered sensitivity in spinal wide dynamic range neurons (Malmberg & Yaksh 1992). This spinal action may be one reason why there is not a clear relationship between the anti-inflammatory and analgesic effects of NSAIDs (McCormack & Brune 1991).

Increasingly, NSAIDs are being used as a component of postoperative pain management because of their acknowledged analgesic actions as well as their anti-inflammatory effects. It is also possible that some NSAIDs may exert at least part of their analgesic effect by inhibiting nitric oxide synthase (NOS) in the CNS (Gordh et al 1995). Chapter 3 provides a more detailed description of the role of nitric oxide in spinal nociceptive processing. Inhibition of NOS and consequent prevention of sensitization may be an important effect of several NSAIDs including diclofenac, ibuprofen and paracetamol/acetaminophen (Bjorkman 1995, Bjorkman et al 1996).

Drugs acting on supraspinal sites

Opioid analgesics

The analgesic actions of opioids in the peripheral tissues and the dorsal horn of the spinal cord have been discussed. However, the most potent analgesic effect occurs with opioid binding at supraspinal opioid receptor sites in the periaquaductal grey (PAG) area and adjacent brain regions (Fig. 16.8). The reader is directed to Chapter 3 for a more detailed explanation of endogenous pain modulatory systems.

Routes of administration will influence the available concentration of drug at supraspinal sites. Oral, sublingual, transdermal and intramuscular administration result in high levels of drug in the peripheral tissues, while epidural and intrathecal administration produce higher levels in the CNS. The most potent route of administration, however, is direct intraventricular infusion, which results in high concentrations of drug at supraspinal sites such as the PAG. This method of treatment is sometimes used in patients with severe pain, due to a terminal illness, who have become relatively tolerant to morphine administered via other routes. In this context it appears to be an effective treatment approach with an acceptable side-effect profile (Karavelis et al 1996).

Paracetamol/acetaminophen

Paracetamol/acetaminophen, although commonly grouped with the non-steroidal anti-inflammatory drugs, has only a weak peripheral anti-inflammatory effect. It has analgesic and antipyretic actions and its antagonistic effect on COX appears to be predominantly central rather than peripheral. It is also thought to have a significant inhibitory effect on NOS, which may be important for its central analgesic effect (Bjorkman 1995).

Tricyclic antidepressants

The tricyclic antidepressants are a class of drugs used primarily in the treatment of depression. Newer agents now exist for treating depression, but these older drugs still play an important role in the management of chronic pain. Noradrenaline and serotonin (5-hydroxytryptamine or 5-HT) are two neurotransmitters involved in the descending pain inhibitory pathways from the midbrain to the spinal cord (see Chapters 2 and 3). The tricyclic antidepressants inhibit the reuptake of these transmitters, thereby increasing the concentration of noradrenaline and 5-HT available to inhibit nociceptive transmission in the spinal cord (Godfrey 1996). The degree to which different drugs inhibit the uptake of noradrenaline, 5-HT and dopamine varies within the group (Baldessarini 1996, Godfrey 1996).

Amitriptyline is the first-line tricyclic antidepressant used in the management of chronic pain, although other agents are also effective, and may be used if patients encounter problems with the side-effects produced by amitriptyline (Godfrey 1996). The recommended approach is to give amitriptyline 25 mg 2–3 hours before bedtime (Godfrey 1996). This approach helps to promote sleep and improve sleep quality, which is an important factor in the management of patients with fibromyalgia and other chronic pain problems. The dose is then titrated over a period of weeks or months to provide an optimal pain-relieving effect while minimizing side-effects (Godfrey 1996).

The tricyclic antidepressants are regarded clinically as a better alternative than using the benzodiazepines, because dependence (both physical and psychological) and tolerance to benzodiazepines tends to occur with chronic therapy (King & Strain 1990). The available drugs in this category include amitriptyline, clomipramine, dothiepin, doxepin, desipramine, imipramine, nortriptyline and trimipramine. There are variations within this group in terms of the ability of individual drugs to block 5-HT re-uptake, which is considered to be an important element in their ability to modulate pain (Godfrey 1996).

It is important for patients to be aware that tricyclic antidepressants will probably not produce an immediate improvement in their condition. It may take between 6 weeks and 3 months before noticeable improvements occur (Godfrey 1996). This is similar to their influence on depression (Baldessarini 1996). This delayed effect has led to suggestions that the mechanism of action of these drugs may be more complex than blockade of neurotransmitter re-uptake (Godfrey 1996).

The main problem with the tricyclic antidepressants is their side-effect profile, which can result in poor patient compliance. Common side-effects include drowsiness, dry mouth, blurred vision, constipation, urinary retention and sweating. More severe adverse effects may include hypotension, hypertension, arrhythmias, heart block, myocardial infarction and stroke. It is also possible for these drugs to produce a variety of psychiatric side-effects. Patients need to be educated about the effects of the drug and encouraged to persist with therapy as the therapeutic effect may take several weeks to be established, and some tolerance to side-effects often occurs over time. Dosage can be titrated or the drug used can be changed in order to minimize the side-effects produced.

There is evidence from clinical trials to support the use of tricyclic antidepressants in the management of fibromyalgia, pain from rheumatoid arthritis, low back pain and other chronic pain states (Frank et al 1988, Godfrey 1996, Tollison & Kriegel 1988, Ward 1986). It appears that these drugs are equally effective whether pain patients exhibit symptoms of depression or not, and it is also apparent that they modify hyperalgesia in these patient populations (Frank et al 1988, Ward 1986).

DRUG THERAPY OF NEUROPATHIC PAIN

Neuropathic pain can be regarded as pain due to an abnormality within the nervous system. Normally this will be related to disease or damage to the nervous system. Endogenous mechanisms for suppressing pain may be relatively ineffective. Common neuropathic pain syndromes include post-herpetic neuralgia (chronic pain following 'shingles' or acute herpes zoster infection), pain related to peripheral neuropathies secondary to various causes, such as diabetes mellitus (diabetic neuropathy), phantom limb pain, stump pain, trigeminal neuralgia and complex regional pain syndromes. The pain is most often described as sharp, lancinating, hot, burning, shocking or searing and it can be intermittent or constant. The syndrome may also involve paraesthesias that are sensed as numbness or tingling in a limb. A more detailed

description of neuropathic pain states is provided in Chapter 18.

Because of the variety of disease processes that can affect the nervous system and because of the individual nature of any nerve damage, patients with neuropathic pain are not a homogeneous group. A treatment that is effective in one patient, may fail in another patient presenting with similar pain symptoms, as the underlying pathophysiological changes within their pain pathways may be different.

A variety of strategies are available to manage neuropathic pain states. In terms of pharmacological management these include treatments for the underlying disease (e.g. improved management of diabetes), topical agents, regional anaesthetic blocks and a variety of systemic drugs with different mechanisms of action (Belgrade 1999). Many of the agents that are proving to have some value in the management of neuropathic pain are membrane-stabilizing drugs, which have been used clinically to manage other disorders, rather than traditional analgesics.

Disease management

Treatment of the underlying disease may be an important factor for some neuropathic pain states. It may also be possible to prevent or limit the development of neuropathic pain by improved management of certain diseases. Examples include improved glucose control in patients with diabetes, which may limit the development of complications such as diabetic neuropathy (The Diabetes Control and Complications Trial Research Group 1993) or the use of surgery and chemotherapy in the management of tumours that impinge on nerve structures.

As with nociceptive pain, drug therapy targets four major sites:

1. Peripheral tissues
2. Peripheral nerve fibres
3. Dorsal horn of the spinal cord
4. Supraspinal sites.

Drugs acting on the peripheral tissues

Capsaicin cream

Capsaicin, derived from the red pepper/capsicum, has the ability to deplete the peripheral C fibres (Fig. 16.8) of various neurotransmitters including substance P. If the cream formulation is applied regularly (initially four times per day), it is sometimes effective in reducing or eliminating constant neuropathic pain. This is particularly true for small areas of allodynia. It is

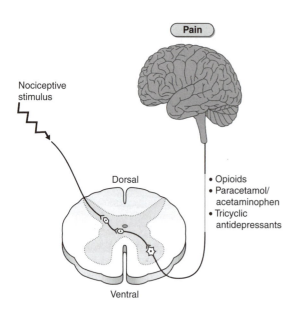

Figure 16.8 Drugs acting at supraspinal sites. Shaded area denotes site of drug action.

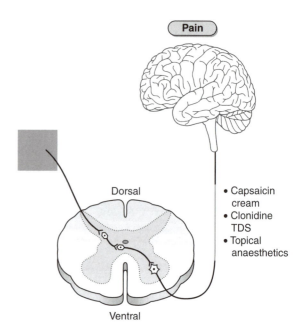

Figure 16.9 Neuropathic pain, drugs acting on the peripheral tissues. Shaded area denotes site of drug action.

indicated for the management of post-herpetic neuralgia, painful diabetic neuropathy, stump pain, osteoarthritis and rheumatoid arthritis.

The response of individual patients may be variable, but randomized clinical trials and meta-analyses suggest that capsaicin is superior to placebo in the management of pain related to diabetic neuropathy and post-herpetic neuralgia (Kingery 1997, Winter et al 1995, Zhang & Li Wan Po 1994). There is also evidence to support the effectiveness of capsaicin cream in reducing pain associated with osteoarthritis (Winter et al 1995, Zhang & Li Wan Po 1994). Side-effects of capsaicin administration are minimal, however the initial burning sensation induced by the drug may limit patient compliance with the treatment (Chren & Bickers 1991). Capsaicin may provide partial or effective pain-relief in some patients with specific disorders.

Clonidine transdermal patch

It has been established that α_2-adrenergic agents such as clonidine inhibit pain in animal models (Yaksh 1985). The possibility of using transdermal delivery of clonidine from a patch system has been investigated in relation to some common neuropathic disorders. It would appear that in relation to painful diabetic neuropathy, transdermal clonidine is not efficacious except for a specific sub-group of patients who represent

approximately 25% of the total population with painful diabetic neuropathy (Byas-Smith et al 1995, Zeigler et al 1992). The specific characteristics of the pain mechanisms in these individuals, that render them responsive to clonidine, have not been identified. Topical clonidine has also been shown to relieve hyperalgesia, in skin areas to which the patch was applied, in some patients with sympathetically maintained pain (Davis et al 1991). It would appear that while topical clonidine may be useful in the treatment of some individuals with neuropathic pain, it does not have universal efficacy.

Adverse effects of clonidine include dry mouth, sedation, sexual dysfunction and bradycardia. It is considered that these effects may be less common with transdermal delivery systems because high peak plasma concentrations are avoided with this delivery method (Hoffman & Lefkowitz 1991).

Drugs acting on peripheral nerve fibres

Local anaesthetics

Local anaesthetics can be administered topically to areas of allodynia. Modest success in the treatment of post-herpetic neuralgia has been demonstrated using lignocaine/lidocaine gel or patch preparations (Rowbotham et al 1995, 1996).

Many options also exist for the administration of local anaesthetics to injured peripheral nerves (Fig. 16.10) using regional block techniques. Regional nerve blocks using local anaesthetics are always worth considering in the management of neuropathic pain. Local anaesthetics have a stabilizing effect on the peripheral nerve membrane. If a regional nerve block is continued for a few days or repeated at regular intervals (e.g. brachial plexus block), the elimination of nociception may have a desensitizing effect on the peripheral and central nervous systems, resulting in prolonged pain relief even after the anaesthetic drug has been ceased (Arner et al 1990, Chabal et al 1992). The local anaesthetics also have a stabilizing effect in diminishing spontaneous activity from neuromas, which may be an important factor contributing to pain in some neuropathic pain states (see Chapter 18).

Drugs in common use include lignocaine/lidocaine, bupivacaine and ropivacaine. Clinical trials investigating the use of intravenous lignocaine/lidocaine have shown positive results in patients with painful diabetic neuropathy (Kastrup et al 1987), post-herpetic neuralgia (Rowbotham et al 1991) and neuropathic pain linked to peripheral nerve injury (Wallace et al 1996). A critical appraisal of the literature concluded that both topical and intravenous lignocaine/lidocaine were effective agents in the management of neuropathic pain (Kingery 1997). Using an alternative method to analyse the available literature, Sindrup and Jensen (1999) also concluded that lignocaine/lidocaine was an effective means of treating painful diabetic neuropathy. Interestingly, the effect of lignocaine/lidocaine does not appear to be dose-dependent but rather represents a precipitous break in pain over a relatively narrow concentration range (Ferrante et al 1996).

Analgesic blocks may be used as a means to promote rehabilitation and restoration of function in some patients and may provide a satisfactory basis for instituting and progressing physiotherapy and occupational therapy interventions.

Anticonvulsants

Anticonvulsant drugs, used routinely in the management of epilepsy, are regarded as one of the most effective forms of treatment for neuropathic pain. They have a particular role in managing lancinating pain in disorders such as trigeminal neuralgia (Belgrade 1999). Lancinating pain is believed to be due to an ectopic discharge within the nerve, arising at the site of irritation or injury (see Chapter 18 for a more specific discussion of the proposed aetiology of trigeminal neuralgia).

The anticonvulsant drugs are normally used in the treatment of epilepsy as they stabilize the neuronal membrane, making an ectopic discharge with associated seizure less likely. Likewise, these drugs stabilize the peripheral neuronal membranes, reducing the incidence and severity of neuralgic pains. Commonly used drugs include gabapentin, carbamazepine, phenytoin and valproic acid. Gabapentin is rapidly becoming established as the drug of choice in the management of a variety of neuropathic pain states (Belgrade 1999).

In addition to its membrane stabilization properties and its potential influence on peripheral neuromas, gabapentin is an analogue of γ-aminobutyric acid (GABA) and may have the capacity to directly inhibit nociceptive transmission in the CNS (Rosenberg et al 1997, Rosner et al 1996, Rowbotham et al 1998).

As a relatively new drug, gabapentin's efficacy in the management of neuropathic pain has not been extensively evaluated, however there is now evidence to support its use in the management of post-herpetic neuralgia and painful diabetic neuropathy. A high-quality randomized controlled trial showed that gabapentin had a significantly greater effect on pain, sleep and measures of well being than placebo (Rowbotham et al 1998). It appears to be equivalent to amitriptyline in the management of diabetic neuropathy

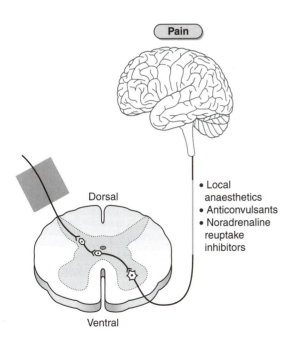

Figure 16.10 Neuropathic pain, drugs acting on the peripheral nerves. Shaded area denotes site of drug action.

pain (Morello et al 1999) and there have been suggestions that it can be effectively combined with amitriptyline to produce an additive effect. Gabapentin is relatively well tolerated. Some of the more common side-effects include sleepiness, dizziness and ataxia (Rowbotham et al 1998).

Other anticonvulsants (carbamazepine and phenytoin) have been investigated, particularly in the management of painful diabetic neuropathy and trigeminal neuralgia. Outcomes of these studies were mixed. A structured review of the literature in this area concluded that there was evidence to support the efficacy of carbamazepine but that evidence in relation to the use of phenytoin was inconclusive (Kingery 1997). Carbamazepine is considered to be particularly useful in the management of trigeminal neuralgia (Belgrade 1999). Two structured reviews provide favourable evidence for the effectiveness of carbamazepine in the management of trigeminal neuralgia (McQuay et al 1996, Sindrup & Jensen 1999).

Noradrenaline re-uptake inhibitors

A number of different drugs with the capacity to depress the activity of sympathetic post-ganglionic neurons can be administered using regional infusion. One of the most commonly used is guanethidine (Breivik et al 1998). Guanethidine initially stimulates the release of noradrenaline, leading to enzymatic breakdown of the available noradrenaline, and it subsequently blocks re-uptake, consequently depleting noradrenaline in post-ganglionic neurons (Gerber & Nies 1991). Despite the popularity of intravenous regional blocks with guanethidine, results of randomized clinical trials have failed to support the use of guanethidine for the management of complex regional pain syndrome (Kingery 1997). Other agents that can be used to block peripheral noradrenergic function include bretylium and reserpine.

Drugs acting on the dorsal horn and supraspinal sites

Local anaesthetics

Local anaesthetics can be administered via the epidural route to patients with neuropathic pain (Belgrade 1999) (Fig. 16.11). They may also be administered in combination with other drugs such as clonidine as outlined above.

Alternatively, systemic administration may have an important influence on nociceptive systems in the dorsal horn of the spinal cord. Because of the prolonged

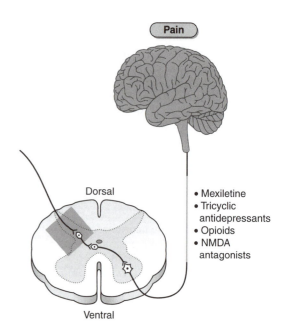

Figure 16.11 Neuropathic pain, drugs acting on the dorsal horn and supraspinal sites. Shaded area denotes site of drug action.

nature of neuropathic pain states, one approach has been to use orally administered lignocaine/lidocaine analogues such as mexiletine in the treatment of neuropathic pain. More commonly used as an anti-arrhythmic agent in the management of ventricular arrhythmias, mexiletine has a chemical structure similar to lignocaine/lidocaine but has a longer duration of action. It is administered orally on a regular basis, two or three times a day, with the dose dependent on the analgesic effect and possible side-effects (such as dizziness, ataxia, nausea and vomiting). Mexiletine does appear to be efficacious in the management of neuropathic pain states (Chabal et al 1992, Tanelian & Brose 1991)

Tricyclic antidepressants

The tricyclic antidepressants, described previously, are frequently useful in the management of neuropathic pain. They have been investigated in a number of studies on patients with post-herpetic neuralgia and painful diabetic neuropathy and they appear to be effective for the treatment of these conditions (McQuay et al 1996, Sindrup & Jensen 1999). Using the meta-analysis technique of calculating the number of patients needed to treat (NNT) before obtaining better than 50% pain-relief in one patient, Sindrup and

Jensen (1999) concluded that the tricyclic antidepressants are among the most effective treatments currently available for neuropathic pain. This finding has also been supported in a similar meta-analysis (McQuay et al 1996).

The major problem associated with use of tricyclic antidepressants is the side-effect profile of these drugs (see above). It is clear that the presence of side-effects and the need to reduce dose in response to side-effects, may reduce the effectiveness of these drugs in clinical practice. Sindrup and Jensen (1999) suggested that by establishing an effective plasma concentration of drug, rather than titrating the dose in response to side-effects, it was possible to improve the NNT figure from 2.4–1.4 individuals, indicating that in practice, management of neuropathic pain patients with tricyclic antidepressants is probably less than optimal. Tricyclic antidepressants remain an important mainstay in the pharmacological management of neuropathic pain.

Opioid analgesics

There has been a good deal of controversy about the use of opioid analgesics (particularly morphine) in the management of neuropathic pain states. A number of studies reported in the 1980s appeared to support the clinical impression that neuropathic pain states are unresponsive to opioid analgesics (Arner & Meyerson 1988). Subsequent investigations have suggested, however, that although patients with neuropathic pain may be less responsive to opioids, and may require higher doses of opioids to produce an adequate clinical response, blanket statements concluding that patients with neuropathic pain do not respond to opioids are not supported by the research evidence (Portenoy et al 1990). Variations in the pathophysiology of individual pain states and inter-individual variation in the pharmacodynamics of opioids may influence the variable response of patients with neuropathic pain to opioid medications (Portenoy et al 1990).

Recent structured reviews have concluded that opioids are effective in the management of certain neuropathic pain states in which they have been investigated (Sindrup & Jensen 1999). There is evidence to support the efficacy of morphine and orally administered oxycodone in the management of post-herpetic neuralgia (Rowbotham et al 1991, Watson & Babul 1998) and fentanyl in the management of a variety of neuropathic pain states (Dellemijn & Vanneste 1997).

In summary, it appears that opioids can be effective in the management of neuropathic pain states but that their effectiveness may not be universal. Additionally, in some cases, due to individual variation or the nature of the pathophysiological mechanisms involved, the response may be less than optimal.

NMDA-receptor antagonists

It has been suggested that NMDA-receptor antagonists such as ketamine may play an important role in the management of neuropathic pain states (Belgrade 1999, Wiesenfeld-Hallin 1998). While side-effects with ketamine are a significant problem, studies suggest that ketamine administration may be efficacious in the management of stump pain in amputees (Nikolajsen et al 1996) and other forms of neuropathic pain (Sang 2000). The efficacy of other NMDA antagonists appears to be more variable (Sindrup & Jensen 1999).

CONCLUSION AND IMPLICATIONS FOR OCCUPATIONAL THERAPISTS AND PHYSIOTHERAPISTS

The pharmacological management of pain is a complex area. No one drug provides effective pain relief for all pain states in every patient. Given the complexity of pain and pain modulation, it is unlikely that any single universal pain-relieving drug will ever emerge. Effective pain management depends on the judicious use and combination of a variety of drugs to provide the most effective treatment for any individual. Therapy should be based on the principles of evidence-based medicine and on sound clinical judgement.

It is important for rehabilitation professionals to be aware of the actions and side-effects of the main groups of analgesic drugs in order to understand the effects that these drugs may have on their patients, and the implications that they may have for other aspects of patient management. Increasingly, it is realised that pain management must occur in combination with restoration of function, and so there is a clear need for judicious combination of pharmacological therapies with physiotherapy and occupational therapy interventions.

Occupational therapists and physiotherapists should be proactive in advocating for effective management of patients' pain, especially in cases where effective pain control would enhance patients' compliance with other aspects of their rehabilitation programme.

Study questions/questions for revision

1. List three major actions of NSAIDs.
2. List five side-effects of opioid drugs.
3. By what mechanism are the tricyclic antidepressant drugs thought to inhibit pain perception?
4. List five side-effects of tricyclic antidepressant drugs.
5. By what mechanism are anticonvulsant drugs thought to inhibit pain perception?
6. List four different methods of administration for opioid drugs.

REFERENCES

Arner S, Lindblom U, Meyerson B A, Molander C 1990 Prolonged relief of neuralgia after regional anesthetic blocks. A call for further experimental and systematic clinical studies. Pain 43: 287–297

Arner S, Meyerson B A 1988 Lack of analgesic effect of opioids on neuropathic and idiopathic forms of pain. Pain 33: 11–23

Baldessarini R J 1996 Drugs and the treatment of psychiatric disorders: psychoses and anxiety. In: Hardman J G, Limbird L E, Molinoff P B, Ruddon R W, Goodman Gilman A (eds) The Pharmacological Basis of Therapeutics, 9th edn, Vol. 1. McGraw-Hill, New York, pp 383–435

Barkas G, Duafala M E 1988 Advances in cancer pain management: a review of patient-controlled analgesia. Journal of Pain and Symptom Management 3: 150–160

Belgrade M J 1999 Following the clues to neuropathic pain. Postgraduate Medicine 106: 127–140

Benson H A E, McElnay J C 1994 Topical non-steroidal anti-inflammatory products as ultrasound couplants. Physiotherapy 80: 74–76

Bjorkman R 1995 Central antinociceptive effects of non-steroidal anti-inflammatory drugs and paracetamol. Experimental studies in the rat. Acta Anaesthesiologica Scandinavica Supplementum 103: 1–44

Bjorkman R, Hallman K M, Hedner J, Hedner T, Henning M 1996 Nonsteroidal antiinflammatory drug modulation of behavioral responses to intrathecal N-methyl-D-aspartate, but not to substance P and amino-methyl-isoxazole-propionic acid in the rat. Journal of Clinical Pharmacology 36: 20S–26S

Breivik H, Cousins M J, Lofstrom J B, Sympathetic neural blockade of upper and lower extremity. In: Cousins M J, Bridenbaugh P O (eds) 1998 Neural Blockade in Clinical Anesthesia and Management of Pain. Lippincott-Raven Publishers, Philedelphia, pp 411–447

British National Formulary Vol. 36 1999 British Medical Association and Royal Pharmaceutical Society of Great Britain

Brownridge P, Cohen S E, Ward M E 1998 Neural blockade for obstetrics and gynaecological surgery. In: Cousins M J, Bridenbaugh P O (eds) Neural Blockade in Clinical Anesthesia and Management of Pain. Lippincott-Raven Publishers, Philadelphia, pp 557–604

Byas-Smith M G, Max M B, Muir J, Kingman A 1995 Transdermal clonidine compared to placebo in painful diabetic neuropathy using a two-stage 'enriched enrollment' design. Pain 60: 267–274

Carr D B, Cousins M J 1998 Spinal route of analgesia – opioids and future options. In: Cousins M J, Bridenbaugh P O (eds) Neural blockade in clinical anesthesia, Lippincott-Raven Publishers, Philadelphia, pp 915–983

Chabal C, Jacobson L, Mariano A, Chaney E, Britell C W 1992 The use of oral mexiletine for the treatment of pain after peripheral nerve injury. Anesthesiology 76: 513–517

Chren M-M, Bickers D R 1991 Dermatological pharmacology. In: Goodman Gilman A, Rall T W, Nies A S, Taylor P (eds) The Pharmacological Basis of Therapeutics, Vol. 2. Pergamon Press, New York, pp 1572–1591

Coggeshall R E, Zhou S, Carlton S M 1997 Opioid receptors on peripheral sensory axons. Brain Research 764: 126–132

Concepcion M 1996 Acute complications and side effects of regional anesthesia. In: Brown D L (ed) Regional Anesthesia and Analgesia. WB Saunders Company, Philadelphia, pp 446–461

Cousins M J, Veering B T 1998 Epidural neural blockade. In: Cousins M J, Bridenbaugh P O (eds) Neural Blockade in Clinical Anesthesia and Management of Pain. Lippincott-Raven Publishers, Philadelphia, pp 243–321

Davis K D, Treede R D, Raja S N, Meyer R A, Campbell J N 1991 Topical application of clonidine relieves hyperalgesia in patients with sympathetically maintained pain. Pain 47: 309–317

De Benedittis G, Lorenzetti A 1996 Topical aspirin/diethyl ether mixture versus indomethacin and diclofenac/diethyl ether mixture for acute herpetic neuralgia and postherpetic neuralgia: a double-blind cross-over placebo-controlled study. Pain 65: 48–53

Dellemijn P L, Vanneste J A 1997 Randomised double-blind active-placebo-controlled crossover trial of intravenous fentanyl in neuropathic pain. Lancet 349: 753–8

Devor M 1995 Periheral and central nervous system mechanisms of sympathetic related pain. Pain Clinic 8: 5–14

Diabetes Control and Complications Trial Research Group 1993 The effect of intensive treatment of diabetes on the development and progression of long-term complications in insulin-dependent diabetes mellitus. New England Journal of Medicine 329: 977–986

Dirig D M, Konin G P, Isakson P C, Yaksh T L 1997 Effect of spinal cyclooxygenase inhibitors in rat using the formalin test and in vitro prostaglandin E2 release, European Journal of Pharmacology 331: 155–160

Dray A 1995 Inflammatory mediators of pain. British Journal of Anaesthesia 75: 125–131

Ferrante F M, Paggioli J, Cherukuri S, Arthur G R 1996 The analgesic response to intravenous lidocaine in the treatment of neuropathic pain. Anesthesia and Analgesia 82: 91–97

Foley K M 1985 The treatment of cancer pain. New England Journal of Medicine 313: 84–95

Frank R G, Kashani J H, Parker J C, Beck N C, Brownlee-Duffeck M, Elliott T R, Haut A E, Atwood C, Smith E, Kay D R 1988 Antidepressant analgesia in rheumatoid arthritis. Journal of Rheumatology 15: 1632–8

Gebhart G F, McCormack K J 1994 Neuronal plasticity. Implication for pain therapy. Drugs 47 Suppl 5: 1–47

Gerber J G, Nies A S 1991 Antihypertensive agents and the drug therapy of hypertension. In: A. Goodman G, Rall T W, Nies A S, Taylor P (eds) The Pharmacological Basis of Therapeutics. Pergamon Press, New York, pp 784–813

Godfrey R G 1996 A guide to the understanding and use of tricyclic antidepressants in the overall management of fibromyalgia and other chronic pain syndromes. Archives of Internal Medicine 156: 1047–1052

Gordh T, Karlsten R, Kristensen J 1995 Intervention with spinal NMDA, adenosine, and NO systems for pain modulation. Annals of Medicine 27: 229–34

Gustafsson L L, Wiesenfeld-Hallin Z 1988 Spinal opioid analgesia. A critical update. Drugs 35: 597–603

Hoffman B B, Lefkowitz R J 1991 Catecholamines and sympathomimetic drugs. In: Goodman Gilman A, Rall T W, Nies A S, Taylor P (eds) Goodman and Gilman's Pharmacological basis of Therapeutics, Vol. 1. Pergamon Press, New York, pp 187–220

Insel P A 1996 Analgesic-antipyretic and antiinflammatory agents and drugs employed in the treatment of gout. In: Hardman J G, Limbird L E, Molinoff P B, Ruddon R W, Gilman A G (eds) Goodman and Gilman's Pharmacological Basis of Therapeutics. McGraw-Hill, New York, pp. 617–657

Jeal W, Benfield P 1997 Transdermal fentanyl. A review of its pharmacological properties and therapeutic efficacy in pain control. Drugs 53: 109–138

Jones R H, Tait C L 1995 Gastrointestinal side-effects of NSAIDs in the community. British Journal of Clinical Practice 49: 67–70

Karavelis A, Foroglou G, Selviaridis P, Fountzilas G 1996 Intraventricular administration of morphine for control of intractable cancer pain in 90 patients. Neurosurgery 39: 57–61

Kastrup J, Petersen P, Dejgard A, Angelo H R, Hilsted J 1987 Intravenous lidocaine infusion – a new treatment of chronic painful diabetic neuropathy? Pain 28: 69–75

Kehlet H 1995 Synergism between analgesics. Annals of Medicine 27: 259–262

King S A, Strain J J 1990 Benzodiazepines and chronic pain. Pain 41: 3–4

Kingery W S 1997 A critical review of controlled clinical trials for peripheral neuropathic pain and complex regional pain syndromes. Pain 73: 123–139

Kopacz D J 1996 Regional anesthesia of the trunk. In: Brown D L (ed) Regional anesthesia and analgesia. WB Saunders Company, Philadelphia, 1996, pp 292–318

Lubenow T 1996 Analgesic techniques. In: Brown D L (ed) Regional Anesthesia and Analgesia. WB Saunders Company, Philedelphia, pp 644–657

Malmberg A B, Yaksh T L 1992 Antinociceptive actions of spinal nonsteroidal anti-inflammatory agents on the formalin test in the rat. Journal of Pharmacology and Experimental Therapeutics 263: 136–146

McCormack K, Brune K 1991 Dissociation between the antinociceptive and anti-inflammatory effects of the nonsteroidal anti-inflammatory drugs. A survey of their analgesic efficacy. Drugs 41: 533–547

McQuay H J, Tramer M, Nye B A, Carroll D, Wiffen P J, Moore R A 1996 A systematic review of antidepressants in neuropathic pain. Pain 68: 217–227

Meidan V M, Walmsley A D, Irwin W J 1995 Phonophoresis – is it a reality?, International Journal of Pharmaceutics 118: 129–149

Melzack R, Wall P D 1965 Pain mechanisms: a new theory. Science 150: 971–979

Morello C M, Leckband S G, Stoner C P, Moorhouse D F, Sahagian G A 1999 Randomized double-blind study comparing the efficacy of gabapentin with amitriptyline on diabetic peripheral neuropathy pain. Archives of Internal Medicine 159: 1931–1937

Nikolajsen L, Hansen C L, Nielsen J, Keller J, Arendt-Nielsen L, Jensen T S 1996 The effect of ketamine on phantom pain: a central neuropathic disorder maintained by peripheral input. Pain 67: 69–77

O'Banion M K 1999 Cyclooxygenase-2: Molecular biology, pharmacology and neurobiology. Crtical Reviews in Neurobiology 13: 45–82

O'Brien C P 1996 Drug addiction and drug abuse. In: Hardman J G, Limbird L E, Molinoff P B, Ruddon R W, Gilman A G (eds) Goodman and Gilman's Pharmacological Basis of Therapeutics. McGraw-Hill, New York, pp 557–577

Orth D N 1995 Cushing's syndrome. New England Journal of Medicine 332: 791–803

Perl E R 1999 Causalgia, pathological pain and adrenergic receptors. Proceedings of the National Academy of Science USA 96: 7664–7667

Pleuvry B J 1983 An update on opioid receptors, British Journal of Anaesthesia 55: 143S–146S

Portenoy R K, Foley K M, Inturrisi C E 1990 The nature of opioid responsiveness and its implications for neuropathic pain: new hypotheses derived from studies of opioid infusions. Pain 43: 273–286

Porter J, Jick H 1980 Addiction rare in patients treated with narcotics. New England Journal of Medicine 302: 123

Rainsford K D 1999 Profile and mechanisms of gastrointestinal and other side effects of nonsteroidal anti-inflammatory drugs (NSAIDs). American Journal of Medicine 107: 27S–35S

Rawal N 1996 Neuraxial administration of opioids and nonopioids. In: Brown D L (ed) Regional Anesthesia and Analgesia. WB Saunders Company, Philadelphia, pp 208–231

Reisine T, Pastarnak G 1996 Opioid analgesics and antagonists. In: Hardman J G, Limbird L E, Molinoff P B, Ruddon R W, Gilman A G (eds) Goodman and Gilman's Pharmacological Basis of Therapeutics. McGraw-Hill, New York, pp 521–555

Rogers J N, Ramamurthy S 1996 Lower extremity blocks. In: Brown D L (ed) Regional anesthesia and analgesia. WB Saunders Company, Philadelphia, pp 254–278

Rosenberg J M, Harrell C, Ristic H, Werner R A, de Rosayro A M 1997 The effect of gabapentin on neuropathic pain. Clinical Journal of Pain 13: 251–255

Rosner H, Rubin L, Kestenbaum A 1996 Gabapentin adjunctive therapy in neuropathic pain states. Clinical Journal of Pain 12: 56–58

Rowbotham M C, Davies P S, Fields H L 1995 Topical lidocaine gel relieves postherpetic neuralgia. Annals of Neurology 37: 246–253

Rowbotham M C, Davies P S, Verkempinck C, Galer B S 1996 Lidocaine patch: double-blind controlled study of a new treatment method for post-herpetic neuralgia. Pain 65: 39–44

Rowbotham M, Harden N, Stacey B, Bernstein P, Magnus-Miller L 1998 Gabapentin for the treatment of post-herpetic neuralgia. Journal of the American Medical Association 280: 1837–1842

Rowbotham M C, Reisner-Keller L A, Fields H L 1991 Both intravenous lidocaine and morphine reduce the pain of postherpetic neuralgia. Neurology 41: 1024–1028

Sang C N 2000 NMDA-receptor antagonists in neuropathic pain: experimental methods to clinical trials. Journal of Pain and Symptom Management 19: S21–25

Sindrup S H, Jensen T S 1999 Efficacy of pharmacological treatments of neuropathic pain: an update and effect related to mechanism of drug action. Pain 83: 389–400

Stein C, Schafer M, Hassan A H S 1995 Peripheral opioid receptors. Annals of Medicine 27: 219–221

Tanelian D L, Brose W G 1991 Neuropathic pain can be relieved by drugs that are use-dependent sodium channel blockers: lidocaine, carbamazepine, and mexiletine. Anesthesiology 74: 949–951

Tollison C D, Kriegel M L 1988 Selected tricyclic antidepressants in the management of chronic benign pain. Southern Medical Journal 81: 562–564

Urmey W F 1996 Upper extremity blocks. In: Brown D L (ed) Regional Anesthesia and Analgesia. WB Saunders, Philadelphia, pp 254–278

Vaile J H, Davis P 1998 Topical NSAIDs for musculoskeletal conditions. Drugs 56: 783–799

Vane J R 1971 Inhibition of prostaglandin synthesis as a mechanism of action for aspirin-like drugs. Nature 231: 232–235

Veering B T 1996 Local anesthetics. In: Brown D L (ed) Regional anesthesia and analgesia, WB Saunders Company, Philadelphia, pp 188–207

Wallace M S, Dyck J B, Rossi S S, Yaksh T L 1996 Computer-controlled lidocaine infusion for the evaluation of neuropathic pain after peripheral nerve injury. Pain 66: 69–77

Ward N G 1986 Tricyclic antidepressants for chronic low-back pain. Mechanisms of action and predictors of response. Spine 11: 661–665

Watson C P, Babul N 1998 Efficacy of oxycodone in neuropathic pain: a randomized trial in postherpetic neuralgia. Neurology 50: 1837–1841

Wiesenfeld-Hallin Z 1998 Combined opioid-NMDA antagonist therapies. What advantages do they offer for the control of pain syndromes? Drugs 55: 1–4

Willingale H L, Gardiner N J, McLymont N, Giblett S, Grubb B D 1997 Prostanoids synthesized by cyclo-oxygenase isoforms in rat spinal cord and their contribution to the development of neuronal hyperexcitability. British Journal of Pharmacology 122: 1593–1604

Winter J, Bevan S, Campbell E A 1995 Capsaicin and pain mechanisms. British Journal of Anaesthesia 75: 157–168

Woolf C J 1995 Somatic pain – pathogenesis and prevention. British Journal of Anaesthesia 75: 169–176

Woolf C J, Mannion R J 1999 Neuropathic pain: aetiology, symptoms, mechanisms, and management. Lancet 353: 1959–1964

Yaksh T L 1985 Pharmacology of spinal adrenergic systems which modulate spinal nociceptive processing. Pharmacology, Biochemistry and Behavior 22: 845–858

Yaksh T L 1988 CNS mechanisms of pain and analgesia. Cancer Surveys 7: 5–28

Yaksh T L 1999 Spinal systems and pain processing: development of novel analgesic drugs with mechanistically defined models. Trends in Pharmacological Sciences 20: 329–337

Zeigler D, Lynch S A, Muir J, Benjamin J, Max M B 1992 Transdermal clonidine versus placebo in painful diabetic neuropathy. Pain 48: 403–408

Zhang W Y, Li Wan Po A 1994 The effectiveness of topically applied capsaicin. A meta-analysis. European Journal of Clinical Pharmacology 46: 517–522

Different pain problems

17

Musculoskeletal pain

*Bill Vicenzino   Tina Souvlis
Anthony Wright*

OVERVIEW

This chapter will consider a range of musculoskeletal pain problems. It will deal with factors contributing to the aetiology of these problems, the underlying mechanisms of pain perception, and in addition the development of sound clinical reasoning skills that students acquire in their clinical training, it will provide the basis from which rational approaches to treatment are derived. The examples of musculoskeletal pains are: acute ankle sprain, osteoarthritis of the knee, low back and lower limb pain, and chronic lateral epicondylalgia. Muscle pains are dealt with in a more generic way due to the nature of some of the chronic muscle pain syndromes (e.g. fibromyalgia and myofascial pain syndrome). The aim will be to assist students in the process of using their knowledge and skills to ensure optimum benefit for their clients.

Not inconceivably, musculoskeletal pain problems will present clinically with a variety of underlying aetiological features. For example, a sprain of a joint such as the ankle joint, if seen initially after injury, presents with different features than if it was a chronically painful or arthritic joint. Pain referred from spinal structures to the upper or lower limb that is somatic in nature differs in aetiology, presenting signs and symptoms and treatment approach, to neurologically referred pain. Muscle and tendon pain following an acute strain injury differs from pain that follows an overuse injury. Muscle pain that is localized to the muscle and that has been caused by an acute or overuse injury differs in aetiology to globally diffuse and chronic muscle pains that are features of conditions such as fibromyalgia and myofascial pain syndromes. Some of the factors that may influence the aetiology of a musculoskeletal pain state, as is reflected in presenting signs and symptoms, are the period of time from injury, the type and nature of injury, other injuries or re-injury, and adequate and appropriate treatment or the lack thereof. Changes to pain-processing mechanisms contribute to musculoskeletal pain. It is therefore important for therapists to carefully examine their clients' pain states before considering the underlying aetiology of the condition and its treatment.

Learning objectives

At the end of this chapter and related chapters the reader will have an understanding that:

1. Musculoskeletal pain following an injury predominantly results from the inflammatory process.
2. Not all musculoskeletal pain is indicative of an inflammatory process.
3. Not all pain is indicative of local pathology underlying the area of pain.
4. Knowledge of pain mechanisms is essential for understanding musculoskeletal pain.
5. Deficits in articular, neural, sensorimotor and motor systems are frequently present in musculoskeletal pain states.
6. The associated articular, neural, sensorimotor and motor deficits are not automatically self-limiting. That is, the deficits do not automatically reverse when pain has subsided below levels of perception.
7. Treatment of musculoskeletal pain:
   - Should address the inflammatory process in acutely injured musculoskeletal tissues.
   - Is not necessarily treatment of inflammation in all instances.
   - Does not always require the application of therapeutic modalities at the site of pain.
   - Requires knowledge of various pain mechanisms.
   - Should be based on sound clinical reasoning skills.
   - Is guided through the interpretation of signs and symptoms elucidated on clinical examination.
8. Presenting signs and symptoms that are carefully discerned from the clinical assessment serve as indicators of underlying pathology.

ACUTE ANKLE SPRAIN

Ankle injuries are a good example of acute joint sprains that are frequently treated in clinical practice because they are common and highlight several key issues pertinent in the understanding of aetiology and management of acute joint injuries. In most cases,

ankle-joint sprains involve rolling the foot into plantarflexion/inversion. This usually occurs when planting the foot on an uneven surface or landing with the foot in plantarflexion while the person is being distracted (e.g. focusing on a ball or another player in sport or talking with someone while walking on uneven surfaces).

A number of ankle and midfoot structures are implicated in this injury, for example the following may be traumatized: anterior talofibular ligament, anterior inferior tibiofibular ligament, calcaneofibular ligament, neurovascular bundle within the sinus tarsi, talar dome, malleoli and the peroneal tendons (Brukner & Khan 1991, 1993). In terms of clinical examination and interpretation of data from that examination, the acute injury is characteristically different from either chronic pain states or referred pain states referred to in latter sections of this chapter, because the location and structural source of the perceived pain are most likely the same. That is, the pain arises from the injured tissue underlying the area of perceived pain, making the cause of the pain reasonably easy to identify on examination.

Aetiological features and clinical implications

Within the 24 hours following an ankle sprain the client will present with a painful and swollen ankle that is warm to touch and possibly red in appearance. The pain and swelling may have spread beyond the local area of the injured tissues. In addition to these signs and symptoms the client will exhibit marked limitation of function, most usually related to a lack of dorsiflexion (e.g. walking down stairs, walking on toes (plantarflexion) or with the entire lower limb externally rotated in order to avoid dorsiflexion). That is, the client presents with the cardinal signs and symptoms of the inflammatory process (pain, swelling, heat, redness and dysfunction). The inflammatory process occurs immediately after the injury, lasts up to 72 hours and is characterized by a set of vascular, cellular and chemical events. In order to appreciate the rationale underpinning the physiotherapy management of an acute injury it is important to first understand the relationship between the presenting signs and symptoms and the underlying aetiological features, and second to understand the associated biological changes that contribute to the healing process.

The pain during and initially after an injury results from the stimulation of nociceptive receptors on group III and IV type afferent fibres by mechanical or chemical means. Mechanical stimulation of the fibres may initially occur by direct stretch of the soft tissues produced by the injury forces, followed by mechanical distortion of soft tissues by the ensuing swelling. Chemical stimulation occurs via potent noxious compounds that are released during the inflammatory phase, such as prostaglandins, leukotrienes, bradykinins, histamine and serotonin (Fantone 1990, Kidd et al 1996). These chemical substances are also responsible for sensitizing the nerve endings so that a number of factors may contribute to the perception of pain (Hargreaves 1990). For example, the chemically sensitized nerve endings may require less mechanical distortion to trigger pain perception, a lower level of previously innocuous stimulation may cause pain perception, or in severe cases the presence of spontaneous ongoing pain in the absence of any external pain provocative stimulation (Sluka 1996).

The preceding brief overview of the pain process following an acute injury infers that the nervous system is a passive entity in the inflammatory process when in fact this may not be the case. The nervous system has been shown to actively participate in the inflammatory process (Basbaum & Levine 1991, Rees et al 1994, Sluka 1996). For example, stimulation of polymodal C fibres can induce plasma extravasation by release from their terminals of substance P and CGRP (Lembeck & Holzer 1979, Morton & Chahl 1980). Confirming the active role of these small-diameter unmyelinated fibres in the inflammatory process are findings that interruption of such nerves will reduce the amount of inflammation (Joris & Hargreaves 1987). Dorsal root reflexes also contribute to the acute inflammation of an inflamed joint (Rees et al 1994). The sympathetic nervous system may also play a role in this acute neurogenically mediated inflammation (Basbaum & Levine 1991), although it would seem not through dorsal-root reflexes (Rees et al 1994).

Disruption of tissue during an injury results in a series of parallel events, all of which have marked effects on the vascularity of the injured body region, ultimately resulting in swelling or oedema, which is a major feature of an acute soft-tissue injury. For example, the breakdown of circulating platelets, leukocytes and mast cells induce endothelial changes that lead to extravasation of intravascular fluids (Fantone 1990). Activation of the platelet coagulation system further contributes to the increase in vascular permeability through the release of potent vasoactive substances such as serotonin, histamine and thromboxane A_2. The platelet coagulation system, which is responsible for maintenance of homeostasis through stimulation and

regulation of clot formation, is an important mechanism through which the injury-induced bleeding is controlled.

In addition, inflammatory mediators such as prostaglandins, leukotrienes, and platelet-activating factor may activate the classic complement system, an integral component of the body's immune system. The complement system produces a number of plasma proteins that further contribute to the inflammatory process. One of the roles of these proteins is to increase vascular permeability by releasing histamine, leukotrienes and platelet-activating factor through mast cell and basophil degranulation.

These mechanisms are largely responsible for the swelling observed following injury. The initial bleeding from ruptured blood vessels is usually minimal in most injuries. It is important to recognize that where there is a rapid onset and a substantial quantity of joint-swelling that there may have been significant disruption of highly vascular structures such as major blood vessels and subchondral bone, which requires urgent medical attention.

The dysfunction observed following injury results from the interruption to normal joint mechanics, sensorimotor function and pain. In the example of the ankle sprain in which the client has suffered a tear of the anterior talofibular ligament following a plantarflexion inversion injury of the ankle, there are a set of reasonably well-recognized biomechanical events that significantly impact on treatment approaches.

Figure 17.1 depicts a biomechanical model for acute injuries to connective tissues such as ligaments and other capsular restraints of joints. When the ankle joint is perturbed into a plantarflexion inversion direction, the anterior talofibular ligament and associated structures undergo changes described by the stress–strain relationship (Bader & Bouten 2000). The stress–strain relationship is initially curvilinear at low loads and then linear with increasing loads to the point where, should sufficient load be experienced, the ligament suffers total disruption. Clinical tests of instability would grade the latter as a grade III instability (Brukner & Khan 1993). A grade I is indicative of little compromise of stability and grade II, which is most common, encompasses the partial tears with varying grades on instability from grades I–III. In the case of a grade II tear there will remain a degree of hysteretic set (Bader & Bouten 2000, Frank 1996) which manifests itself in an altered length of ligament, resulting in altered joint mechanics (Figure 17.1). Further creep and hysteresis under normal loading may occur as a result of this altered joint mechanics, increasing the likelihood of repetitive microtrauma, inflammation, abnormal loading of joint nociceptors and ongoing pain (Figure 17.1).

For this cycle to be interrupted it is crucial that appropriate joint mechanics are established soon after the injury. This is usually accomplished by specific manual therapy to obtain adequate motion, followed up by therapeutic exercise and taping or bracing to maintain and integrate the restored joint mechanics into normal functional movement patterns. This mechanical model of ligament restraint and control of joint movement and function understates the sensory function of ligaments. It is well established that injury of ankle ligaments results in marked deficits in proprioception (e.g. joint-position sense, balance ability, movement-detection sense, vibration sense) and protective muscle reaction timing (Bullock-Saxton 1994, Fernandes et al 2000, Lentell et al 1995, Pope et al 1998, Wilkerson & Nitz 1994, Wilkerson et al 1997). The impact on the sensorimotor and motor systems is not only local, with deficits being identified in hip-muscle function (Bullock-Saxton 1994). Interestingly, the effect of ankle sprains on muscle strength has not been conclusively established, with divided opinions and research findings (Lentell et al 1995, McKnight & Armstrong 1997, Wilkerson et al 1997).

The impact of injury and pain on sensorimotor and muscle system function has also been reported in a number of body regions in humans and in animal models (Hodges & Richardson 1998, 1999, Indahl et al 1997, Richardson, 1987, Svensson et al 1998, Valeriani et al 1999a, 1999b, Zedka et al 1999). The sensorimotor and motor deficits contribute to abnormal joint function which delays resolution of injury, promotes ongoing musculoskeletal pain, and predisposes to recurrent injuries (see Figure 17.1).

The inflammatory response is regarded as the preliminary phase of the healing process, lasting some 72 hours following injury. Following on from the acute inflammatory reaction is the cellular and matrix proliferation phase lasting several weeks, which leads into the remodelling and maturation phases that may take 12–24 months (Andriacchi et al 1987, Martinez-Hernandez & Amenta 1987).

In the proliferative phase, there is a continuation of the hypercellularity that commenced in the inflammatory phase by the recruitment of neutrophils, monocytes and lymphocytes at the injury site, most likely due to the release of chemotactic factors such as C5a, a plasma protein from the complement system.

The cellular and matrix proliferation phase is characterized by increased concentration of monocytes, macrophages and fibroblasts. The monocytes and macrophages are actively involved in phagocytosis of the cellular debris and clot that resulted in the inflammatory stage. The fibroblasts are largely responsible for producing the scar tissue that replaces the injured connective tissue structures (i.e. ligaments).

Morphologically, this phase is associated with organization of the original blood-clot early and then by vascular granulation tissue comprising of endothelial buds which communicates as a diffuse vascular network (Andriacchi et al 1987). Immature scar tissue also forms with increased total collagen content and a matrix of an amorphous ground substance surrounding the emerging collagen fibrils. Reflecting these morphological changes are peaks in type III collagen, DNA

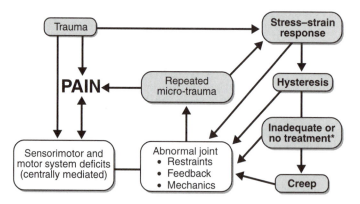

Figure 17.1 This diagram explains how the mechanical sequelae to injury may contribute to pain, especially ongoing pain following injury. It includes characteristics of connective tissues such as the stress–strain relationship and the properties of hysteresis and creep, which contribute to abnormal joint mechanics, which along with sensorimotor and motor system deficits may predispose to delayed resolution of the injury and further injury and pain. *Optimum treatment includes a check against harmful elongation stresses of the remaining ligament fibres, immature scar tissue and pain receptors.

levels, glycosaminoglycans, as well as increasing quantities of type I collagen as the scar moves to a more mature status and a reduction in water content as the oedema subsides (Martinez-Hernandez & Amenta 1987).

The signs and symptoms reflective of the cellular and proliferative phase are a reduction in swelling and pain and an improvement in function such as weight-bearing gait, despite persistent structural and functional instability on specific stress tests. Over the ensuing weeks the proliferative phase gives way to a remodelling and maturation phase. The remodelling phase is characterized by a reduction in hypercellularity, especially in the fibroblasts and macrophages, which parallels a reduction in vascularity as well as an increase in collagen fibril diameter and the density of the scar collagen matrix. The maturation phase of the healing scar tissue may last months or years, even though function is achieved in a much shorter time-frame (Andriacchi et al 1987, Martinez-Hernandez & Amenta 1987).

Many factors are considered to influence the healing process, both local and systemic (Martinez-Hernandez & Amenta 1987). Some of the local factors are the severity and extent of the initial trauma and any recurrent trauma, poor local vascularity, and infection. Some of the systemic ones relate either to nutrients such as vitamin C, zinc and proteins or systemic conditions such as diabetes or the sequelae of catabolic steroid usage.

Treatment approach and its rationale

The treatment approach for most acute sprains of joints is usually considered in at least three phases: emergency management phase (acute inflammatory phase), the early post-injury phase (cellular and matrix proliferation phase) and the rehabilitation phase (cellular and matrix proliferation through to the remodelling and maturation).

Emergency management phase

In the emergency management phase, which lasts from 2–24 hours, the emphasis is on containing the sequelae of the inflammatory response, that is, limiting swelling and pain. This is achieved by resting the injured part, especially from any activity involving the injury mechanism. For example, in the plantarflexion/inversion sprain of the ankle, dorsiflexion and eversion are encouraged and plantarflexion and inversion are discouraged. To this end, the therapist has a responsibility to advise and educate the client and pro-

vide some form of protection against injuring stresses, such as taping or bracing. There is evidence that demonstrates that taping or bracing is effective at limiting motion at the ankle and is beneficial in the treatment and prevention of ankle injuries (Cordova et al 2000, Thacker et al 1999).

As well as protecting the injured structures with relative rest, and taping or bracing, a common recommendation is the application of ice, compression and elevation (ICE) in order to retard and help reverse the effects of the inflammatory process. There is some evidence of the effects of elevation and compression on swelling (Sims 1986, Wilkerson 1985). Ice is frequently advocated, for which there is some evidence for its efficacy. Combined intermittent pulsed compression and ice has been recommended as it seems beneficial in reducing swelling and pain while also improving movement (Quillen & Rouillier 1982).

Various electrotherapy modalities have been advocated for their anti-inflammatory or healing capabilities, although many remained unproven. Although ultrasound and laser therapy have both been shown to exert in vitro effects that appear commensurate with an effect on the inflammatory process (Dyson 1987, Harvey et al 1975, Shimizu et al 1995, Young & Dyson 1990), their clinical efficacy in ankle treatment has been questioned by the results of several randomized clinical trials (de Bie et al 1998, Nyanzi et al 1999). High-voltage stimulation has also been shown to exert a significant anti-swelling effect in in vivo animal studies (Bettany et al 1990a, 1990b).

Early post-injury phase

The early post-injury phase starts within the first 24–48 hours, when the active inflammatory phase is subsiding, and extends over the next several weeks. It is essential that, as early as the second day after injury, motion in directions that do not stretch the injured tissues (i.e. safe directions), such as dorsiflexion for example, are encouraged. Encouraging early safe movement assists in the removal of swelling, the early regeneration of functional scar tissue and possibly most importantly, in the restoration of functional movement patterns.

It is well documented that complete immobilization is extremely detrimental to connective tissues and healing tissue, resulting in structurally weaker and morphologically poorer scar tissue (Andriacchi et al 1987). Interestingly, a recent study of rehabilitation following reconstructive surgery of ankle injuries has demonstrated that mobilized ankles performed far better on outcome measures such as range of motion, functional abilities, radiographic stress tests, than did immobilized ankles (Karlsson et al 1999). The healing scar tissue depends upon functional activities to mechanically guide and stimulate the architectural arrangement and orientation of the connective tissue fibrils and their interrelationships with matrix and neighbouring collagen fibrils (DeLee 1990, Andriacchi et al 1987).

The sensorimotor and motor system deficits, such as proprioceptive deficits and reduced reaction times, are targeted as early as 48–72 hours, first in a non-stressful limited weight-bearing situation and progressed to more stimulating and demanding tasks as function improves and pain subsides. This primarily involves extensive use of specific therapeutic exercises and adjunctive measures such as motor biofeedback techniques and instruments, facilitatory procedures, tape or braces and manual therapy (e.g. soft-tissue massage and joint manipulation).

The rehabilitation phase

The rehabilitation phase has actually commenced in the early post-injury phase and should theoretically last for another 6–12 months if morphological features of healing connective tissue structures are taken into consideration. Unfortunately, it usually only lasts as long as it takes for the client to successfully return to their desired level of participation.

There are two major components of this phase. The first involves the progression of the therapeutic exercise programme commenced in the early post-injury phase to higher-level physical activities that reflect the functional requirements of the client's desired type and level of participation in work and recreational activities.

The other component of this phase consists of the implementation of strategies that may prevent further injury either to the injured joint or to other related joints and structures, that is, the tertiary level of pain and injury prevention. For example, in ankle injuries it has been shown that ongoing limitations in dorsiflexion range of motion, proprioceptive deficits and certain activities (e.g. playing football, basketball or netball) contribute significantly to a higher risk of re-injury (Pope et al 1998, Wilkerson & Nitz 1994). So it would be important to address these risk-factors in the rehabilitation programme by using specific stretching and mobilizing exercises, therapeutic exercises to retrain the sensorimotor system, and protective sports tape or braces. The use of wobble-boards or ankle discs have been shown to improve sensorimotor deficits (Gauffin et al 1988, Hoffman & Payne 1995, Sheth et al 1997, Wester et al 1996) and should be strongly encouraged in rehabilitation of an injury and prevention of re-injury.

Summary

- Acute joint sprains resulting in pain present with a characteristic pattern of signs and symptoms, including a readily identifiable traumatic event, and a classic inflammatory response profile of pain, swelling, redness, heat and dysfunction within the first 24–48 hours.
- Pain is usually perceived locally over the injured structures (i.e. primary hyperalgesia).
- The pain process involved in acute joint injury is predominantly based in the periphery.
- Inflammatory-phase treatment involves the application of elevation, compression and ice, and most importantly protection of the injured ligament from harmful stresses. The latter is facilitated with tape and bracing.
- A healing process that has a number of phases (proliferation, maturation and remodelling) usually follows the inflammatory process.
- The fibrous scar tissue, which results from the healing process, is fashioned in response to stresses placed upon it. Hence, it is important to protect against harmful stresses and encourage functional stresses.
- There is a characteristic biomechanical response to the injurious movements and stresses. Understanding the properties of the stress–strain curve, hysteresis and creep facilitates an understanding of protective and appropriate functional stresses required in optimal treatment.
- A consistent associated feature of acute joint pain is deficits in the muscle and sensorimotor systems, involving muscle inhibition, spasm and altered proprioception.
- Treatment of all musculoskeletal pain and injury, including ankle injury, must address deficits of the sensorimotor and muscle systems.
- Prevention of ankle joint re-injury involves proprioceptive retraining, as well as gaining and maintaining adequate ankle-joint dorsiflexion. Use of protective taping and braces is also helpful.

OSTEOARTHRITIS OF THE KNEE

Osteoarthritis is a condition encountered frequently by therapists. Primary osteoarthritis results from an idiopathic onset of symptoms and signs whereas as secondary osteoarthritis is commonly thought to result from injury to joint structures or abnormal stresses acting on the joint, and consequent degeneration of the articular cartilage. Clients may report functional limitations associated with joint stiffness or instability and muscle weakness, however, one of the primary symptomatic features of this condition is pain. There are many potential causes for the pain associated with osteoarthritis and this section will use the example of a client presenting with osteoarthritis of the knee to highlight the possible sources of pain.

The structure most commonly at fault in osteoarthritis is the articular cartilage. The morphological features of this condition are fibrillation or flaking of cartilage, as well as resultant sclerosis of subchondral bone and formation of cysts within the bone. Microfractures can also be seen in the subchondral bone. In extreme cases where the articular cartilage has completely eroded, the exposure of bone surfaces may result (Stockwell, 1991). Osteophyte formation can occur at the joint margins where proliferating cartilage ossifies.

It must be remembered that the osteoarthritis under consideration in this section does not refer to the common presence of minor articular cartilage degeneration during aging, which is often not associated with pain and dysfunction.

Aetiological features of osteoarthritic knee-joint pain

The presentation of the client will depend on the stage of the condition. In the early phase the predominant feature is joint pain, which is often described as an ache deep in the joint. The pain may be situated in the medial or lateral compartments of the joint depending on structures and the area of the joint involved. Frequently the client will describe pain following movement (particularly at the extremes of range of flexion and extension) or following periods of weight-bearing, which rest may relieve. However, spontaneous pain at rest may also be present without movement, especially in severe cases.

Pain is characteristically experienced at the end of the day and commonly is worse during the night, whereas stiffness is present on arising in the morning and following periods of inactivity. The client may describe functional limitations related to the pain and loss of range of movement and may often minimize movement and activity and adopt antalgic or pain-relieving positions of the joint such as flexion, especially during periods of pain exacerbation.

On physical examination, there may be a joint effusion, thickening of the joint and capsular thickening due to recurrent effusions, or formation of osteophytes (later in the course of the condition). The joint may be tender and warm to palpation, and crepitus may be evident on movement of the joint. Loss of joint movement is common, with the extreme of range being lost in the early stages of the condition progressing to more loss as the condition progresses. Muscle inhibition and weakness can occur very quickly after the onset of pain and joint effusion, leading to rapid atrophy of the quadriceps muscle (Slemender et al 1997). Often associated with the stiffness and muscle weakness is joint deformity, but deformity following injury may actually occur as a precursor to the condition.

Interestingly, the main structure involved in the pathophysiology of osteoarthritis – the articular cartilage – does not have pain receptors and as such is not sensitive to pain-producing stimuli (Kellgren 1983). This suggests pain from the arthritic joint arises from other structures and mechanisms. Initially, there was also little evidence to suggest that the synovium, which becomes highly inflamed during osteoarthritis, is pain-sensitive (Kellgren & Samuel 1950). However, more recent studies have demonstrated the presence of neuropeptides involved in neurogenic inflammation in this area, suggesting afferent innervation (Schaible & Grubb 1993). Breakdown of cartilage and bone causes the release of inflammatory mediators that can cause this synovial inflammation, causing an increase in its thickness and the volume of the intra-articular synovial fluid, leading to an increase in pressure within the joint capsule.

As was discussed in the acute sprained ankle example, presence of inflammation can cause sensitization of the peripheral, spinal and supraspinal structures involved with nociceptive processing. Under normal conditions normal joint movement does not activate high-threshold mechanosensitive afferents located within the joint structures (group III and IV afferents) (Grigg et al 1986). They only become activated at the extremes of range to signal potential joint damage. However, as has been highlighted in other conditions, the inflammatory state and the release of inflammatory mediators (e.g. prostaglandins, bradykinin) which occurs within the joint sensitizes the afferents, so that they become responsive to movement within normal range. The receptive field of the afferents is expanded and afferents exhibit a tonic discharge that may account for resting pain in the arthritic joint (Schaible & Schmidt 1985).

In addition, there exists a group of mechanoinsensitive fibres that are not activated by noxious mechanical stimulation of normal joints. These afferents can become active or sensitized to movement following inflammation and as such can be considered 'silent nociceptors' (Schaible & Grubb 1993), adding to the upregulation or propagation of pain. Pressure increases within the joint, along with the inflammatory changes, may also activate the nociceptors as the receptors are now under increased stress within the tissue (Schaible & Grubb 1993).

In addition to sensitization of the peripheral afferent fibres, release of neuropeptides such as substance P from unmyelinated afferent terminals can lead to an increase in the inflammatory response (i.e. neurogenic inflammation), with resultant plasma extravasation leading to further joint oedema (Zimmerman 1989).

Dorsal horn mechanisms also contribute to the pain associated with osteoarthritis. Stimulation studies of spinal-cord neurons demonstrate convergence of receptive fields of cutaneous and muscle with the joint input (Schaible & Grubb 1993). As such these second-order neurons would respond to input from these cutaneous and muscular structures and account for pain that is usually perceived on the surface and deep within the muscles surrounding the joint (i.e. cutaneous and muscle hyperalgesia). As well, spinal-cord neurons demonstrate sensitization, again demonstrating decreased threshold and increased response to stimulation and an increase in receptive fields, such that previously innocuous movement and touch in areas around and outside the involved joint cause activation and therefore potentially the perception of pain (Farrell et al 2000).

Interestingly it has been demonstrated that the tonic descending inhibitory influences are increased during acute inflammation. It appears that supraspinal activity counteracts to some extent the increase in spinal and peripheral excitability (Sluka & Rees 1997). In addition to this central effect, it has been demonstrated that there is an increase in peripheral receptors for opioids, which mediate pain relief in response to inflammation. These receptors have been located in synovia and it has been suggested that opioids are released from inflamed tissue and activate the receptors to decrease the level of pain (Stein et al 1999). Thus both central and peripheral nervous system activity is present to decrease the level of pain experienced in the inflamed arthritic joint.

Adjunct to the pain involved in osteoarthritis is dysfunction of the muscle and sensorimotor systems. As described, the client will adopt pain-relieving postures and refrain from painful activity. This may be in part a conscious effort by the client but also reflects the effect of joint afferents on motor reflexes. Intra-articular inflammation can produce an increase of the flexor withdrawal response (Ferrell et al 1988), which may in part be responsible for the characteristic flexion deformity of the arthritic knee. Alternatively, there appears to be a reduced capacity of the muscle to contract in the presence of pain and joint swelling (Lund et al 1991), even if minor, resulting in inhibition of the quadriceps muscles.

Proprioception is reduced in osteoarthritic knees (Garsden & Bullock-Saxton 1999) and the proprioceptive deficits are bilateral in unilateral osteoarthritic knee joints, inferring the involvement of central control mechanisms of joint proprioception (Sharma et al 1997).

Compounding the situation is the loss of joint control that occurs as a result of pain and injury-induced deficits in motor control (Hodges & Richardson 1996). The pattern of motor activity is altered in the presence of pain leading to delay in activation of key stabilizing muscles. Therefore, in this condition it is important to determine the effect of pain on the individual client's performance of activity.

Treatment approach and its rationale

Treatment of the client with an osteoarthritic knee must be tailored to the findings of the physical examination, the level of pain and to the client's functional abilities and requirements. Pain- and inflammation-relieving measures may include anti-inflammatory medications and the application of ice during the active inflammatory stages in the presence of heat and swelling. Long-standing pain and swelling may also be alleviated by the application of heat and other physical modalities such as TENS (Nicholas 1994).

Active exercise for improving muscle and sensori-motor system function is important (McCarthy & Oldham 1999) and a recent study has shown that manual physical therapy and therapeutic exercise combined provides a benefit to subjects with knee arthritis (Deyle et al 2000). Physical therapy remains relatively uninvestigated as a treatment of arthritis when compared to drug and surgical interventions (Chard et al 2000), leaving clinicians to apply sound clinical reasoning skills in managing their clients.

It is important to note that there is a fine balance between pain regulation and function of the motor system that must be appreciated by the therapist. It is important to ensure proper activation of the muscles in order to maintain joint stability and facilitate normal function, however the influence of movement on pain must always be taken into account during treatment and in the performance of home exercise programmes. It is rarely appropriate to exacerbate pain during therapeutic exercise programmes for osteoarthritis, especially protracted or delayed-onset pain.

Summary

- Pain is one of the main presenting features of osteoarthritis of the knee.
- Loss of range of movement, joint changes and deformity, as well as muscle weakness, accompany pain.
- Pain may be mediated peripherally due to inflammation within the joint, pressure from synovial effusion and oedema, as well as changes in the subchondral bone.
- Inflammation will cause both peripheral and central sensitization leading to increased sensitivity to movement and touch and to spontaneous pain without movement.
- Sensorimotor deficits and changes in the neuromuscular control of the joint can also occur.
- Treatment should be based on the findings of the individual client and directed towards pain relief and amelioration of sensorimotor system deficits, with an emphasis on maintaining function and active participation in life. Therapeutic exercise and manual therapy serve this purpose.

BACK AND LOWER LIMB PAIN: RADICULAR OR SOMATIC REFERRAL

Back and lower limb pain commonly occur in modern society and are frequently treated by therapists. Pain that is referred from the back is important to recognize, because the site at which the client is reporting the pain to be located is not necessarily the source of the pain, and most importantly is not always the area to which treatment will be most effectively directed.

Low back pain with referral to the lower limb was once considered to be only a consequence of nerve-root entrapment and compromise of neural function. Recently it has become appreciated that although nerve-root entrapment is a cause of referred pain, it is not the only possible causative factor. Any structure which is innervated can potentially generate referred pain and because these structures are not neural the term somatic referred pain was introduced (Bogduk 1984). However, spinal-nerve root pathology, especially that which compromises neural motor and sensory function, must not be misdiagnosed, overlooked or ignored, as the consequences of such dysfunction impact significantly on the client's ability to pursue function normally.

The possible aetiological mechanisms of spinal-nerve root pathology and referred pain will be covered in this section. Low back and leg pain caused by radiculopathy at the L5–S1 motion segment will be used as a case example for spinal-nerve root pathology, while leg pain with or without concomitant low back pain but without radiculopathy at L5–S1 will serve as an example of somatic referred pain.

Aetiological features of S1 radiculopathy

A client suffering from this condition will report pain that radiates from the lower back into the leg, most likely in a discreet dermatomal distribution, and characteristically felt more distally in the dermatome. The pain may be sharp or shooting in quality and may be increased by movement or by touch. The client will present with increased mechanosensitivity of the nerve root and movement of the low back and of the leg can exacerbate pain.

Radicular pain is typically severe in nature with compression of the nerve root producing associated symptoms such as paraesthesia, anaesthesia, motor weakness and a decreased response to reflex testing. Signs and symptoms of motor involvement such as weakness in muscles innervated by S1 are diagnostic of compression to this nerve root. That is, weakness of the ankle evertors, with or without weakness of extensors of the distal great toe phalanx and ankle plantar flexors, would confirm the presence of S1 compressive radiculopathy. The Achilles tendon reflex may also be diminished.

Symptoms and signs of sensory deficits, manifesting as areas of numbness or paraesthesia in the S1 dermatome, when present in combination with motor deficits, lend support to the diagnosis. Indeed, changes in nerve-conduction properties, which can be demonstrated by either clinical and/or electrodiagnostic testing, need to be present for a definitive diagnosis of compression to be made.

Low back pain, which radiates into the leg, is commonly known as 'sciatica'. It was thought that pain in the leg most commonly resulted from compression of the nerve root and so was termed 'radicular pain'. Nerve roots provide the link between the central and peripheral nervous systems and differ from peripheral nerves in that they lack epineurium and perineurium and as such may be more susceptible to damage by compressive forces than peripheral nerves. They have a complex structure consisting of a motor and sensory root as well as the dorsal root ganglion, and are surrounded by cerebrospinal fluid, which provides nutrition and may afford some protection from compression (Rydevik 1984).

Several structures in the lumbar spine can cause compression of the nerve root including herniated intervertebral discs and degenerative osteophytic changes in the intervertebral foramen. It was original-ly thought that pain experienced was also related to the compression or mechanical deformation of the nerve root. However, it has been demonstrated both in animal and human studies that compression can exist without painful consequences. For example, when the peroneal nerve is compressed by sitting with legs crossed, paraesthesia and anaesthesia and a sensation of muscle weakness may result, which is not accompa-nied by pain. The presence of inflammation of the nerve root was necessary before mechanical deforma-tion, such as compression or traction on the nerve root, produced pain (Howe et al 1977).

Damage to the nerve root by compression may be accompanied by compromise in nerve-root circulation and subsequent ischaemia leading to inflammation and oedema (Rydevik et al 1984). This inflammation can also be mediated by the nervi nervorum which innervates the connective tissue of the nerves (Ashbury & Fields 1984). This plexus has a nociceptive function and may be responsible for the spread of pain and sen-sitivity along the length of an affected nerve (Bove & Light 1997).

Nerve-root compression and damage can also lead to demyelination and the formation of neuromas, which in turn can cause hyperexcitability of the nerve roots, causing them to discharge spontaneously and to become sensitive to mechanical stimuli (Devor 1994). As a consequence, nerve movement, which normally accompanies spinal movement, as well as nerve root compression, becomes a source of pain.

Disc lesions allowing herniation of the nucleus pul-posus may result in the nerve root being exposed to irri-tant substances, which can also sensitize the nerve root and make compression or traction on the root painful (Boulu & Benoist 1996). Intact annular fibres prevent exposure of the nerve roots to nuclear material, which is reported to be an irritant, so disc degeneration or injury allowing extrusion of the nucleus pulposus can expose the nerve root to chemical irritation.

Also significant in the pathophysiology of this painful condition are the changes occurring within the central nervous system as a result of continuous input from the painful site to dorsal horn and supraspinal structures. As well as the increase in mechanosensitiv-ity of the peripheral nociceptors, activation of specific receptors within the spinal cord by sustained release of neurotransmitters involved with nociception (e.g. Substance P and excitatory amino acids) contributes to the ongoing pain response that follows nerve injury and inflammation (Mao et al 1995).

Hypersensitivity to touch (allodynia) can also result due to reorganization of the dorsal horn, whereby large myelinated fibres can now access second-order neurones that previously were accessed only by noci-ceptive afferents (Cervero & Laird 1996). Noxious afferent input from deep structures also increases flex-or reflexes, possibly contributing to the decrease in straight-leg raise test due to the protective function of the hamstring muscles (Hall & Elvey 1999).

Although radiculopathy is primarily a dysfunction of the neural system, changes of the local muscular and articular systems will also be present (O'Sullivan et al 1997a). Studies in acute and chronic recurrent low back pain have documented evidence of changes in the local muscle system about the injured motion seg-ment (Hides et al 1994, Hodges & Richardson 1996, 1999). Inhibition of the multifidus muscle function occurs after the first episode of low back pain and is present in recurrent back pain (Hides 1994, 1996). It is thought to be causative of chronic back problems.

The compression of the nerve root may have result-ed from an acute injury or repetitive microtrauma to the intervertebral disc and zygapophyseal joints of the L5–S1 motion segment. Depending on the time-course from the original injury and the severity of the injury, clinical testing may reveal articular dysfunction, which could be either instability at the motion seg-ment or specific restrictions of motion. The instability may arise from rupture of annular fibres or joint cap-sule, not unlike the sequelae to an acute ankle sprain. Restriction of motion may result from organization of scar tissue following inflammation. Degenerative changes in the intervertebral foramina can occur as late-stage consequences of injury.

Aetiological features of non-radicular somatic S1 pain

Dysfunction of the L5–S1 segment may result from pathology to the vertebral body, intervertebral disc, zygapophyseal joint, interspinous ligaments or mus-cles in the area. The patient may present with local low back symptoms as well as pain referred into the lower limb. This referred pain may be difficult to localize and will not present in a specific pattern of dermatomal distribution (Bogduk 1984, Kellgren 1939). Clients with this type of presentation may report perceiving sensory disturbance or motor weakness in the lower limb, but are unlikely to demonstrate them on clinical tests or on electrodiagnostic testing.

There is evidence that stimulation of the disc, zygapophyseal joint, ligaments and muscles can pro-duce pain that radiates into the lower limb (Bogduk 1984, Kellgren 1938a, 1939, Lewis 1937). Conversely, it has also been demonstrated that injection of these structures with local anaesthetic can relieve referred pain. Interestingly, the area into which different spinal levels and structures refer demonstrates considerable overlap (Grieve 1994). Tenderness (hyperalgesia) and allodynia may also occur in the area of referral as well as at the source of the symptoms, providing further difficulties with establishing the structure or mechanism at the source of the symptoms. Therefore, skill in assessment of potential sources of pain is important in differential diagnosis.

The mechanisms for somatic referred pain are not fully understood. However, it is generally recognized that changes in central nervous system function are responsible for the onset of referred pain. It is much more likely to be triggered by deep somatic tissue (such as muscles or joints) or viscera, rather than by cutaneous input (Mense et al 1997). The following are some of the possible mechanisms for the perception of referred symptoms:

1. Pain may be referred to areas having the same segmental innervation and which converge on the same second-order neurons within the dorsal horn. An example of this is the referral of cardiac pain to the left shoulder. This mechanism may explain superficial referred pain as neurons receiving information from deep somatic tissue also receiving input from cutaneous afferents. However, convergence between muscle and other deep afferents is unlikely (Hoheisel et al 1993).

2. Intense nociceptive input following tissue or nerve damage can lead to increases in the excitability of the dorsal-horn neurons, termed sensitization. This in turn leads to the development of expanded receptive fields so that pain is perceived outside the original area of the injury. It has been suggested that the development of referred pain may be reliant on the intensity and duration of the initiating stimulus (Arendt-Nielsen et al 1999). It appears that the greater the initial stimulus, the larger the area and intensity of the remote pain site.

3. The sympathetic nervous system may also contribute to referred symptoms as changes in outflow, mediated either spinally or supraspinally, can produce trophic changes in the area of referral. Nociceptors can also develop sensitivity to noradrenaline, such that normal sympathetic activity involving noradrenaline as a transmitter can now produce pain.

4. Supraspinal regions such as the thalamus and cortex have demonstrated changes, which may mediate an increase in response to stimulation by movement or touch, of areas remote from the source of symptoms. In addition, a decrease in descending inhibitory control, possibly resulting from continued afferent nociceptive input, may cause widespread musculoskeletal symptoms such as are evident in the condition of fibromyalgia (Graven-Nielsen et al 1999).

Two possible scenarios for the referral of symptoms to a remote source have been presented and it may be tempting to consider that these conditions exist separately as described. However, if the mechanisms for pain referral are considered, it is possible to see that both types of mechanisms can coexist. The client with a herniated disc compressing the S1 nerve root may experience both sharp, shooting dermatomally distributed pain as well as a deep ache within the buttock, as the pain may be both somatic and neural in origin. Somatic referral from the disc and nerve-root compression induced sensory and motor signs.

As mentioned at the outset, referred pain presents a diagnostic challenge, both to localize the source of the pain and to develop an understanding of the underlying aetiology. The skilled practitioner takes into account all presenting signs and symptoms and attempts to organize them into a clinical picture which reflects an understanding of the possible pathophysiological mechanisms of the structures involved, as well as the pain-processing systems.

Treatment approach and its rationale

It is important when considering treatment of the patient with back and lower limb pain that a complete physical examination is performed to determine the cause of the pain and associated symptomatology. In cases where there is significant neurological deficit such as motor weakness, it is appropriate to refer the client for further investigation, as surgical decompression of the nerve root or pharmacological management may be the required treatment.

With other cases of low back and lower limb pain in which the accurate identification of neural and somatic components of the symptoms is less clear-cut, the musculoskeletal therapist is required to employ clinical-reasoning skills in the examination of the client, to devise a customized treatment programme. For example, if there is evidence of instability then there is evidence of the efficacy of applying a specific therapeutic exercise programme (O'Sullivan et al 1997a, 1997b). In the presence of hypomobility of the intervertebral motion segments, manual physical therapy is indicated (Maitland et al 2000).

Altered neurodynamics if present can be addressed with specific manual-therapy treatment techniques and exercises (Butler 1991, Hall & Elvey 1999). In the lumbar spine, there is a body of evidence that indicates that pain interferes with the proper functioning of the sensorimotor, motor and muscle systems and that the judicious application of specific therapeutic exercises not only ameliorates these deficits and pain but also lessens recurrence (Hides et al 1996, McLain et al 1999, O'Sullivan et al 1997a, 1997b, 1998, Richardson et al 1999, Sullivan et al 2000). Interestingly, this phenomenon of altered sensorimotor-system functioning in response to pain and injury occurs in many if not all other body regions, emphasizing the need for adequate examination and therapeutic intervention for this system.

Advice on the nature of the problem and back care, as well as the importance of encouraging pain-free movement, is also necessary to reassure the patient and prevent the sequelae of damaging effects of inactivity.

Summary

- Related spinal and limb pain may arise from either neural compression and irritation (e.g. nerve root), somatic structures (e.g. disc, ligaments, joints), or a combination of all these potential sources.
- Nerve-root pain is characteristically a sharp shooting pain that is dermatomally distributed and often worse distally.
- Somatic referred pain is characteristically a deep aching sensation that is not dermatomally distributed:
- Both mechanical and biochemical factors are important in the initial pathophysiology of nerve-root compression.
- True nerve-root compression is accompanied by changes in nerve conductivity, such as motor weakness or decreased reflexes.
- Changes to central nervous system function also contribute to this painful condition.
- Radicular pain may also result from increased mechanosensitivity of nerves following inflammation mediated by nervi nervorum.
- In addition to neural system changes, dysfunction of the muscular and articular systems contribute to the clinical picture. Sensorimotor deficits are usually present.
- Treatment will be directed by the examination findings related to the types of dysfunction that are present.

CHRONIC LATERAL EPICONDYLALGIA

Chronic lateral epicondylalgia, or as it is commonly referred to but not always appropriately so, 'tennis

elbow', occurs in about 3% of the general population and as much as 15% in high-risk populations (e.g. tennis, fish processing, repetitive manual industries).

There is no scientifically validated test to determine if it is chronic or acute, but it is generally accepted that it is chronic after 4–6 weeks from its onset. This condition is used as an example because it typifies a type of overuse or chronic musculotendinous pain that occurs throughout the body (e.g. patellar and Achilles tendonopathy).

The primary reason that these conditions are important to cover in a chapter on musculoskeletal pain is the stark contrast between the ease with which they can be identified or diagnosed on clinical examination and the difficulty in identifying the underlying aetiology. Also, they are usually very difficult to treat and interfere with normal function.

A simple uncomplicated case of lateral epicondylalgia presents with local pain over the lateral elbow region with or without some spread into the forearm and possibly into the wrist in some clients. The pain is usually intermittent, meaning that it is not present at rest, and is aggravated by manual tasks that require gripping actions.

Key physical examination signs are pain reproduction on direct manual palpation over the lateral epicondyle and with grip-strength testing (Haker 1991). Pain-free grip strength is almost always markedly limited in chronic lateral epicondylalgia (Stratford et al 1993, Vicenzino et al 1996, 1998). Other signs relate to pain with muscle stretches and contractions of the wrist extensors and in particular extensor carpi radialis brevis (Haker 1991, Stratford et al 1993). Note that the clinical presentation, although reported by the client as being predominantly a painful one, almost always manifests as a motor dysfunction. This simple clinical presentation is in stark contrast to the inconclusive understanding of this condition's aetiology.

Aetiological features and clinical implications

Studies conducted on biopsy material taken at the time of surgical treatment for lateral epicondylalgia have not identified any signs of inflammatory process. Instead there have been signs of connective-tissue degeneration (Nirschl 1989, Regan et al 1992, Verhaar et al 1993). However, these findings are confounded by the prior administration of numerous corticosteroid injections into the site of pain.

This finding of degenerative collagen changes in chronic tendonopathies has been shown at other common problem sites (Khan & Cook 2000, Khan et al

2000, Nirschl 1989). Khan and Cook's (2000) review on the subject of tendonopathies, which focuses on the patellar and Achilles tendons, provides a treatise of this matter. In terms of studying the aetiology of chronic lateral epicondylalgia, another approach has been taken, in which qualitative sensory and motor testing has been conducted in order to characterize the pain condition and to develop an understanding of possible pain mechanisms at play.

Quantitative sensory testing has indicated that the pain mechanism of lateral epicondylalgia may be that of secondary hyperalgesia (Smith & Wright 1993, Wright et al 1992, 1994). The mechanism of secondary hyperalgesia is one of central sensitization rather than peripheral sensitization through exposure of C-fibre polymodal nociceptors to algogenic substances such as those produced by inflammation. Central sensitization refers to the increased excitatory or decreased inhibitory influences on central nervous system neurons in the dorsal horn and at higher centres (Sluka 1996, Sluka & Rees 1997). This process is one of nociceptive system dysfunction that has also been proposed as a possible underlying mechanism for other chronic pain states (see other sections and (Cohen et al 1992, Cohen & Quintner 1993, Meyer et al 1994)).

One of the characteristics of secondary hyperalgesia is that it is found in an area that is neurologically related, but not directly over the site of the injured tissue. A potential source of chronic lateral epicondylalgia is any of the structures of the cervical spine. A case series study of treatment of the cervical spine of chronic lateral epicondyle sufferers who had failed conservative and in some cases surgical treatments resulted in an amelioration of the painful condition (Gunn & Milbrandt 1976). In our laboratory, in which all subjects with chronic lateral epicondylalgia have a complete physical examination prior to admission into a study, we found that most of subjects who have not experienced neck pain have signs of abnormal joint, muscle and neural function (Vicenzino et al 1996, 1998).

Randomized, double blind, placebo-controlled studies have shown that manual therapy treatment of the neck produces an initial reduction in pain thresholds at the elbow, thereby concurring with the concept that lateral epicondylalgia may well be a secondary hyperalgesia (Vicenzino et al 1996, 1998). Further research is required to accurately determine the role of cervical spine structures in the pain experienced in chronic lateral epicondylalgia.

Two other features of lateral epicondylalgia point to central nervous system involvement. They are dysfunction of the motor and neural systems (Pienimaki et al 1997; Vicenzino & Wright 1996, Vicenzino et al 1995, 1998 Wright et al 1994, Yaxley & Jull 1993). Pienimaki et al (1997) demonstrated that the affected arm in subjects with chronic lateral epicondylalgia had reduced performance on a number of tasks of reaction time, speed of movement and coordination. Most insightful was the finding that the unaffected side also displayed motor deficits when compared to a normal control group, possibly implicating a central motor control problem.

The neural system dysfunction usually manifests itself as positive neurodynamic tests (Wright et al 1994, Yaxley & Jull 1993). Interpretation of positive neurodynamic tests is not without problem, with two competing models that seek to explain the presence of such a test; the peripheral or local neural tissue and the central pain-processing models. The peripheral model explains the positive test in terms of mechanical restriction of gliding motion of the nerve within the surrounding tissues, whereas the central model explains a positive test as a manifestation of the flexor withdrawal response, implying altered central nervous system processing (Butler 1991, Vicenzino & Wright 1996).

At this stage, no definitive statement can be made about which model applies to chronic lateral epicondylalgia, but the presence of such a positive test, like deficits in motor processing and grip-strength tests, serve as guidelines to the management of the condition.

The preceding discussion has assumed that the case example was a relatively simple one, site of pain presentation over the lateral epicondyle. This is not always the case. There are some clients who will have concomitant neck and radicular pain either of somatic or neural origin. In this case of a complicated neck–arm pain and lateral epicondylalgia the clinician needs to identify by physical examination the most appropriate and expedient manner in which to control the pain and improve function.

Treatment approach and its rationale

Labelle et al (1992) attempted a meta-analysis of treatments for this condition and reported that it was not possible, mainly due to the poor methodological quality of the research. Subsequent to Labelle's publication, two randomized clinical trials have examined therapeutic exercise (Pienimaki et al 1996) and manual therapy (Drechsler et al 1997).

Pienimaki et al (1996) studied the efficacy of a progressive and slowly graduated programme of strengthening and stretching exercises and found it to be superior to ultrasound. This study was of a high methodological rating and corroborates the clinical notion that treatment should focus on addressing the presenting physical impairments, which in chronic lateral epicondylalgia are predominantly deficits of motor control and the muscular system. Pain is the other major presenting feature of this condition.

Drechsler et al (1997) showed that manipulation of the radiohumeral joint and radial nerve provided greater improvements in pain and function than did massage, exercise and ultrasound. A new manual-therapy treatment technique called mobilization with movement has also been shown to improve grip strength and reduce pain in a single case study (Vicenzino & Wright 1995) and a case series study (Abbott et al 2000).

Manual therapy is often used clinically to relieve pain and there is a growing evidence-base of its efficacy (see chapter on physical treatments). Note the approach is again one based on using specifically applied physical activity through a programme of therapeutic exercise as a stimulus to resolve the chronic musculoskeletal pain.

Summary

- Pain and motor system dysfunction is a characteristic of conditions such as chronic lateral epicondylalgia.
- Inflammation is not a feature of chronic lateral epicondylalgia or in many other chronic tendinopathies.
- The pain and possibly the dysfunction of chronic lateral epicondylalgia appear to result from the altered pain processing of secondary hyperalgesia.
- Motor-system impairment is a strong feature of chronic lateral epicondylalgia.
- Treatment must address motor system deficits while providing pain relief.

MUSCLE PAIN

Muscle is highly innervated and can be a source of pain and dysfunction. There are several types of muscle pain that will bring the client to a physical or occupational therapist. They can be thought of in two broad categories: the acute localized muscle injury with a defined precipitating incident and the insidious multiple-muscle pain which is usually chronic and complex in its presentation and aetiology.

In the acute muscle injury the client will usually describe an injurious event, either a sudden rapid movement or a repetitive microtraumatic movement, in which the muscle was overloaded to the extent that

some or all of its fibres were disrupted. The pain and injury is usually restricted to one muscle or at least a group of muscles that have synergistic functions about the same joint or motion segment.

The other type of muscle pain is usually generalized to a number of body regions and systems (e.g. immune, articular, psychological), has an insidious onset and is usually longstanding in nature. These muscle pain syndromes have attracted various labels over time, such as fibromyalgia syndrome, myofascial pain syndrome, fibrositis, muscular rheumatism, myalgia, myofascitis, fibromyalgia rheumatism and tension rheumatism (Cantu & Grodin 1992, Salter 1999). They have been associated with unknown aetiology, negative results from traditional medical diagnostic tests and by a process of elimination frequently attributed a predominant psychological basis. Currently fibromyalgia syndrome and myofascial pain syndrome are the terms used to describe two loose groupings of signs and symptoms of the globally spread muscle aches and pains of long-standing duration.

Cantu and Grodin (1992) have further classified muscle pain by describing a continuum of the complexity of such pain states. In their schema, fibromyalgia syndrome is at the very complex end of the continuum (Carli et al 2000), mechanical or acute-onset muscle pains at the least complex end of the continuum and myofascial pain syndrome somewhere in-between. They propose that the best approach to management of these pain states is to consider where along the continuum the pain syndrome is located. This section will provide a brief overview of the aetiological features pertaining to clinical presentations of muscle pain and its treatment.

There are two other forms of muscle pain that will likely present to a therapist's clinic. One is muscle pain that is referred, usually from spinal structures or viscera. The phenomenon of referred pain and visceral pain has been covered in other sections of this chapter and book. The other pain that may present to a clinic is delayed-onset muscle soreness or DOMS, which is usually a transient muscle soreness that occurs after a bout of unaccustomed exercise, especially that which involves novel eccentric contractions. This soreness is usually transient and will not be covered herein. The reader is referred to the sports medicine and exercise literature for information regarding DOMS.

As elaborated elsewhere in this and other chapters, the muscle and motor systems are frequently involved in musculoskeletal pain states that originate from other structures (i.e. articular, ligaments, capsule, nerve, tendon). Muscles become inhibited and eventually weak in response to pain and swelling. They may also become overactive or facilitated following injury and in the presence of pain. Both these inhibited and facilitated states may predispose the muscles to injury and pain, making it essential to include a thorough investigation of the muscle and motor systems in any client presenting with musculoskeletal pain.

Aetiological features of acute-onset muscle pain and clinical implications

Much like the acute ankle sprain described above, the client will present to the clinic with reasonably classic signs and symptoms and a recollection of a definite event that precipitated the muscle pain. The area of pain is most likely to be localized deep in the muscle that was injured, although muscle referral patterns beyond the area of the injured muscle and the mechanism of such referral have been reported (Andersen et al 2000, Arendt-Nielsen 1999, Kellgren 1938a, 1938b, Torebjork et al 1984). Associated with the pain are the other classic signs of the inflammatory response to injury, namely swelling, redness, heat and dysfunction, the underlying aetiological features being similar to that described in the section on the acute inflammatory response to the ankle injury.

The location of the swelling should be noted for several reasons. Widespread oedema beyond the location of the injured muscle, often distal to the muscle as a result of gravitation of the oedema, is often associated with pain and dysfunction from structures bathed in the oedema (e.g. nerves, tendons, and joints), as well as the injured muscle. Localization of the swelling to the site of injury within a muscle compartment is indicative of an intramuscular injury. It is important to identify intramuscular swelling which is considerable, tense and under pressure as this may be a precursor to a compartment syndrome.

If the swelling follows a severe injury and is rapid in onset and progressively increasing, medical referral is strongly recommended, as this may result in compromise of the neurovascular supply to the region and subsequent tissue-death.

In severe muscle tears there may be a total disruption of muscle fibres and an observable gap and discontinuity in the muscle. Often this is associated with a bunching-up of the torn fibres proximal to the tear site or gap.

The dysfunction that occurs following an injury to muscle usually involves either a restriction of extensibility of the muscle and resultant reductions in the relevant joint motion, weakness on muscle-strength testing, or both.

The healing process that follows the inflammatory response to trauma is very similar to that described with the acute ankle sprain, but with the distinct difference that muscle fibre may regenerate in the appropriate environment, unlike connective tissue such as ligaments and capsules, which heal by fibrous scar (Caplan et al 1987, Grounds 1991).

Muscle contusions that occur following a direct blow to the muscle are aetiologically similar to the acute muscle tear, in that there is the initial inflammatory response followed by the healing processes outlined above. The treatment is much the same as described for muscle tears, with the resolution usually being uneventful except in rare cases, in which the resolution of the healing haematoma is retarded by the replacement of fibroblasts by osteoblasts and the subsequent laying down of bone in the muscle (Brukner & Khan 1993).

In these cases the muscle pain does not settle within the first several weeks as occurs normally. Persistent pains at night, on awaking in the morning and during physical activity are key clinical symptoms. On examination there is marked dysfunction of the muscle with a consolidating haematoma present on palpation. Radiographic examination between 3 and 6 weeks reveals the formation of bone at the site of injury and confirms a diagnosis of myositis ossificans (Brukner & Khan 1993, Sanders & Nemeth 1996). The condition should resolve if the client does not aggravate it and treatment usually involves rest from aggravating activities and pain relief.

Treatment approach for acute muscle pain and injury and its rationale

The treatment of acute muscle injuries is much the same in principle as it is for the acute ankle sprain. That is, there is an initial focus on combating the deleterious effects of the inflammatory process, that is then followed by an active approach to facilitating the restoration of function. Therapeutic exercise and massage are two invaluable physical treatments for muscle pain and injury. As is the case with any musculoskeletal pain, the clinical-reasoning process employed in the examination of the client's problem and the evaluation of the signs and symptoms underpins the treatment approach.

In terms of clinical management of muscle injuries there are two patterns of clinical presentation that are noteworthy. For simplicity's sake, they are termed the 'stretch' and 'contraction' muscle injuries. The major difference between the two is based on the mechanism of injury and findings from tests of muscle length and strength.

The muscle stretch injury usually occurs following an activity in which the client has over-stretched the muscle and presents with markedly reduced muscle length and good if not normal muscle strength. For example, this could occur in a football player who has raised his leg well beyond his normal range of motion.

In contrast, the contraction-type muscle injury occurs following a sudden explosive contraction as in sprinting or sudden acceleration during running and presents with good muscle length and marked weakness on muscle-strength tests, especially eccentric contraction.

It is hypothesized that the stretch injury involves the connective-tissue framework of the muscle but not the contractile components, whereas the contraction-type tear has had a limited impact on the connective-tissue framework and a substantial impact on the contraction mechanism. The contraction tear appears also to manifest as impairment in the coordination of the eccentric to concentric contraction switch-over during rapid movements.

Although these two types of patterns of muscle injury signs occur commonly as separate entities, they may also occur concurrently. The significance of identifying differences in clinical presentation is evident during management of the muscle pain, especially after the initial anti-inflammatory treatment phase. Stretch-type injuries require treatment approaches that increase muscle length (e.g. PNF, heat, stretching exercises, relaxation exercises), whereas contraction-type tears require re-education of the contraction mechanism and strengthening (e.g. specific therapeutic exercise, especially coordination of eccentric-concentric coupling, progressive resistance exercise programmes).

Stanton and Purdam (1989) present an example of the clinical rationale required to address a hamstring contraction-type injury with an eccentric-concentric coupling contraction-type dysfunction. Most notably, the therapeutic exercises that are used should mimic elements of the hamstring contraction during sprinting activities, such as hip and knee angles, hamstring contraction type, and speed of the movement (Stanton & Purdham 1989).

Aetiological features of diffuse muscle pain states and clinical implications

In stark contrast to the relatively uncomplicated clinical presentation of muscle pain following an injury, the diffuse aches and pains of fibromyalgia and myofascial pain syndromes have provoked considerable debate and controversy (Bennett 1999, 2000, Cantu &

Grodin 1992, Cohen 1999, Cohen & Quintner 1993, 1998, Goldenberg 1999, Norregaard et al 1999, Quintner & Cohen 1994, 1999, Tunks et al 1995).

This is especially so for fibromyalgia syndrome, which has been classified by the American College of Rheumatology as the presence of widespread aching and pain that has been present for at least 3 months (Wolfe et al 1990) and there should be tenderness to manual palpation of approximately 4 kg cm^{-2} pressure over at least 11 of a possible nine paired (18) sites across the body. These sites are located at the:

- Insertion of nuchal muscles into occiput
- Intertransverse ligament of C5–C7
- Upper border of trapezius
- Supraspinatus muscle belly
- Pectoralis major muscle 2 cm from the sternum over the second rib
- About 2 cm below the lateral epicondyle of the elbow
- Proximal lateral gluteal area
- Over the muscle insertion into the greater trochanter
- Medial femoral epicondyle.

However, the clinical relevance of this classification of fibromyalgia and indeed of the existence of the syndrome itself has recently been questioned (Bennett 1999, Cohen 1999, Cohen & Quintner 1998, Quintner & Cohen 1999). As well as the widespread muscle pain, clients frequently experience significant sleep disorders, awaking unrefreshed and physically fatigued in the morning, and they often experience anxiety and depression (Cantu & Grodin 1992). Associated with this disorder are physiological, biochemical and psychosocial abnormalities, such as altered central nervous system processing of pain, and abnormal levels of substance P, excitatory amino acids and certain neurohormones (Bennett 1999, 2000, Carli et al 2000, Goldenberg 1999, Graven-Nielsen et al 1999, Larson et al 2000, Russell et al 1996, 1999b, Sorensen et al 1998, Tunks et al 1995). Interestingly, Carli et al (2000) showed that the severity of the disease is related to the number of tender points and their reactivity to pressure–pain tests, which seems to contradict the condition's largely unknown but apparently complex aetiology.

Myofascial pain syndrome is believed to differ from fibromyalgia syndrome in at least two ways, although the two syndromes are also thought to exist along a continuum of complexity and severity with some overlap of diagnostic features (Cantu & Grodin 1992). The pain is more localized to a region (neck–head and face, neck–arm, trunk–chest/abdomen, back–thigh/

leg) and the palpation examination identifies a clinical phenomenon called trigger points.

Trigger points are defined as a focus of hyperirritability in a muscle or its fascia that contributes to dysfunction of the muscle (e.g. tightness, weakness and altered proprioception). A trigger point is always tender as is the tender point of fibromyalgia syndrome, but different in that the trigger point should also be tight or taught, refer pain in a characteristic pattern and sometimes exhibit a local twitch on palpation. Travell and Simons (1983, 1992), in their comprehensive textbooks of this condition, have described the referral patterns of trigger points. The reader is referred to their texts for further technical details.

Despite what appears superficially to be a clear entity with distinct features this condition is also somewhat contentious, as the pathophysiology of the trigger point has not been agreed upon. A peripherally based mechanism of pain generation in myofascial pain syndrome at the trigger points has been postulated (Travell & Simons 1983, 1992).

It has been postulated that there are two stages of trigger-point development. The first occurs early in the development of the condition and is one of neuromuscular dysfunction and the second stage, the musculodystrophic stage, involves the development of local structural changes in the muscle. Interestingly, the research into the pathology at the local trigger point has not produced consistent findings that would corroborate these stages and their underlying aetiological significance. However, the regional distribution, referral patterns of trigger points, and the lack of any evidence of pathological processes in the muscle, favour a central mechanism. Quintner and Cohen (1994) have argued that secondary hyperalgesia originating from peripheral nerves may better explain the underlying mechanism of myofascial pain syndrome. Often there are concomitant dysfunctions of the articular and neural systems, and associated postural and movement imbalances, adding to the concept that the disorder involves more than just the muscle system.

Treatment approach for fibromyalgia and myofascial pain syndromes and its rationale

Not unlike the approach for many musculoskeletal pain disorders, it would appear that the optimum treatment approach for these conditions is one that involves a graduated and progressive therapeutic exercise programme of physical activity that is based on a thorough clinical examination.

Meta-analysis of treatment trials of fibromyalgia syndrome indicates that treatments that should be favoured are non-pharmacological treatments such as exercise and cognitive–behavioural therapy, in conjunction with appropriate pharmacological management of pain and depression, should it be a feature of the presentation (O'Malley et al 1999, 2000, Rossy et al 1999). Moderate to high-intensity exercise was found to be slightly more efficacious than mind–body therapy in a systematic review of mind–body therapies (Hadhazy et al 2000).

Other treatments that have been used in the treatment of this condition are the administration of low doses of human interferon alpha (Russell et al 1999a), zinc (Russell et al 2000), anti-inflammatory medication (Russell et al 1991) and acupuncture (Berman et al 1999).

Much has been written about the treatment of myofascial pain syndrome and in particular trigger points, but it appears that systematic reviews have not been conducted. A problem confronting researchers is the difficulty in finding a homogeneous subject group. Treatments for myofascial pain syndrome aim to reduce myofascial pain and restore function. Travell and Simmons (1983, 1992), in their landmark textbooks, described several approaches to the management of trigger points in myofascial pain syndrome, notably spray and stretch, and inject and stretch techniques of the muscles containing the trigger points. The spray and inject techniques offer pain relief while the myofascial tissue is stretched.

Massage techniques such as ischaemic pressures and myofascial massage were also advocated as alternative approaches. There is some level of support in the literature for the use of injection therapy (Fischer 1999, Hong 1994) but not all research is supportive of it (McMillan & Blasberg 1994). Ischaemic pressures and stretching exercises have been shown to be of benefit in subjects with neck and upper back pain (Hanten et al 2000).

Other approaches that have been advocated, although not by all (Hong 1994, McMillan et al 1997), are autogenic relaxation (Banks et al 1998), TENS (Graff Radford, et al 1989, Hsueh et al 1997), neuroreflexotherapy (Kovacs et al 1997) and dry needling (Hesse et al 1994).

Electrotherapy modalities such as ultrasound (Gam et al 1998) and LASER (Simmons 2000, Simunovic et al 1998) seem not to be of benefit, whereas exercise and massage exert a small beneficial effect (Gam et al 1998). However, caution must be used when interpreting the results of some of the LASER therapy studies as this treatment may exert beneficial effects that are masked by poor study methodology (Beckerman et al 1992).

Summary

- As Cantu and Grodin (1992) have stated, muscle pain seems to exist along a continuum of complexity in clinical presentation and aetiology, with simple uni-muscle pains at one end and complex multi-muscle pains at the other end of the continuum.
- Muscle pain following a defined traumatic event is usually localized to that muscle with or without some referral, and has a characteristic and reasonably simple underlying aetiology.
- Early after the injury there is an inflammatory response, which over several days resolves, being taken over by the healing response much like the healing process following an ankle injury (see above).
- Referred muscle pain appears to be a feature of severity and chronicity.
- Longstanding muscle pain that is spread across a number of muscles and body regions appears to have a complex underlying pathophysiology that is not fully understood. Two such muscle pains are fibromyalgia and myofascial pain syndromes.
- The aetiology of chronic muscle pain involves an active involvement of the central nervous system in the form of changes in central processing of somatosensory information and disordered nociceptive system function.

- Treatment of all muscle pains should address the inevitable impairments in muscle and motor function and encourage active participation. Therapeutic exercise is the modality of choice, but with due respect for the pain experienced by the client.

Study questions/questions for revision

1. Explain the processes that occur immediately after an injury and how they contribute to the pain experienced by the client. Use an acute injury of the medial collateral ligament of the knee as an example.
2. Outline the stages that are involved in healing following injury, the pain mechanisms involved and implications for therapy.
3. What are some of the mechanisms by which the area of perceived pain may not be the source of the pain?
4. Describe the changes that may occur to other systems in the presence of musculoskeletal pain and how they may influence treatment planning.
5. Describe the aetiology of the following conditions and briefly outline implications for treatment approach:
   - Hip osteoarthritis
   - Neck and upper limb pain (e.g. brachialgia, cervico-brachialgia)
   - Achilles tendinosis
   - Acute quadriceps muscle strain, highlighting differences between contraction- and stretch-type injuries.

REFERENCES

Abbott J, Patla C, Jensen R 2000 Grip strength changes immediately following elbow mobilisation with movement in subjects with lateral epicondylalgia. Proceedings of the 7th Scientific Conference of the IFOMT in conjunction with the MPAA, Perth, Australia

Andersen O K, Graven-Nielsen T, Matre D, Arendt-Nielsen L, Schomburg E D 2000 Interaction between cutaneous and muscle afferent activity in polysynaptic reflex pathways: a human experimental study. Pain 84(1): 29–36

Andriacchi T, Sabiston P, Dehaven K, Dahners L, Woo S, Frank C, Oakes B, Brand R, Lewis J 1987 Ligament: injury and repair. In: Woo S, Buckwalter J (eds) Injury and Repair of the Musculoskeletal Soft Tissues. American Academy of Orthopaedic Surgeons, Illinois, pp 103–128

Arendt-Nielsen L, Graven-Nielsen T, Svensson P 1999 Assessment of muscle pain in humans – Clinical and experimental aspects. Journal of Musculoskeletal Pain 7(1–2): 25–41

Ashbury A, Fields H 1984 Pain due to peripheral nerve damage: an hypothesis. Neurology 34: 1587–1590

Bader D, Bouten, C 2000 Biomechanics of soft tissues. In: Dvir Z (ed) Clinical Biomechanics. Churchill Livingstone, New York, pp 35–64

Banks S L, Jacobs D W, Gevirtz R, Hubbard D R 1998 Effects of autogenic relaxation training on electromyographic activity in active myofascial trigger points. Journal of Musculoskeletal Pain 6(4): 23–32

Basbaum A I, Levine J D 1991 The contribution of the nervous-system to inflammation and inflammatory disease. Canadian Journal of Physiology and Pharmacology 69(5): 647–651

Beckerman H, Debie R A, Bouter L M, Decuyper H J, Oostendorp R A B 1992 The efficacy of laser therapy for musculoskeletal and skin disorders – a criteria-based metaanalysis of randomized clinical trials. Physical Therapy 72(7): 483–491

Bennett R M 1999 Fibromyalgia review. Journal of Musculoskeletal Pain 7(4): 85–102

Bennett R M 2000 Fibromyalgia review. Journal of Musculoskeletal Pain 8(3): 93–110

Berman B M, Ezzo J, Hadhazy V, Swyers J P 1999 Is acupuncture effective in the treatment of fibromyalgia? Journal of Family Practice 48(3): 213–218

Bettany J A, Fish D R, Mendel F C 1990a High-voltage pulsed direct current: effect on edema formation after hyperflexion injury. Archives of Physical Medicine and Rehabilitation 71(9): 677–681

Bettany J A, Fish D R, Mendel F C 1990b Influence of high voltage pulsed direct current on edema formation following impact injury. Physical Therapy 70(4): 219–224

Bogduk N 1984 The rationale for referred patterns of neck and back pain. Patient Management, August: 13–21

Boulu P, Benoist M 1996 Recent data on the pathophysiology of nerve root compression and pain. Revue Du Rhumatisme 63(5): 358–363

Bove G M, Light A R 1997 The nervi nervorum – Missing link for neuropathic pain? Pain Forum 6(3): 181–190

Brukner P, Khan K 1991 The difficult ankle. Australian Family Physician 20(7): 919–930

Brukner P, Khan K 1993 Clinical Sports Medicine. McGraw-Hill Book Company, Sydney

Bullock-Saxton J E 1994 Local sensation changes and altered hip muscle function following severe ankle sprain. Physical Therapy 74(1): 17–31

Butler D 1991 Mobilisation of the Nervous System. Churchill Livingstone, Melbourne

Cantu R, Grodin A 1992 Myofascial Manipulation: Theory and Clinical Application. Aspen Publishers, Gaithersburg, Maryland

Caplan A, Carlson B, Faulkner J, Fischman D, Garrett W J 1987 Skeletal Muscle. In: Woo S, Buckwalter J, (eds) Injury and Repair of the Musculoskeletal Soft Tissues. American Academy of Orthopaedic Surgeons, Illinois, pp 213–291

Carli G, Suman A, Badii F, Bachiocco V, Di Piazza G, Biasi G, Castrogiovanni P, Marcolongo R 2000 Differences between patients with fibromyalgia and patients with chronic musculoskeletal pain. In: Devor M, Rowbotham M, Wiesenfeld-Hallin Z, (eds) Proceedings of the 9th World Congress on Pain, Vol. 16. IASP Press, Seattle, pp 1031–1037

Cervero F, Laird J M A 1996 Mechanisms of touch-evoked pain (allodynia): A new model. Pain 68(1): 13–23

Chard J A, Tallon D, Dieppe P A 2000 Epidemiology of research into interventions for the treatment of osteoarthritis of the knee joint. Annals of the Rheumatic Diseases 59(6): 414–418

Cohen M L 1999 Is fibromyalgia a distinct clinical entity? The disapproving rheumatologist's evidence. Best Practice & Research in Clinical Rheumatology 13(3): 421–425

Cohen M L, Quintner J L 1993 Fibromyalgia syndrome, a problem of tautology. Lancet 342(8876): 906–909

Cohen M L, Quintner J L 1998 Fibromyalgia syndrome and disability: a failed construct fails those in pain. Medical Journal of Australia 168(8): 402–404

Cohen M L, Arroyo J F, Champion G D, Browne C D 1992 In search of the pathogenesis of refractory cervicobrachial pain syndrome. A deconstruction of the RSI phenomenon. Medical Journal of Australia 156(6): 432–436

Cordova M L, Ingersoll C D, LeBlanc M J 2000 Influence of ankle support on joint range of motion before and after

exercise: A meta-analysis. Journal of Orthopaedic & Sports Physical Therapy 30(4): 170–177

de Bie R A, de Vet H C W, Lenssen T F, van den Wildenberg F, Kootsra G, Knipschild P G 1998 Low-level laser therapy in ankle sprains: A randomized clinical trial. Archives of Physical Medicine and Rehabilitation 79(11): 1415–1420

DeLee J 1990 Tissue remodelling and response to therapeutic exercise. In Leadbetter W, Buckwalter J, Gordon S, (eds), Sports-induced Inflammation. American Academy of Orthopaedic Surgeons, Illinois, pp 547–554

Devor M 1994 The pathophysiology of damaged peripheral nerves. In: Melzack R, Wall P (eds) The Textbook of Pain pp 79–100

Deyle G D, Henderson N E, Matekel R L, Ryder M G, Garber M B, Allison S C 2000 Effectiveness of manual physical therapy and exercise in osteoarthritis of the knee. A randomized, controlled trial. Annals of Internal Medicine 132(3): 173–181

Drechsler W I, Knarr J F, SnyderMackler L 1997 A comparison of two treatment regimens for lateral epicondylitis: A randomized trial of clinical interventions. Journal of Sport Rehabilitation 6(3): 226–234

Dyson M 1987 Mechanisms involved in therapeutic ultrasound. Physiotherapy 73: 116–120

Fantone J 1990 Basic concepts in inflammation. In: Leadbetter W, Buckwalter J, Gordon S (eds) Sports-induced Inflammation. American Academy of Orthopaedic Surgery, Illinois, pp 47–48

Farrell M, Gibson S J, McMeeken J M, Helme R D 2000 Increased movement pain in osteoarthritis of the hands is associated with A beta-mediated cutaneous mechanical sensitivity. Journal of Pain 1(3): 229–242

Fernandes N, Allison G T, Hopper D 2000 Peroneal latency in normal and injured ankles at varying angles of perturbation. Clinical Orthopaedics and Related Research (375): 193–201

Ferrell W R, Wood L, Baxendale R H 1988 The effect of acute joint inflammation on flexion reflex excitability in the decerebrate, low-spinal cat. Quarterly Journal of Experimental Physiology, 73(1): 95–102

Fischer A A 1999 Treatment of myofascial pain. Journal of Musculoskeletal Pain 7(1–2): 131–142

Frank C 1996 Ligament injuries: Pathophysiology and healing. In: Zachewski J, Magee D J, Quillen W S (ed) Athtetic Injuries and Rehabilitation. WB Saunders Company, Philadelphia, pp 9–25

Gam A N, Warming S, Larsen L H, Jensen B, Hoydalsmo O, Allon I, Andersen B, Gotzsche N E, Petersen M, Mathiesen B 1998 Treatment of myofascial trigger-points with ultrasound combined with massage and exercise – a randomised controlled trial. Pain 77(1): 73–79

Garsden L R, Bullock-Saxton J E 1999 Joint reposition sense in subjects with unilateral osteoarthritis of the knee. Clinical Rehabilitation 13(2): 148–155

Gauffin H, Tropp H, Odenrick P 1988 Effect of ankle disk training on postural control in patients with functional instability of the ankle joint. International Journal of Sports Medicine 9(2): 141–144

Goldenberg D L 1999 Fibromyalgia syndrome a decade later – What have we learned? Archives of Internal Medicine 159(8): 777–785

Graff Radford S B, Reeves J L, Baker R L, Chiu D 1989 Effects of transcutaneous electrical nerve stimulation on myofascial pain and trigger point sensitivity. Pain 37(1): 1–5

Graven-Nielsen T, Sorenson J, Henriksson K G, Bengtsson M, Arendt-Nielsen L 1999 Central hyperexcitability in fibromyalgia. Journal of Musculoskeletal Pain 7(1–2): 261–271

Grieve G P 1994 Referred pain and other clinical features. In Boyling G D, Palastanga N (eds) Grieve's Modern Manual Therapy: The Vertebral Column, 2nd edn. Churchill Livingstone, Edinburgh, pp 271–292

Grigg P, Schaible H G, Schmidt R F 1986 Mechanical sensitivity of group III and IV afferents from posterior articular nerve in normal and inflamed cat knee. Journal of Neurophysiology 55(4): 635–643

Grounds M D 1991 Towards understanding skeletal-muscle regeneration. Pathology Research and Practice 187(1): 1–22

Gunn C, Milbrandt W 1976 Tennis elbow and the cervical spine. Canadian Medical Association Journal 114: 803–809

Hadhazy V A, Ezzo J, Creamer P, Berman B M 2000 Mind–body therapies for the treatment of fibromyalgia. A systematic review. Journal of Rheumatology 27(12): 2911–2918

Haker E 1991 Lateral epicondylalgia (tennis elbow): A diagnostic and therapeutic challenge. Akademisk Avhandling 8: 9–33

Hall T M, Elvey R L 1999 Nerve trunk pain: physical diagnosis and treatment. Manual Therapy 4(2): 63–73

Hanten W P, Olson S L, Butts N L, Nowicki A L 2000 Effectiveness of a home program of ischemic pressure followed by sustained stretch for treatment of myofascial trigger points. Physical Therapy 80(10): 997–1003

Hargreaves K 1990 Mechanisms of pain sensation resulting from inflammation. In: Leadbetter W, Buckwalter J, Gordon S (eds) Sports-induced inflammation. American Academy of Orthopaedic Surgeons, Illinois, pp 383–392

Harvey W, Dyson M, Pond J, Grahame R 1975 The 'in-vitro' stimulation of protein synthesis in human fibroblasts by therapeutic levels of ultrasound. Paper presented at the Proceedings of 2nd European Congress on Ultrasonics in Medicine

Hesse J, Mogelvang B, Simonsen H 1994 Acupuncture versus metoprolol in migraine prophylaxis – a randomized trial of trigger point inactivation. Journal of Internal Medicine 235(5): 451–456

Hides J A, Stokes M J, Saide M, Jull G A, Cooper D H 1994 Evidence of lumbar multifidus muscle wasting ipsilateral to symptoms in patients with acute subacute low-back-pain. Spine 19(2): 165–172

Hides J A, Richardson C A, Jull G A 1996 Multifidus muscle recovery is not automatic after resolution of acute, first-episode low back pain. Spine 21(23): 2763–2769

Hodges P W, Richardson C A 1996 Inefficient muscular stabilization of the lumbar spine associated with low back pain – A motor control evaluation of transversus abdominis. Spine 21(22): 2640–2650

Hodges P W, Richardson C A 1998 Delayed postural contraction of transversus abdominis in low back pain associated with movement of the lower limb. Journal of Spinal Disorders 11(1): 46–56

Hodges P W, Richardson C A 1999 Altered trunk muscle recruitment in people with low back pain with upper limb movement at different speeds. Archives of Physical Medicine and Rehabilitation 80(9): 1005–1012

Hoffman M, Payne V 1995 The effects of proprioceptive ankle disk training on healthy subjects. Journal of Orthopaedic and Sports Physical Therapy 21(2): 90–93

Hoheisel U, Mense S, Simons D G, Yu X M 1993 Appearance of new receptive-fields in rat dorsal horn neurons following noxious stimulation of skeletal muscle – a model for referral of muscle pain. Neuroscience Letters 153(1): 9–12

Hong C Z 1994 Lidocaine injection versus dry needling to myofascial trigger point – the importance of the local twitch response. American Journal of Physical Medicine & Rehabilitation 73(4): 256–263

Howe J F, Loeser J D, Calvin W H 1977 Mechanosensitivity of dorsal root ganglia and chronically injured axons: a physiological basis for the radicular pain of nerve root compression. Pain 3: 25–41

Hsueh T C, Cheng P T, Kuan T S, Hong C Z 1997 The immediate effectiveness of electrical nerve stimulation and electrical muscle stimulation on myofascial trigger points. American Journal of Physical Medicine & Rehabilitation 76(6): 471–476

Indahl A, Kaigle A M, Reikeras O, Holm S H 1997 Interaction between the porcine lumbar intervertebral disc, zygapophysial joints, and paraspinal muscles. Spine 22(24): 2834–2840

Joris J, Hargreaves K 1987 Involvement of the peripheral nerve system in the development of carrageenan-induced inflammation. Society of Neuroscience 13: 1017

Karlsson J, Lundin O, Lind K, Styf J 1999 Early mobilization versus immobilization after ankle ligament stabilization. Scandinavian Journal of Medicine & Science in Sports 9(5): 299–303

Kellgren J H 1938a Observation on referred pain arising from muscle. Clinical Sciences 3: 175–190

Kellgren J H 1938b A preliminary account of referred pains arising from muscle. British Medical Journal 12: 325–327

Kellgren J 1939 On the distribution of pain arising from deep somatic structures with charts of segmental pain areas. Clinical Sciences 4: 35–46

Kellgren J 1983 Pain in osteoarthritis. Journal of Rheumatology (Suppl.) 2) 18: 108–109

Kellgren J H, Samuel E P 1950 Sensitivity and innervation of articular capsule. Journal of Bone and Joint Surgery 32B: 84–92

Khan K, Cook J 2000 Overuse tendon injuries: where does the pain come from? In: Dilworth Cannon W, DeHaven K (eds) Sports Medicine and Arthroscopy Review, Vol. 8. Lippincott Williams & Wilkins, Philadelphia, pp 17–31

Khan K M, Cook J L, Maffulli N, Kannus P 2000 Where is the pain coming from in tendinopathy? It may be biochemical, not only structural, in origin. British Journal of Sports Medicine 34(2): 81–83

Kidd B, Morris V, Urban L 1996 Pathophysiology of joint pain. Annals of the Rheumatic Diseases 55(5): 276–283

Kovacs F M, Abraira V, Pozo F, Kleinbaum D G, Beltran J, Mateo I, deAyala C P, Pena A, Zea A, GonzalezLanza M, Morillas L 1997 Local and remote sustained trigger point therapy for exacerbations of chronic low back pain – A randomized, double-blind, controlled, multicenter trial. Spine 22(7): 786–797

Labelle H, Guibert R, Joncas J, Newman N, Fallaha M, Rivard C 1992 Lack of scientific evidence for the treatment of lateral epicondylitis of the elbow. An attempted meta-analysis. Journal of Bone and Joint Surgery 74B(5): 646–651

Larson A A, Giovengo S L, Russell I J, Michalek J E 2000 Changes in the concentrations of amino acids in the cerebrospinal fluid that correlate with pain in patients with fibromyalgia: implications for nitric oxide pathways. Pain 87(2): 201–211

Lembeck F, Holzer K 1979 Substance P as a neurogenic mediator of antidromic vasodilation and neurogenic plasma extravasation. Naunym Schmiedebergs Archives of Pharmacology 310: 175–183

Lentell G, Baas B, Lopez D, McGuire L, Sarrels M, Snyder P 1995 The contributions of proprioceptive deficits, muscle function, and anatomic laxity to functional instability of the ankle. Journal of Orthopaedic & Sports Physical Therapy 21(4): 206–215

Lewis T 1937 The nocifensive system of nerves and its reactions. British Medical Journal 194: 431–435: 491–494

Lund J, Donga R, Stohler C 1991 The pain-adaptation model: a discussion of the relationship between chronic musculoskeletal pain and motor activity. Canadian Journal of Physiology and Pharmacology 69: 683–694

Maitland G, Hengeveld E, Banks K, English K 2000 Maitland's Vertebral Manipulation, 6th edn. Butterworth-Heinemann, Sydney

Mao J, Price D D, Mayer D J 1995 Experimental mononeuropathy reduces the antinociceptive effects of morphine: implications for common intracellular mechanisms involved in morphine tolerance and neuropathic pain. Pain 61(3): 353–364

Martinez-Hernandez A, Amenta P 1987 Basic concepts in wound healing. In: Woo S, Buckwalter J (eds) Injury and Repair of the Musculoskeletal Soft Tissues. Illinois: American Academy of Orthopaedic Surgeons, pp 55–101

McCarthy C J, Oldham J A 1999 The effectiveness of exercise in the treatment of osteoarthritic knees: a critical review. Physical Therapy Reviews 4: 241–250

McKnight C M, Armstrong C W 1997 The role of ankle strength in functional ankle instability. Journal of Sport Rehabilitation 6(1): 21–29

McLain K, Powers C, Thayer P, Seymour R J 1999 Effectiveness of exercise versus normal activity on acute low back pain: An integrative synthesis and meta-analysis. Online Journal of Knowledge Synthesis for Nursing 6(7): U1–U8

McMillan A S, Blasberg B 1994 Pain-pressure threshold in painful jaw muscles following trigger point injection. Journal of Orofacial Pain 8(4): 384–390

McMillan A S, Nolan A, Kelly P J 1997 The efficacy of dry needling and procaine in the treatment of myofascial pain in the jaw muscles. Journal of Orofacial Pain 11(4): 307–314

Mense S, Hoheisel U, Kaske A, Reinert A 1997 Muscle pain: Basic mechanisms and clinical correlates. Paper presented at the 8th World Conference on Pain, Seattle

Meyer R, Campbell J, Raja S 1994 Peripheral neural mechanisms of nociception. In: Wall P, Melzack R (eds) Textbook of Pain, 3rd edn. Edinburgh: Churchill Livingstone, pp 13–44

Morton C, Chahl L 1980 Pharmacology of the neurogenic oedema response to electrical stimulation of the saphenous nerve in the rat. Naunym Schmiedebergs Archives of Pharmacology 314: 271–276

Nicholas J J 1994 Physical modalities in rheumatological rehabilitation. Archives of Physical Medicine and Rehabilitation 75(9): 994–1001

Nirschl R 1989 Patterns of failed healing in tendon injury. In: Leadbetter W, Buckwalter J, Gordon S (eds) Sports-induced Inflammation. Illinois: American Academy of Orhtopaedic Surgeons, pp 577–585

Norregaard J, Jacobsen S, Kristensen J H 1999 A narrative review on classification of pain conditions of the upper extremities. Scandinavian Journal of Rehabilitation Medicine 31(3): 153–164

Nyanzi C S, Langridge J, Heyworth J R C, Mani R 1999 Randomized controlled study of ultrasound therapy in the management of acute lateral ligament sprains of the ankle joint. Clinical Rehabilitation 13(1): 16–22

O'Malley P G, Jackson J L, Santoro J, Tomkins G, Balden E, Kroenke K 1999 Antidepressant therapy for unexplained symptoms and symptom syndromes. Journal of Family Practice 48(12): 980–990

O'Malley P G, Balden E, Tomkins G, Santoro J, Kroenke K, Jackson J L 2000 Treatment of fibromyalgia with antidepressants – A meta-analysis. Journal of General Internal Medicine 15(9): 659–666

O'Sullivan P, Twomey L, Alison G 1997a Dysfunction of the neuro-muscular system in the presence of low back pain: Implications for physical therapy management. Journal of Manual and Manipulative Therapy 5(1): 20–26

O'Sullivan P, Twomey L, Alison G 1997b Evaluation of specific stabilising exercise in the treatment of chroic low back pain with radiologic diagnosis of spondylosis or spondylolisthesis. Spine 22: 2959–2967

O'Sullivan P, Twomey L, Alison G 1998 Altered abdominal muscle recruitment in patients with chronic back pain following a specific exercise intervention. Journal of Orthopaedic & Sports Physical Therapy 27(2): 114–124

Pienimaki T, Tarvainen T, Siira P, Vanharanta H 1996 Progressive strengthening and stretching exercises and ultrasound for chronic lateral epicondylitis. Physiotherapy 82(9): 522–530

Pienimaki T T, Kauranen K, Vanharanta H 1997 Bilaterally decreased motor performance of arms in patients with chronic tennis elbow. Archives of Physical Medicine and Rehabilitation 78(10): 1092–1095

Pope R, Herbert R, Kirwan J 1998 Effects of ankle dorsiflexion range and pre-exercise calf muscle stretching on injury risk in Army recruits. Australian Journal of Physiotherapy 44(3): 165–172

Quillen W S, Rouillier L H 1982 Initial management of acute ankle sprains with rapid pulsed compression and cold. Journal of Orthopaedic and Sports Physical Therapy 4(1): 39–43

Quintner J L, Cohen M L 1994 Referred pain of peripheral nerve origin: an alternative to the 'myofascial pain' construct. Clinical Journal of Pain 10(3): 243–251

Quintner J L, Cohen M L 1999 Fibromyalgia falls foul of a fallacy. Lancet 353(9158): 1092–1094

Rees H, Sluka K A, Westlund K N, Willis W D 1994 Do dorsal root reflexes augment peripheral inflammation? Neuroreport 5(7): 821–824

Regan W, Wold L E, Coonrad R, Morrey B F 1992 Microscopic histopathology of chronic refractory lateral epicondylitis. American Journal of Sports Medicine 20(6): 746–749

Richardson C 1987 Atrophy of vastus medialis in patello-femoral pain syndrome. Paper presented at the Proceedings 10th International Congress World Confederation for Physical Therapy, Sydney

Richardson C, Jull G, Hodges P, Hides J 1999 Therapeutic Exercise for Spinal Segmental Stabilisation. Scientific basis and practical techniques. Edinburgh: Churchill Livingstone

Rossy L A, Buckelew S P, Dorr N, Hagglund K J, Thayer J F, McIntosh M J, Hewett J E, Johnson J C 1999 A meta-analysis of fibromyalgia treatment interventions. Annals of Behavioral Medicine 21(2): 180–191

Russell I J, Fletcher E M, Michalek J E, McBroom P C, Hester G G 1991 Treatment of primary fibrositis fibromyalgia syndrome with ibuprofen and alprazolam – a double-blind, placebo-controlled study. Arthritis and Rheumatism 34(5): 552–560

Russell I J, Vipraio G A, Fletcher E M, Lopez Y M, Orr M D, Michalek J E 1996 Characteristics of spinal fluid (CSF) substance P (SP) and calcitonin gene related peptide (CGRP) in fibromyalgia syndrome (FMS). Arthritis and Rheumatism 39(9): 1485–1485

Russell I J, Michalek J E, Kang Y K, Richards A B 1999a Reduction of morning stiffness and improvement in physical function in fibromyalgia syndrome patients treated sublingually with low doses of human interferon-alpha. Journal of Interferon and Cytokine Research 19(8): 961–968

Russell I J, Vipraio G A, Michalek J E, Craig F E, Kang Y K, Richards A B 1999b Lymphocyte markers and natural killer cell activity in fibromyalgia syndrome: Effects of low-dose, sublingual use of human interferon-alpha. Journal of Interferon and Cytokine Research 19(8): 969–978

Russell I J, Older S, Seal L A, Merrill G A, Michalek J E, Ayala E, Vipraio G, Kang Y K, Fletcher E, Haynes W, Flores Y, Walters D 2000 The role of zinc in fibromyalgia [FMS] pain – A pilot study. Arthritis and Rheumatism 43(9): 880

Rydevik B L, Brown M D, Lundborg G 1984 Pathoanatomy and pathophysiology of nerve root compression. Spine 9(1): 7–15

Salter R 1999 Textbook of Disorders and Injuries of the Musculoskeletal System, 3rd edn. Lippincott Williams & Wilkins, Philadelphia

Sanders B, Nemeth W 1996 Hip and thigh injuries. In: Zachewski J, Magee D, Quillen W (eds) Athtetic Injuries and Rehabilitation (pp. 605). Philadelphia: WB Saunders Company

Schaible H G, Grubb B D 1993 Afferent and spinal mechanisms of joint pain. Pain 55(1): 5–54

Schaible H G, Schmidt R F 1985 Effects of an experimental arthritis on the sensory properties of fine articular afferent units. Journal of Neurophysiology 54(5): 1109–1122

Sharma L, Pai Y C, Holtkamp K, Rymer W Z 1997 Is knee joint proprioception worse in the arthritic knee versus the unaffected knee in unilateral knee osteoarthritis? Arthritis and Rheumatism 40(8): 1518–1525

Sheth P, Yu B, Laskowski E R, An K N 1997 Ankle disk training influences reaction times of selected muscles in a simulated ankle sprain. American Journal of Sports Medicine 25(4): 538–543

Shimizu N, Yamaguchi M, Goseki T, Shibata Y, Takiguchi H, Iwasawa T, Abiko Y 1995 Inhibition of prostaglandin E(2) and interleukin-1-beta production by low-power laser irradiation in stretched human periodontal-ligament cells. Journal of Dental Research 74(7): 1382–1388

Simmons D 2000 Myofascial pain syndromes – trigger points. Journal of Musculoskeletal Pain 8(3): 111–117

Sims D 1986 Effects of positioning on ankle edema. Journal of Orthopaedic and Sports Physical Therapy 8(1): 30–33

Simunovic Z, Trobonjaca T, Trobonjaca Z 1998 Treatment of medical and lateral epicondylitis – tennis and golfer's elbow – with low level laser therapy: A multicenter double blind, placebo-controlled clinical study on 324 patients. Journal of Clinical Laser Medicine & Surgery 16(3): 145–151

Slemender C, Brandt K D, Heilman M S, Mazzuca S A, Braunstein E M, Katz B P, Wolinsky F D 1997 Quadriceps weakness and osteoarthritis of the knee. Annals of Internal Medicine 127: 97–104

Sluka K A 1996 Pain mechanisms involved in musculoskeletal disorders. Journal of Orthopaedic and Sports Physical Therapy 24(4): 240–254

Sluka K A, Rees H 1997 The neuronal response to pain. Physiotherapy Theory and Practice 13(1): 3–22

Smith J, Wright A 1993 The effect of selective blockade of myelinated afferent neurons on mechanical hyperalgesia in lateral epicondylalgia. The Pain Clinic 6(1): 9–16

Sorensen J, Graven-Nielsen T, Henriksson K G, Bengtsson M, Arendt-Nielsen L 1998 Hyperexcitability in fibromyalgia. Journal of Rheumatology 25(1): 152–155

Stanton P, Purdham C 1989 Hamstring injuries in sprinting: The role of eccentric exercises. The Jounral of Orthopaedic and Sports Physical Therapy 10: 343–349

Stein C, Cabot P, Schafer M 1999 Peripheral opioid analgesia: Mechanisms and clinical implications. Opioids in Pain Control: Basic and Clinical Aspects. Cambridge University Press, USA

Stockwell R A 1991 Cartilage failure in osteoarthritis: Relevance of normal structure and function. A review. Clinical Anatomy 4: 161–191

Stratford P, Levy D, Gowland C 1993 Evaluative properties of measures used to assess patients with lateral epicondylitis at the elbow. Physiotherapy Canada 45(3): 160–164

Sullivan P, Chan R, DeMuth N, Chuang Y 2000 Efficacy of lumbar stability program for persons with recurrent low back dysfunction. Paper presented at the Proceedings of the 7th Scientific Conference of the IFOMT in conjunction with the MPAA, Perth, Australia

Svensson P, Arendt-Nielsen L, House L 1998 Muscle pain modulates mastication: An experimental study in humans. Journal of Orofacial Pain 12(1): 7–16

Thacker S B, Stroup D F, Branche C M, Gilchrist J, Goodman R A, Weitman E A 1999 The prevention of ankle sprains in sports – A systematic review of the literature. American Journal of Sports Medicine 27(6): 753–760

Torebjork H E, Ochoa J L, Schady W 1984 Referred pain from intraneural stimulation of muscle fascicles in the median nerve. Pain 18(2): 145–156

Travell J, Simons D 1983 Myofascial Pain and Dysfunction: The trigger point manual, Vol. 1. Baltimore: Williams & Wilkins

Travell J, Simons D 1992 Myofascial pain and dysfunction: The trigger point manual: The lower extremities, Vol 2. Baltimore: Williams & Wilkins

Tunks E, McCain G A, Hart L E, Teasell R W, Goldsmith C H, Rollman G B, McDermid A J, DeShane P J 1995 The reliability of examination for tenderness in patients with myofascial pain, chronic fibromyalgia and controls. Journal of Rheumatology 22(5): 944–952

Valeriani M, Restuccia D, Di Lazzaro V, Franceschi F, Fabbriciani C, Tonali P 1999a Clinical and neurophysiological abnormalities before and after reconstruction of the anterior cruciate ligament of the knee. Acta Neurologica Scandinavica 99(5): 303–307

Valeriani M, Restuccia D, Di Lazzaro V, Oliviero A, Profice P, Le Pera D, Saturno E, Tonali P 1999b Inhibition of the human primary motor area by painful heat stimulation of the skin. Clinical Neurophysiology 110(8): 1475–1480

Verhaar J, Walenkamp G, Kester A, van Mameren H, van der Linden T 1993 Lateral extensor release for tennis elbow. A prospective long-term follow-up study. Journal of Bone and Joint Surgery 75(7): 1034–1043

Vicenzino B, Wright A 1995 Effects of a novel manipulative physiotherapy technique on tennis elbow: a single case study. Manual Therapy 1(1): 30–35

Vicenzino B, Wright A 1996 Lateral epicondylalgia I: a review of epidemiology, pathophysiology, aetiology and natural history. Physical Therapy Reviews 1(1): 23–34

Vicenzino B, Collins D, Wright A 1995 Cervical mobilisation: Immediate effects on neural tissue mobility, mechanical hyperalgesia and painfree grip strength in lateral epicondylitis. Paper presented at the Clinical Solutions, Ninth Biennial Conference of the Manipulative Physiotherapists Association of Australia, Gold Coast, Queensland

Vicenzino B, Collins D, Wright A 1996 The initial effects of a cervical spine manipulative physiotherapy treatment on the pain and dysfunction of lateral epicondylalgia. Pain 68(1): 69–74

Vicenzino B, Collins D, Benson H, Wright A 1998 An investigation of the interrelationship between manipulative therapy induced hypoalgesia and sympathoexcitation. Journal of Manipulative and Physiological Therapeutics 21(7): 448–453

Wester J U, Jespersen S M, Nielsen K D, Neumann L 1996 Wobble board training after partial sprains of the lateral ligaments of the ankle: A prospective randomized study. Journal of Orthopaedic & Sports Physical Therapy 23(5): 332–336

Wilkerson 1985 External compression for controlling traumatic edema. The Physician and Sports Medicine 13(6): 97–106

Wilkerson G, Nitz A 1994 Dynamic ankle stability: mechanical and neuromuscular interrelationships. Journal of Sport Rehabilitation 3: 43–57

Wilkerson G B, Pinerola J J, Caturano R W 1997 Invertor vs evertor peak torque and power deficiencies associated with lateral ankle ligament injury. Journal of Orthopaedic & Sports Physical Therapy 26(2): 78–86

Wolfe F, Smythe H A, Yunus M B, Bennett R M, Bombardier C, Goldenberg D L, Tugwell P, Campbell S M, Abeles M, Clark P, Fam A G, Farber S J, Fiechtner J J, Franklin C M, Gatter R A, Hamaty D, Lessard J, Lichtbroun A S, Masi A T, McCain G A, Reynolds W J, Romano T J, Russell I J, Sheon R P 1990 The American College of Rheumatology criteria for the classification of fibromyalgia – report of the Multicenter Criteria Committee. Arthritis and Rheumatism 33(2): 160–172

Wright A, Thurnwald P, Smith J 1992 An evaluation of mechanical and thermal hyperalgesia in patients with lateral epicondylalgia. The Pain Clinic 5(4): 221–227

Wright A, Thurnwald P, O'Callaghan J, Smith J, Vicenzino B 1994 Hyperalgesia in tennis elbow patients. Journal of Musculoskeletal Pain 2(4): 83–97

Yaxley G, Jull G 1993 Adverse tension in the neural system. A preliminary study in patients with tennis elbow. Australian Journal of Physiotherapy 39(1): 15–22

Young S R, Dyson M 1990 The effect of therapeutic ultrasound on angiogenesis. Ultrasound in Medicine and Biology 16(3): 261–269

Zedka M, Prochazka A, Knight B, Gillard D, Gauthier M 1999 Voluntary and reflex control of human back muscles during induced pain. Journal of Physiology 520(2): 591–604

Zimmerman M 1989 Pain mediators and mechanisms in osteoarthritis. Seminars in Arthritis and Rheumatism (Suppl. 2) 18: 22–29

18

Neuropathic pain

Anthony Wright

OVERVIEW

Neuropathic pain is a common clinical problem that has proved difficult to manage (see Box 18.1 for classifications). Standard analgesics such as non-steroidal anti-inflammatory drugs and opioids may fail to control neuropathic pain and consequently many patients experience significant pain and suffering. Recent improvements in our knowledge of the pathophysiological processes that contribute to the development of neuropathic pain states have highlighted the multiple mechanisms that may be involved, and provided some indication as to why standard analgesic drugs may not be effective in controlling neuropathic pain.

This chapter provides an outline of current knowledge in relation to the pathophysiology of neuropathic pain, and then presents information on a number of common neuropathic pain states in terms of their pathophysiology, and common approaches to their management. Anticonvulsant and tricyclic antidepressant drugs are the main pharmacological agents used to manage neuropathic pain, in combination with topical treatments such as capsaicin, and regional blocks with local anaesthetics, where appropriate. Physical and psychological treatment interventions are considered important in the management of some neuropathic pain problems, however they are rarely described in detail in the literature and there is little research to support their use.

The chapter will discuss five common peripheral neuropathic pain disorders (post-herpetic neuralgia, diabetic neuropathy, trigeminal neuralgia, phantom limb pain and complex regional pain syndrome). The evidence-base to support various interventions for each of the conditions is discussed, however in many cases the level of evidence available is poor. This chapter attempts to provide a summary of the best available evidence in relation to the management of each condition, and to suggest what the optimal approach might be to management. In general, a multifaceted

---

Box 18.1 Key terms defined

Allodynia – Pain due to a stimulus that does not normally provoke pain.

Anaesthesia dolorosa – Pain in an area or region that is anaesthetic.

Central pain – Pain associated with a lesion of the central nervous system.

Formication – The sensation of insects (ants) crawling over the skin.

Hyperaesthesia – Increased sensitivity to stimulation, excluding special senses.

Insulin-dependent diabetes mellitus – A chronic condition in which the pancreas makes little or no insulin because the beta cells have been destroyed. The body is then not able to use glucose (blood sugar) for energy. The disorder usually comes on abruptly, although the damage to the beta cells may begin much earlier. The signs are a great thirst, hunger, a need to urinate often, and loss of weight. To treat the disease the person must inject insulin, follow a diet plan, exercise daily, and test blood glucose several times a day.

Neuroma – A benign tumour of nervous tissue. May form at the distal end of a transected nerve.

Neuropathic pain – Any pain syndrome in which the predominating mechanism is a site of aberrant somatosensory processing in the peripheral or central nervous system. Some clinical neuroscientists restrict this definition to pain originating in peripheral nerves and nerve roots.

Non-insulin-dependent diabetes mellitus – The most common form of diabetes mellitus; it affects about 90–95% of people who have diabetes. Unlike the insulin-dependent type of diabetes, in which the pancreas makes no insulin, people with non-insulin dependent diabetes produce some insulin, sometimes even large amounts. However, either their bodies do not produce enough insulin or their body cells are resistant to the action of insulin.

Phenotype – The total characteristics displayed by an organism or tissue under a particular set of environmental factors, regardless of the actual genotype of the organism or tissue. Results from interactions between the genotype and the environment.

---

approach is recommended, including preventive strategies, pharmacological therapies, physical therapies and psychological interventions. There is a clear need for further research in this area, in order to determine the optimum treatment regimes for all of the conditions discussed.

Learning objectives

Having studied this chapter students will:

1. Have an understanding of the pathophysiological mechanisms contributing to the development of neuropathic pain states.
2. Understand the distinction between central and peripheral neuropathic pain states.
3. Have an understanding of current knowledge in relation to the pathophysiological basis of each of the neuropathic pain states described.
4. Have an understanding of current approaches to management of the pain states described.
5. Have an understanding of the limited evidence-base for many of the treatments described.
6. Have an understanding of the need to develop a multifaceted approach to managing neuropathic pain states.
7. Have an understanding of the possible role of physical and psychological interventions for some of the conditions described.

8. Understand the need for further research to determine the optimal treatment regimes for many of the conditions described.

NEUROPATHIC PAIN

Neuropathic pain represents a significant healthcare problem. Relief of symptoms following treatment is often only moderate and pain may persist indefinitely, despite multiple interventions. The increased incidence of neuropathic pain states in the elderly, their persistence, and the cost of medication and other interventions, mean that neuropathic pain represents a considerable healthcare problem, resulting in significant disability and expense.

Neuropathic pain states are those in which the nociceptive system itself has been injured or damaged, either as a result of direct trauma, disease processes or mechanical impingement on the nervous system (Belgrade 1999). In the case of chronic neuropathic pain, the initial cause of injury may have resolved, but pain continues (Braune & Schady 1993). In such conditions, the pathological process exists within the nervous system itself and pain can be regarded as a pathological state.

Some neuropathic pain states may be due to damage to central nervous system structures as a result of stroke, other disease processes or trauma. These are described as central pain states. Others arise as a result of injury or disease affecting peripheral nervous system structures; these are peripheral neuropathic pain states. The emphasis of this chapter will be on the latter category of neuropathic pain states.

Five basic pathophysiological mechanisms appear to be associated with the development of neuropathic pain (Belgrade 1999). These are direct stimulation of pain-sensitive neurons, automatic firing of damaged nerves, central sensitization and nervous system reorganization due to deafferentation, disruption of endogenous pain inhibitory systems and sympathetically mediated pain (Belgrade 1999). Neuropathic pain states in different individuals may involve one or more of these processes.

Many forms of trauma and a variety of disease states can result in damage to the nervous system, and the development of peripheral neuropathic pain. Some common examples include post-herpetic neuralgia (infection), painful diabetic neuropathy (metabolic disturbance), trigeminal neuralgia (vascular anomaly), phantom limb pain (trauma) and complex regional pain syndrome type II (trauma).

Despite the different aetiologies of neuropathic pain states, the clinical manifestations of these conditions may be similar. Patients frequently present with burning pain; they may also suffer from lancinating or shooting pains. The pain may be constant or intermittent. Such patients will commonly exhibit allodynia to touch and they may exhibit other forms of altered sensation; for example, cold stimuli may evoke a sensation of burning pain. In some cases there will be a complete lack of sensation in the area but pain will nevertheless be experienced in that region of the body; this is known as anaesthesia dolorosa (see Box 18.1). Burning pain, lancinating pain and altered sensation are the three cardinal features of most clinical presentations.

In addition to pain, other changes may include localized hyperhidrosis, altered skin temperature, and trophic changes to the nails, skin, muscles and bones.

Neuropathic pain mechanisms

A number of different mechanisms may contribute to the development of neuropathic pain, and the mechanistic basis of a patient or client's pain state may vary depending on the underlying pathophysiology and inter-individual variations (Woolf & Mannion 1999).

Many of the changes in nociceptive system function that may contribute to neuropathic pain states have been described in Chapter 3. In summary, these changes include: alterations in the phenotype of peripheral neurons, the development of central

sensitization and structural reorganization of cells in the dorsal horn of the spinal cord and other regions of the central nervous system (Woolf & Costigan 1999, Woolf & Mannion 1999).

Another mechanism that may contribute to some neuropathic pain states is a structural reorganization of sympathetic innervation and an acquired sensitivity to noradrenaline (Woolf & Mannion 1999).

Neuroma formation

One important mechanism that can contribute to neuropathic pain is the development of a neuroma at the site of nerve injury. Formation of a neuroma can contribute to the development of ectopic stimuli (Govrin-Lippmann & Devor 1978, Wall & Gutnick 1974). Spontaneous activity from the neuroma is perceived as pain, and may be interpreted by the central nervous system as arising from the area of innervation.

The development of ectopic discharges involves anterograde axoplasmic transport of cellular constituents, such as receptors and chemical mediators, from the cell body to the periphery. As the peripheral portion of the nerve has been severed, the transported mediators accumulate at the site of injury and contribute to the development of a neuroma (Laduron 1987). The nerve membrane in this region attempts to regenerate and in the process becomes highly excitable, leading to the generation of ectopic signals.

Impulse generation can result from hypersensitivity of the neuroma to mechanical stimuli, chemical changes, metabolic changes, ischaemia, inflammation, cold stimuli or circulating catecholamines. Alternatively, spontaneous discharges can occur as a result of the development of a pacemaker region in the nerve membrane (Devor 1991).

Phenotype change

It has been suggested that nerve injury results in a change of phenotype in the peripheral nerve, to a state more like that of early pre-natal and neonatal development (McCormack 1999, Woolf & Costigan 1999, Woolf & Mannion 1999). The resultant increased expression of voltage-sensitive calcium channels and protein kinase C may be important factors contributing to neuroma formation and increased excitability of peripheral neurons (McCormack 1999).

Change in phenotype may mean that myelinated afferent fibres adopt characteristics that are similar to those of C fibres, including the ability to generate central sensitization (Woolf & Costigan 1999).

Genetic variability and diversity of phenotype may account for individual variation in the development of neuropathic pain states such as post-herpetic neuralgia, because not all persons who experience herpes zoster infection go on to develop post-herpetic neuralgia (Woolf & Mannion 1999).

Central sensitization

Central nervous system changes are clearly of considerable importance in the development of neuropathic pain states. The process of central sensitization has been strongly implicated as an important factor contributing to the development of neuropathic pain (Woolf & Mannion 1999).

This process has been described in some detail in Chapter 3. In summary, it involves release of glutamate and neuropeptides such as substance P from primary afferent neurons, increased intracellular calcium concentration and activation of protein kinase C with consequent phosphorylation of the N-methyl-D-aspartate (NMDA) receptor (Woolf & Costigan 1999, Woolf & Mannion 1999). Phosphorylation of the NMDA receptor results in removal of the magnesium ion that provides a physical block to the receptor's ion channel, and subsequent activation of the NMDA receptor leading to increased excitability of postsynaptic spinal cord neurons (See Fig. 18.1).

Consequences of central sensitization include: alterations in the receptive fields of spinal cord cells (Devor & Wall 1981a, 1981b, Wall & Devor 1983), increased responses to supra-threshold stimuli and responses evoked by previously sub-threshold stimuli (Woolf & Costigan 1999, Woolf & Mannion 1999).

Neuroanatomical reorganization

Neuroanatomical reorganization within the central nervous system is another important consideration in most forms of neuropathic pain. In situations where there is complete transection of peripheral nerves, dorsal horn cells, which previously received inputs from the denervated region, begin to respond to stimulation of other body regions. They will often develop receptive fields in more proximal, innervated regions of the affected limb, or other regions of the body (Devor & Wall 1978, 1981a, 1981b, Hylden et al 1987).

This process is generally thought to occur as a result of up-regulation of existing synapses due to central sensitization, although there is also evidence to indicate that axonal sprouting in dorsal horn cells may lead to the establishment of new synaptic connections. Myelinated axons that normally terminate in laminae III and IV of the dorsal horn have been shown to sprout into lamina II of the dorsal horn (See Fig. 18.2), potentially developing synaptic connections with intrinsic neurons involved in the transmission of nociceptive afferent inputs (Woolf et al 1992). It has been postulated that this may constitute a mechanism whereby normally innocuous afferent input could contribute to nociception (Woolf & Mannion 1999), and provide a neuroanatomical basis for the development of allodynia.

Another form of neuroanatomical reorganization has been demonstrated following a constriction injury

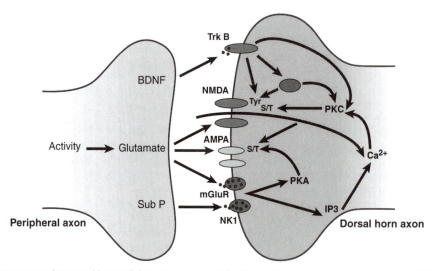

Figure 18.1 Neurotransmitters and intracellular processes contributing to the development of central sensitization in dorsal horn neurons (from Woolf and Costigan, Transcriptional and posttranslational plasticity and the generation of inflammatory pain. Proceedings of the National Academy of Sciences of the USA 96: 7723–7730. © 1999, National Academy of Sciences, USA with kind permission).

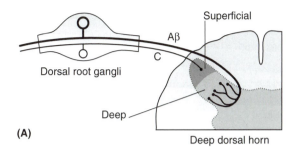

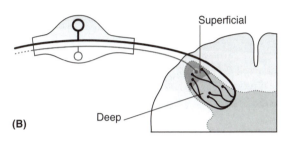

(A)

(B)

Figure 18.2 Sprouting of A-beta afferents into the superficial laminae of the dorsal horn following transection of a peripheral nerve (from Woolf & Mannion, Neuropathic pain: aetiology, symptoms, mechanisms and management. The Lancet 353: 1959–1964. © The Lancet Ltd. 1999).

to a peripheral nerve (McLachlan et al 1993). These authors found that following sciatic nerve ligation in rats, noradrenergic perivascular axons sprout into dorsal root ganglia and form basket-like structures around large-diameter sensory neurons. The noradrenergic terminals located around the dorsal root ganglia somata may be responsible for sympathetically-mediated paraesthesia, as a result of initiating afferent activity during ongoing and evoked sympathetic postganglionic discharges (McLachlan et al 1993).

Pain might be generated if central nociceptive neurons become sensitized to activity in large-diameter afferent fibres, or if there is an alteration in the phenotype of the relevant myelinated afferents. Activity in large dorsal root ganglion cells, initiated by the release of noradrenaline, might therefore be converted to nociceptive signals within the central nervous system (McLachlan et al 1993).

Disinhibition

Firing of dorsal horn projection neurons is influenced not only by excitatory inputs from the periphery but also by inputs from the brain that may be either inhibitory or excitatory. Peripheral nerve injury may result in disinhibition of spinal cord neurons through various mechanisms (Woolf & Mannion 1999). Dorsal horn content of gama-aminobutyric acid (GABA) is reduced and GABA and opioid receptors are down-regulated in neuropathic pain states (Woolf & Mannion 1999).

In addition, the expression of cholecystokinin, an endogenous opioid inhibitor, is up-regulated in injured sensory neurons and excitotoxic mechanisms may result in the death of inhibitory interneurons in the dorsal horn (Woolf & Mannion 1999). These mechanisms in combination result in decreased tonic inhibition of spinal cord neurons, which may be an important pathophysiological mechanism in many neuropathic pain states.

Summary

It is clear that many different mechanisms could be involved in the development of neuropathic pain. In most cases, multiple mechanisms will contribute to the development of a specific pain state. The concept of providing treatment for patients with neuropathic pain based on the mechanisms contributing to their pain state, rather than their disease process, is an approach that is gaining significant momentum and may represent an important new initiative in the management of these conditions (Woolf & Mannion 1999).

Neuropathic pain therapy

Treatment of neuropathic pain is difficult, and it is widely accepted that current therapies do not provide optimal outcomes. There is, however, considerable optimism that improved methods of treatment may become available in the future (Fields 1994, Woolf & Mannion 1999). A number of different drugs may be useful in the management of neuropathic pain states. In addition, clinical algorithms have been established for the treatment of neuropathic pain using a combination of existing pharmacological, physiological and psychological therapies (Belgrade 1999) (See Fig. 18.3). However, evidence-based approaches to the management of many individual disorders still require further substantiation. In general, pharmacological therapies provide the mainstay for the management of neuropathic pain states, with relatively little emphasis on surgery or physical therapies, although in specific conditions such as phantom limb pain and complex regional pain syndrome, an increasingly important role for physical therapies is now emerging.

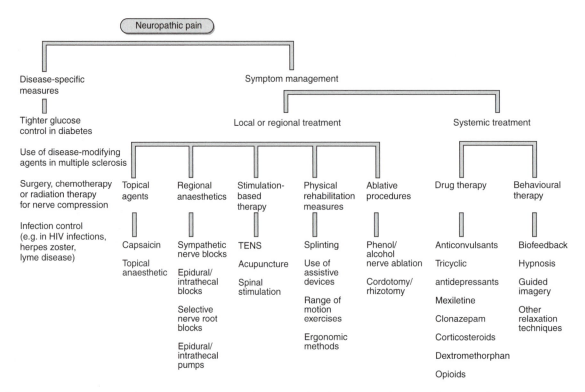

Figure 18.3 Algorithm for the treatment of neuropathic pain (reprinted, with permission from Belgrade MJ 1999 Following the clues to neuropathic pain. Postgraduate Medicine 106(6): 127–140. © 1999, The McGraw-Hill Companies).

Where possible, improved management of underlying disorders such as diabetes is recommended as a means of preventing neuropathic pain (Belgrade 1999).

When a neuropathic pain state has become established, the tricyclic antidepressants such as amytriptyline and imipramine are frontline therapies, in conjunction with the anticonvulsant drugs such as gabapentin, carbamazepine and sodium valproate, and the sodium channel blocker mexiletine.

Limited use is made of opioid analgesics since there is still considerable controversy about the value of opioid analgesics in the management of neuropathic pain states (Arner & Meyerson 1988, Portenoy et al 1990). Chapter 16 provides a more detailed synopsis of drug therapies for the management of neuropathic pain states.

Physiologically based therapies, such as transcutaneous electrical nerve stimulation and acupuncture have been considered as methods of treating neuropathic pain, and a range of physiotherapy and occupational therapy approaches may be important to minimize disability associated with chronic neuropathic pain.

The importance of functional use of an affected limb (or residual limb) is being increasingly emphasized in conditions such as phantom limb pain, and complex regional pain syndrome. Approaches to the management of a range of neuropathic pain states are discussed below.

NEUROPATHIC PAIN STATES

Post-herpetic neuralgia

Post-herpetic neuralgia is one of the most common forms of neuropathic pain. It is defined as pain that persists or recurs 1 month or more following the initial eruption of herpes zoster infection. It is considered that post-herpetic neuralgia is a complication of herpes zoster infection, rather than a symptom of continued infection.

Patients usually describe severe aching and burning sensations in the affected dermatome; the most commonly affected regions are the thoracic dermatomes and the trigeminal distribution (Watson et al 1988).

The area of pain can be associated with a sensory deficit (anaesthesia dolorosa). Loss of sensation does not usually occur in those patients with herpes zoster who fail to develop post-herpetic neuralgia. Chronic symptoms are often associated with shooting, stabbing pains; in many cases the intensity of pain subsides with time, although it may not completely resolve. Where spontaneous resolution does occur, it usually takes place within 3–6 months of the initial infection.

The risk of developing post-herpetic neuralgia subsequent to a herpes zoster infection increases substantially with age. Persons over the age of 60 have both an increased risk of herpes zoster infection, and an increased risk that they will develop post-herpetic neuralgia (Bowsher 1994, Hope-Simpson 1975, Watson et al 1988). The chance of developing sustained post-herpetic neuralgia is approximately 50% in this age-group (Watson et al 1988).

The pain of post-herpetic neuralgia is both intense and constant. It is often associated with unpleasant sensations and the skin may be hyper- or hypoaesthetic and itchy. The contact of clothing against the affected area, changes in temperature, movement of the skin when walking and emotional states, are all likely to trigger allodynia. The disorder is frequently associated with social withdrawal and depression.

There is still considerable debate about the mechanistic basis of post-herpetic neuralgia (Rowbotham et al 1999). It has been suggested that there may in fact be at least two different forms of post-herpetic neuralgia, resulting from different mechanisms (Rowbotham et al 1999). In patients who exhibit allodynia it is suggested that infection may result in partial nerve injury, with associated sensitization of nociceptors and recruitment of large-diameter afferent inputs to contribute to nociception (Rowbotham et al 1999).

It has also been suggested that a smaller group of patients have complete deafferentation and develop anaesthesia dolorosa. In approximately 15% of patients there is no evidence of allodynia (Nurmikko & Bowsher 1990), and it has been suggested that in these cases the predominant pain mechanisms may be deafferentation-induced hypersensitivity of central nervous system neurons, with disinhibition and reorganization of spinal cord neurons (Rowbotham et al 1999).

Evidence from quantitative sensory testing suggests that some patients have enhanced sensitivity to thermal stimuli and it has been proposed that this may be evidence of sensitization of C nociceptors (Fields 1994, Rowbotham & Fields 1996). Other researchers have suggested that the presence of a generalized subclinical A fibre polyneuropathy may be an important predisposing factor to the development of post-herpetic neuralgia (Baron et al 1997). These findings are not necessarily contradictory; they may simply reflect very complex disturbances of sensory function, as a result of the variable influence of herpes zoster infection on sensory neurons.

Examination of peripheral nerve, dorsal root ganglia and dorsal horn tissue samples failed to identify clearcut differences in pathology between those individuals in which herpes zoster resolved without further complication, and those who went on to develop post-herpetic neuralgia (Watson et al 1991).

In summary, there is still considerable doubt about what pathological changes contribute to the development of post-herpetic neuralgia after herpes zoster infection, and what distinguishes those individuals who developed post-herpetic neuralgia from those individuals who exhibit complete resolution after herpes zoster infection.

Primary prevention

Preventing the development of neuropathic pain is always a preferred option. While the development of anti-viral drugs has impacted on the treatment of herpes zoster, the ability of anti-viral medications to prevent the development of post-herpetic neuralgia remains controversial, and on balance it seems that they have limited prophylactic benefit in preventing post-herpetic neuralgia.

Systemic anti-viral drugs administered in the prodromal period of the infection can have a positive effect on healing and prevention of complications in immunocompromised patients (Wagstaff et al 1994). However, whether systemic anti-virals can prevent, or significantly reduce, the incidence of post-herpetic neuralgia in immunocompetent individuals is still a matter of considerable debate. Conflicting evidence has been presented; some data suggests benefit from anti-viral administration (McKendrick et al 1989), although findings to the contrary have also been presented (Mandal et al 1988, Wagstaff et al 1994).

It is possible that there may be differences in effectiveness depending on the body area affected. Harding (1995) suggests that acyclovir treatment may be more effective in controlling herpes zoster opthalmicus, and in that group it may have a beneficial effect on both acute pain and the occurrence of post-herpetic neuralgia. However, acyclovir treatment seems to be of limited benefit for the general population of post-herpetic pain sufferers as a means of preventing the development of this painful condition.

Since herpes zoster infection results in an inflammatory response within the nerve and dorsal root ganglia, another preventative approach might be to limit the initial inflammation using corticosteroids. However, a study using prednisolone failed to demonstrate any reduction in the development of post-herpetic neuralgia (Esmann et al 1987).

In general, it appears that while the option of preventing post-herpetic neuralgia with more effective management of the initial herpes zoster outbreak or the associated inflammation is intuitively sensible, there is little real evidence that this approach is effective in actually preventing the development of the disorder.

Pharmacological therapies

A wide variety of pharmacological treatments have been used to manage post-herpetic neuralgia. These include anticonvulsants, tricyclic antidepressants, sodium channel blockers and steroids. Their success is variable between individuals and no treatment is universally efficacious.

Several topical treatments have also been used to treat post-herpetic neuralgia. These include capsaicin, aspirin and local anaesthetics (De Benedittis et al 1992, Rowbotham & Fields 1989, Watson et al 1988). It is increasingly being suggested that treatment should be mechanistically based, and that in many cases, combinations of therapies that address different mechanisms will be required (Fields 1994).

The tricyclic antidepressant amitriptyline is one of the primary treatments for post-herpetic neuralgia. It has analgesic efficacy in patients who are not clinically depressed, and it has been suggested that drugs of this group are most effective against constant burning pain. Other drugs in this group, including imipramine, nortriptyline and desipramine have also been shown to be effective (Watson 1988). Chapter 16 provides a more detailed description of the actions and effects of tricyclic antidepressants.

Unfortunately, the tricyclic antidepressants have quite marked side-effects that may affect patient/client compliance. The dose of amitriptyline is individually titrated to the patient's requirements to allow for response, and to minimize side-effects. In controlled clinical trials, administration of amitriptyline nightly has proven successful in pain reduction (Max et al 1988, Watson & Evans 1985; Watson et al 1982, 1992). It is important to note, however, that amitriptyline rarely eliminates pain. Most commonly, the effect is to convert severe pain to moderate or mild pain. The onset of effect is often delayed, and so therapy is maintained for at least 3

months. If a beneficial effect is demonstrated it is then slowly reduced over a period of months. It is possible that nortriptyline may be as effective as amitriptyline (Watson et al 1998) and it would appear that amitriptyline is more effective than the benzodiazepines such as lorazepam (Max et al 1988).

Anticonvulsant drugs have also been used in the management of post-herpetic neuralgia. Early studies with carbamazepine, phenytoin and valproic acid suggested that there was little clinical benefit from this class of drugs. However, more recently a major multi-centre randomized controlled trial of gabapentin in the management of post-herpetic neuralgia provided convincing evidence for the effectiveness of gabapentin in reducing pain and improving quality-of-life measures in this patient population (Rowbotham et al 1998).

A variety of topical treatments have been investigated in patients with post-herpetic neuralgia; these include capsaicin cream, lignocaine or lidocaine gel and topical aspirin.

Capsaicin is a natural product extracted from hot chilli peppers. When applied, it causes the release of substance P and other neuropeptides from the terminals of slow-conducting unmyelinated C fibres. Initial application of capsaicin cream to the skin causes burning and hyperalgesia, as a result of substance P release. This eventually diminishes as substance P becomes depleted from C-fibre terminals. In randomized clinical trials capsaicin has been shown to be more effective than placebo in controlling post-herpetic neuralgia (Rains & Bryson 1995). Meta-analysis of data from published trials suggests that capsaicin is an effective treatment for post-herpetic neuralgia provided that it has been applied for at least 6 weeks (Sindrup & Jensen 1999, Zhang & Li Wan Po 1994).

A major limiting factor in the use of capsaicin is the burning sensation produced by initial administration; in some patients with post-herpetic neuralgia this may prove to be intolerable. Another limitation is that the cream must be applied to the entire affected area four times per day. These factors may limit compliance for many patients/clients.

Topical application of lignocaine/lidocaine (Rowbotham & Fields 1989) and topical application of aspirin appear to have a beneficial effect on post-herpetic neuralgia (De Benedittis et al 1992). Aspirin applications are beneficial in limiting the pain of acute herpes zoster infection, as well as post-herpetic neuralgia (De Benedittis et al 1992). To date, only preliminary investigations have been published. Further research is required to establish a firm evidence-base for these topical treatments. The main limitation of topical treatments is the need to maintain patient compliance with treatments that must be regularly re-applied for a prolonged period of time.

Although the role of opioids in the management of neuropathic pain remains a matter of some controversy (see Chapter 16), several researchers have evaluated the efficacy of opioids in the management of post-herpetic neuralgia (Pappagallo & Campbell 1994, Rowbotham et al 1991, Watson & Babul 1998). A recent randomized, controlled trial using orally administered oxycodone demonstrated significant benefit in terms of reduced pain ratings and improved quality-of-life ratings in patients with post-herpetic neuralgia (Watson & Babul 1998). This study, in addition to evidence of pain relief with intravenous morphine (Rowbotham et al 1991), suggests that opioid medications may be beneficial in patients with post-herpetic neuralgia.

In the study reported by Rowbotham and colleagues (1991) slow intravenous infusion of morphine produced greater benefit that infusion of lignocaine/ lidocaine. Combination of opioids with clonidine has also been recommended as a method of management (Fields 1994).

Physical therapies

Other potential treatments for post-herpetic neuralgia include transcutaneous electrical nerve stimulation (TENS), biofeedback, ultrasound and acupuncture. Despite some early studies presenting encouraging data in relation to the effects of TENS (Nathan & Wall 1974), a strong evidence-base has not emerged to support the efficacy of any physical therapy in the management of post-herpetic neuralgia (Lewith et al 1983, Payne 1984). There is a distinct lack of research in this area, however data from early studies do not provide encouragement that larger, controlled studies would yield positive outcomes.

Summary

Outcome measurement in post-herpetic neuralgia studies is difficult, due to variability of the condition and the possibility that a number of distinct mechanisms may be responsible for pain in this population. However, there is mounting evidence advocating early administration of a tricyclic antidepressant and possible co-administration of an antiviral agent as the most effective way to manage this condition. Anticonvulsants such as gabapentin provide a useful alternative to the tricyclic antidepressants. There is minimal evidence to support the use of physical therapies such as TENS.

Diabetic neuropathy

Diabetes is a disorder affecting the metabolism of sugar that results in abnormally high glycaemic levels, among other metabolic changes. Diabetic neuropathy is a relatively common complication of diabetes. It is reported to affect more than 50% of individuals with diabetes of more than 25 years duration (Pirart et al 1978). It is suggested that approximately 7.5% of patients being treated at a diabetes clinic present with neuropathic pain (Chan et al 1990).

It should be noted that not all forms of diabetic neuropathy result in neuropathic pain. There are several distinct forms of diabetic neuropathy (See Box 18.2) and although they do not all result in pain, they may be associated with other severe complications (i.e. cardiovascular autonomic neuropathy).

It is clear, however, that the most common complication associated with diabetes, particularly in the elderly, is peripheral neuropathy (Sima & Greene 1995). There is no difference in prevalence of neuropathy between those suffering insulin-dependant diabetes mellitus, and those suffering non-insulin-dependant diabetes mellitus (Fedele & Giugliano 1997, Pirart et al 1978). However, there is evidence that the mechanisms involved in the development of neuropathy may be different in these two groups (Sima & Greene 1995); diabetic neuropathy appears to be predominantly linked to uncontrolled hyperglycaemia.

The most common form of diabetic neuropathy is distal symmetrical sensorimotor polyneuropathy or diabetic peripheral neuropathy. This condition is associated with progressive nerve-fibre loss, tissue atrophy and neuropathic pain. The clinical symptoms of diabetic

---

Box 18.2 Classification of diabetic neuropathy (reprinted from American Journal of Medicine 107 Greene et al, Diabetic neuropathy: scope of the syndrome, 2–8. © 1999 with permission from Excerpta Medica Inc).

Diffuse
  Distal symmetric sensorimotor polyneuropathy
  Autonomic neuropathy
  — Sudomotor
  — Cardiovascular
  — Gastrointestinal
  — Genitourinary
  Symmetric proximal lower limb neuropathy
  (amyotrophy)

Focal
  Cranial neuropathy
  Radiculopathy/plexopathy
  Entrapment neuropathy
  Asymmetric lower limb motor neuropathy
  (amyotrophy)

neuropathy are progressive insensitivity to external painful stimuli, damage and deformity to the limb, and the development of chronic neuropathic pain (Boulton 1994). A variety of pathological changes may occur in the peripheral nerves and there is controversy as to which of these changes contributes to pain production.

It is apparent that hyperglycaemia plays an important role and it seems that a number of mechanisms may work together to produce diabetic neuropathy (Fedele & Giugliano 1997, Greene et al 1999). Abnormal metabolism of glucose leads to the build-up of sorbitol in nerves, that in turn leads to other metabolic changes resulting in delayed nerve conduction. Metabolic changes may contribute to secondary vascular changes and disease, resulting in ischaemia in nerves and further impairing nerve conduction (Greene et al 1999).

Loss of neurotrophic factors such as nerve growth factor appears to be another effect of diabetes that contributes to the development of neuropathy. This then interacts with metabolic and vascular changes because neurotrophic factors are important in protecting nerves against oxidative stress. The absence of neurotrophic factors such as nerve growth factor means that the cell is more vulnerable to damage as a result of the metabolic and vascular changes that occur.

In combination, these factors contribute to the development and progression of diabetic neuropathy (Greene et al 1999). Box 18.3 provides a summary of these mechanisms.

Primary prevention

It is clear that the most effective therapy for diabetic neuropathy, as well as other complications of diabetes, is glycaemic control (Santiago 1993). Rigorous glycaemic control includes regular self-monitoring of blood-glucose concentration and adherence to insulin or oral hypoglycaemic regimens. An appropriate diet, weight control, cigarette-smoking cessation and regular exercise are also important.

A large multicentre clinical trial conducted by the diabetes control and complications group provided convincing evidence that the incidence of neuropathy could be significantly reduced by meticulous control of blood-glucose levels (DCCT Research group 1993). Research also suggests that intensive insulin therapy reduces the incidence of diabetic neuropathy in later life by up to 60% (Feldman & Stevens 1994). Unfortunately, there is no clear evidence to suggest that intensive insulin therapy reduces existing neuropathy. Unlike post-herpetic neuralgia, there does appear to be clear evidence that primary prevention strategies are effective in reducing the incidence of diabetic neuropathy.

Pharmacological therapies

A specific approach to the treatment of diabetic neuropathy has been to use drugs that limit the negative metabolic consequences of poor glycaemic control. The main class of drug that has been used for this purpose is the aldose reductase inhibitors.

Aldose reductase is an enzyme that converts glucose to sorbitol (Greene et al 1999). As outlined above, sorbitol then builds up in nerve tissue, leading ultimately to the development of neuropathy. Aldose reductase inhibitors reduce the flux of glucose through this metabolic pathway, preventing tissue accumulation of sorbitol and fructose and potentially limiting the development of neuropathy (Vinik 1999). To date few of the drugs tested have demonstrated significant improvements in patients with diabetic neuropathy (Vinik 1999). Studies with the aldose reductase inhibitor tolrestat showed significant improvements in patients after 1 year of treatment, and a meta-analysis concluded that patients had a reduced risk of developing nerve-function loss (Nicolucci et al 1996). However, recent large-scale studies failed to demonstrate any benefit from tolrestat administration, and following the deaths of three patients due to drug-related hepatic failure the drug was withdrawn from the market (Fedele & Giugliano 1997).

It appears that there is limited benefit from using aldose reductase inhibitors to minimize or reverse some of the metabolic changes contributing to neuropathy. A range of other metabolism-modifying drugs may be useful in treating neuropathy (Fedele & Giugliano 1997, Vinik 1999). Most of these approaches are still in the early stages of development.

Box 18.3 Pathophysiological mechanisms of nerve damage in diabetics (from Fedele & Giugliano 1997, Drugs 54(3): 414–421 with kind permission from Adis International)

- Excessive polyol pathway activity with increased sorbitol content in nerve and altered myoinositol and phosphoinositide
- Increased non-enzymatic glycation of structural proteins with formation of advanced glycated end-products (AGE)
- Impaired essential fatty acid metabolism
- Oxidative stress
- Vascular changes with endoneurial hypoxia
- Impairment in trophic or growth factors

In terms of conventional therapies to provide symptomatic control of painful diabetic neuropathy, the tricyclic antidepressants represent one of the main forms of treatment. Amitriptyline and imipramine have been the drugs most commonly investigated in the diabetic neuropathy population (McQuay et al 1996). Desipramine, a relatively selective noradrenaline reuptake inhibitor, has also been shown to be efficacious in the management of diabetic neuropathy, with fewer side-effects than amitriptyline (Max et al 1991). In a comparative study Max et al (1991) demonstrated that desipramine and amitriptyline were equally effective in reducing pain and that there was less sedation and fewer anticholinergic side-effects with desipramine, leading them to suggest that desipramine is the drug of choice to manage painful diabetic neuropathy.

Both drugs were superior to the serotonin-selective reuptake inhibitor fluoxetine, suggesting that inhibition of noradrenaline reuptake is more important than inhibition of serotonin reuptake (Max et al 1992). However, the selective serotonin inhibitor paroxetine has been shown to have a modest positive impact on painful diabetic neuropathy in clinical trials (Sindrup et al 1990).

Anticonvulsants such as carbamazepine have also been recommended for treatment of painful diabetic neuropathy (Belgrade & Lev 1991). More recent studies using gabapentin have suggested that this drug is effective in relieving neuropathic pain in diabetic patients. Backonja and Galer (1998) titrated the dose for each individual to produce an efficacious effect with minimal side-effects. Gabapentin does appear to have fewer side-effects than the tricyclic antidepressants, although dizziness, somnolence and confusion can be significant adverse effects with gabapentin treatment (Backonja & Galer 1998). It is possible that gabapentin could be used in combination with a tricyclic, but to date no studies have been reported that evaluate this combination.

Other treatments for diabetic neuropathy include lignocaine/lidocaine and other local anaesthetics. It has been shown that intravenous infusion of lignocaine/lidocaine reduces pain in chronic painful diabetic neuropathy and that the effects are sustained for between 3 and 21 days beyond the period of infusion (Bach et al 1990, Kastrup et al 1987). It is possible that multiple infusions may lead to sustained benefit.

The orally administered lignocaine/lidocaine analogue mexiletine has also been tested in patients with diabetic neuropathy (Stracke et al 1992). While the difference between mexiletine and placebo for overall pain ratings did not quite reach statistical significance, several sub-groups of patients with particular pain characteristics showed significant differences between treatment and placebo conditions. In particular those patients with stabbing pain, heat sensations and formication showed the most benefit from this form of treatment (Stracke et al 1992). Given that the primary action of mexiletine is membrane stabilization, it is probably not surprising that it might influence specific aspects of sensation where ectopic activity in affected neurons might be a contributing factor.

Topical application of capsaicin has been used in the management of diabetic neuropathy pain. Results of randomized controlled trials have been variable, however a meta-analysis of the available studies concluded that capsaicin was effective in relieving diabetic neuropathy pain (Zhang & Li Wan Po 1994).

Transdermal clonidine has also been used to treat painful diabetic neuropathy (Byas-Smith et al 1995). While it was found that clonidine was not effective for the entire population of diabetic neuropathy sufferers, there was a sub-group of patients (approximately 25%) who showed a significant improvement in pain scores with this form of treatment (Byas-Smith et al 1995). It is apparent that diabetic neuropathy involves a number of different pain mechanisms, and so there may be sub-populations of patients who will respond to specific interventions that influence their predominant pain mechanism.

An interesting approach to the management of diabetic neuropathic pain has been proposed by Pfeifer et al (1993). These authors proposed that painful diabetic neuropathy involves multiple mechanisms and may manifest as several distinctly different types of pain. They categorize these as deep pain, superficial pain and muscle pain, and propose a management regime that involves different treatments to address each of these types of pain when they appear in any given patient.

If a patient presents with a superficial dysaesthetic type of pain associated with burning, allodynia and predominantly perceived in the skin, they recommend using capsaicin. If a patient presents with a deep nerve-trunk type of pain associated with pins and needles or electric-shock type sensations, then they recommend treatment with the tricyclic antidepressant imipramine. If imipramine is unsuccessful they recommend replacing it with mexiletine or combining it with mexiletine.

Muscle pain is described as a cramping aching muscle tenderness, or a drawing sensation. They recommend that muscular pain should be treated with stretching exercises and a muscle relaxant. If that does not produce sufficient improvement then they suggest the addition of a non-steroidal anti-inflammatory drug

(Pfeifer et al 1993). Figure 18.4 provides a description of this treatment approach. Unfortunately, the nature of the stretching exercises is not clearly defined.

Individual patients might present with one, two or three different forms of pain and receive treatment based on the corresponding treatment regimes. After a 3-month treatment period, pain scores for each type of pain and total pain scores were significantly reduced by this comprehensive treatment protocol compared to an untreated control group. With such an individualized treatment protocol it is difficult to provide a placebo control group and so results must be interpreted with caution. Nevertheless, this seems to represent a sensible and effective approach to the treatment of diabetic neuropathy that might be of potential benefit in other forms of neuropathic pain.

Physical therapies

A variety of physical therapies including TENS, acupuncture, relaxation and biofeedback have been recommended as adjunctive therapies in the management of painful diabetic neuropathy (Belgrade & Lev 1991). TENS has been shown to be effective in the management of diabetic neuropathy following stimulation of the distal limbs (Armstrong et al 1997, Kumar &

Marshall 1997) and following stimulation of the lumbar region (Somers & Somers 1999). Studies supporting the use of acupuncture in the management of diabetic neuropathy have also been published (Abuaisha et al 1998).

Further research is required before a substantial evidence-base can be established to support the use of physical therapies in the management of diabetic neuropathy.

Summary

The mainstays of painful diabetic neuropathy treatment are normoglycaemic control with the addition of a tricyclic antidepressant. Other medications may be included if required (James & Page 1994).

A comprehensive approach addressing multiple pain mechanisms (Pfeifer et al 1993) has been proposed and appears to have some merit. This approach includes the use of physical treatments to address the muscular pain component of the disorder.

Unfortunately, in many cases long-term sensory deficit manifests as foot ulceration and ultimately amputation, potentially leading to further neuropathic pain problems.

Trigeminal neuralgia

Trigeminal neuralgia or tic douloureux is possibly the most excruciating of the neuropathic pain syndromes. It is most common in elderly people. Periods of pain usually occur in cycles that may be separated by pain-free periods, possibly lasting several years.

Trigeminal neuralgia is characterized by certain specific features that provide the differential diagnosis between it and atypical facial pain, another affliction of the face. It involves brief stabbing pains followed by pain-free periods. Pain is triggered abruptly, usually by a non-noxious stimulus, and it normally occurs unilaterally. A light touch on the cheek by a hand or scarf may send the patient into a painful spasm. Pain triggered by chewing may prevent the patient from enjoying a proper diet, and they may stop eating altogether to prevent attacks. Pain can be precipitated by a cool breeze, thus preventing the patient from going outdoors. Pain occurs in the distribution of the trigeminal nerve, normally involving the third or mandibular division, possibly in combination with the second or maxillary division. Trigeminal neuralgia is not usually associated with a sensory deficit of the affected area (Loeser 1994).

The pathology of trigeminal neuralgia is thought to involve neurovascular compression of the trigeminal

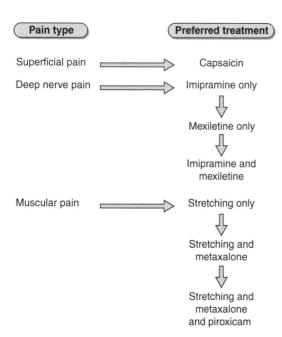

Figure 18.4 Comprehensive treatment approach for painful diabetic peripheral neuropathy (from Pfeifer et al 1993, Diabetes Care 16(8): 1103–1115. © American Diabetes Association with kind permission).

nerve as it leaves the brain stem. A number of vascular structures may lie in close proximity to the root entry zone of the trigeminal nerve (Tash et al 1989), although the most common source of pathology appears to be the superior cerebellar artery (van Loveren et al 1982). Contact between the trigeminal nerve and vascular structures appears to be relatively normal (30% of pain-free individuals), however it seems that in pathological situations where trigeminal neuralgia develops there is some degree of deformity of the vascular and neural structures (Tash et al 1989). Contact between the trigeminal nerve and vascular structures has been documented preoperatively by magnetic resonance tomographic angiography and confirmed at subsequent surgery (Meaney et al 1995).

A small group of patients can develop trigeminal neuralgia symptoms as a result of other compression events, e.g. posterior fossa tumours (Barker et al 1996a). Other causative pathologies may involve focal demyelination within the nerve root or the root entry zone (Bederson & Wilson 1989), which may be linked to multiple sclerosis or may occur spontaneously.

Trigeminal neuralgia is one of the few neuropathic pain states in which there appears to be a consensus in relation to optimal treatment approaches. Microvascular decompression surgery is a well-established treatment approach, and carbamazepine seems to be well established as the drug therapy of choice.

Primary prevention

Given the idiopathic nature of trigeminal neuralgia and the insidious onset of the problem, primary prevention of the disorder is probably not possible. It is clear, however, that early investigation of patients, using the most current imaging procedures, would be helpful in identifying those patients who might benefit from surgical management and early surgical intervention. This might help to limit the morbidity and cost associated with the condition.

Surgery

Trigeminal neuralgia is one of the few neuropathic pain complaints where surgery is indicated as a primary intervention. Neurovascular compression lends itself to surgical decompression procedures. Microvascular decompression involves removal of the implicated vessel or separating the vessel from the nerve root with a sponge pledget. Studies have shown that decompression surgery has a profound long-term effect on trigeminal neuralgia with severe adverse events occurring at frequencies comparable to those witnessed following other surgical procedures (Barker et al 1996b).

A large, long-term prospective study of trigeminal neuralgia patients following microvascular decompression found the procedure to be safe and effective in the treatment of trigeminal neuralgia with long-term amelioration of pain (Barker et al 1996b). Approximately 70% of patients showed significant pain relief 10 years following the procedure. In those who did not obtain a satisfactory outcome, female gender and failure to obtain a significant clinical improvement immediately after surgery were the main factors predicting a poor outcome.

In an extensive series Bederson and Wilson (1989) reported a good (8%) or excellent (75%) outcome following decompression and partial sensory rhizotomy in 83% of patients treated. The duration of symptoms before surgery and prior surgical procedures were factors that contributed to poor outcomes for some patients (Bederson & Wilson 1989). Major adverse events ranging from trigeminal nerve complications and hearing loss to brainstem infarction and death can be associated with posterior fossa surgery.

The incidence of adverse events ranges from 0.1% (Barker et al 1996b) to 1% (Sidebottom & Maxwell 1995). Previous surgical procedures significantly increase the risk of developing trigeminal nerve complications such as dysaesthesia and analgesia dolorosa (Bederson & Wilson 1989). Figure 18.5 shows the surgical procedure for decompressive surgery.

A number of percutaneous techniques have been developed to treat trigeminal neuralgia. These include radiofrequency rhizotomy, glycerol rhizotomy and balloon compression (Taha & Tew 1996). It appears that percutaneous radiofrequency rhizotomy is the most successful of the percutaneous techniques. Figure 18.6 shows the surgical procedure for percutaneous radiofrequency rhizotomy. A comprehensive review suggests that this procedure is as successful as microvascular decompression and that the risk of death and major intracranial complications is much lower (Taha & Tew 1996).

Sweet (1988) recommends that the initial surgical procedure for any patient should be a percutaneous procedure. This of course is at odds with the finding that previous surgery reduces the likelihood of obtaining a successful outcome with microvascular decompression surgery. Improved imaging techniques and careful selection of patients for surgical procedures may help to resolve the issue of which surgical procedure represents the treatment of choice for any given patient.

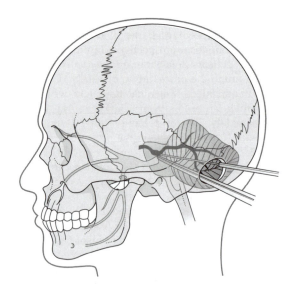

Figure 18.5 Surgical procedure for decompression surgery in trigeminal neuralgia (from Tew and van Loveren 1985, reprinted with permission from the Mayfield Clinic).

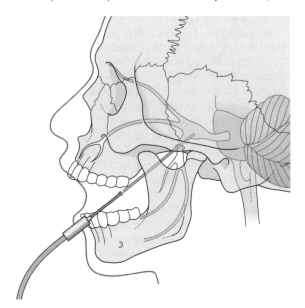

Figure 18.6 Surgical procedure for percutaneous readiofrequency rhizotomy in trigeminal neuralgia (from Tew and van Loveren 1985, reprinted with permission from the Mayfield Clinic).

Pharmacological therapies

Pharmacotherapy of trigeminal neuralgia usually involves the use of an anticonvulsant such as carbamazepine, sodium valproate or phenytoin.

Since the early 1960s, carbamazepine has been the drug treatment of choice for trigeminal neuralgia

(Amols 1970). Carbamazepine is chemically related to the tricyclic antidepressant imipramine. It has the ability to raise the threshold of activation of peripheral nerves, to reduce action potential amplitude, depress repetitive action potentials and generally reduce excitability. It also acts to suppress synaptic transmission in the trigeminal nucleus and spinal cord (Amols 1970). Chapter 16 provides further information on the uses and actions of carbamazepine.

The success of carbamazepine in treating trigeminal neuralgia has been attributed to its sodium-channel blocking function, and consequent membrane-stabilizing ability. This may cause inhibition of the lancinating pain that is characteristic of the condition. The drug has a rapid onset of effect, with 93% of patients obtaining pain relief within 48 hours. The degree of pain relief is related to the dosage and plasma concentration of the drug (Tomson et al 1980). Effective plasma concentrations ranged from 5.7–10.1 $\mu g\ ml^{-1}$.

Doses of carbamazepine are generally titrated to produce an efficacious effect with the minimum of side-effects; these effects tend to occur at plasma concentrations in excess of 7.9 $\mu g\ ml^{-1}$ (Tomson et al 1980). The most common side-effects are dizziness, drowsiness, nausea, skin reactions, generalized weakness, appetite loss, ataxia, gastrointestinal disorders and haematological abnormalities (Umino et al 1993). Unfortunately, side-effects experienced with carbamazepine may lead to withdrawal of the drug from the pain control regimen. The most common side-effect is central nervous system depression, which is experienced mainly in elderly patients.

It is also clear that the efficacy of carbamazepine may decline over time. Taylor and colleagues (1981) suggest that the mean time-period for developing late resistance to the drug is approximately 4 years; in their series 44% of patients ultimately required an alternative treatment because of lack of efficacy from carbamazepine.

Because of the side-effect profile of carbamazepine, attempts have been made to evaluate the efficacy of the active metabolite of carbamazepine (carbamazepine-10,11-epoxide) and carbamazepine analogues such as oxcarbazepine (Farago 1987, Tomson & Bertilsson 1984). While these drugs may have comparable efficacy to carbamazepine, they have not gained widespread acceptance. Preliminary trials have also been conducted using newer anti-epileptic drugs such as lamotrigine with promising results (Zakrzewska et al 1997).

Carbamazepine may be replaced by phenytoin if side-effects are considerable, or if the condition is not adequately controlled. The side-effect profile of phenytoin is as significant as carbamazepine, therefore transferring a patient to phenytoin may not be advantageous. In some instances, the two anticonvulsants may be administered concomitantly to allow a reduction in the dose of both.

Other anticonvulsants used include valproic acid, clonazepam and gabapentin. A systematic review on the use of anticonvulsants to manage pain has been reported by McQuay et al (1995). The available studies appear to support the use of anticonvulsants in the management of trigeminal neuralgia.

Physical therapies

While surgery provides the most effective means of controlling trigeminal neuralgia, other methods including transcutaneous electrical nerve stimulation and acupuncture may be considered as primary treatments in high-risk patients (Guo et al 1995, Holt et al 1995). The efficacy of these procedures is not well established. The role of occupational therapy or physiotherapy in the management of this disorder is limited, however, if the pain interferes with activities of daily living, then advice on dressing and personal grooming, among other things, may be required.

Summary

The aetiology of trigeminal neuralgia remains a matter of some controversy. In those patients for whom imaging studies provide a clear indication of neurovascular deformity, early microvascular decompression surgery would seem to be appropriate. For those patients in whom there is not a clear indication of an anatomical anomaly, or in whom the risk of surgery is too great, then the first-line treatment will often be carbamazepine. For those patients who do not respond to carbamazepine, or whose response diminishes over time, or who experience intolerable side-effects, then percutaneous surgery and radiofrequency rhizotomy would appear to be the best option.

Phantom pain

Reports of amputees experiencing pain and sensation from their amputated limbs can be traced back hundreds of years. Battleground surgeons, such as Mitchell in the American Civil War, reported that the majority of amputees complained of pain or sensation from limbs that clearly no longer existed (Mitchell 1871, Patterson 1988). Today, these phenomena are categorized as phantom sensation (non-painful sens-

ations referred to the amputated limb), stump pain (pain at the amputation site) and phantom pain (pain referred to the amputated limb or body part) (Davis 1993a). Phantom sensations and phantom pain are not confined to the limbs, and can occur with amputation of other body parts such as the teeth, the tongue, the bladder, the rectum, the genitalia and the breast (Davis 1993a).

Precise epidemiological statistics on the incidence and prevalence of phantom pain are difficult to collate due to unreliable reporting of the existence of pain in an amputated limb, and the fact that the pain may be of variable severity and duration. While psychological wellbeing is an important aspect in the treatment of amputee patients there is no clear evidence that a psychological disorder is responsible for the development of phantom limb pain (Katz 1992a, 1992b). It is suggested, however, that the psychological status of the patient affects the manner of pain reporting (Sherman 1980). Reports suggest that most amputees experience phantom sensation and that as many as 85% of amputees suffer from phantom pain of variable severity (Sherman & Sherman 1983).

Phantom limb pain may vary substantially in terms of intensity, frequency and the nature of the sensation, with some patients reporting relatively constant burning pain and others reporting episodic electric-shock type sensations (Davis 1993a). The location of the pain may also vary with some patients reporting that the whole limb is involved, while for others the pain is restricted to a particular part of the limb, usually the hand or foot (Jensen et al 1985).

Stump pain may also be quite variable in terms of its nature and provoking factors (Davis 1993a). The majority of patients experience significant lifestyle changes following limb amputation, with pain being a major contributor to these changes (Jones & Davidson 1995).

Most individuals with phantom pain experience pain in the first week following surgery, however some instances may not occur for several months (Davis 1993a). Pain may decrease over the first 6 months, however if pain is still present after 6 months it becomes a relatively constant phenomenon that is difficult to relieve (Davis 1993a, Jensen et al 1985). Initially phantom pain may resemble the preoperative pain in the leg, but after a few years that association becomes weaker as the nature of the phantom pain changes (Jensen et al 1985).

Stump pain, on the other hand, is more common in the early stages after amputation, with approximately 57% of patients affected, but by 2 years post-surgery it has declined to approximately 21% of patients affected

(Jensen et al 1985). Causes of stump pain include ill-fitting prostheses, neuroma formation, joint pain and referred pain from proximal regions such as the lumbar spine (Davis 1993a).

Katz (1992a) suggests that pain experienced in the limb prior to amputation correlates with the degree of pain in the phantom. He proposes that afferent nociceptive information from the stump is being processed by regions in the cortex that were once responsible for receiving input from the amputated limb, thus referring pain to the phantom.

With the development of cortical mapping, researchers are able to test this theory. Case studies have been reported indicating that patients experience referred phenomena in a phantom limb following stimulation of other areas of the upper body, suggesting cortical reorganization (Halligan et al 1993). Altered cortical mapping of face and proximal limb regions to encompass the area normally linked to the distal limb has been demonstrated by Yang et al (1994), using magnetoencephalography, in upper limb amputees.

Also using neuromagnetic-imaging techniques, Flor et al (1995) observed that the amount of cortical reorganization and the degree of phantom limb pain were correlated. The degree of cortical reorganization was significantly higher in patients suffering painful phantom sequelae than those suffering non-painful sequelae (Flor et al 1995). Techniques to measure cerebral bloodflow have demonstrated increased bloodflow in relevant cortical regions during periods of increased phantom pain (Liaw et al 1998).

It is apparent that cortical reorganization is highly plastic, and that it can be rapidly reversed following the administration of a regional anaesthetic block (Birbaumer et al 1997). The capacity to reverse cortical reorganization, even after significant periods of time, provides hope that highly effective treatments for phantom limb pain can ultimately be developed.

It is likely that the development of stump pain and phantom pain are due to a variety of factors that are present to varying degrees in different individuals, and that treatment of these conditions should address the multifactorial nature of the problem.

The management of stump pain and phantom limb pain reflects the diverse nature of the clinical picture, with a multiplicity of approaches being used. Sherman (1980) identified 43 different treatments for phantom limb pain that had been reported in the literature and suggested that many more unreported treatments were in use. The treatment approaches included surgery, pharmacological therapies, physical therapies and psychological interventions. In common with many other forms of neuropathic pain, there is no well-established treatment that is considered to be efficacious in the management of phantom pain.

Primary prevention

An increased awareness of the importance of central sensitization, and the link between pre-amputation pain and the development of phantom limb pain, has prompted researchers to consider aggressive pre-amputation pain control as a means of preventing the development of phantom limb pain. This approach is of limited value in relation to traumatic amputations, but it does have a potential role in relation to elective amputations as a result of peripheral vascular disease, diabetes or cancer.

Iacono et al (1987) suggest a comprehensive approach to the preoperative management of phantom limb pain, which includes psychological preparation (particularly addressing the issue of grief), aggressive preoperative pain control, careful attention to technical aspects of the amputation surgery, in order to avoid stump complications, and rapid postoperative mobilization (Iacono et al 1987).

Several studies have been conducted investigating pre-emptive analgesia and aggressive postoperative pain control as a means of preventing the development of phantom limb pain. While early reports suggested that pre-emptive analgesia might be effective in reducing phantom limb pain (Bach et al 1988, Jahangiri et al 1994), later studies have failed to demonstrate any benefit from lumbar epidural blockade (Nikolajsen et al 1997a), perineural infusion (Pinzur et al 1996) or continuous regional infusion (Elizaga et al 1994). A number of factors may account for the disparity of results to date: different treatment regimes have been used, including different drugs, different routes of administration and different time-periods of pre-emptive analgesia; it is possible that some regimes may be more effective than others. Katz (1997) has suggested that all treatment options have not yet been investigated. Nevertheless, pre-emptive analegesia does not appear to be as beneficial in preventing phantom limb pain as many of its original proponents would have expected.

Surgery

Historically, the mainstay of surgical intervention involved transection of neuromas formed as a consequence of the initial injury or surgery. The proximal end of the cut nerve is then implanted into a nearby anatomical site. This procedure may only provide short-term pain relief, as a subsequent neuroma can develop at the transection site. In reviewing a variety of surgical procedures for the management of phantom limb pain, Sherman (1980) concluded that there is no evidence to support the effectiveness of any ablative procedure.

An alterative surgical approach has been to implant electrodes to stimulate endogenous pain control mechanisms (dorsal column stimulation); this approach has been more successful (Sherman 1980). More recently, sophisticated stimulation paradigms using an array of electrodes placed over the motor cortex have shown beneficial effects in treating refractory phantom limb pain (Saitoh et al 2000). There seems little evidence to support the use of surgical procedures that attempt to cut or ablate the pain pathways, however surgical implantation of electrodes to stimulate the spinal cord and various parts of the brain may be of some value in treating patients with phantom limb pain that is not responsive to any other form of treatment.

Pharmacological therapies

Pharmacotherapy of phantom limb pain is similar to that of the other neuropathic pain problems discussed in this chapter. Initial drug therapy may involve tricyclic antidepressants and anticonvulsants (Iacono et al 1987). Other more conventional analgesics such as opioids may be considered. Regional blocks with local anaesthetics or epidural administration of local anaesthetics e.g. lignocaine/lidocaine, and narcotic analgesics, e.g. fentanyl, may also be used in the treatment of phantom limb pain. On occasions, a local anaesthetic and a narcotic analgesic are infused in combination, allowing the dose of both the narcotic and local anaesthetic to be reduced (Jahangiri et al 1994).

Various treatments may also be used to manage stump pain. There are comparatively few large scale, randomized, controlled trials and no meta-analyses of drug treatments for phantom pain or stump pain. The evidence-base is largely composed of small-scale, open-label trials and case series. This makes it difficult to arrive at clear conclusions about what represents the best approach to treating phantom pain and stump pain.

Capsaicin has been suggested as a topical treatment for persistent stump pain. The evidence to support its use is limited and conflicting (Rayner et al 1989, Weintraub et al 1990), however, given that capsaicin has been shown to be valuable in other neuropathic pain states, it may be useful in the management of stump pain characterized by significant allodynia.

An innovative approach to phantom limb pain treatment has been developed in the form of local anaes-thetic injection into areas of the contralateral limb corresponding to areas of maximum pain in the phantom limb. This has been shown to be of some benefit in a limited case series, but does not appear to have been subjected to a randomized controlled trial (Gross 1982).

Regional nerve blocks may be effective in controlling phantom and stump pain, and pain relief may outlast the period of infusion. Beneficial effects of brachial plexus block using ropivacaine and mepivacaine in upper-limb amputees have been demonstrated in small-scale trials (Birbaumer et al 1997, Lierz et al 1998).

Epidural and intrathecal blocks have also been used to manage phantom pain and stump pain, particularly in lower limb amputees. Administration of various opioids has proven effective in limited studies. Omote et al (1995) reported two cases where phantom pain was successfully controlled by the intrathecal administration of the synthetic opioid buprenorphine and subsequent management using buprenorphine suppositories. Intrathecal administration of fentanyl and epidural administration of morphine also seem to be effective in the management of phantom limb pain (Jacobson et al 1989) and prolonged stump pain (Jacobson et al 1990). In the case of stump pain, administration of the opioid fentanyl was significantly more effective than administration of the local anaesthetic lignocaine/lidocaine (Jacobson et al 1990).

In many cases it seems that the effect of regional, epidural or intrathecal block significantly outlasts the duration to the block, suggesting that these procedures can have a long-term modulatory influence on the mechanisms responsible for phantom limb pain or prolonged stump pain.

A wide variety of oral medications have been used to manage phantom limb pain and stump pain. These include tricyclic antidepressants such as amitriptyline (Urban et al 1986), opioids such as methadone (Urban et al 1986), benzodiazepines such as clonazepam (Bartusch et al 1996), antiarrhythmics such as mexiletine (Davis 1993b), anticonvulsants such as carbamazepine (Patterson 1988), antipsychotics such as chlorpromazine (Logan 1983), peptides such as calcitonin (Kessel & Worz 1987, Wall & Heyneman 1999) and NMDA-receptor antagonists such as ketamine (Nikolajsen et al 1997b). All of these medications have been reported as successful in small-scale studies and case reports.

In a number of cases, judicious combinations of medications such as amitriptyline and methadone (Urban et al 1986) and mexiletine and clonidine (Davis 1993b) have demonstrated very encouraging results.

This is an area that would benefit from further research using large-scale randomized clinical trials to assist in identifying the optimum medication, or combination of medications, to manage phantom pain.

Physical therapies

A wide variety of treatments have been used in managing stump and phantom limb pain (Berger 1980). The evidence-base to support these treatments is also limited to small-scale uncontrolled studies and case reports. One of the most common approaches has been the use of TENS for symptomatic relief. In an early study, Winnem and Amundsen (1982) demonstrated satisfactory reduction of pain using TENS in approximately 50% of the patients studied.

An innovative approach has been to use TENS applied to the contralateral normal limb in the same area in which pain is perceived in the phantom limb (Carabelli & Kellerman 1985); very encouraging responses to this form of treatment were demonstrated in this small case series. It is interesting to note that TENS applied in the postoperative period actually improves stump healing and limits the need for re-amputation, as well as reducing phantom pain at 4 months but not at 1 year follow-up (Finsen et al 1988).

Acupuncture has also been used as a means of producing symptomatic relief in patients with phantom limb pain (Monga & Jaksic 1981, Xing 1998).

Recently, more active physical treatments and use of the affected limb have been shown to be beneficial (Lotze et al 1999, Weiss et al 1999). In particular, active use of a functional upper limb prosthesis is effective in reducing phantom pain (Weiss et al 1999). Activity of the limb seems to contribute to reversal of the cortical reorganization that may provide the neurophysiological basis for phantom limb pain (Lotze et al 1999, Weiss et al 1999).

These results are very encouraging and suggest that rapid progression of patients to prosthesis use and redirection of attention to active use of the limb may be beneficial in managing or preventing phantom pain.

Another approach that has received some consideration is imagined exercise or movement of the phantom (Sherman 1980), although there do not appear to be any published studies related to the benefits of this approach.

Psychological therapies

Psychological approaches to the management of phantom limb pain have been investigated and it is well recognized that psychological issues such as grief related to the loss of a body part must be recognized and addressed when managing patients with phantom limb pain (Pucher et al 1999).

It is apparent that coping reactions may influence the occurrence of phantom pain (Pucher et al 1999). Catastrophizing, and 'hoping and praying' strategies appear to increase pain (Hill et al 1995). There seems to be some potential to improve pain by developing alternative coping strategies, however this has not been extensively investigated.

Hypnosis has also been used as a means of managing phantom pain with some evidence of success in limited case series (Muraoka et al 1996, Siegel 1979).

Summary

Stump pain and phantom pain are common problems for amputees, which are difficult to manage effectively. The pathophysiological basis of phantom pain still requires further elucidation, although recent studies show that cortical reorganization is a very important factor in producing this pain state.

A multiplicity of treatments have been used to relieve persistent stump pain and phantom pain, however none have gained universal acceptance and the evidence-base to support the efficacy of any therapy is limited.

Recent research suggests that active use of an amputated limb is important to relieve pain and reverse or modify cortical reorganization. This has important implications for physiotherapists and occupational therapists in terms of promoting early active rehabilitation and prosthesis use in amputees.

It is likely that a multifaceted approach to pain management will provide optimum efficacy for individuals with both phantom pain and stump pain. Much more research is required in this area to establish effective treatment protocols for a common and difficult clinical problem.

Complex regional pain syndromes

The group of conditions that are described under the heading complex regional pain syndrome were previously known as reflex sympathetic dystrophy and causalgia. The 2nd edition of the IASP Classification of Chronic Pain Syndromes (Merskey & Bogduk 1994) recognizes two distinct types of complex regional pain syndrome. Type I, formerly known as reflex sympathetic dystrophy, does not involve a nerve lesion, whereas type II, formerly known as causalgia, refers to the condition where a describable nerve injury has occurred.

Replacement of the terms reflex sympathetic dystrophy and causalgia resulted from their misuse. It has become clear that pain in these disorders is not always dependent on the presence of sympathetic hyperactivity. While tissues may become hypersensitive to noradrenaline release from sympathetic efferents, sympathetic nervous system activity may be either normal or reduced.

While the nature of the initial insult is different between the two types of complex regional pain syndrome, both conditions have similar features. These include spontaneous pain, pain that extends beyond the innervation boundaries of a single peripheral nerve, allodynia or hyperalgesia that is disproportionate to the original insult, oedema, skin bloodflow abnormalities, bone demineralization and altered sudomotor activity (Wong & Wilson 1997).

The pain is often described as an intense burning sensation, sometimes in combination with stabbing paroxysms. Dysaesthesia may also be a feature of the disorder and motor dysfunction is more common than previously suggested; such motor features include tremor, dystonia, poor coordination, decreased endurance and restricted motion (Bushnell & Cobo-Castro 1999, Wong & Wilson 1997).

Complex regional pain syndrome type I involves deep diffuse pain brought on by minor injury or resulting from a variety of causes including inflammation, surgery, infection, bone fracture, myocardial infarct, stroke, degenerative joint disease, surgical trauma, plaster cast application, frostbite and burns (Hendler & Raja 1994, Payne 1986).

Complex regional pain syndrome type II is always related to nerve injury and diagnosis is typically made 5–6 weeks following pain onset (Payne 1986). This disorder was previously termed causalgia. The areas of the body affected are almost invariably the hand and foot, as the most common nerves involved are the median, ulnar, sciatic, and tibial nerves, however, pain can spread to involve the entire limb.

Some authorities recognize three distinct stages in the progression of the disorder (Bushnell & Cobo-Castro 1999). These stages are outlined in Box 18.4. It is clear however, that there is little evidence to support a progression of patients through each of these stages, and so they may simply be distinct presentations linked to the same underlying disorder (Veldman et al 1993).

Complex regional pain syndrome type II persists for more than 6 months in 85% of cases and continues for more than 1 year in 25% of cases (Payne 1986). The condition can have a major impact on the patient's life.

A positive response to sympathetic blockade does not form part of the differential diagnosis of complex

---

> **Box 18.4** Hypothesized stages of complex regional pain syndrome (from Bushnell and Cobo-Castro 1999, with kind permission)
>
> **First stage** – acute or warm phase
> This stage occurs immediately after the pain starts. Generally the limb is warm and swollen and there may be increased nail and hair growth, spontaneous burning pain, hyperpathia and allodynia.
>
> **Second stage** – instability or dystrophic phase
> Classically begins 3 months after the precipitating event. The pain now occurs in an extended area, and limitation of movements and joint stiffness become significant features. Osteoporosis and muscle wasting are usually evident at this point
>
> **Third stage** – Atrophic phase
> Generally occurs 6 months after first symptoms if the condition remains untreated. Pain may actually decrease or cease to be the most significant symptom for the patient. The skin is cool, cyanotic, smooth and glossy

---

regional pain syndrome. While sympathetic hyperactivity may be an aspect of the condition, its reversal is not a requirement for diagnosis. It is possible that sympathetic nervous system activity may contribute to pain in a variety of ways (see Chapter 3 for a more detailed discussion of the relevant neurophysiology). The concepts of sympathetically maintained pain and sympathetically independent pain have been devised to differentiate those patients who do and do not respond to sympathetic blocks. Box 18.4 provides a diagrammatic representation of the complex interaction between factors contributing to complex regional pain syndromes.

The concept that sympathetic hyperactivity, or conversely the development of hypersensitivity to circulating noradrenaline, might provide a pathophysiological basis for this disorder has been a matter of considerable dispute, as strong scientific evidence to support either of these proposals has failed to emerge.

More recently, an old concept of this disorder has begun to re-emerge. This suggests that complex regional pain syndrome is, in effect, an exaggerated inflammatory response to injury of some form (van der Laan & Goris 1997). Changes in venous oxygen saturation, arterial flow and lactate levels suggest that complex regional pain syndrome is characterized by the paradox of high oxygen supply and tissue hypoxia, due to some impairment of oxygen diffusion (van der Laan & Goris 1997). This paradoxical combination is also found in other disorders associated with marked inflammation, such as burns, varicose ulcers, malignant tumours, ischaemia and diabetes.

The concept of complex regional pain syndrome as an exaggerated inflammatory state has resulted in the development of alternative treatment approaches that do not hinge on disruption of sympathetic nervous system function. These treatments are discussed below.

Primary prevention

Several authors have highlighted the need for early intervention to minimize the pain and disability of complex regional pain syndrome. Ramamurthy and Hoffman (1995) conducted a trial to test the effect of regional intravenous guanethidine block in patients with both upper and lower limb complex regional pain syndrome type I, of less than 3 months duration (average 1.6 months). Guanethidine was administered in saline and combined with lignocaine/lidocaine to prevent the burning sensation that guanethidine induces. Control blocks using saline and lignocaine/lidocaine alone were also administered.

All groups showed a significant improvement over the 6 months of the study. No difference between the guanethidine blocks and the control blocks could be demonstrated. Unfortunately, the study did not include a no-treatment control and so it is not clear whether the improvements represent the natural history of the disorder or a true treatment effect.

While it is possible that early intervention may be beneficial, further research is required to demonstrate the value of early interventions and to determine what the optimal intervention might be.

Pharmacological therapies

Management of complex regional pain syndrome depends on the severity and progression of the condition. Initial treatment may involve a sympathetic block targeted at the stellate or lumbar sympathetic ganglia. Local anaesthetics, such as bupivacaine, provide short-term pain relief of approximately 3–4 hours when injected directly into the ganglion. A phentolamine test may also be carried out to determine the extent to which the pain is responsive to sympathetic blockade.

As an alternative to ganglion blocks, intravenous regional sympathetic blockade can be performed. This procedure involves isolating the affected limb with a tourniquet and administering an adrenergic blocking agent, such as guanethidine, intravenously (Hannington-Kiff 1979). The tourniquet remains in place for 20 minutes following the administration of guanethidine, to keep the agent localized in the limb, thus preventing systemic side-effects, e.g. hypotension.

Guanethidine acts to block nerve function by depleting intraneural vesicles of noradrenaline. It causes an initial release of noradrenaline, which eventually subsides as it occupies adrenergic vesicles; this inhibits nerve-impulse transmission.

The effectiveness of regional blockade with guanethidine has been questioned in some studies (Kaplan et al 1996, Ramamurthy & Hoffman 1995). Findings from a structured review of controlled clinical trials suggest that, while regional sympathetic blockade may be used quite frequently, there is little evidence to support its efficacy (Kingery 1997). It is also apparent that this procedure may produce significant side-effects (Kaplan et al 1996).

There has been a good deal of debate about the value of guanethidine blocks, with many authorities increasingly recognizing the limited evidence-base to support the use of this treatment (Schott 1998, Valentin 1996). Others, however, continue to argue in favour of the treatment (Lamacraft et al 1998). One of the difficulties that arise is that most clinicians administer guanethidine in combination with lignocaine/lidocaine, and so there may be some benefit from administering the local anaesthetic.

Intravenous regional blocks have also been carried out with other drugs that affect peripheral noradrenergic function, including reserpine and bretylium. Beneficial effects have been demonstrated in one small-scale trial with bretylium (Hord et al 1992). Reserpine was not significantly different to guanethidine or a lignocaine/lidocaine control condition, with only a small proportion of patients gaining relief with either drug (Rocco et al 1989). It is clear that there is limited benefit from regional sympathetic blockade in most patients, however it is possible that there may be a subgroup of 20–25% of patients who benefit from this treatment; to date, criteria for clearly identifying these patients have not been established.

Iontophoresis provides an alternative method of administering guanethidine without the discomfort of the regional block technique. Iontophoresis increases tissue penetration of charged molecules, delivered across the skin by the application of a weak electric field. Positive results in complex regional pain syndrome type I patients have been demonstrated following iontophoretic administration of guanethidine (Bonezzi et al 1994).

The alpha-adrenergic antagonist phentolamine has also been investigated as a means of managing complex regional pain syndrome. The phentolamine test has been suggested as a way to determine the potential value of sympathetic blockade in the management of individual patients. Trials have produced conflicting results, with some authors suggesting that phentolamine produces demonstrable pain relief (Raja et al 1991), while others suggest that response to the test is largely based on placebo (Verdugo & Ochoa 1994, Verdugo et al 1994). Phentolamine has not been considered as a long-term treatment for complex regional pain syndrome because of the cardiovascular effects of intravenous infusion.

It is interesting to note that while a structured review of treatments for complex regional pain syndrome failed to provide evidence to support treatments that attempted to modify sympathetic nervous system function, it did conclude that there was evidence from a number of studies that corticosteroids are effective in providing pain relief in patients with early complex regional pain syndrome (Kingery 1997). Treatment with both prednisone (Christensen et al 1982) and methylprednisolone (Braus et al 1994) was effective in producing pain relief in short-term trials.

The limitations of this approach are that the doses of corticosteroid required are relatively high, and that they need to be used for a prolonged period with associated risk of severe adverse effects (van der Laan & Goris 1997).

Alternative approaches to managing complex regional pain syndrome, based on the concept that the disorder represents an exaggerated inflammatory response, have been developed. A combination of intravenous infusion of mannitol and topical application of dimethylsulfoxide (DMSO) has shown some value in managing complex regional pain syndrome (van der Laan & Goris 1997). DMSO treatment alone has also been shown to be beneficial by other researchers (Zuurmond et al 1996). The concept is that these drugs enhance free-radical scavenger function and help to limit the inflammatory response. Mannitol therapy resulted in decreased arterial flow and decreased venous oxygen saturation, suggesting improved tissue oxygen extraction.

In complex regional pain syndrome patients with a predominantly cold presentation van der Lann and Goris (1997) recommend initial treatment with a vasodilator such as verapamil, before moving to the mannitol/DMSO regime. These authors also recommend the inclusion of physical therapies into the treatment regime, although they caution against the use of vigorous techniques because these tend to exacerbate the problem. This approach to managing complex regional pain syndrome shows considerable potential and warrants further investigation by other groups.

An alternative and perhaps unusual approach to treating complex regional pain syndrome has been to administer the hormone calcitonin. The initial rationale for this approach was to treat the osteoporosis that is a significant feature of this disorder once it becomes well established. It has been noted, however, that administration of calcitonin can significantly reduce pain and many of the other clinical features of the disorder (Doury et al 1975). The method of delivery for calcitonin appears to be important, with nasal administration being relatively ineffective (Bickerstaff & Kanis 1991). A combination of calcitonin and regional block with guanethidine has also been used in a case study, with apparent success (McKay et al 1977).

Other pharmacological treatments for complex regional pain syndrome include tricyclic antidepressants, anticonvulsants and non-steroidal anti-inflammatory drugs.

Physical therapies

A number of physical therapies have been advocated in the management of complex regional pain syndrome. These include intermittent pneumatic compression, contrast baths, desensitization, splinting, TENS and continuous passive motion (Bengtson 1997, Headley 1987).

Regional blockade is often combined with physical therapies to address the dystrophic changes in connective tissue and the movement limitations that are part of the condition (Wilder et al 1992). Active movement, particularly with an emphasis on functional movements and weight-bearing through the affected limb are important components of the treatment (Wilder et al 1992). Gentle massage and intermittent compression may be helpful in reducing oedema (Headley 1987).

Acupuncture has also been used as a method of treatment with some evidence of benefit (Fialka et al 1993). While the combination of physical therapy and regional sympathetic block has been strongly advocated by a number of authors, there have been no well-controlled studies evaluating the combined intervention, and there is little evidence available to suggest which specific physical therapies might be of value.

In many pain centres the aim of treatment is to return function to the affected limb. A recent study provided an interesting comparison between physiotherapy and occupational therapy management of patients with complex regional pain syndrome (Oerlemans et al 1999). This study suggested that there was some beneficial effect of both therapeutic approaches compared with a control but that improvement in pain measures was faster and more sustained with physiotherapy management. There is a distinct lack of controlled studies to evaluate the effects of specific physical therapies in the management of complex regional pain syndromes.

Psychological therapies

It has been suggested that particular personality traits or psychological disturbances may predispose to the development of complex regional pain syndrome, however there appears to be little evidence to support such suggestions (Didierjean 1997). Nevertheless, it is clear that the pain and suffering that most patients with this disorder experience have inevitable psychological consequences.

Patients with complex regional pain syndrome may exhibit more depression, have greater feelings of inadequacy and be more anxious than patients with a comparable disorder such as carpal tunnel syndrome (Geertzen et al 1994). It also appears that clients with complex regional pain syndrome are more likely to have experienced a significant life-event in conjunction with the onset of the disorder, suggesting that psychological factors may be important in triggering this syndrome (Geertzen et al 1994).

It is possible that a variety of psychologically based interventions may be beneficial for individuals suffering from this problem, however, there are few trials that have investigated specific psychological interventions in this disorder.

Psychotherapy, cognitive–behavioural therapy and hypnotherapy have all been described as beneficial in the management of this disorder in small-scale studies (Didierjean 1997, Gainer 1992, Lebovits et al 1990). Further studies are required to evaluate the efficacy of specific psychological interventions for patients, or sub-groups of patients, with complex regional pain syndrome.

Summary

Complex regional pain syndrome remains an elusive clinical problem. The aetiology and pathophysiology of the disorder are not well understood. The role of the sympathetic nervous system in maintaining the disorder remains a matter of substantial controversy.

As a consequence of our lack of understanding of the pathophysiology of the disorder there remains significant controversy about the optimal approach to management. Sympathetic blocks have been used extensively as a means of treating this disorder for several decades yet this approach has fallen

into disrepute in recent years. More research is required to determine if there is a sub-population of patients who clearly benefit from regional sympathetic block.

New approaches to treatment are emerging based on a model of complex regional pain syndrome as an exaggerated inflammatory response. These approaches warrant further investigation.

It is very clear that pharmacological interventions alone are not likely to be effective with most clients. Consequently, there is a clear need to better define the role of physical therapies and psychological therapies. Further research to expand the evidence-base for these interventions is urgently required.

CONCLUSION AND IMPLICATIONS

Neuropathic pain states constitute a very significant clinical problem that results in significant distress for individuals and significant costs for healthcare systems. Neuropathic pain can become a chronic problem that will impact on every aspect of a sufferer's life.

Our knowledge of the pathophysiological processes that may contribute to the development of neuropathic pain states is improving and it has become apparent that multiple processes may be involved in the development of different pain states. It is also increasingly recognized that management of these problems must be multifaceted in order to address the complex pathophysiology.

In general terms, management should consider options to prevent the development of neuropathic pain, a range of pharmacological therapies, and, where appropriate, the use of both physical and psychological therapies. The scope of the management program depends on the nature of the individual disorder and the specifics of each patient's presentation.

There is an urgent need to undertake further research in relation to many of the interventions used to treat neuropathic pain. Currently the evidence-base to support a variety of widely used interventions is very poor. Physiotherapists and occupational therapists could contribute to improving this situation by conducting research to evaluate a range of interventions that are within the scope of practice of each of these professions.

In particular, further research in relation to the management of painful diabetic neuropathy, phantom limb pain, stump pain and complex regional pain syndrome is urgently required and would contribute significantly to providing evidence-based management of these painful disorders.

Study questions/questions for revision

1. What are the two distinct mechanisms that researchers have suggested might lead to the development of pain in post-herpetic neuralgia?
2. Describe the treatment approach to managing painful diabetic neuropathy that addresses several potential mechanisms for producing pain in this disorder.
3. What are the two main surgical approaches used to treat trigeminal neuralgia?
4. What are the distinctions between phantom sensation, phantom pain and stump pain?
5. Describe the potential benefits of physical therapies in the management of complex regional pain syndrome.

REFERENCES

Abuaisha B B, Costanzi J B, Boulton A J 1998 Acupuncture for the treatment of chronic painful peripheral diabetic neuropathy: a long-term study. Diabetes Research and Clinical Practice 39: 115–121

Amols W 1970 Facial pain. Treatment with carbamazepine. New York State Journal of Medicine 70: 2429–2432

Armstrong D G, Lavery L A, Fleischli J G, Gilham K A 1997 Is electrical stimulation effective in reducing neuropathic pain in patients with diabetes? Journal of Foot and Ankle Surgery 36: 260–263

Arner S, Meyerson B A 1988 Lack of analgesic effect of opioids on neuropathic and idiopathic forms of pain. Pain 33: 11–23

Bach F W, Jensen T S, Kastrup J, Stigsby B, Dejgard A 1990 The effect of intravenous lidocaine on nociceptive processing in diabetic neuropathy. Pain 40: 29–34

Bach S, Noreng M F, Tjellden N U 1988 Phantom limb pain in amputees during the first 12 months following limb amputation, after preoperative lumbar epidural blockade. Pain 33: 297–301

Backonja M M, Galer B S 1998 Pain assessment and evaluation of patients who have neuropathic pain. Neurology Clinics 16: 775–790

Barker F G, Jannetta P J, Babu R P, Pomonis S, Bissonette D J, Jho H D 1996a Long-term outcome after operation for trigeminal neuralgia in patients with posterior fossa tumors. Journal of Neurosurgery 84: 818–825

Barker F G, Jannetta P J, Bissonette D J, Larkins M V, Jho H D 1996b The long-term outcome of microvascular decompression for trigeminal neuralgia. New England Journal of Medicine 334: 1077–1083

Baron R, Haendler G, Schulte H 1997 Afferent large fiber polyneuropathy predicts the development of postherpetic neuralgia. Pain 73: 231–238

Bartusch S L, Sanders B J, D'Alessio J G, Jernigan J R 1996 Clonazepam for the treatment of lancinating phantom limb pain. Clinical Journal of Pain 12: 59–62

Bederson J B, Wilson C B 1989 Evaluation of microvascular decompression and partial sensory rhizotomy in 252 cases of trigeminal neuralgia. Journal of Neurosurgery 71: 359–367

Belgrade M J 1999 Following the clues to neuropathic pain. Distribution and other leads reveal the cause and the treatment approach. Postgraduate Medicine 106: 127–132, 135–140

Belgrade M J, Lev B I 1991 Diabetic neuropathy. Helping patients cope with their pain. Postgraduate Medicine 90: 263–270

Bengtson K 1997 Physical modalities for complex regional pain syndrome. Hand Clinics 13: 443–454

Berger S M 1980 Conservative management of phantom-limb and amputation-stump pain. Annals of the Royal College of Surgeons of England 62: 102–105

Bickerstaff D R, Kanis J A 1991 The use of nasal calcitonin in the treatment of post-traumatic algodystrophy. British Journal of Rheumatology 30: 291–294

Birbaumer N, Lutzenberger W, Montoya P, Larbig W, Unertl K, Topfner S, Grodd W, Taub E, Flor H 1997 Effects of regional anesthesia on phantom limb pain are mirrored in changes in cortical reorganization. Journal of Neuroscience 17: 5503–5508

Bonezzi C, Miotti D, Bettaglio R, Stephen R 1994 Electromotive administration of guanethidine for treatment of reflex sympathetic dystrophy: a pilot study in eight patients. Journal of Pain and Symptom Management 9: 39–43

Boulton A J 1994 End-stage complications of diabetic neuropathy: foot ulceration. Canadian Journal of Neurological Sciences 21: S18–S22

Bowsher D 1994 Post-herpetic neuralgia in older patients. Incidence and optimal treatment. Drugs and Aging 5: 411–418

Braune S, Schady W 1993 Changes in sensation after nerve injury or amputation: the role of central factors. Journal of Neurology, Neurosurgery and Psychiatry 56: 393–399

Braus D F, Krauss J K, Strobel J 1994 The shoulder-hand syndrome after stroke: a prospective clinical trial. Annals of Neurology 36: 728–733

Bushnell T G, Cobo-Castro T 1999 Complex regional pain syndrome: becoming more or less complex? Manual Therapy 4: 221–218

Byas-Smith M G, Max M B, Muir J, Kingman A 1995 Transdermal clonidine compared to placebo in painful diabetic neuropathy using a two-stage 'enriched enrollment' design. Pain 60: 267–274

Carabelli R A, Kellerman W C 1985 Phantom limb pain: relief by application of TENS to contralateral extremity. Archives of Physical Medicine and Rehabilitation 66: 466–467

Chan A W, MacFarlane L A, Bowsher D R, Wells J C, Bessex C, Griffiths K 1990 Chronic pain in patients with diabetes mellitus; comparison with non-diabetic population. Pain Clinic 3: 147–159

Christensen K, Jensen E M, Noer I 1982 The reflex dystrophy syndrome response to treatment with systemic corticosteroids. Acta Chirurgica Scandinavica 148: 653–655

Davis R W 1993a Phantom sensation, phantom pain, and stump pain. Archives of Physical Medicine and Rehabilitation 74: 79–91

Davis R W 1993b Successful treatment for phantom pain. Orthopedics 16: 691–695

DCCT Research Group 1993 The effect of intensive treatment of diabetes on the development and progression of long-term complications in insulin-dependent diabetes mellitus. New England Journal of Medicine 329: 977–986

De Benedittis G, Besana F, Lorenzetti A 1992 A new topical treatment for acute herpetic neuralgia and post-herpetic neuralgia: the aspirin/diethyl ether mixture. An open-label study plus a double-blind controlled clinical trial (published erratum appears in Pain 50(2): 245) Pain 48: 383–390

Devor M 1991 Neuropathic pain and injured nerve: peripheral mechanisms. British Medical Bulletin 47: 619–630

Devor M, Wall P D 1978 Reorganisation of spinal cord sensory map after peripheral nerve injury. Nature 276: 75–76

Devor M, Wall P D 1981a Plasticity in the spinal cord sensory map following peripheral nerve injury in rats. Journal of Neuroscience 1: 679–684

Devor M, Wall P D 1981b Effect of peripheral nerve injury on receptive fields of cells in the cat spinal cord. Journal of Comparative Neurology 199: 277–291

Didierjean A 1997 Psychological aspects of algodystrophy. Hand Clinics 13: 363–366

Doury P, Pattin S, Delahaye R P, Metges P J, Batisse R 1975 Thyrocalcitonin in the treatment of algodystrophia. Nouvelle Presse Medicale 4: 2527–2528

Elizaga A M, Smith D G, Sharar S R, Edwards W T, Hansen S T, Jr, 1994 Continuous regional analgesia by intraneural block: effect on postoperative opioid requirements and phantom limb pain following amputation. Journal of Rehabilitation Research and Development 31: 179–187

Esmann V, Geil J P, Kroon S, Fogh H, Peterslund N A, Petersen C S, Ronne-Rasmussen J O, Danielsen L 1987 Prednisolone does not prevent post-herpetic neuralgia. Lancet 2: 126–129

Farago F 1987 Trigeminal neuralgia: its treatment with two new carbamazepine analogues. European Journal of Neurology 26: 73–83

Fedele D, Giugliano D 1997 Peripheral diabetic neuropathy. Current recommendations and future prospects for its prevention and management. Drugs 54: 414–421

Feldman E L, Stevens M J 1994 Clinical testing in diabetic peripheral neuropathy. Canadian Journal of Neurological Sciences 21: S3–S7

Fialka V, Resch K L, Ritter-Dietrich D, Alacamlioglu Y, Chen O, Leitha T, Kluger R, Ernst E 1993 Acupuncture for reflex sympathetic dystrophy. Archives of Internal Medicine 153: 661, 665

Fields H 1994 Pain modulation and the action of analgesic medications. Annals of Neurology 35: S42–S45

Finsen V, Persen L, Lovlien M, Veslegaard E K, Simensen M, Gasvann A K, Benum P 1988 Transcutaneous electrical nerve stimulation after major amputation. Journal of Bone and Joint Surgery 70: 109–112

Flor H, Elbert T, Knecht S, Wienbruch C, Pantev C, Birbaumer N, Larbig W, Taub E 1995 Phantom-limb pain as a perceptual correlate of cortical reorganization following arm amputation. Nature 375: 482–484

Gainer M J 1992 Hypnotherapy for reflex sympathetic dystrophy. American Journal of Clinical Hypnosis 34: 227–232

Geertzen J H, de Bruijn H, de Bruijn-Kofman A T, Arendzen J H 1994 Reflex sympathetic dystrophy: early treatment and psychological aspects. Archives of Physical Medicine and Rehabilitation 75: 442–446

Govrin-Lippmann R, Devor M 1978 Ongoing activity in severed nerves: source and variation with time. Brain Research 159: 406–410

Greene D A, Stevens M J, Feldman E L 1999 Diabetic neuropathy: scope of the syndrome. American Journal of Medicine 107: 2S–8S

Gross D 1982 Contralateral local anaesthesia in the treatment of phantom limb and stump pain. Pain 13: 313–320

Guo J, Kang X, Zhang S 1995 Treatment of primary trigeminal neuralgia with acupuncture at the sphenopalatine ganglion. Journal of Traditional Chinese Medicine 15: 31–33

Halligan P W, Marshall J C, Wade D T, Davey J, Morrison D 1993 Thumb in cheek? Sensory reorganization and perceptual plasticity after limb amputation. Neuroreport 4: 233–236

Hannington-Kiff J G 1979 Relief of causalgia in limbs by regional intravenous guanethidine. British Medical Journal 2: 367–368

Harding S P 1995 Acyclovir and post-herpetic neuralgia. The balance of available evidence supports its use. British Medical Journal 310: 1005

Headley B 1987 Historical perspective of causalgia. Management of sympathetically maintained pain. Physical Therapy 67: 1370–1374

Hendler N, Raja S N 1994 Reflex sympathetic dystrophy and causalgia. In: C D Tollinson (ed), Handbook of Pain Management. Williams & Wilkins, Baltimore, pp 484–496

Hill A, Niven C A, Knussen C 1995 The role of coping in adjustment to phantom limb pain. Pain 62: 79–86

Holt C R, Finney J W, Wall C L 1995 The use of transcutaneous electrical nerve stimulation (TENS) in the treatment of facial pain. Annals of the Academy of Medicine, Singapore 24: 17–22

Hope-Simpson R E 1975 Postherpetic neuralgia. Journal of the Royal College of General Practitioners 25: 571–575

Hord A H, Rooks M D, Stephens B O, Rogers H G, Fleming L L 1992 Intravenous regional bretylium and lidocaine for treatment of reflex sympathetic dystrophy: a randomized, double-blind study. Anesthesia and Analgesia 74: 818–821

Hylden J L, Nahin R L, Dubner R 1987 Altered responses of nociceptive cat lamina I spinal dorsal horn neurons after chronic sciatic neuroma formation. Brain Research 411: 341–350

Iacono R P, Linford J, Sandyk R 1987 Pain management after lower extremity amputation. Neurosurgery 20: 496–500

Jacobson L, Chabal C, Brody M C 1989 Relief of persistent postamputation stump and phantom limb pain with intrathecal fentanyl. Pain 37: 317–322

Jacobson L, Chabal C, Brody M C, Mariano A J, Chaney E F 1990 A comparison of the effects of intrathecal fentanyl and lidocaine on established postamputation stump pain. Pain 40: 137–141

Jahangiri M, Jayatunga A P, Bradley J W, Dark C H 1994 Prevention of phantom pain after major lower limb amputation by epidural infusion of diamorphine, clonidine and bupivacaine. Annals of the Royal College of Surgeons of England 76: 324–326

James J S, Page J C 1994 Painful diabetic peripheral neuropathy. A stepwise approach to treatment. Journal of the American Podiatric Medicine Association 84: 439–447

Jensen T S, Krebs B, Nielsen J, Rasmussen P 1985 Immediate and long-term phantom limb pain in amputees: incidence, clinical characteristics and relationship to pre-amputation limb pain. Pain 21: 267–278

Jones L E, Davidson J H 1995 The long-term outcome of upper limb amputees treated at a rehabilitation centre in Sydney, Australia. Disability and Rehabilitation 17: 437–442

Kaplan R, Claudio M, Kepes E, Gu X F 1996 Intravenous guanethidine in patients with reflex sympathetic dystrophy, Acta Anaesthesiologica Scandinavica 40: 1216–1222

Kastrup J, Petersen P, Dejgard A, Angelo H R, Hilsted J 1987 Intravenous lidocaine infusion – a new treatment of chronic painful diabetic neuropathy? Pain 28: 69–75

Katz J 1992a Psychophysical correlates of phantom limb experience. Journal of Neurology, Neurosurgery and Psychiatry 55: 811–821

Katz J 1992b Psychophysiological contributions to phantom limbs. Canadian Journal of Psychiatry 37: 282–298

Katz J 1997 Phantom limb pain. Lancet 350: 1338–1339

Kessel C, Worz R 1987 Immediate response of phantom limb pain to calcitonin. Pain 30: 79–87

Kingery W S 1997 A critical review of controlled clinical trials for peripheral neuropathic pain and complex regional pain syndromes. Pain 73: 123–139

Kumar D, Marshall H J 1997 Diabetic peripheral neuropathy: amelioration of pain with transcutaneous electrostimulation. Diabetes Care 20: 1702–1705

Laduron P M 1987 Axonal transport or presynatic receptors. In: Smith R S, Bisby M (eds) Axonal Transport. Liss, New York, pp 347–363

Lamacraft G, Price C M, Prosser A S, Rogers P D, Pounder D 1998 Interrupting the sympathetic outflow in causalgia and reflex sympathetic dystrophy. Intravenous regional guanethidine blockage is a safe and effective treatment [letter; comment]. British Medical Journal 317: 752–753

Lebovits A H, Yarmush J, Lefkowitz M 1990 Reflex sympathetic dystrophy and post traumatic stress disorder. Multidisciplinary evaluation and treatment. Clinical Journal of Pain 6: 153–157

Lewith G T, Field J, Machin D 1983 Acupuncture compared with placebo in post-herpetic pain. Pain 17: 361–368

Liaw M Y, You D L, Cheng P T, Kao P F, Wong A M 1998 Central representation of phantom limb phenomenon in amputees studied with single photon emission computerized tomography. American Journal of Physical Medicine and Rehabilitation 77: 368–375

Lierz P, Schroegendorfer K, Choi S, Felleiter P, Kress H G 1998 Continuous blockade of both brachial plexus with ropivacaine in phantom pain: a case report. Pain 78: 135–137

Loeser J D 1994 Tic douloureux and atypical face pain. In: Wall P D, Melzack R (eds) Textbook of Pain. Churchill Livingstone, Edinburgh

Logan T P 1983 Persistent phantom limb pain: dramatic response to chlorpromazine. Southern Medical Journal 76: 1585

Lotze M, Grodd W, Birbaumer N, Erb M, Huse E, Flor H 1999 Does use of a myoelectric prosthesis prevent cortical reorganization and phantom limb pain? Natural Neusoscience 2: 501–502

Mandal B K, Dunbar E M, Ellis M E, Ellis J, Dowd P 1988 A double-masked, placebo-controlled trial of acyclovir cream in immunocompetent patients with herpes zoster. Journal of Infection 17: 57–63

Max M B, Kishore-Kumar R, Schafer S C, Meister B, Gracely R H, Smoller B, Dubner R 1991 Efficacy of desipramine in painful diabetic neuropathy: a placebo-controlled trial. Pain 45: 1–9

Max M B, Lynch S A, Muir J, Shoaf S E, Smoller B, Dubner R 1992 Effects of desipramine, amitriptyline, and fluoxetine on pain in diabetic neuropathy [see comments]. New England Journal Medicine 326: 1250–1256

Max M B, Schafer S C, Culnane M, Smoller B, Dubner R, Gracely R H 1988 Amitriptyline, but not lorazepam, relieves postherpetic neuralgia. Neurology 38: 1427–1432

McCormack K 1999 Fail-safe mechanisms that perpetuate neuropathic pain. Pain Clinical Updates 7: 1–4

McKay N N S, Woodhouse N J Y, Clarke A K 1977 Post-traumatic reflex sympathetic dystrophy syndrome (Sudeck's atrophy): effects of regional guanethidine infusion and salmon calcitonin. British Medical Journal 1: 1575–1576

McKendrick M W, McGill J I, Wood M J 1989 Lack of effect of acyclovir on postherpetic neuralgia. British Medical Journal 298: 431

McLachlan E M, Janig W, Devor M, Michaelis M 1993 Peripheral nerve injury triggers noradrenergic sprouting within dorsal root ganglia. Nature 363: 543–546

McQuay H, Carroll D, Jadad A R, Wiffen P, Moore A 1995 Anticonvulsant drugs for management of pain: a systematic review. British Medical Journal 311: 1047–1052

McQuay H J, Tramer M, Nye B A, Carroll D, Wiffen P J, Moore R A 1996 A systematic review of antidepressants in neuropathic pain. Pain 68: 217–227

Meaney J F, Eldridge P R, Dunn L T, Nixon T E, Whitehouse G H, Miles J B 1995 Demonstration of neurovascular compression in trigeminal neuralgia with magnetic resonance imaging. Comparison with surgical findings in 52 consecutive operative cases. Journal of Neurosurgery 83: 799–805

Merskey H, Bogduk N 1994 Classification of Chronic Pain: descriptions of chronic pain syndromes and definitions of pain terms. IASP Press, Seattle

Mitchell S W 1871 Phantom limbs. Lippincott's Magazine of Popular Literature and Science 8: 563–569

Monga T N, Jaksic T 1981 Acupuncture in phantom limb pain. Archives of Physical Medicine and Rehabilitation 62: 229–231

Muraoka M, Komiyama H, Hosoi M, Mine K, Kubo C 1996 Psychosomatic treatment of phantom limb pain with post-traumatic stress disorder: a case report. Pain 66: 385–388

Nathan P W, Wall P D 1974 Treatment of post-herpetic neuralgia by prolonged electric stimulation. British Medical Journal 3: 645–647

Nicolucci A, Carinci F, Graepel J G, Hohman T C, Ferris F, Lachin J M 1996 The efficacy of tolrestat in the treatment of diabetic peripheral neuropathy. A meta-analysis of individual patient data. Diabetes Care 19: 1091–1096

Nikolajsen L, Hansen P O, Jensen T S 1997b Oral ketamine therapy in the treatment of postamputation stump pain. Acta Anaesthesiologica Scandinavica 41: 427–429

Nikolajsen L, Ilkjaer S, Christensen J H, Kroner K, Jensen T S 1997a Randomised trial of epidural bupivacaine and morphine in prevention of stump and phantom pain in lower-limb amputation. Lancet 350: 1353–1357

Nurmikko T, Bowsher D 1990 Somatosensory findings in postherpetic neuralgia. Journal of Neurology, Neurosurgery and Psychiatry 53: 135–141

Oerlemans H M, Oostendorp R A, de Boo T, Goris R J 1999 Pain and reduced mobility in complex regional pain syndrome I: outcome of a prospective randomised controlled clinical trial of adjuvant physical therapy versus occupational therapy. Pain 83: 77–83

Omote K, Ohmori H, Kawamata M, Matsumoto M, Namiki A 1995 Intrathecal buprenorphine in the treatment of phantom limb pain. Anesthesia and Analgesia 80: 1030–1032

Pappagallo M, Campbell J N 1994 Chronic opioid therapy as alternative treatment for postherpetic neuralgia. Annals of Neurology 35: S54–56

Patterson J F 1988 Carbamazepine in the treatment of phantom limb pain. Southern Medical Journal 81: 1100–1102

Payne C 1984 Ultrasound for post-herpetic neuralgia. A study to investigate the results of treatment. Physiotherapy 70: 96–97

Payne R 1986 Neuropathic pain syndromes, with special reference to causalgia and reflex dystrophy. Clinical Journal of Pain 2: 59–73

Pfeifer M A, Ross D R, Schrage J P, Gelber D A, Schumer M P, Crain G M, Markwell S J, Jung S 1993 A highly successful and novel model for treatment of chronic painful diabetic peripheral neuropathy. Diabetes Care 16: 1103–1115

Pinzur M S, Garla P G, Pluth T, Vrbos L 1996 Continuous postoperative infusion of a regional anesthetic after an amputation of the lower extremity. A randomized clinical trial. Journal of Bone and Joint Surgery 78: 1501–1505

Pirart J, Lauvaux J P, Rey W 1978 Blood sugar and diabetic complications. New England Journal of Medicine 298: 1149

Portenoy R K, Foley K M, Inturrisi C E 1990 The nature of opioid responsiveness and its implications for neuropathic pain: new hypotheses derived from studies of opioid infusions. Pain 43: 273–286

Pucher I, Kickinger W, Frischenschlager O 1999 Coping with amputation and phantom limb pain. Journal of Psychosomatic Research 46: 379–383

Rains C, Bryson H M 1995 Topical capsaicin. A review of its pharmacological properties and therapeutic potential in post-herpetic neuralgia, diabetic neuropathy and osteoarthritis. Drugs and Aging 7: 317–328

Raja S N, Treede R D, Davis K D, Campbell J N 1991 Systemic alpha-adrenergic blockade with phentolamine: a diagnostic test for sympathetically maintained pain. Anesthesiology 74: 691–698

Ramamurthy S, Hoffman J 1995 Intravenous regional guanethidine in the treatment of reflex sympathetic dystrophy/causalgia: a randomized, double-blind study. Guanethidine Study Group. Anesthesia and Analgesia 81: 718–723

Rayner H C, Atkins R C, Westerman R A 1989 Relief of local stump pain by capsaicin cream. Lancet 2: 1276–1277

Rocco A G, Kaul A F, Reisman R M, Gallo J P, Lief P A 1989 A comparison of regional intravenous guanethidine and reserpine in reflex sympathetic dystrophy. A controlled, randomized, double-blind crossover study. Clinical Journal of Pain 5: 205–209

Rowbotham M, Harden N, Stacey B, Bernstein P, Magnus-Miller L 1998 Gabapentin for the treatment of postherpetic neuralgia: a randomized controlled trial. Journal of the American Medical Association 280: 1837–1842

Rowbotham M C, Fields H L 1989 Topical lidocaine reduces pain in post-herpetic neuralgia. Pain 38: 297–301

Rowbotham M C, Fields H L 1996 The relationship of pain, allodynia and thermal sensation in post-herpetic neuralgia. Brain 119: 347–354

Rowbotham M C, Petersen K L, Fields H L 1999 Is postherpetic neuralgia more than one disorder? IASP Newsletter 3–7

Rowbotham M C, Reisner-Keller L A, Fields H L 1991 Both intravenous lidocaine and morphine reduce the pain of postherpetic neuralgia. Neurology 41: 1024–1028

Saitoh Y, Shibata M, Hirano S, Hirata M, Mashimo T, Yoshimine T 2000 Motor cortex stimulation for central and peripheral deafferentation pain. Report of eight cases. Journal of Neurosurgery 92: 150–155

Santiago J V 1993 Lessons from the Diabetes Control and Complications Trial. Diabetes 42: 1549–1554

Schott G D 1998 Interrupting the sympathetic outflow in causalgia and reflex sympathetic dystrophy. British Medical Journal 316: 792–793

Sherman R A 1980 Published treatments of phantom limb pain. American Journal Physical Medicine 59: 232–244

Sherman R A, Sherman C J 1983 Prevalence and characteristics of chronic phantom limb pain among American veterans. Results of a trial survey. American Journal Physical Medicine 62: 227–238

Sidebottom A, Maxwell S 1995 The medical and surgical management of trigeminal neuralgia. Journal of Clinical Pharmacy and Therapeutics 20: 31–35

Siegel E F 1979 Control of phantom limb pain by hypnosis. American Journal of Clinical Hypnosis 21: 285–286

Sima A A, Greene D A 1995 Diabetic neuropathy in the elderly. Drugs and Aging 6: 125–135

Sindrup S H, Gram L F, Brosen K, Eshoj O, Mogensen E F 1990 The selective serotonin reuptake inhibitor paroxetine is effective in the treatment of diabetic neuropathy symptoms. Pain 42: 135–144

Sindrup S H, Jensen T S 1999 Efficacy of pharmacological treatments of neuropathic pain: an update and effect related to mechanism of drug action. Pain 83: 389–400

Somers D L, Somers M F 1999 Treatment of neuropathic pain in a patient with diabetic neuropathy using transcutaneous electrical nerve stimulation applied to the skin of the lumbar region. Physical Therapy 79: 767–775

Stracke H, Meyer U E, Schumacher H E, Federlin K 1992 Mexiletine in the treatment of diabetic neuropathy. Diabetes Care 15: 1550–1555

Sweet W H 1988 Percutaneous methods for the treatment of trigeminal neuralgia and other faciocephalic pain; comparison with microvascular decompression. Seminars in Neurology 8: 272–279

Taha J M, Tew J M, Jr 1996 Comparison of surgical treatments for trigeminal neuralgia: reevaluation of radiofrequency rhizotomy. Neurosurgery 38: 865–871

Tash R R, Sze G, Leslie D R 1989 Trigeminal neuralgia: MR imaging features. Radiology 172: 767–770

Taylor J C, Brauer S, Espir M L 1981 Long-term treatment of trigeminal neuralgia with carbamazepine. Postgraduate Medicine Journal 57: 16–18

Tew J M, van Loveren H 1985 Surgical treatment for trigeminal neuralgia. American Family Physician 31: 143–150

Tomson T, Bertilsson L 1984 Potent therapeutic effect of carbamazepine-10,11-epoxide in trigeminal neuralgia. Archives Neurology 41: 598–601

Tomson T, Tybring G, Bertilsson L, Ekbom K, Rane A 1980 Carbamazepine therapy in trigeminal neuralgia: clinical effects in relation to plasma concentration. Archives Neurology 37: 699–703

Umino M, Ohwatari T, Shimoyama K, Nagao M 1993 Long-term observation of the relation between pain intensity and serum carbamazepine concentration in elderly patients with trigeminal neuralgia. Journal of Oral and Maxillofacial Surgery 51: 1338–1344

Urban B J, France R D, Steinberger E K, Scott D L, Maltbie A A 1986 Long-term use of narcotic/antidepressant medication in the management of phantom limb pain. Pain 24: 191–196

Valentin N 1996 Reflex sympathetic dystrophy treated with guanethidine. Time for a change of name and strategy. Acta Anaesthesiologica Scandinavica 40: 1171–1172

van der Laan L, Goris R J 1997 Reflex sympathetic dystrophy. An exaggerated regional inflammatory response? Hand Clinics 13: 373–385

van Loveren H, Twe J M, Keller J T, Nurre M A 1982 A 10-year experience in the treatment of trigeminal neuralgia. Journal of Neurosurgery 57: 757–764

Veldmand P H, Reynen H M, Arntz I E, Goris R J 1993 Signs and symptoms of RSD: prospective study of 829 patients. Lancet 342: 1012–1016

Verdugo R J, Campero M, Ochoa J L 1994 Phentolamine sympathetic block in painful polyneuropathies. II. Further questioning of the concept of 'sympathetically maintained pain'. Neurology 44: 1010–1014

Verdugo R J, Ochoa J L 1994 'Sympathetically maintained pain' I. Phentolamine block questions the concept. Neurology 44: 1003–1010

Vinik A I 1999 Diabetic neuropathy: pathogenesis and therapy. American Journal of Medicine 107: 17S–26S

Wagstaff A J, Faulds D, Goa K L 1994 Aciclovir. A reappraisal of its antiviral activity, pharmacokinetic properties and therapeutic efficacy. Drugs 47: 153–205

Wall G C, Heyneman C A 1999 Calcitonin in phantom limb pain. Annals of Pharmacotherapy 33: 499–501

Wall P D, Devor M 1983 Sensory afferent impulses originate from dorsal root ganglia as well as from the periphery in normal and nerve injured rats. Pain 17: 321–339

Wall P D, Gutnick M 1974 Properties of afferent nerve impulses originating from a neuroma. Nature 248: 740–743

Watson C P, Babul N 1998 Efficacy of oxycodone in neuropathic pain: a randomized trial in postherpetic neuralgia. Neurology 50: 1837–1841

Watson C P, Chipman M, Reed K, Evans R J, Birkett N 1992 Amitriptyline versus maprotiline in postherpetic

neuralgia: a randomized, double-blind, crossover trial. Pain 48: 29–36

Watson C P, Deck J H, Morshead C, Van der Kooy D, Evans R J 1991 Post-herpetic neuralgia: further post-mortem studies of cases with and without pain. Pain 44: 105–117

Watson C P, Evans R J 1985 A comparative trial of amitriptyline and zimelidine in post-herpetic neuralgia. Pain 23: 387–394

Watson C P, Evans R J, Reed K, Merskey H, Goldsmith L, Warsh J 1982 Amitriptyline versus placebo in postherpetic neuralgia. Neurology 32: 671–673

Watson C P, Evans R J, Watt V R 1988a Post-herpetic neuralgia and topical capsaicin. Pain 33: 333–340

Watson C P, Evans R J, Watt V R, Birkett N 1988b Post-herpetic neuralgia: 208 cases. Pain 35: 289–297

Watson C P, Vernich L, Chipman M, Reed K 1998 Nortriptyline versus amitriptyline in postherpetic neuralgia: a randomized trial. Neurology, 51: 1166–1171

Weintraub M, Golik A, Rubio A 1990 Capsaicin for treatment of post-traumatic amputation stump pain [letter]. Lancet 336: 1003–1004

Weiss T, Miltner W H, Adler T, Bruckner L, Taub E 1999 Decrease in phantom limb pain associated with prosthesis-induced increased use of an amputation stump in humans. Neuroscience Letters 272: 131–134

Wilder R T, Berde C B, Wolohan M, Vieyra M A, Masek B J, Micheli L J 1992 Reflex sympathetic dystrophy in children. Clinical characteristics and follow-up of seventy patients. Journal of Bone and Joint Surgery (Am) 74: 910–909

Winnem M F, Amundsen T 1982 Treatment of phantom limb pain with TENS. Pain 12: 299–300

Wong G Y, Wilson P R 1997 Classification of complex regional pain syndromes. New concepts. Hand Clinics 13: 319–325

Woolf C J, Costigan M 1999 Transcriptional and posttranslational plasticity and the generation of inflammatory pain. Proceedings of the National Academy of Sciences of the USA 96: 7723–7730

Woolf C J, Mannion R J 1999 Neuropathic pain: aetiology, symptoms, mechanisms, and management. Lancet 353: 1959–1964

Woolf C J, Shortland P, Coggeshall R E 1992 Peripheral nerve injury triggers central sprouting of myelinated afferents. Nature 355: 75–78

Xing G 1998 Acupuncture treatment of phantom limb pain – a report of 9 cases. Journal of Traditional Chinese Medicine 18: 199–201

Yang T T, Gallen C, Schwartz B, Bloom F E, Ramachandran V S, Cobb S 1994 Sensory maps in the human brain. Nature 368: 592–593

Zakrzewska J M, Chaudhry Z, Nurmikko T J, Patton D W, Mullens E L 1997 Lamotrigine (lamictal) in refractory trigeminal neuralgia: results from a double-blind placebo controlled crossover trial. Pain 73: 223–230

Zhang W Y, Li Wan Po A 1994 The effectiveness of topically applied capsaicin. A metanalysis. European Journal of Clinical Pharmacology 46: 517–522

Zuurmond W W, Langendijk P N, Bezemer P D, Brink H E, de Lange J J, and van Loenen A C 1996 Treatment of acute reflex sympathetic dystrophy with DMSO 50% in a fatty cream. Acta Anaesthesiologica Scandinavica 40: 364–367

19

Pain in the acute care setting

Stephan A. Schug
Deborah S. B. Watson

OVERVIEW

Acute pain is seen in patients in a multitude of clinical situations – in the postoperative and post-trauma setting, following burns, in acute medical diseases (e.g. pancreatitis, myocardial infarction) and as obstetric pain. Postoperative pain is the most common form of acute pain (and of major relevance for therapists), and the focus of this chapter will be directed towards management of patients with postoperative pain.

This chapter focuses on the importance of effective management of acute pain. It incorporates the most important pharmacological and non-pharmacological modalities of analgesia in the treatment of acute pain. Reference will be made to comparisons of efficacy, benefits and side-effects of these modalities. Some of the newer techniques used have accumulated substantial evidence demonstrating an improvement not only in quality of analgesia and patient satisfaction, but also in short- and long-term morbidity, and potentially, even mortality.

However, despite the theoretical availability of a wide range of appropriate agents and techniques (see Box 19.1), the cause of poor acute pain management is often the insufficient, inappropriate or unsupervised

---

Box 19.1 Key terms defined

PCA (patient-controlled analgesia) – A technique using a programmable infusion device that can be activated by the patient to deliver small bolus doses of iv morphine on demand.
Pre-emptive analgesia – Any method of providing analgesia prior to surgical trauma with the goal of preventing pain.
Epidural analgesia – Drugs administered into the epidural space outside the spinal meninges.
Intrathecal analgesia – Drugs administered into the intrathecal space inside the meninges.

application of such agents and techniques. Therefore the chapter would be incomplete without a discussion of appropriate organizational structures to provide acute pain relief, i.e. the concept and the role of the Acute Pain Service.

There is widespread agreement in the literature on the inadequacy of acute pain management. On the other hand, there is also a wide body of evidence which suggests that relief of acute pain is not only an integral part of humane healthcare, but can also have profound effects on patient outcomes.

Only over the last decade has a considerable amount of scientific and clinical effort been put into providing the patient in acute pain with the best quality analgesia, and at the same time ensuring safety from potentially life-threatening adverse events for each modality of analgesia. In this chapter, the principles of acute pain management will be outlined.

Given that pharmacological management is a mainstay of acute pain management, emphasis will be given in this chapter to the pharmacological methods of pain relief.

Learning objectives

On completion of this chapter, students will:

1. Be able to describe the principles of acute pain management.
2. Be able to identify conditions where acute pain management is required.
3. Describe the place of systemic opioids in acute pain management.
4. Understand the place of systemic non-opioid analgesics and other systemic agents.
5. Be aware of the place of epidural and intrathecal analgesia.
6. Be able to identify non-pharmacological methods for acute pain management.

PRINCIPLES OF ACUTE PAIN MANAGEMENT

Postoperatively, up to 75% of patients experience moderate to severe pain (Oden 1989). 77% of adults believe that postoperative pain is to be expected and 60% regard it as their primary fear before surgery (Warfield & Kahn 1990).

Psychological factors, e.g. expectation of pain, fear of death and associated sleep deprivation, influence postoperative pain control, and therefore attention must be given to individual patient differences, which may lead to an improved outcome.

Traditionally, postoperative pain has been managed using fixed doses of intramuscularly (im) administered opioids on an as-needed basis. This treatment approach has lead to unrelieved pain in more than 50% of postoperative patients (Austin et al 1980, Oden 1989). The major problem with this approach is explained by the huge interindividual variation in dose requirements, which can vary more than 10-fold for patients of similar age and weight having the same operation. Furthermore, opioid concentrations following im bolus doses exhibit a pronounced peak and trough pattern with periods of inadequate analgesia, but also the associated risk of delayed overdose.

A more appropriate approach to acute pain should therefore consider a much wider array of techniques for its management. These include the following pharmacological options:

- Systemic opioids (intravenous (iv), subcutaneous (sc), im, and oral (po) on a regular and/or 'as required' basis, or via patient-controlled analgesia (PCA)
- Non-opioid analgesics (paracetamol acetaminophen), non-steroidal anti-inflammatory drugs-(NSAIDs)
- Other systemic agents that have uses in particular settings, such as nitrous oxide (Entonox), adrenergic drugs, tricyclic antidepressants and anticonvulsants
- Neuraxial analgesia (epidural or intrathecal administration of opioid and/or local anaesthetic drugs)
- Intermittent or continuous peripheral neural blockade with local anaesthetic drugs.

Besides these, there are many non-pharmacological options, which are often under-utilized despite their simplicity and effectiveness:

- Explanation, reassurance and discussion of analgesic options
- Cognitive–behavioural interventions such as relaxation, distraction and imagery, which can be taught preoperatively
- Various physical interventions such as splints, massage, application of heat or cold and transcutaneous electrical nerve stimulation (TENS).

The majority of this chapter focuses on the pharmacological options, discussing the efficacy, benefits, side-effect profiles and combination therapy with other analgesic agents.

PHARMACOLOGICAL MODALITIES
Systemic opioids

Systemic opioids are the treatment of choice in the management of moderate to severe acute pain. They include the 'gold-standard' morphine, as well as drugs such as pethidine, fentanyl, codeine and methadone. They all bind to opioid receptors within and outside the central nervous system (CNS), with the μ-receptor being the most important because of morphine's affinity for it.

While this receptor activation explains the analgesic effect of opioids, it also explains most of the adverse effects of these agents, intrinsically linked to their analgesic effect. The most common side-effects are nausea and vomiting, sedation, pruritus, slowing of gastrointestinal function (constipation), urinary retention and sometimes (surprisingly) dysphoria (see Chapter 16 for more details).

The most serious, but rare, complication of opioid usage is respiratory depression and subsequent hypoxia, which can be potentially life-threatening or even fatal (Schug et al 1992).

Systemic opioids can be given by a wide variety of different routes (see Chapter 16). The decision on which route to use is dependent on the individual situation of the patient, the acuteness of the pain, and the infrastructure of the hospital. The traditional routes of opioid administration were po, sc and im, however, there is an increasing trend towards iv administration, in particular following opioid protocols or via PCA devices.

Other routes of administration, e.g. by inhalation or transdermally, are under investigation.

Oral opioids

Oral opioids are an option only after return of gastric motility, i.e. when the patient is able to tolerate fluids freely. Evidence suggests that oral opioids are as effective as parenteral opioids in appropriate doses, and should be used as soon as oral medication is tolerated in such a scenario, this is the route of choice for acute pain management.

Codeine is used widely, however it might not be the drug of choice, as its efficacy is limited and some patients (ca. 10%) lack the enzyme which is needed to generate its active metabolite, morphine.

Morphine itself is a preferable option, initially used in immediate (ca. 20 minutes to onset) and short-acting preparations such as morphine elixir or immediate-release tablets. Once an ongoing need for oral morphine is established, in particular in the post-operative and more commonly the post-trauma rehabilitation period, sustained-release formulations are useful to provide long-term analgesia.

An alternative currently under investigation is the agent tramadol, a centrally acting analgesic with a mixed mechanism of action (opioid, noradrenergic, serotinergic). This mechanism of action explains its different side-effect profile from classic opioids, in particular with regard to sedation, constipation and respiratory depression (Houmes et al 1992, Vickers et al 1992).

Intramuscular opioids

As mentioned above, intramuscular opioids have, until recently, been the mainstay of postoperative pain management using opioids. Traditionally, standard doses (commonly '10 mg for everyone') were administered by intermittent im injections, usually no more frequently than every 4 hours, hence the infamous prescription: '10 mg morphine im, prn 4-hourly'. Such a 'one-dose-fits-all' approach leads to some patients being left in extreme pain and others at risk of suffering from major side-effects such as respiratory depression. The incidence of respiratory depression using this route is ~0.9% (Miller & Greenblatt 1976).

In addition, intramuscular injections are painful, disliked by patients, and carry the risk of tissue damage (e.g. nerves) and infection (abscesses).

Finally, absorption from an intramuscular injection site is slow, unpredictable and delayed by physical factors such as hypothermia, hypovolaemia and immobility, commonly encountered in the early postoperative period.

Therefore, the current recommendation and standard practice is to avoid this route if at all possible. If for organizational, political or training (rather, lack of training) reasons, im injections are the only parenteral route of administration permitted or (inappropriately) deemed safe in a certain environment, then the dose used should be based on age and medical condition, and the administration interval should be shortened to at least 2-hourly prn, to increase flexibility (Macintyre & Ready 1996).

Subcutaneous opioids

Opioids can be given intermittently or as a low-volume continuous infusion via the subcutaneous route. The absorption profile is similar to that of im administration (Semple et al 1997), and both routes have similar analgesic and side-effect profiles. However, patients prefer the sc route, in particular if used via an indwelling sc cannula, for obvious reasons (Cooper 1996).

The approach has been shown to be beneficial as a continuous infusion (volumes < 1–2 ml hr^{-1}) in severe cancer pain, and in postoperative patients in whom iv access is not (or not easily) available.

Morphine and hydromorphone are used preferentially as they are low irritants to the subcutaneous tissue. In patients with an indwelling iv line (i.e. most early postoperative patients), there are no advantages, but some disadvantages (delayed onset of analgesia, second access) of the sc route in comparison to the iv route.

Intravenous opioids

Opioids can be given as boluses (0.5–4 mg every 5 minutes as directed by a formal iv protocol), as a continuous infusion or via PCA devices by the iv route. The iv route is the route of choice following major surgery: However, there is a risk of respiratory depression with inappropriate dosing, and therefore close monitoring and safety precautions are required.

Intermittent iv boluses They provide a rapid, predictable and observable response compared to other parenteral routes. This is the rationale behind use of iv PCA. The iv route is particularly useful in the following situations:

- To obtain initial and rapid pain relief such as in the immediate postoperative period and in acute trauma
- In patients who are hypovolaemic and/or hypotensive and will absorb im/sc opioids in a delayed and unpredictable fashion
- To treat so called 'incident pain' caused by events such as dressing changes, mobilization and physiotherapy.

Intermittent boluses are also an ideal way to titrate pain relief in the recovery room, and bridge times of severe pain, until medical review and/or more appropriate analgesic methods become accessible. Most commonly, nurse-administered bolus doses, prescribed according to a protocol or algorithm are used. Such protocols specify (or permit some flexibility with regard to) bolus size, assessments and 'lock-out' time (Schug 1999).

Continuous iv infusion avoids the 'peaks and troughs' in blood concentrations associated with intermittent administration, but it has proven difficult to 'predict' the required individual blood concentration for optimal analgesia. A continuous infusion requires reliable infusion devices and frequent assessment and monitoring by staff, who are trained and authorized to adjust the infusion rate and give bolus doses.

To provide adequate analgesic blood concentrations can take up to 20 hours (five half-lives). Consequently, if analgesia is inadequate, a bolus is given as well as the rate being increased.

The risk of respiratory depression using a continuous morphine infusion (up to 1.65%) is the highest of all parenteral routes. This needs to be considered carefully, as fatal outcomes are reported, in particular in sleeping or sedated patients (Schug & Torrie 1993).

Patient controlled analgesia (PCA) was introduced to overcome the variability in individual morphine dose requirements and the problems associated with insufficient analgesia and potentially serious adverse outcomes.

A PCA device is a sophisticated, programmable infusion device that can be activated by the patient to self-administer small bolus doses of iv morphine on demand, separated by a lock-out period, during which the device does not respond to further activation. As such, the PCA concept overcomes the interindividual variation in opioid requirements, and allows the patient to adjust the level of analgesia to their own desired level of comfort, balanced to an individually acceptable severity of side-effects.

It has been demonstrated that a bolus dose of 1 mg morphine with a 5-minute lock-out period is ideal for most patients. Other programmes are associated with either inadequate analgesia or sedation and increased respiratory compromise (Owen et al 1989a). However, some patients might need different programmes, depending on age, comorbidity, pain intensity and previous opioid exposure, therefore regular review by experienced personnel of all patients using PCA devices is mandatory for a good outcome.

Following surgery the average patient will require PCA for 2–4 days. Consumption of drug is maximal within the first 24 hours and thereafter rapidly declines. Use after abdominal surgery tends to be increased and relatively prolonged (Sidebotham et al 1997). This reflects the major physiological insult and the additional pain associated with mobilization and physiotherapy. Women use 20–30% less morphine than men (Sidebotham et al 1997), and at 80 years of age, morphine consumption drops to less than 30% of that at 30 years. However, there is little correlation between weight and consumption (Burns et al 1989).

Using a PCA technique, patients control their own analgesia. It can be used via the sc route, but the more common route is iv. The technique provides good, steady analgesia and is popular with patients. It requires special infusion pumps and staff education. In addition, patients require instructions preoperatively to be able to understand the principles underlying the PCA technique and how/when to activate it.

Although the safest way of administering systemic opioids, there still remains a small risk of respiratory depression (incidence in the range of 0.2%) (Baird & Schug 1996). This risk is much smaller than that associated with continuous iv infusion or intermittent im injection. This advantage with regard to safety is due to the fact that acute pain causes stimulation of respiratory centres in the brain and consequently respiratory depression does not occur simultaneously with acute pain. As patients use the PCA device by titrating opioids to effect, there is less likelihood of respiratory depression; even more so as the sedated patient will stop using the device. In the rare cases of respiratory depression, the causes are commonly:

- Operator error (e.g. inappropriate prescription, incorrect programming of PCA device, incorrect dilution of medication)
- Patient-related error (e.g. relatives using PCA button instead of the patient)
- Equipment failure (e.g. cracked syringes with gravity siphoning of opioid solution (rare)).

Other side-effects associated with PCA administration of opioids are nausea and vomiting in 35% of cases (Quinn et al 1994), occurring mainly on the first postoperative day, and sedation in 18% and confusion in 12% of cases (Schug & Fry 1994). These problems occur with similar incidence to other methods of opioid administration and are not reduced by the PCA approach.

If a continuous low-dose iv infusion is given together with a PCA, this has been shown to increase the risk of side-effects (Notcutt & Morgan 1990, Schug & Torrie 1993), without significantly improving analgesia (Owen et al 1989b, Smythe et al 1996). The incidence of respiratory depression is 5–8 times higher than PCA alone, as the inherent safety concept of PCA is violated. Hence, the only patients that should be prescribed a background opioid infusion are those already receiving opioids as they already have some degree of opioid tolerance and increased requirements (e.g. chronic pain, recreational abuse, methadone substitution) (Hansen et al 1991).

All routes of opioid administration, especially parenteral routes, need to be carefully monitored for side-effects, notably respiratory depression. Specific protocols are written for each route of administration

so that patients receive optimal analgesia while always being safeguarded against respiratory depression, and monitored for other side-effects of opioids. Safe and appropriate use of a PCA requires frequent and informed monitoring by nurses who have undergone relevant education and accreditation in the management of these devices. Standard orders and drug dilutions are suggested to maximize the effectiveness of the PCA and minimize complications (Schug & Haridas 1993).

The risk of opioid addiction is often cited as a reason for provision of inadequate analgesia. It has been demonstrated that addiction to opioids is rare when used in the treatment of acute pain. Patients choose not to fully relieve their pain, despite free access to drugs, and demands tend to be conservative with patients choosing to remain alert and in a small amount of discomfort (Keeri-Szanto 1979, Tamsen et al 1982). There is at present no evidence that opioid use in the management of acute pain leads to opioid dependence or addiction (Chapman & Hill 1989, Schug & Torrie 1993).

Summary Opioids delivered via a PCA device provide greater analgesic efficacy, higher patient satisfaction and reduced risk of respiratory compromise compared to conventional routes of administration (McArdle 1987). PCA is preferred over other parenteral routes by patients, probably because it provides them with a degree of control over their pain management (Egan & Ready 1994). However, although the incidence of respiratory depression is lower using PCA there is no reduction in the incidence of other side-effects and no proven effect on outcome from surgery or shortening of hospital stay (Ballantyne et al 1993).

PCA, although currently the optimal parenteral method of opioid administration, is not without its problems, notably side-effects, which include nausea and vomiting, sedation, hypoxaemia and delayed recovery of bowel function. It provides incomplete analgesia at rest and on movement. About 40% of patients using a PCA have a pain score > 3/10 at rest, 1 day postoperatively. The occurrence of unpleasant side-effects by increased opioid usage may be responsible for some of this inadequate analgesia, which prevents 20% of patients from complying with physiotherapy at 1 day postoperatively (Schug & Fry 1994, Sidebotham et al 1997).

To improve pain relief by PCA and to reduce these side-effects, other drugs can be used in conjunction with opioids. These include anti-emetics, nonsteroidal anti-inflammatory drugs, paracetamol, clonidine or ketamine.

Systemic non-opioid analgesics

Paracetamol/acetaminophen

Paracetamol/acetaminophen has analgesic and anti-pyretic effects, but is not anti-inflammatory (See Chapter 16). It has been shown to be extremely useful on its own in cases of mild to moderate pain. For the elderly population, where the use of non-steroidal anti-inflammatory drugs carries a high risk of adverse effects, paracetamol/acetaminophen and/or low-dose opioid, is probably safer for non-inflammatory conditions, and low-dose steroid may be more appropriate for inflammatory conditions (Roth 1989).

Paracetamol/acetaminophen co-administration with opioids via PCA has been shown to reduce pain intensity and the period of time that a PCA device is needed postoperatively, and also to increase patient satisfaction with analgesic control (Schug et al 1998). Regular intake of 1 g 4-hourly is strongly recommended in this setting.

Non-steroidal anti-inflammatory drugs (NSAIDs)

NSAIDs are effective in the management of mild to moderate acute pain, but not powerful enough to be used alone for severe pain. Clinical trials have confirmed their usefulness as components of multimodal analgesia (Cepeda et al 1995, Pavy et al 1995, Power et al 1990).

These drugs reduce the levels of inflammatory mediators generated at the site of tissue injury and it has been suggested that they are more effective if commenced preoperatively, thus having a pre-emptive role when used as a sole analgesic agent. This is the subject of current investigations, as clinical studies to date have not yet justified their pre-emptive use (Buggy et al 1994, Espinet et al 1996).

Some examples of NSAIDs that are useful in the treatment of postoperative pain are indometacin, tenoxicam and ketorolac, the latter two also being available for parenteral administration.

When given as an adjunct to opioids there is clear evidence that they have a significant opioid dose-sparing effect of 15–60%. Some studies demonstrate improved pain relief when these drugs are given together, compared to either class alone (Pavy et al 1995, Power et al 1994), in addition to a reduction in opioid side-effects (Liu et al 1995).

However, although they do not cause sedation or respiratory depression, there are other extremely important, potentially serious side-effects, with a higher incidence in the elderly, which must be considered before prescribing these drugs.

Renal complications Renal prostaglandins are important in maintaining renal function in the perioperative period and NSAIDs disrupt this balance at the time of surgery (Power et al 1992). In particular, ketorolac has been associated with cases of unexplained renal dysfunction (Smith et al 1993).

Factors that are likely to contribute to the development of renal dysfunction are age (older patients have a higher incidence of pre-existing limitation of renal function), concomitant use of nephrotoxic antibiotics (gentamicin), poor perioperative fluid management, and raised intra-abdominal pressure (as at laparoscopy).

Effects on haemostasis NSAIDs inhibit platelet function by preventing the production of thromboxanes, and thus impair haemostasis. For most patients this does not produce a clinical bleeding problem, even though the bleeding time (a test to assess platelet function) is prolonged (Power et al 1990). Indeed, this effect may be of some benefit if thromboembolic prophylaxis is desired (Anonymous 1994). However, for patients with pre-existing clotting or platelet disorders, and/or concomitant use of anticoagulation, this effect can be problematic.

Effects on bone and wound healing Prostaglandins are required for adequate healing and theoretically this is delayed if NSAIDs are used.

Gastrointestinal effects There is an increased risk of bleeding from a known peptic ulcer if NSAIDs are used (Strom et al 1996).

Aspirin-induced asthma This can occur in susceptible individuals (Power 1993), e.g. development of wheezing with any NSAID.

Due to these potential side-effects, NSAIDs should only be used with caution and following appropriate guidelines. Research is currently underway to develop NSAIDs that specifically have an anti-inflammatory and analgesic role with reduced life-threatening side-effects. Such so called COX-2 inhibitors have just reached the market in form of celecoxib and rofecoxib (Malmstrom et al 1999). At least the gastrointestinal rate of side-effects for these novel drugs is identical to placebo, and significantly better than those of older NSAIDs (for details see Chapter 16).

Other systemic agents

Entonox

Entonox is a mixture of 50% oxygen and 50% nitrous oxide. It provides a safe way to administer the analgesic inhalational anaesthetic nitrous oxide in a sub-anaesthetic concentration. The agent is usually given by self-administration via a face-mask or mouth-piece. Self-administration enhances safety, as the patient will stop usage in the unlikely case of loss of consciousness. Entonox is particularly useful as a safe short-term analgesic with a rapid onset of action. Therefore it is commonly used for painful procedures such as dressing changes or passive mobilization (Baskett 1972, Parbrook 1972).

Clonidine

Clonidine is an alpha-2 receptor agonist and thus potentiates the descending inhibitory pathways within the spinal cord that act on pain transmission at the dorsal horn. It reduces opioid requirement and is therefore potentially useful as an adjunct to a PCA (Park et al 1996). It also reduces the incidence of opioid-induced nausea and vomiting and does not cause respiratory depression per se. Sedation and hypotension can be problems with its use. Its administration in neuraxial analgesia techniques (Paech et al 1997) and peripheral nerve blocks (Singelyn et al 1996) is also useful.

Ketamine

Ketamine is an antagonist at the N-methyl-D-aspartate (NMDA) receptor within the central nervous system. This receptor is involved with the production of 'wind-up' during excitation of the dorsal horn with repetitive pain impulses. Ketamine has been shown to reduce opioid consumption when given preoperatively (Roytblat et al 1993) and improve pain control, but only in certain patients, probably those who already have an element of central sensitization occurring, which is indicated clinically by hyperalgesia and allodynia. It has been shown to be particularly useful in the management of neuropathic pain and acute pain in patients with preceding long-standing chronic pain problems (Gehling & Tryba 1998).

Tricyclic antidepressants and membrane stabilizers

Tricyclic antidepressants and membrane stabilizers are commonly used in chronic pain management (where their role is discussed more extensively – see Chapters 16 and 18). However, they play a minor role in the management of acute and subacute neuropathic pain, i.e. sciatica, pain caused by nerve or spinal-cord injury and stroke.

A typical 'emergency' medication here is the use of intravenous lignocaine in anti-arrhythmic doses, followed by continuous infusion, if needed. This agent can provide immediate and convincing pain relief, in particular in situations unresponsive to aggressive opioid medication (Boas et al 1982). Similarly clonazepam, an anticonvulsant, can be useful in such situations (Swerdlow & Cundill 1981).

Neuraxial analgesia

The two types of neuraxial analgesia used in acute care are:

- Epidural (extradural) analgesia – drugs are administered into the epidural space
- Intrathecal analgesia – drugs are administered into the intrathecal space.

The epidural space lies outside the spinal meninges (dura mater) and the intrathecal space lies inside the meninges, which hold the cerebrospinal fluid (CSF). The spinal nerve roots traverse both spaces. As they pass through the epidural space, they are surrounded by a cuff of dura. The neuraxial route provides access to nerve roots supplying the thorax, abdomen, pelvic organs, perineum and lower limbs. Drugs administered by this route can affect pain transmission in the dorsal horn of the spinal cord, the somatic afferent (sensory) and efferent (motor) nerve roots, and the sympathetic efferent nerves.

Intrathecal analgesia

Intrathecal analgesia is usually given preoperatively as a 'single-shot' technique which involves insertion of a spinal needle through a lumbar intervertebral space, gentle advancement of the needle until CSF back-flow occurs through the needle, and subsequent injection of local anaesthetic with or without opioid. This method provides good surgical anaesthesia for up to 4 hours, but a long-acting opioid can provide ongoing postoperative analgesia for 12–24 hours and more (Boezaart et al 1999).

The technique is often used for urological and orthopaedic operations, as it covers primarily the pelvis and the lower limbs. The use of continuous intrathecal techniques is an option, primarily in cancer pain management, and only in an experimental state for provision of postoperative analgesia.

Epidural analgesia

If analgesia is required for a prolonged period postoperatively, notably following upper abdominal surgery or thoracic surgery, it is better to have a continuous infusion as opposed to a 'single-shot'. Under these circumstances, epidural analgesia is commonly employed. A needle is inserted into the epidural space, which is usually identified by a 'loss-of-resistance' technique, and a catheter is fed into the space allowing longer-term infusion or repeated bolus doses of analgesic agents.

Drugs that are commonly given by the spinal route are:

- Local anaesthetics, e.g. bupivacaine, lignocaine, ropivacaine
- Opioids, e.g. morphine, fentanyl, pethidine, diamorphine.

Local anaesthetics

Local anaesthetics block axonal conduction and hence prevent transmission of nociceptive (pain) impulses into the dorsal horn of the spinal cord (see Chapter 16). Dependent on which level is selected for the insertion of the epidural catheter (dermatomal level), they preferentially block those dermatomes closer to the site of catheter insertion. Hence, lumbosacral epidural catheters are inserted for lower limb surgery, low-thoracic epidurals for lower abdominal surgery and mid-thoracic for upper abdominal surgery. Local anaesthetic drugs are the only drugs to provide good analgesia for mobilization and coughing, and also offer benefits as a result of sympathetic blockade.

As local anaesthetic agents block axonal conduction in all nerves to some extent, most of their side-effects (see Chapter 16), when used spinally, are basically an extension of this property:

- Inadvertent overdose or injection into an epidural vessel which can lead to local anaesthetic toxicity, the most serious consequences being central nervous system toxicity (convulsions and coma) and cardiovascular toxicity (fatal arrhythmias)
- Urinary retention
- 'Total spinal anaesthesia' as a result of an excess of local anaesthetic being inadvertently administered directly into the CSF, i.e. intrathecally, rather than into the epidural space. This blocks the sympathetic outflow from the spinal cord and constitutes an emergency situation – the patient rapidly develops total body paralysis and is unable to breath, followed by cardiovascular collapse, loss of consciousness and, if untreated, death
- Variable haemodynamic effects of sympathetic blockade, commonly resulting in hypotension as a result of vasodilatation. This is often requires

treatment with vasoconstrictors and/or increased volumes of intravenous fluid
- Motor blockade, which can impair mobilization, and, in combination with sensory blockade, may contribute to the development of pressure areas, if nursing care is inadequate.

Opioids

Opioids administered neuraxially block opioid receptors in the dorsal horn of the spinal cord. Lower doses than those needed for systemic analgesia are required for provision of neuraxial analgesia and as a result opioid side-effects may be reduced. Epidural opioids can cause analgesia by:

- Diffusion through the dural membrane of the spinal root cuffs into the CSF and then to the opioid receptors in the dorsal horn and to the brain (cephalad spread)
- Direct transfer from the epidural space to the spinal cord via spinal arteries (Bernards 1993)
- Vascular uptake into the bloodstream, thus providing systemic analgesia.

If morphine or other hydrophilic (water-soluble) opioids are used, they stay in the CSF for a longer period of time and are more commonly associated with cephalad migration. The advantage of a single dose providing analgesia for 12–24 hours are traded off by the potential to cause delayed respiratory depression 12–24 hours after the dose is administered as a result of cephalad migration to the respiratory centres in the brain.

Fentanyl and other lipophilic (fat-soluble) opioids conversely do not stay in the CSF as long, and consequently provide a shorter duration of analgesia and less risk of respiratory depression. As such, epidural fentanyl can and should be given as an infusion.

Other side-effects of neuraxial opioids, particularly morphine, are pruritus, nausea and urinary retention.

Epidural opioids are rarely given as the sole analgesic agent, as it has been demonstrated that there is no clear advantage of using spinal opioids over intravenous opioids: both provide the same quality of analgesia and the same risk of side-effects. However, it has been demonstrated that if local anaesthetic drugs are used in combination with opioids in the epidural space, they reduce the requirement for opioids and therefore the risk of opioid side-effects (opioid-sparing). They may in fact improve the quality of analgesia and reduce the incidence of patchy/unilateral blocks. Such a combination of low-dose epidural opioid and local anaesthetic allows low concentrations of local anaesthetic to be used, providing good quality analgesia with minimal motor blockade, seen as limb weakness and inability to mobilize, and less sympathetic blockade. Continuous infusions of these combinations are currently the most common way to provide epidural analgesia.

Complications and advantages of neuraxial techniques

In addition to the adverse effects of drugs, neuraxial techniques have other potential complications related to insertion of an epidural needle and subsequent presence of an epidural catheter (Baird & Schug 1996).

Dural puncture is the inadvertent puncturing of the dural membrane during insertion of an epidural catheter, allowing leakage of CSF into the epidural space. This occurs during ~1% of epidural catheter insertions. There is a high chance of developing a post-dural puncture headache following this, in particular, if the patient is young and mobilizing soon after epidural insertion.

Neurological deficit with regional numbness as a consequence of nerve injury by needle or catheter has an incidence of ~1 in 10 000. These are usually temporary deficits and complete recovery occurs, at least within 3 months.

Epidural haematoma can result in neurological deficit due to compression of the spinal cord. Unless surgical intervention (decompression) occurs within hours of first symptoms, permanent neurological injury in the form of paraplegia can be the outcome. Fortunately this complication is an extremely rare event with an estimated incidence in the range of 1 in 150 000.

Epidural abscess or meningitis can be the result of contamination on insertion or haematogenic colonization of the indwelling catheter. This is another extremely rare complication requiring antibiotic treatment and possibly surgical intervention. The incidence can be reduced by maintenance of appropriate asepsis during catheter placement and handling, as well as careful consideration of risks and benefits in septic patients.

Many different drugs have been mistakenly administered into epidural catheters, commonly as a result of nursing error or system failure. Consequences depend on the type of drug injected, but can be severe.

Epidural analgesia is used after a large variety of surgical operations ranging from thoracic surgery to vascular surgery on the lower limbs. It can also be used for acute pain secondary to medical disease, e.g. angina or pancreatitis. In comparison to PCA, continuous epidural analgesia provides significantly better-quality analgesia (Eisenach et al 1988, Schug & Fry 1994). Incidence of rest pain greater than 3 in 10 on the first postoperative day is reduced from 40% on PCA to 20% on epidural analgesia, and ability to comply with physiotherapy increased from 76% to 93%.

There is also a reduced incidence of adverse effects, e.g. nausea and vomiting, sedation, confusion, respiratory depression, pruritus (Schug & Fry 1994).

In contrast to systemic opioid administration, there is increasing evidence that epidural analgesia offers the potential for improved outcome, i.e. reduced morbidity and possibly mortality (Ballantyne et al 1998, de Leon-Casasola et al 1995). Data on such results show the following benefits.

Preservation of gastrointestinal function Epidurals significantly reduce the incidence of ileus (reduced gut motility) (Liu et al 1995), allowing early oral feeding, and reduce the incidence of breakdown of surgical bowel anastomoses. Also, they reduce the breakdown of body protein and energy sources (catabolism) and thus prevent protein loss.

Preservation of pulmonary function Epidurals significantly reduce the incidence of pulmonary infections, atelectasis and hypoxaemia (Ballantyne et al 1998).

Reduced incidence of thromboembolic complications Epidurals reduce the incidence of deep venous thrombosis (DVT) (Jorgensen et al 1991), pulmonary embolism (PE), and graft thrombosis after vascular reconstruction.

Reduced neuroendocrine response to surgery This is a physiological response (stress) due to surgery and occurs as a result of hormones (catecholamines) and cytokines released during surgical trauma (Kehlet 1989). This forces the body into a catabolic state (increased metabolic rate) whereby the body's nutritional state is depleted, it makes the blood clot more readily, increasing the risk of DVT and PE, and it may contribute to immunosuppression and increased risk of infection. An epidural is extremely effective in abolishing the stress response following lower abdominal and lower limb surgery, with a variable effect following upper abdominal and lower limb surgery, with a variable effect following upper abdominal and thoracic surgery.

Providing protection of the heart Epidurals reduce the oxygen requirement of the heart and increase its blood supply. It has recently been demonstrated that epidurals reduce the incidence of fatal arrhythmias and myocardial ischaemic events and prevent myocardial infarction following upper abdominal surgery (de Leon-Casasola 1996).

Modification of surgical and nursing protocols to ensure early oral feeding, improved nutrition and active mobilization is required to maximize the effects of neural blockade on pain, the stress response, and organ dysfunction. A multidisciplinary approach, which incorporates all aspects of perioperative rehabilitation, is likely to offer the best chances of improving outcome, reducing hospital stay and ensuring cost–benefit advantages (Kehlet 1997).

Peripheral neural blockade

Neuraxial analgesia is just one method by which local anaesthetics can be used to provide analgesia. Other types of peripheral neural blockade, which are commonly used, improve analgesia with minimal adverse effects and reduce the requirements for opioid analgesia and thus the incidence of opioid side-effects.

Wound infiltration is an extremely simple technique, usually performed by the surgeon at the end of the operation. Use of long-acting local anaesthetics such as bupivacaine and ropivacaine can provide good analgesia, lasting for many hours after surgery. It is a particularly useful technique following minor surgery such as hernia repair (Erichsen et al 1995), paediatric surgery or trauma. After major surgery its benefit is less certain, although some trials show benefit where large volumes of local anaesthetic were infiltrated into deeper wound structures rather than just subcutaneously (Dahl et al 1994).

Femoral nerve block can be performed as a single-shot technique with a long-acting local anaesthetic. Alternatively, a catheter can be placed in the fascial sheath of the femoral nerve and analgesia provided by bolus injections or continuous infusion of local anaesthetics. This technique is useful for relief of pain and muscle spasm following knee surgery, arthroplasty and fractures of the neck of femur.

Similarly for brachial plexus block, a single-shot injection or a catheter can be placed near the brachial plexus. Access is possible through the axilla, around the clavicle or interscalene by use of a variety of techniques. Depending on access and catheter position, analgesia covers nearly the entire upper limb, also providing sympathetic blockade with resulting vasodilatation. This is a desired effect in plastic surgery (skin flaps, retransplantations, etc) and in vascular surgery (e.g. shunt formation). The block is also useful for orthopaedic surgery to the arm and the shoulder, in particular when early mobilization is required.

Repeat injections or a catheter placed in one of the intercostal spaces can provide intercostal nerve blocks. One block can cover the innervation of 3–4 ribs and is thus useful for treatment of rib fractures, enabling pain-free respiration and facilitating physiotherapy. Long-lasting intercostal nerve blocks can also be performed with a cryoprobe (to –65°C) after thoracotomy, resulting in lower postoperative pain scores and a 50% reduction in analgesic medication requirements compared with controls (Seino et al 1985).

For inter-pleural blocks, a catheter is placed in the pleural space, between the parietal and visceral layer of the pleura. This can be done under direct vision during thoracotomy or with a Tuohy needle by use of a loss-of-resistance technique. Bolus injections or continuous infusions of a local anaesthetic result in widespread unilateral intercostal nerve block, a partial brachial plexus block and often a bilateral splanchnic nerve block. The technique is therefore useful for pain relief after multiple rib fractures, thoracotomies and in visceral pain (e.g. caused by acute pancreatitis). Compared with systemic opioids alone, this block can improve respiratory function (Frenette et al 1991) and is opioid-sparing.

NON-PHARMACOLOGICAL MODALITIES

These techniques are used to *supplement* pharmacological modalities, but can sometimes be sufficient on their own, and are listed in Box 19.2.

Although evidence for the efficacy of non-pharmacological modalities in acute pain management is largely at the expert opinion level, certain patients may derive benefit from them as a result of reducing drug therapy, and also if they are likely to experience a prolonged interval of pain (see Chapters

---

Box 19.2   Non-pharmacological modalities

Physical
- Superficial heat or cold
- Massage
- Exercise
- Immobilization
- Electroanalgesia, e.g. TENS

Cognitive
- Behavioural approaches
- Preparatory information
- Simple relaxation
- Imagery
- Hypnosis
- Biofeedback

9 and 11 for a more complete description of the effects of physical and cognitive therapies).

Physical treatments

Physical modalities may provide comfort, correct physical dysfunction, alter physiological responses, and reduce fears associated with pain-related immobility or activity restriction.

In general, modalities may be used with or without pharmocological support in musculoskeletal pain.

In the postoperative pain setting, where techniques are always used in conjunction with pharmocological agents, commonly used treatments include heat and cold application, mobilization, exercise, TENS, support (i.e. abdominal, thoracic cage) and massage.

Heat or cold application

Applications of heat or cold are commonly used as adjuncts to other therapies with the aim of reducing pain, muscle spasm and congestion in an injured area, often involving the musculoskeletal system.

Ice therapy to produce analgesia (cryoanalgesia) seems to be more effective than heat, but each significantly raises the normal pain threshold (Benson & Copp 1974). In both the effect declines within 30 minutes. Cold application following trauma, e.g. after sports injury, often in combination with pressure (elastic bandage) is beneficial as it reduces pain perception and also reduces bleeding and oedema formation due to vasoconstriction (Kay 1985). Later heat may help with healing and haematoma resolution (Lehmann et al 1983).

In acute surgical trauma patients, cold application causes a reduction in swelling and has been shown to reduce the amount of opioid required. It has also been shown to reduce the need for pain medication after anterior cruciate ligament repair.

Heat is contraindicated in an acute deep-seated inflammatory reaction as it increases hyperaemia, oedema, pain and acceleration of abscess formation. Heat can be applied locally or at a distance. Locally, it produces changes in neuromuscular activity, blood-flow, capillary permeability, enzymatic activity and pain threshold.

When applied at a distance, heat produces its effects via a reflex action. Heat also involves reflexogenic changes in smooth muscle activity in the gastrointestinal tract and uterus, hence heat application to the abdominal wall causes blanching of the mucous membrane with reduced gastric acid production, and marked reduction in peristalsis of the gut. The reverse occurs with cold application, so that pain resulting from spasm of smooth muscle of the gastrointestinal tract or in the uterus, e.g. viral enteritis or menstrual cramps, may be relieved.

TENS

The aim of TENS is to activate sensory myelinated fibres without producing muscle contraction or uncomfortable sensations (see Chapter 11). Its use in the management of acute pain is limited, as it is not indicated for most minor trauma pain which is of short duration, and it has a very limited place in the analgesic treatment of major trauma with multiple injuries – systemic analgesia is the appropriate treatment here.

However, sports injuries (torn ligaments, pulled muscles, back strain) can benefit from TENS. It has also been shown to be effective in certain other situations e.g. fractured ribs (Myers et al 1977), acute orofacial pain due to peridontal infection (Black 1986), acute arthritis or myalgia, myofascial syndrome, labour pain (Nesheim 1981) and primary dysmenorrhoea. TENS tends to reduce pain but not eliminate it.

Postoperative pain was the first form of acute pain to be successfully treated with TENS (Hymes et al 1973). Subsequently, TENS use in this area increased with electrode-placement adjacent to the incision at the end of an operation. It has been used for abdominal and thoracic surgery (Cooperman et al 1977), total hip replacement (Pike 1978), lumbar spine operations, hand operations and for post Caesarean section pain (Smith et al 1986).

The major advantage with TENS is that there is no respiratory depression/sedation, no reduced bowel motility and it produces continuous analgesia.

However, it has been reported that both TENS therapy and application of electrodes without transmission of electric current (sham-TENS) significantly reduced analgesic use and subjective reports of pain; no significant differences were found between TENS therapy and sham-TENS (Hargreaves & Lander 1989).

More recently, there has been a review of all the trials using TENS in the treatment of postoperative pain. The findings were that, in 15 out of 17 randomized controlled trials of TENS in postoperative pain, there was no benefit compared with placebo (Carroll et al 1996). In addition, in the excluded non-randomized studies there was an over-estimation of treatment effects. Therefore, the use of TENS as a sole postoperative analgesic modality is not recommended, although its role as an adjunct to other modalities postoperatively may be beneficial in some patients.

A further advantage of TENS is that its use and the settings of intensity are under control of the patient, thus enabling him/her to use it as felt appropriate.

Mobilization

Exercise, activation and early mobilization are important components of management in the postoperative period, aimed at achieving rapid return to normal function and life after surgery, with as little as possible deconditioning of physical function. The aim is the establishment of a normal routine for postoperative patients as quickly as possible, allowing pain relief prior to intervention and scheduled rest, but with a consistent approach encouraging restoration of function and clear guidelines as to how to mobilize out of bed, how far to mobilize, and how frequently to mobilize.

Cognitive–behavioural therapy

Cognitive–behavioural therapies are psychological methods that aim to give patients greater control over their pain (see Chapter 9). They are usually combined with all the other approaches. The simplest method is provision of psychological support and reassurance. It has been demonstrated that education of the patient, by providing sensory (explaining what sensations may be expected during/after surgery) and procedural information, and instruction aimed at reducing activity-related pain, is effective for reduction of pain. It reduces analgesic requirements (Egbert et al 1964) and requires about 5–15 minutes of staff time. It appears that the more actively the information is relayed, the more potential it has to reduce pain.

Modelling is a variant of the provision of procedural information that can reduce pain and anxiety by presenting (by videotape) a patient experiencing pain but displaying effective pain-relieving strategies that may be copied.

Coping skills training teach patients specific coping behaviours in order to reduce pain perception during procedures or postoperatively. Examples are distraction, imagery, dissociation and re-interpreting painful stimuli. Imagery has been shown to be effective in reducing mild to moderate pain but requires skilled personnel to instruct patients.

Simple relaxation involving jaw relaxation, progressive muscle relaxation and simple imagery has been shown to be effective in reducing anxiety and mild to moderate pain, and as an adjunct to analgesic drugs for severe pain. It is useful for the patient who expresses an interest in relaxation and requires 3–5 minutes of staff time for instructions. The techniques are easy to learn and carry out. They should be commenced preoperatively and continued after surgery. Also music (patient-preferred or 'easy-listening') is effective in reducing mild to moderate pain.

Complex relaxation, which incorporates biofeedback and imagery, is an approach that should be initiated preoperatively. Biofeedback is effective in reducing mild to moderate pain and operative-site muscle tension. It requires skilled personnel and special equipment.

Desensitization presents a graded 'hierarchy' of feared events and allows patients to tackle each one before moving up the ladder of these unpleasant or feared events.

In all this, it should be remembered that for patients with high levels of anxiety, giving too much information or asking them to make too many decisions can exacerbate fear and pain.

THE CONCEPT OF 'PRE-EMPTIVE ANALGESIA'

As described in Chapter 3, pain is characterized by peripheral sensitization from inflammatory mediators and also by central sensitization, which occurs by means of an increased excitability of neurones in the dorsal horn of the spinal cord. This results in a number of changes, including an increase in area of the periphery provoking a response in the dorsal horn neurones, an increase in duration of the response and a lowering of threshold-to-activation. The resultant psychophysical phenomena are hyperalgesia and allodynia (see Chapter 3).

The mechanism(s) of long-lasting changes in excitability of spinal neurones seem to relate at least partially to stimulation of NMDA receptors, leading to resultant changes in levels of calcium, cyclic AMP, and diacylglycerol intracellularly, triggering prolonged changes (Woolf 1989). Progressing further, there is evidence from recent studies that prolonged changes in the nociceptive response of the dorsal horn neurones may be associated with gene induction, notably the protooncogene c-fos. This gene encodes for an altered pattern of enhanced responsiveness of dorsal horn neurones (Munglani et al 1996).

With the identification of the mechanisms that underlie injury-evoked changes in the spinal cord has come the development of new treatment strategies to reduce or prevent the barrage of nociceptive impulses on the dorsal horn. Preclinical research has mainly been directed at use of local anaesthetic drugs prior to or immediately following surgery, for prevention of both postoperative pain and the development of the excitable state within the central nervous system. In theory, by administering local anaesthetic pre-operatively, this prevents the spinal cord from 'experiencing' the injury and also prevents the laying down of a 'memory' trace of the injury.

Pre-emptive analgesia is the term used to describe any pharmacological method of preventing transmission of nerve impulses from the nociceptive input along Aδ and C fibres to the spinal cord. Consequently, this interference in transfer of noxious input prevents the development of the hyperexcitable state within the spinal cord (Wall 1988).

In animal studies, simple comparisons of pre- and postoperative administration of opioids and local anaesthetics suggest a pre-emptive effect of the preoperative administration. However, most clinical studies with similar design have been unable to confirm these impressive results in the postoperative setting (McQuay 1995). Reasons for this failure may include poor study design and involuntary use of pre-emptive measures in the control group. However, there is also increasing recognition that postoperative pain in a clinical setting might be more complex (Kissin 1996). In particular, there is the notion that a short-lasting preoperative intervention will not prevent nociceptive barrage of the spinal cord in the extended postoperative period, thereby enabling sensitization to develop later on.

On the basis of these considerations, pre-emptive analgesia in a wider sense might mean the aggressive pre- and postoperative relief of pain preventing the development of chronic pain states later on.

Studies to date suggest that more aggressive and possibly pre-emptive approaches to the management of early postoperative pain may reduce the transition to ongoing postoperative pain, first described in phantom pain (Bach et al 1988). Local anaesthetics and NMDA-receptor antagonists (Rice & McMahon 1994) are the most promising agents here. A study which followed-up patients for 18 months after thoracotomy, found that the only predictor of continued post-thoracotomy pain was severe pain in the early postoperative period (Katz et al 1996).

THE ACUTE PAIN SERVICE

Acute pain is an area of growing interest in all specialities involved with in-patient care. As shown above, the benefits that the patient receives from effective analgesia extend beyond patient comfort into areas that often result in reduced morbidity.

An increasing body of knowledge covering the mechanism of acute pain and its effects on the dorsal horn of the spinal cord has emerged. This has resulted in an increased availability of better and more sophisticated techniques to treat acute pain, i.e. regional blockade and PCA. However, until recently, provision of optimal analgesia for acute pain has been moving at a much slower pace. Before the late-1980s, most surveys demonstrated that 60–80% of postoperative patients suffered considerable pain in the early postoperative period (Marks & Sachar 1973). Even in 1991, many patients were still dissatisfied with their postoperative analgesia (Semple & Jackson 1991). This was in part due to a large number of traditionally held (incorrect) beliefs concerning the provision of effective analgesia, such as the common idea that pain is merely a symptom and not harmful in itself, the mistaken impression that analgesia makes accurate diagnosis difficult or impossible (Attard et al 1992), and fear of the potential for addiction to opioids and concerns about respiratory depression and other opioid-related side-effects such as nausea and vomiting.

Another reason for provision of inadequate analgesia was that, although more sophisticated methods of providing analgesia were being introduced, such as regional blockade and PCA, there was a lack of appropriate organizational structures to use this equipment effectively and safely. As evidence of shortened hospital stay, reduced morbidity and mortality, and increased patient satisfaction was being reported in association with effective pain relief using these new analgesic techniques, this led to increased medical and public awareness of the importance of effectively managing acute pain. There was a need for a service to manage acute pain patients, hence the introduction of acute pain services.

In 1986, Ready set up the first 'anesthesiology-based postoperative pain management service' in Seattle, USA (Ready et al 1988), with the rapid subsequent development of other similar services worldwide (for further descriptions see Macintyre et al 1990, Schug & Haridas 1993, Wheatley et al 1991).

The Royal Australasian College of Surgeons summarised the following topics as prerequisites for effective pain control:

- Patient education
- Assessment of pain
- Appropriate prescribing
- Use of special techniques
- Individualization of treatment.

In order to provide the above services, a coordinated, organized team approach is necessary. This team should include anaesthetists, surgeons, nurses and pharmacists, not to mention a multitude of other specialists such as physiotherapists, occupational therapists, infection-control specialists and psychologists – an acute pain service (APS).

Recommendations were made that acute pain teams be established in all major hospitals and that there should be a formal, team approach to the management of acute pain with 'clear lines of responsibility'. In summary the role of an APS is to:

- Provide education about pain management as well as more specialized analgesic techniques
- Introduce the newer and more specialized methods of pain relief (epidural and PCA) and guidance to improve the more traditional methods
- Provide and standardize orders, procedures and methods of pain assessment for all methods of pain relief, as well as ongoing improvement to these based on the results of audit activity
- Provide daily supervision and 24-hour cover for patients under the care of the APS, as well as for patients with any other acute pain management problems
- Undertake audit and clinical research activity.

Thus, the management of acute pain has really only been fully addressed over the last 10 years. As more scientific evidence emerges outlining the benefits and safety of the more recently introduced analgesic techniques, together with the establishment of APS, the occurrence of inadequate relief of acute pain should eventually become a less frequent event.

As for any newly-established service, there has to be research carried out to ascertain the cost–benefit of running an APS. Some preliminary results show that there is little difference in direct costs comparing management of more advanced, expensive techniques of analgesia (epidural or PCA) to pre-APS-managed pain ('4-hourly prn im morphine') (Schug & Large 1993). The reduced nursing workload achieved by these newer techniques does offset some of the cost. Therefore, in order to justify the use of more sophisticated methods of analgesia other potential beneficial aspects must be considered.

Although the following require more thorough investigation and evidence is slender, they all may contribute to the cost-effectiveness of newer techniques compared to more traditional approaches to acute pain management:

- Reduced complications
- Reduced morbidity and mortality
- Reduced duration of hospital stay.

Also, with regard to safety of these newer, more aggressive techniques of pain control, most assessments involving the performance of an APS give results that identify APS management as being superior to routine 'pre-APS' pain management (Rawal & Allvin 1996, Ready et al 1991, Schug & Torrie 1993). A study demonstrating this assessed the safety outcome of > 3000 postoperative patients under the care of an APS, using a wide range of relatively invasive techniques (Schug & Torrie 1993). The results showed that potentially severe complications occurred rarely (0.5%), but had no sequelae and compared favourably to the incidence of complications using more traditional techniques. Also, the incidence of complications for epidural and systemic opioids occurred at similar rates.

In summary, an anaesthesiology-based APS can provide postoperative pain relief using a wide range of relatively invasive techniques without endangering patient safety.

Study questions/questions for revision

1. What is the major problem associated with intramuscularly administered opioids on an as-needed basis?
2. What are treatments of choice for managing moderate to severe acute pain?
3. Describe how PCA can be used in the post-operative setting, including its benefits and risks.
4. What are the side-effects of NSAIDs?
5. Describe five physical modalities which can assist in acute pain management.
6. Describe six cognitive methods, which can aid in acute pain management.

ACKNOWLEDGEMENTS

We are grateful for the constructive criticism of the manuscript, which we received from Samantha Bond and other members of the Physiotherapy Department of Auckland Hospital.

REFERENCES

Anonymous 1994 Collaborative overview of randomised trials of antiplatelet therapy – III: Reduction in venous thrombosis and pulmonary embolism by antiplatelet prophylaxis among surgical and medical patients. Antiplatelet Trialists' Collaboration. British Medical Journal 308(6923): 235–246

Attard A R, Corlett M J, Kidner N J, Leslie A P, Fraser I A 1992 Safety of early pain relief for acute abdominal pain. British Medical Journal 305(6853): 554–556

Austin K L, Stapleton J V, Mather L E 1980 Multiple intramuscular injections: A major source of variability in analgesic response to meperidine. Pain 8(1): 47–62

Bach S, Noreng M F, Tjellden N U 1988 Phantom limb pain in amputees during the first 12 months following limb amputation, after preoperative lumbar epidural blockade. Pain 33(3): 297–301

Baird M B, Schug S A 1996 Safety aspects of postoperative pain relief. Pain Digest 6(4): 219–225

Ballantyne J C, Carr D B, Chalmers T C, Dear K B, Angelillo I F, Mosteller F 1993 Postoperative patient-controlled analgesia: meta-analyses of initial randomized control trials. Journal of Clinical Anesthesia 5(3): 182–193

Ballantyne J C, Carr D B, deFerranti S, et al 1998 The comparative effects of postoperative analgesic therapies on pulmonary outcome: cumulative meta-analyses of randomized, controlled trials. Anesthesia & Analgesia 86(3): 598–612

Baskett P J 1972 The use of Entonox by nursing staff and physiotherapists. Nursing Mirror Midwives Journal 135(11): 30–32

Benson T B, Copp E P 1974 The effects of therapeutic forms of heat and ice on the pain threshold of the normal shoulder. Rheumatology & Rehabilitation 13(2): 101–104

Bernards C M 1993 Flux of morphine, fentanyl, and alfentanil through rabbit arteries in vivo. Evidence supporting a vascular route for redistribution of opioids between the epidural space and the spinal cord. Anesthesiology 78(6): 1126–1131

Black R R 1986 Use of transcutaneous electrical nerve stimulation in dentistry. Journal of the American Dental Association 113(4): 649–652

Boas R, Covino B, Shahnarian A 1982 Analgesic responses to IV lignocaine. British Journal of Anaesthesia 54: 501–505

Boezaart A P, Eksteen J A, Spuy G V, Rossouw P, Knipe M 1999 Intrathecal morphine. Double-blind evaluation of optimal dosage for analgesia after major lumbar spinal surgery. Spine 24(11): 1131–1137

Buggy D J, Wall C, Carton E G 1994 Preoperative or postoperative diclofenac for laparoscopic tubal ligation. British Journal of Anaesthesia 73(6): 767–770

Burns J W, Hodsman N B, McLintock T T, Gillies G W, Kenny G N, McArdle C S 1989 The influence of patient characteristics on the requirements for postoperative analgesia. A reassessment using patient-controlled analgesia. Anaesthesia 44(1): 2–6

Carroll D, Tramer M, McQuay H, Nye B, Moore A 1996 Randomization is important in studies with pain outcomes: systematic review of transcutaneous electrical nerve stimulation in acute postoperative pain. British Journal of Anaesthesia 77(6): 798–803

Cepeda M S, Vargas L, Ortegon G, Sanchez M A, Carr D B 1995 Comparative analgesic efficacy of patient-controlled analgesia with ketorolac versus morphine after elective intra-abdominal operations. Anesthesia & Analgesia 80(6): 1150–1153

Chapman C R, Hill H F 1989 Prolonged morphine self-administration and addiction liability. Evaluation of two theories in a bone marrow transplant unit. Cancer 63(8): 1636–1644

Cooper I M 1996 Morphine for postoperative analgesia. A comparison of intramuscular and subcutaneous routes of administration. Anaesthesia & Intensive Care 24(5): 574–578

Cooperman A M, Hall B, Mikalacki K, Hardy R, Sardar E 1977 Use of transcutaneous electrical stimulation in the control of postoperative pain. American Journal of Surgery 133(2): 185–187

Dahl J B, Moiniche S, Kehlet H 1994 Wound infiltration with local anaesthetics for postoperative pain relief. Acta Anaesthesiologica Scandinavica 38(1): 7–14

de Leon-Casasola O A, Lema M J, Karabella D, Harrison P 1995 Postoperative myocardial ischemia: epidural versus intravenous patient-controlled analgesia. A pilot project. Regional Anesthesia 20(2): 105–112

de Leon-Casasola O A 1996 Clinical outcome after epidural anesthesia and analgesia in high-risk surgical patients. Regional Anesthesia 21(6 Suppl): 144–148

Egan K J, Ready L B 1994 Patient satisfaction with intravenous PCA or epidural morphine. Canadian Journal of Anaesthesia 41(1): 6–11

Egbert L, Battit G, Welch C E A 1964 Reduction of postoperative pain by encouragement and instruction of patients. New England Journal of Medicine 270: 825

Eisenach J C, Grice S C, Dewan D M 1988 Patient-controlled analgesia following cesarean section: a comparison with epidural and intramuscular narcotics. Anesthesiology 68(3): 444–448

Erichsen C J, Vibits H, Dahl J B, Kehlet H 1995 Wound infiltration with ropivacaine and bupivacaine for pain after inguinal herniotomy. Acta Anaesthesiologica Scandinavica 39: 67–70

Espinet A, Henderson D J, Faccenda K A, Morrison L M 1996 Does pre-incisional thoracic extradural block combined with diclofenac reduce postoperative pain after abdominal hysterectomy? British Journal of Anaesthesia 76(2): 209–213

Frenette L, Boudreault D, Guay J 1991 Interpleural analgesia improves pulmonary function after cholecystectomy. Canadian Journal of Anaesthesia 38(1): 71–74

Gehling M, Tryba M 1998 New aspects of ketamine in postoperative pain management. Acute Pain 1(5): 22–34

Hansen L A, Noyes M A, Lehman M E 1991 Evaluation of patient-controlled analgesia (PCA) versus PCA plus continuous infusion in postoperative cancer patients. Journal of Pain & Symptom Management 6(1): 4–14

Hargreaves A, Lander J 1989 Use of transcutaneous electrical nerve stimulation for postoperative pain. Nursing Research 38(3): 159–161

Houmes R J, Voets M A, Verkaaik A, Erdmann W, Lachmann B 1992 Efficacy and safety of tramadol versus morphine for moderate and severe postoperative pain with special regard to respiratory depression. Anesthesia & Analgesia 74(4): 510–514

Hymes A C, Raab D E, Yonehiro E G, Nelson G D, Printy A L 1973 Electrical surface stimulation for control of acute postoperative pain and prevention of ileus. Surgical Forum 24: 447–449

Jorgensen L N, Rasmussen L S, Nielsen P T, Leffers A, Albrecht-Beste E 1991 Antithrombotic efficacy of continuous extradural analgesia after knee replacement. British Journal of Anaesthesia 66(1): 8–12

Katz J, Jackson M, Kavanagh B P, Sandler A N 1996 Acute pain after thoracic surgery predicts long-term post-thoracotomy pain. Clinical Journal of Pain 12(1): 50–55

Kay D B 1985 The sprained ankle: current therapy. Foot & Ankle 6(1): 22–28

Keeri-Szanto M 1979 Drugs or drums: what relieves postoperative pain? Pain 6(2): 217–230

Kehlet H 1989 Surgical stress: the role of pain and analgesia. British Journal of Anaesthesia 63(2): 189–195

Kehlet H 1997 Modification of responses to surgery by neural blockade: clinical implications. In: Cousins M, Bridenbaugh P (eds) Neural Blockade in Clinical Anaesthesia and Management of Pain. JB Lippincott, Philadelphia

Kissin I 1996 Preemptive analgesia. Why its effect is not always obvious [editorial]. Anesthesiology 84(5): 1015–1019

Lehmann J F, Dundore D E, Esselman P C, Nelp W B 1983 Microwave diathermy: effects on experimental muscle hematoma resolution. Archives of Physical Medicine & Rehabilitation 64(3): 127–129

Liu S S, Carpenter R L, Mackey D C et al 1995 Effects of perioperative analgesic technique on rate of recovery after colon surgery. Anesthesiology 83(4): 757–765

Macintyre P, Ready L 1996 Acute Pain Management: a Practical Guide. W B Saunders, London

Macintyre P E, Runciman W B, Webb R K 1990 An acute pain service in an Australian teaching hospital: the first year. Medical Journal of Australia 153(7): 417–421

Malmstrom K, Daniels S, Kotey P, Seidenberg B C, Desjardins P J 1999 Comparison of rofecoxib and celecoxib, two cyclooxygenase-2 inhibitors, in postoperative dental pain: a randomized, placebo- and active- comparator-controlled clinical trial. Clinical Therapies 21(10): 1653–1663

Marks R M, Sachar E J 1973 Undertreatment of medical inpatients with narcotic analgesics. Annals of Internal Medicine 78(2): 173–181

McArdle C 1987 Continuous and patient controlled analgesic infusions. In: Doyle 1986 International Symposium on Pain Control. Royal Society of Medicine International Congress and Symposium, 17–22

McQuay H J 1995 Pre-emptive analgesia: a systematic review of clinical studies. Annals of Medicine 27: 249–256

Miller R, Greenblatt D 1976 Drug Effects in Hospitalized Patients. John Wiley, New York

Munglani R, Fleming B G, Hunt S P 1996 Rememberance of times past: the significance of c-fos in pain (Editorial). British Journal of Anaesthesia 76: 1–3

Myers R A, Woolf C J, Mitchell D 1977 Management of acute traumatic pain by peripheral transcutaneous electrical stimulation. South African Medical Journal 52(8): 309–312

Nesheim B I 1981 The use of transcutaneous nerve stimulation for pain relief during labor. A controlled clinical study. Acta Obstetricia et Gynecologica Scandinavica 60(1): 13–16

Notcutt W G, Morgan R J 1990 Introducing patient-controlled analgesia for postoperative pain control into a district general hospital. Anaesthesia 45(5): 401–406

Oden R 1989 Acure postoperative pain: incidence, severity and etiology of inadequate treatment. Anesthesiology Clinics of North America 7: 1–5

Owen H, Plummer J L, Armstrong I, Mather L E, Cousins M J 1989a Variables of patient-controlled analgesia: 1. bolus size. Anaesthesia 44: 7–10

Owen H, Szekely S M, Plummer J L, Cushnie J M, Mather L E 1989b Variables of patient-controlled analgesia. 2. Concurrent infusion. Anaesthesia 44(1): 11–13

Paech M J, Pavy J G, Orlikowski E P, Lim W, Evans S F 1997 Postoperative epidural infusion: a randomized, double-blind, dose-finding trial of clonidine in combination with bupivacaine and fentanyl. Anesthesia & Analgesia 84: 1323–1328

Parbrook G D 1972 Entonox for post-operative analgesia. Proceedings of the Royal Society of Medicine 65(1): 8–9

Park J, Forrest J, Kolesar R, Bhola D, Beattie S, Chu C 1996 Oral clonidine reduces postoperative PCA morphine requirements. Canadian Journal of Anaesthesia 43(9): 900–906

Pavy T J, Gambling D R, Merrick P M, Douglas M J 1995 Rectal indomethacin potentiates spinal morphine analgesia after caesarean delivery. Anaesthesia & Intensive Care 23(5): 555–559

Pike P M 1978 Transcutaneous electrical stimulation. Its use in the management of postoperative pain. Anaesthesia 33(2): 165–171

Power I 1993 Aspirin-induced asthma [editorial]. British Journal of Anaesthesia 71(5): 619–621

Power I, Noble D W, Douglas E, Spence A A 1990 Comparison of i.m. ketorolac trometamol and morphine sulphate for pain relief after cholecystectomy. British Journal of Anaesthesia 65(4): 448–455

Power I, Cumming A D, Pugh G C 1992 Effect of diclofenac on renal function and prostacyclin generation after surgery. British Journal of Anaesthesia 69(5): 451–456

Power I, Bowler G M, Pugh G C, Chambers W A 1994 Ketorolac as a component of balanced analgesia after thoracotomy. British Journal of Anaesthesia 72(2): 224–226

Quinn A C, Brown J H, Wallace P G, Asbury A J 1994 Studies in postoperative sequelae. Nausea and vomiting – Still a problem. Anaesthesia 49(1): 62–65

Rawal N, Allvin R 1996 Epidural and intrathecal opioids for postoperative pain management in Europe – a 17-nation questionnaire study of selected hospitals. Euro Pain Study Group on Acute Pain. Acta Anaesthesiologica Scandinavica 40(9): 1119–1126

Ready L B, Oden R, Chadwick H S, et al 1988 Development of an anesthesiology-based postoperative pain management service. Anesthesiology 68: 100–106

Ready L B, Loper K A, Nessly M, Wild L 1991 Postoperative epidural morphine is safe on surgical wards. Anesthesiology 75(3): 452–456

Rice A S C, McMahon B 1994 Pre-emptive intrathecal administration of an NMDA receptor antagonist (AP-5) prevents hyper-reflexia in a model of persistent visceral pain. Pain 57: 335–340

Roth S H 1989 Merits and liabilities of NSAID therapy. Rheumatic Diseases Clinics of North America 15(3): 479–498

Roytblat L, Korotkoruchko A, Katz J, Glazer M, Greemberg L, Fisher A 1993 Postoperative pain: the effect of low-dose ketamine in addition to general anesthesia. Anesthesia & Analgesia 77(6): 1161–1165

Schug S A 1999 Intramuscular opioids – the slow extinction of a dinosaur. Acute Pain 2(2): 56–59

Schug S A, Fry R A 1994 Continuous regional analgesia in comparison with intravenous opioid administration for routine postoperative pain control. Anaesthesia 49(6): 528–532

Schug S, Haridas R 1993 Development and organizational structure of an acute pain service in a major teaching hospital. Australian & New Zealand Journal of Surgery 63(1): 8–13

Schug S A, Large R G 1993 Economic considerations in pain management. Pharmaco Economics 3(3): 260–267

Schug S, Torrie J 1993 Safety assessment of postoperative pain management by an acute pain service. Pain 55(3): 387–391

Schug S, Zech D, Grond S 1992 Adverse effects of systemic opioid analgesics. Drug Safety 7(3): 200–213

Schug S A, Sidebotham D A, McGuinnety M, Thomas J, Fox L 1998 Acetaminophen as an adjunct to morphine by patient-controlled analgesia in the management of acute postoperative pain. Anesthesia Analgesia 87(2): 368–372

Seino H, Watanabe S, Tanaka J, et al 1985 [Cryoanalgesia for postthoracotomy pain]. Masui – Japanese Journal of Anesthesiology 34(6): 842–845

Semple P, Jackson I J 1991 Postoperative pain control. A survey of current practice. Anaesthesia 46(12): 1074–1076

Semple T J, Upton R N, Macintyre P E, Runciman W B, Mather L E 1997 Morphine blood concentrations in elderly postoperative patients following administration via an indwelling subcutaneous cannula. Anaesthesia 52(4): 318–323

Sidebotham D, Dijkhuizen M, Schug S 1997 The safety and utilization of patient-controlled analgesia. Journal of Pain & Symptom Management 14(4): 202–209

Singelyn F J, Gouverneur J M, Robert A 1996 A minimum dose of clonidine added to mepivacaine prolongs the duration of anesthesia and analgesia after axillary brachial plexus block. Anesthesia & Analgesia 83(5): 1046–1050

Smith C M, Guralnick M S, Gelfand M M, Jeans M E 1986 The effects of transcutaneous electrical nerve stimulation on post-cesarean pain. Pain 27(2): 181–193

Smith K, Halliwell R M, Lawrence S, Klineberg P L, O'Connell P 1993 Acute renal failure associated with intramuscular ketorolac. Anaesthesia & Intensive Care 21(5): 700–702

Smythe M A, Zak M B, O'Donnell M P, Schad R F, Dmuchowski C F 1996 Patient-controlled analgesia versus patient-controlled analgesia plus continuous infusion after hip replacement surgery. Annals of Pharmacotherapy 30(3): 224–227

Strom B L, Berlin J A, Kinman J L, et al 1996 Parenteral ketorolac and risk of gastrointestinal and operative site bleeding. A postmarketing surveillance study. Journal of the American Medical Association 275(5): 376–382

Swerdlow M, Cundill J G 1981 Anticonvulsant drugs used in the treatment of lancinating pain. A comparison. Anaesthesia 36(12): 1129–1132

Tamsen A, Hartvig P, Fagerlund C 1982 Patient-controlled analgesic therapy: Clinical experience. Acta Anaesthesiologica Scandinavica 20(Suppl)

Vickers M D, O'Flaherty D, Szekely S M, Read M, Yoshizumi J 1992 Tramadol: pain relief by an opioid without depression of respiration. Anaesthesia 47(4): 291–296

Wall P D 1988 The prevention of postoperative pain. Pain 33: 289–290

Warfield C A, Kahn C H 1990 Acute pain management: Programs in US hospitals and experiences and attitudes among US adults. Anesthesiology 83(5): 1090–1094

Wheatley R G, Madej T H, Jackson I J, Hunter D 1991 The first year's experience of an acute pain service. British Journal of Anaesthesia 67(3): 353–359

Woolf C J 1989 Recent advances in the pathophysiology of acute pain. British Journal of Anaesthesia 63(2): 139–146

20

Chronic pain problems

Jenny Strong

OVERVIEW

In earlier chapters of this book, we have seen that chronic pain is a phenomenon that is distinct from acute pain. Some of the mechanisms by which complex pain problems develop have been explained. It is argued that clients with chronic pain need to be managed with paradigms different from acute pain management paradigms. Hopefully in future, therapists will see fewer people with chronic pain problems because early intervention when the pain is acute will be successful in reducing the development of chronicity. But for the present, there are many people with chronic pain in our communities.

In this chapter, chronic pain will be described and approaches to management will be discussed. In addition to providing a definition of chronic pain, characteristics of the chronic pain syndrome will be described.

Chronic pain conditions frequently seen by occupational therapists and physiotherapists will be briefly discussed. The literature that examines why some people develop chronic pain will then be considered. Finally, differentiation will be made between people with persistent pain (who seek occasional professional help for pain but largely self-manage their pain) and patients with chronic pain syndromes (who require major assistance from multidisciplinary pain clinics) (see Box 20.1 for definitions). A careful individual assessment needs to be made by the physiotherapist or occupational therapist to ensure that the client receives the optimal management programme.

Learning objectives

At the end of this chapter, students will:

1. Recognize the characteristics of the chronic pain syndrome
2. Identify some factors which may contribute to the development of pain chronicity

> **Box 20.1   Key terms defined**
>
> **Acute pain** – Pain lasting less than 3 months duration. It is characterized by tissue damage, and is associated with anxiety. Interventions are designed to prevent further tissue injury, promote tissue healing and eliminate pain.
>
> **Chronic pain** – Pain which lasts beyond the expected point of tissue healing, longer than 3 months duration.
>
> **Persistent pain** – The type of ongoing pain problem which typically results in individual taking anti-inflammatory medication, and/or seeing a physiotherapist or other health practitioner on an as-needed basis, and getting on with normal activities.
>
> **Chronic pain syndrome** – The type of ongoing pain problem where the individual is severely affected, in many aspects of functioning. The pain may be unbearable and may interfere with activities of daily living and vocations. The individual seeks help from multiple treatment providers, undergoes multiple procedures, has mood changes, loses self-esteem, comes into conflict with others, and has increased incapacity, due to disuse.
>
> **Multidisciplinary pain clinic** – A healthcare facility, run by physicians from different specialities and other non-physician health professionals, which specializes in the diagnosis and management of patients with chronic pain (Loeser 1991).

3. Understand the problems faced by patients with persistent pain
4. Understand distinctions between persistent pain and chronic pain
5. Understand the rationale for management of patients with chronic pain.

THE CONDITION OF CHRONIC PAIN

Chronic pain is a major problem in our communities (Bonica 1984, Pinsky et al 1979, Turk & Melzack 1992). It is a condition that has been hard to understand, hard to eradicate and hard to live with. Patients, health professionals, insurers and the courts all find the condition problematic.

• Its problematic nature may be understood, in part, by considering that it is a phenomenon that our traditional health training has explained poorly. It was the pain of conditions such as phantom limb pain that showed the inadequacy of specificity stimulus and response models of pain (Melzack & Wall 1982). In the acute pain situation, pain serves as a useful biological warning to the person to remove him or herself from danger. In the chronic pain situation, this is not the

case. Chronic pain usually serves no useful biological function. When acute pain becomes chronic pain, it must be managed differently (Sullivan et al 1991).

• Our best efforts at eliminating chronic pain have not worked especially well. The symptomatic relief of chronic pain, and multiple, sequential consultations with different health professionals, has provided minimal benefit for people with chronic pain conditions. The establishment of multidisciplinary pain clinics was seen as a way of providing better management.

• Pain can never be totally understood or experienced by another. It is a subjective phenomenon. We have seen in Chapter 19 how even acute pain, that can be totally expected after surgical procedures, is not well managed. More so the pain that people report which we cannot attribute to a direct cause or injury. We may doubt its authenticity, its magnitude and its quality. We need to remember that pain is what the person says it is.

• Its problematic nature may also be understood, in part, by considering the complexity of the nociceptive system and the enormous plasticity inherent in that system (see Chapter 3). The influence of higher brain centres on all aspects of pain processing, and the numerous cellular mechanisms that can alter processing of nociceptive information, all have the potential to function abnormally and maintain an up-regulated state of the nociceptive system. We expect pain to resolve and the nociceptive system to return to its normal quiescent state, but considering the complexity of the system it is not surprising that this does not always occur.

Pain is the main reason people seek help from health professionals (Crue 1985, Turk & Melzack 1992). When such pain persists, constantly or intermittently, it can have a profound effect on a person's life (and the lives of their family members). Relentless chronic pain can impact on a person's fears and emotions, their interpersonal relationships, their physical and psychological wellbeing, their social situation, their vocational status and their economic circumstances. Craig (1994) observed that, 'Recognition that pain and a disrupted lifestyle may have to be long endured takes its toll, and despondency and a sense of hopelessness become likely outcomes'.

As one patient with chronic low back pain of 26 years duration commented, 'Pain is such a terribly personal thing. And you sort of sit there and you think oh my god I wish it'd go away. Ah, and you start to feel a bit depressed' (quoted in Strong 1992).

It can be useful to consider the cluster of circumstances that are often found in clients with chronic pain conditions. Such a cluster has been called 'the chronic pain syndrome' (Pinsky et al 1979). Characteristics of the syndrome include:

- Multiple surgical and/or pharmacological treatments (Pinsky et al 1979)
- Poor response to conventional analgesic regimes (Sternbach 1974)
- Reduction in normal adaptive defence mechanisms (Sternbach 1974)
- Increased feelings of helplessness, hopelessness and meaningless (Melzack & Wall 1982, Sternbach 1974)
- Mood and affect changes (Pinsky et al 1979)
- Escalating psychosocial withdrawal (Pinsky et al 1979)
- Decrease in self-esteem
- Reduced occupational role performance (Roy 1984, Strong 1989)
- Decreased physical capacity due to disuse (Pinsky et al 1979)
- Interpersonal conflicts (Crue 1985)
- Conflicts with healthcare providers (Pinsky 1979).

It is certainly useful for therapists to remember that when a client attends a physiotherapist or occupational therapist for assistance with chronic pain, the pain impacts on all aspects of that person's life. As Rey (1993) commented, chronic pain affects the person as a whole.

THE USUAL RESPONSE TO ENDURING PAIN

A number of factors may predispose people to have difficulty managing the psychosocial disruption that follows chronic pain and disability (see Reflective exercise 20.1). These factors include:

- Early childhood deprivation, neglect and abuse (Goldberg et al 1999)
- Psychosocial deprivation
- Poor education (Fishbain et al 1993)
- Limited vocational skills (particularly manual workers)
- Isolation (geographical and/or personal)
- Past personal or family ill-health
- Past difficulty coping, particularly with substance abuse, depression, anxiety
- Lack of social support
- Ongoing conflict, notably including multiple medical opinions, and third-party conflicts.

Reflective exercise 20.1

One way of understanding the experience of a patient with chronic pain is to imagine yourself arriving for work, expecting not only a normal day, but also a normal future, only to be told by a stranger that you are never again allowed to work, ever, in any capacity for which you are trained.

Most people in this situation would initially dismiss this as untrue, unbelievable, and try to ignore it. However when it became evident that not only were you not allowed to work, but also you were unable to dress easily, sit, stand, or work in comfort, you could manage only basic household tasks with difficulty and discomfort, you could not concentrate to read, you could not maintain sufficient activity and interest to sustain friendships, and you had to move out of your house to different accommodation more suitable because of physical and financial reasons, then this would start to 'hurt'.

Most people would vigorously and energetically try to identify the cause of such a catastrophe to reverse it, to return to their normal lifestyle, to fulfil the hopes, dreams and expectations they held for themselves, their family, and friends.

When no cause or explanation can be identified, even after considerable effort, it is not unreasonable to consider such a situation as unreasonable, unfair, and undeserved. Most people would be very distressed, angry, confused and apprehensive, and not confident about what to do next. This is a grief reaction to the multitude of losses involved.

If, during one's life, there had been similar losses and/or hardships, the current events may trigger one to remember, and to re-experience, various aspects of those previous difficulties. The connection may be obscure because the association is usually highly variable; while the concepts involved are the same (loss, deprivation, injustice, powerlessness, etc), one's experience of it may be highly individual. For example, a divorce may mean devastation to one person, and release to another. The recall of these past associations may be only partial. Perhaps it may be experienced only by similar emotions rather than a clear, readily identifiable picture of thoughts, ideas, and images, such that the reasons for one being so upset may not be immediately apparent, either to the therapist, or to oneself.

After many struggles, trials, disappointments and frustrations, the search for an answer may give way to acceptance that there is none. The ability of a person to negotiate this difficult course is very reliant upon him or her having developed sufficient skills, knowledge, confidence, and supports to cope with such problems earlier in life.

Essentially, anything that has interfered with a person's ability to access and use information and experiences and to develop life skills, or that adds extra pressure to the person's current overall personal 'workload', will predispose to difficulty managing a painful disorder. The person is more likely to have difficulty tolerating the pain, and to seek help from others.

These factors, many of which occurred well before any injury or illness, may be major contributors to determining whether a person will develop a chronic pain syndrome.

Development of pain chronicity

The question of why some patients will develop an incapacitating chronic pain syndrome while others manage to live productive lives, despite pain, has been frequently asked (see Main & Watson 1995, Pither & Nicholas 1991, Strong & Large 1995). A number of factors have been proposed to explain the variability in patient outcomes from seemingly similar pathologies, including:

- Inappropriate treatment behaviour by health professionals
- The existence of a history of sexual and/or physical abuse in patients who develop chronic pain problems
- The existence of psychological factors
- The presence of work-related or medicolegal factors.

One factor that has been discussed in terms of the development of chronicity, is that of inappropriate treatment behaviour. Pither and Nicholas (1991) examined the existence of inappropriate use of analgesics, inappropriate prescription of hypnotic tranquillizers, over-investigation or over-treatment, prescription of rest as the cure, oversimplified explanations of pain, or referral to a psychiatrist, in 89 patients referred to a pain clinic. They found that only three patients had none of these inappropriate treatments.

Rainville and his colleagues (1995) explored the idea that patients' disability may result in part from the projected attitudes and beliefs held by treating health professionals. Using the Health Care Providers' Pain and Impairment Relationship Scale, they found that significant differences in beliefs about pain were found between health professionals working in the community and in a functional restoration programme. Causal relationships have not been established between health professional's beliefs and patients outcomes, in terms of developing chronic pain, but therapists should be mindful of their attitudes.

Loeser and Sullivan (1995) have suggested that disability in patients with chronic low back pain may be iatrogenic, with factors such as proscription of activity, inappropriate surgery and medication prescription and delivery on an as needed basis (prn) raised as possible contributors. The issues of abnormal illness behaviour and abnormal treatment behaviour are discussed further in Chapter 22.

The association between a history of sexual and/or physical abuse and the occurrence of chronic pain syndromes has received attention in the literature (Goldberg et al 1999, Rapkin et al 1990, Toomey et al 1995, Williams et al 1999). Toomey et al (1995) found that 28% of their consecutive sample of outpatients at a Pain Clinic reported a history of abuse. This finding needs to be considered in relation to the frequency of abuse reported by the wider population (with estimates ranging from 6–62% in the normal population).

Williams et al (1999) examined the incidence of childhood abuse and dissociative disorder in chronic regional pain syndrome (CRPS) Type I patients attending a pain clinic. In this small study, of only 18 CRPS subjects, the patients were found not to be dissociative, and had childhood abuse rates no higher than the general population.

Similarly, Ciccone et al (1997) found no unique psychological traits or history of abuse in CRPS Type I patients as compared to patients with back pain or neuropathic pain. The authors had tested the hypothesis that patients with CRPS Type I and patients with back pain (with symptoms which may not be able to be reconciled to objective pathology) would differ from patients with neuropathic pain (which was circumscribed and of a known organic cause). The finding of no difference by the authors led them to suggest that psychological factors and abuse were not a factor in the development of CRPS Type I. In a recent study by Goldberg et al (1999) of patients with facial pain, myofascial pain, fibromyalgia and a heterogeneous pain group; all had a history of abuse exceeding 48%.

Considerable attention has been directed towards the development of chronic pain in injured workers (see Main & Watson 1995, Polatin & Mayer 1996).

Whether or not an individual becomes chronically incapacitated depends not only on his actual and perceived clinical status, but also on the socioeconomic system within which he finds himself. (Main & Watson 1995; p 214)

Job satisfaction, receipt of workers' compensation benefits, work skill level and psychological variables have all been advanced as possible factors in the development of chronicity (Burns et al 1995). Some of these factors are discussed further in Chapter 22.

The picture regarding aetiological factors is far from clear. Therapists must not be judgemental of people who do develop chronic pain conditions. It is wise for occupational therapists and physiotherapists to be mindful of them as possible contributing factors in individual patients.

The continuum of chronic pain

Early work has clearly described an all-pervasive, downward-spiralling chronic pain syndrome, in which patients typically experience poor response to regular analgesia, multiple treatments, adverse effects of medications, conflicts with healthcare providers, interpersonal difficulties, occupational role dysfunction, escalating physical incapacity and reduced self-esteem (Pinsky et al 1979, Strong 1989).

Clearly, patients with chronic pain syndromes require comprehensive, multidisciplinary management, which has a primary aim of helping patients to learn to live with pain. While many patients with such problems do get referred to a multidisciplinary pain facility, some do not, and may be seen by physiotherapists or occupational therapists in other settings, such as out-patient departments or private practice rooms.

People with chronic pain do not form a homogeneous group. The management of one client with chronic pain may need to be vastly different from the management required for another client with chronic pain. It can be helpful for students and therapists to consider people with chronic pain as fitting at some point along a pain continuum, as in Figure 20.1. At one end of the continuum is the person with chronic pain who stoically gets on with it, and totally self-manages their pain. At the other end of the continuum is the person who is severely disabled by their pain, who eventually may be referred to a Pain Clinic, some years after the onset of the chronic pain problem. Such people with chronic pain appear to have enormous difficulty coping with the pain and maintaining a reasonable quality of life.

Many researchers have investigated the severely disabled, depressed, dysfunctional group of patients with chronic pain in Pain Clinics (Klapow et al 1993, Sanders & Brena 1993, Strong et al 1994, Talo 1992, Turk & Rudy 1988, 1990). Such patients typically present with multiple problems. In essence, these patients have become invalided by their pain. The pain overwhelms them, interfering with their performance of activities across the work, self-care, rest and play continuums. Attendant problems of financial difficulties, interpersonal conflicts, social isolation, physical deconditioning and despair are common.

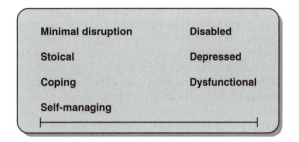

Figure 20.1 The chronic pain continuum.

In recent times, however, researchers have begun to look more closely at people with chronic pain who do not require management of their pain problems by tertiary referral centres, such as Pain Clinics (see Large & Strong 1997, Reitsma & Maijler 1997, Strong & Large 1995, Zitman et al 1992). Zitman et al (1992) compared a group of 46 patients with chronic pain who were attending a Pain Clinic with 40 non-patients who had pain for more than a year but had not consulted a physician for their pain in the previous year. These non-patients were recruited from a newspaper advertisement, and underwent an interview and filled in a battery of questionnaires. They were less depressed, less functionally impaired, and took fewer analgesics than did patients at the Pain Clinic. They also expected less assistance from external resources.

The authors of this study commented, 'these data suggest that the non-consumers responding to our call have as much pain as pain [clinic] patients, but it does not bother them as much. They indeed live a better life than pain [clinic] patients' (Zitman et al 1992).

Reitsma & Meijler (1997) compared patients attending a university hospital multidisciplinary pain centre with people who responded to a newspaper advertisement. While these respondents completed a pack of questionnaires and returned them by mail (i.e. were never seen by a pain physician to determine authenticity of pain by physical examinations and/or other medical tests), the results are interesting. The non-consumers (non-patients) reported less pain distress, fewer distorted cognitions, higher activity levels and greater internal orientation than did the patients. The non-consumers also had higher levels of education.

Strong and Large (1995, Large & Strong 1997) recruited what were described as 'copers' – individuals living with chronic low back pain, who were not undergoing tertiary management for their pain. Nineteen volunteers were recruited following a media release in Auckland, New Zealand. These individuals reported being in pain for an average duration of 14 years. Their average pain intensity (3.36 out of 10) was significantly lower than that of patients attending the Auckland Regional Pain Service. Focus group discussions and repertory grid interviews were used to obtain detailed information about each individual participant.

Repertory grid interviews are a method of eliciting detailed data about how an individual views the world as seen through Personal Construct Theory (Kelly 1963). Through such interviews, the interviewer obtains a view of the personal constructs of the individual as seen through their own eyes.

The participants were found to have successfully acknowledged that they would always have pain, and had carried on with their lives. They used a variety of strategies to provide pain relief and avoid exacerbating their pain, and lived their lives around this planned management. These people with pain had adopted an approach to living that required a somatic focus, attending closely to their bodies and their pain levels, and acting accordingly.

This does not mean that they forsook their occupational roles and life goals. Rather, they had to plan activities more carefully, evaluate consequences of participation and commit to action. They took a very active approach to the management of their lives and their pain. A number of people commented that they managed better, 'once I took charge of myself'. They learned the value of regular exercising (e.g. going to the gym or swimming), and learned to pace themselves (e.g. 'I have learnt to keep pacing myself when I do things like working in the garden. I stop and don't go on for another 10 minutes, because then I will need to go to the physio the next day if I don't stop').

There clearly exist in the community people who live day-to-day with chronic pain problems. These people seem to have a reasonable quality of life. If they had their choice, they would prefer to be pain-free. But since this is not a possibility for them, they get on with enjoying their lives. These people are not typical of those attending multidisciplinary pain clinics. They might be termed persistent pain patients, who live with chronic pain in the suburbs and manage their pain on an as-needed basis. The pain may be constant, or intermittently recurrent. People with persistent pain clearly have ongoing pain problems. They do not have acute pain. Yet they seem to have better coping skills, less emotional distress, and less impairment as a result of their pain.

The case example in Box 20.2 illustrates the problems faced by people with persistent pain who may present to a physiotherapist.

At the other end of the continuum are to be found people with chronic pain who have enormous difficulty coping with the pain and maintaining a reasonable quality of life. The case example in Box 20.3 is illustrative of the complexity of problems that such individuals can face.

MANAGING CHRONIC PAIN

John J Bonica is considered to have been the 'father' of multidisciplinary pain clinics (Loeser 1994). Such clinics were established to overcome the failure of more conventional medical management approaches for patients with chronic pain (Hartman & Ainsworth 1980, Roberts 1983). In 1990, Loeser noted, 'Facilities for the treatment of patients with chronic pain have developed rapidly in the past fifteen years'. The International Association for the Study of Pain (IASP) established a set of characteristics it regarded as desirable for pain treatment facilities. The IASP has classified pain treatment facilities into four different types:

Multidisciplinary Pain Centres – facilities with healthcare professionals and scientists who are involved with patient care, teaching and research. Staff may include physicians, psychologists, nurses, physical therapists, occupational therapists, social workers, vocational counsellors, and others who contribute to patient diagnosis and management.

Multidisciplinary Pain Clinics – facilities with physicians of different specialities plus other health professionals who specialize in the diagnosis and management of patients who have chronic pain.

Pain Clinics – facilities that focus upon the diagnosis and management of patients with chronic pain. These clinics may be staffed by a single physician.

Modality-oriented Clinics – facilities that do not provide comprehensive assessment or management but focus on a particular type of treatment, such as acupuncture or nerve blocks (Loeser 1991).

In 1994, Sanders alerted the pain management community to an image problem with pain clinics. Some of the reasons for such a view were the high cost of pain programs, the lack of measurable effectiveness of pain clinics, inadequate screening and selection of patients, variability in quality of pain clinics, and variability among programs in the attention given to rehabilitation (Sanders 1994). Sanders (1994) urged all pain clinics to therefore demonstrate cost-effectiveness, to individualize the selection and treatment of patients, to emphasize goal-directed rehabilitation, to establish standards of care, to improve disability management and to emphasize education about pain management.

Box 20.2   Case example – Mr MJ

Presentation

Mr MJ was a 69-year-old man who was referred to physiotherapy by his general medical practitioner for assistance with his long-standing low back pain. He was a retired professional man who was still very actively engaged on a number of government and university committees. Radiographs of his lumbar spine, taken 5 years previously, revealed marked and generalized degenerative joint disease.

History

Mr MJ reported that he had suffered from low back pain for approximately 15 years. The onset of pain was insidious and his condition was characterized by semi-constant, central low back pain and stiffness with exacerbations following any type of heavy work or lifting and carrying. Low back pain fluctuated over the years but Mr MJ has never been totally free of pain. Stiffness of his back had always been a feature. His pain had remained consistently in the low back region and had never spread distally. He knows he has a poor standing posture, which has always been related to being very tall. He has managed his condition to this time with exercises, which he

performs every morning. These exercises included prone-lying leg extension, mini trunk curls, double knee to chest presses and crook-lying lumbar rotation exercises.

Recently, Mr MJ reported that his back had become terribly stiff and painful, particularly in the mornings, and he was having great difficulty getting going. His bed was only 3 years old and over the past few weeks he had the pain and marked stiffness in the mornings, regardless of which bed he slept in at home or on business trips. He reported difficulty with any flexion activity. He was unable to pick up the newspaper from the ground in the morning, and could not bend over a bathroom basin to clean his teeth without leaning on one hand for support. His usual morning exercises were not having an effect. During his work meetings, he had increased pain if he had to sit for any length of time, and had difficulty standing up after sitting. He felt he could not trust his back, and it felt vulnerable.

Further questioning revealed that there had been no incident to precipitate this episode. There had been no particular change in his work or leisure activities (gardening and the theatre). He was now doing very little in the garden.

Box 20.3   Case example – Mr JD

Presentation

Mr JD was a 47-year-old man referred to an occupational therapist for a Rehabilitation Program 3 years after his discharge from the Armed Services. He presented with complex and multiple disabilities all relating to his term in the Armed Forces. Symptomatology had worsened over the time Mr JD had unsuccessfully searched for employment.

History

Mr JD had recently undergone bilateral carpal tunnel surgery at time of referral. He also presented with left-sided rotator cuff syndrome, low back pain, left-sided ankle instability, chondromalacia patella of the left knee, right-sided knee pain and hip pain. He had not received any therapeutic intervention other than surgery at time of referral. Mr JD was 20 kg overweight.

Mr JD lived with his wife who suffered from severe health problems (asthma, rheumatoid arthritis and duodenal ulcer) and his two teenage daughters, both of whom were not able to maintain employment and were receiving counselling.

Prior to developing multiple pain problems, Mr JD had been a very active man, participating in sports (soccer, long-distance running, etc) and coaching children's sports. His working life had been very physical and he had prided himself on his high level of participation in a variety of life areas. He expressed distress relating to his pain, loss of function, loss of life roles and altered relationships in his life. He related significant symptoms of depression.

Examination

Assessment of activities of daily living and functional tolerances revealed a man whose functional tolerances for sitting, standing, walking, twisting, lifting and manipulating were all significantly reduced. He had difficulty with most physical tasks including opening doors, getting on and off his lounge chair, getting in and out of his car and walking up and down stairs. His home had stairs at both the front and back entrances.

He had difficulty dressing (pulling shirts on and off over shoulders), showering (needed assistance to wash hair and under his left arm, used a tap turner, lost balance while washing his feet), had difficulty preparing food and sometimes needed assistance eating.

He had difficulty sleeping and woke with pain daily. Pain prevented Mr JD from engaging in sexual relations with his wife. He reported this as a barrier to their being able to express the level of intimacy that they valued.

He could drive for 45 minutes maximum before needing to break for 15 minutes. He was unable to participate in most leisure activities and could no longer help around the home (e.g. fix the car, mow the lawn). He had been unemployed for 3 years.

Mr JD suffered severe levels of pain that interfered significantly with his ability to perform normal daily functions, as well as his ability to perform self-care tasks, work and socialize.

It is generally agreed that for many patients with chronic non-cancer pain, multidisciplinary pain management is the preferred healthcare approach. A truly multidisciplinary approach is required, where the team works cooperatively with the patient to assist them to improve their functioning and quality of life.

Staff working in such a facility should be skilful and up-to-date in their respective disciplines, be dedicated and committed to the job, be aware of self and open to patients and their unique problems, be competent communicators, be able to explain concepts clearly to patients, and be able to gain the patient's trust (Schaefer 1985). Such are the hallmarks of a good therapist.

Frequently seen chronic pain conditions

There are a number of chronic pain conditions that occupational therapists and physiotherapists will frequently see, including back pain and other forms of musculoskeletal pain. There are also a number of chronic pain conditions that are less widely seen by occupational therapists and physiotherapists, but which need to be clearly recognized and correctly managed, such as complex regional pain syndrome (CRPS) Type I and phantom pain.

The incidence of chronic pain in the community has been reported as ranging from 16–82% (Brattberg et al 1989, Croft et al 1993, Crook et al 1984, Cunningham & Kelsey 1984, Jacobsson et al 1989, James et al 1991). The cost of chronic pain in the USA is 20–50 billion dollars annually (Wilson 1996). Many of these conditions have been described in previous chapters.

Sole-practitioner or multidisciplinary management

A question that should arise is when a client with chronic pain should be referred on for multidisciplinary pain rehabilitation. Not all clients need to be referred on for management by multidisciplinary pain clinics. Conversely, not all clients should be managed by a solo health professional.

Various researchers have developed screening tools, and the identification of 'red flags' or 'yellow flags' (see Kendall et al 1997, Waddell et al 1984). Physiotherapists and occupational therapists need to carefully integrate their assessment data and look for inconsistencies, or pointers to more complex issues. The following may be useful indicators of the need for referral on, or more comprehensive management for clients:

- If a client reports a particular location of pain with particular qualitative features, and this seems incompatible with reported functional limitations.
- If the client appears to have magnified illness behaviour. Waddell et al (1984) used this term to describe the presentation of a number of inappropriate symptoms and signs in clients with low back pain, including tail-bone pain, whole leg pain, whole leg numbness, whole leg giving way, no pain-free periods, intolerance to treatments, and hospital emergency admissions, superficial tenderness, tenderness in non-anatomical areas, axial loading, simulated rotation, straight leg raising when distracted, regional weakness, and over-reaction to examination.
- If the client reports multiple problems arising from the pain in multiple domains, for example, interfering with work performance, simple activities of daily living and intimacy (such as in the case of Mr JD reported in Box 20.3).
- If therapy is not resulting in expected functional gains.
- If the client appears to make gains in therapy, but then plateaus (see Box 20.4).
- If the client reports being overwhelmed by it all. Living with chronic disability can place enormous stress upon an individual. The incidence of depression in people with pain is around 10–30%. The risk of suicide is a real one, and therapists need to be aware of this when working with clients with chronic pain. Immediate referral on may be required. The issues of depression and suicide are covered in more detail in Chapter 22.
- If the client develops a post-traumatic stress disorder. The case outlined in Box 20.5 is illustrative of a client with neck pain who would require referral on if seen in a physiotherapy practice.

Having successfully determined who may best be managed by a multidisciplinary pain management programme rather than by a single health professional, there may still be issues with the client's readiness to accept a rehabilitative multidisciplinary pain programme.

While all clients want to be pain-free (Large & Strong 1997), some accept this ideal may not become reality and begin to work hard on rehabilitation. Others still hold out for the complete cure, and are resistant to rehabilitation. Given the resourcing issues and long waiting lists which can exist for admission to some pain clinics, is there some way of determining which clients should be referred on? Whether or not clients are ready to undergo a rehabilitative approach can be a useful thing to determine.

Box 20.4   Case example – Mrs AS

Presentation

Mrs AS is a 52-year-old woman who presented to physiotherapy for treatment of her persistent back and left leg pain. She undertakes home duties and is in good general health, with the exception of her constant back and leg pain. She has three married children and one grandchild. Both her and her husband's recreational passion is playing golf.

History

Mrs AS's back and leg pain began gradually 6 years ago, while she and her husband were living overseas. Six months previously she had fallen down some stairs and landed heavily on her left buttock, but suffered no immediate symptoms. However, she could recall no other incident that may have caused her pain syndrome. The burning pain in the lateral lower leg was, and continues to be, the worst feature but she also suffered associated left buttock and groin pain. The leg pain increased markedly over the next few weeks to a severe level. She had 'every investigation and treatment known' over the next 2 years including medication, facet joint injections, manipulative therapy to her low back and sacroiliac joint, TENS and acupuncture. Nothing substantially changed her leg pain.

She gave up seeking treatment and resolved to living with the pain, attempting not to let it stop her from doing normal physical activity.

Mrs AS and her husband returned to Australia approximately 2 years ago. Once settled, she decided to gradually increase her physical activity level and returned to golf. Her leg pain increased and again she felt that she should not have to live with the level of pain and sought medical advice.

She was referred to a rheumatologist, who consistent with others, diagnosed her pathology as an L5 nerve root problem. X-rays showed some osteoarthroses in the left L4–5, L5–S1 zygapophyseal joints. The rheumatologist referred her for a trial of physiotherapy management.

Mrs AS consulted a physiotherapy colleague. Manual therapy treatment was directed towards the left L4–5 zygapophyseal joint and the joint/neural interface and an active joint stabilization programme was undertaken. The pain did reduce over a 3-month period with the treatment and the specific exercises but improvement then plateaued.

As the patient had been encouraged by the pain-relief to date, she was hopeful of further improvement and in consequence, the physiotherapist referred her on for a second physiotherapy opinion and treatment if deemed appropriate.

Box 20.5   Case example – Mr BF

Mr BF was a 32-year-old man who was seriously injured as the result of a car accident. He had been a passenger in the car, which was being driven by a workmate after a staff barbecue. He had clear recall of the entire accident, which had resulted in chest injuries and a fractured femur. He also had severe neck pain that was overlooked by the hospital staff because of the seriousness of his chest injuries.

He had daily physiotherapy to clear his chest, and began dreading this because of the excruciating neck pain he experienced at each treatment. Some days later, he was noted to have a cervical vertebral fracture and was put in a neck brace. On referral to the pain clinic 3 years later, he had ongoing neck pain and had been unable to return to work. His chest and leg injuries had healed and were pain-free.

Psychiatric assessment revealed frequent intrusive memories in which he had vivid recollections of the accident, but more especially of the initial days in hospital and the regular chest physiotherapy. He tried to put the face of the physiotherapist out of his mind, but could not. He had regular nightmares about this, often waking from sleep sweating and screaming in panic and pain.

He was overtly anxious, sweaty, easily startled and at times a little vague and disconnected, as if preoccupied. He had the classical presentation of a post-traumatic stress disorder and was strongly kinesiophobic and afraid to move his neck in particular.

Treatment involved the use of a serotonin-specific re-uptake inhibitor antidepressant medication to reduce his anxiety and to treat the incidental depression. He was enrolled in a pain management programme, and gradually gained confidence about moving his neck. He also underwent a specific deconditioning programme for his intrusive memories using hypnotic imagery and EMDR (eye-movement desensitization and reprogramming).

Kerns and colleagues (1997, 2000) have described the Pain Stages of Change Questionnaire (PSOCQ), which looks at the readiness of clients to adopt a self-management approach to dealing with their pain. The PSOCQ is a 30-item, self-report questionnaire de-signed to assess a client's readiness to take up a self-management approach to pain (Kerns et al 1997). Preliminary data are available supporting the stability and reliability of the PSOCQ. This might be a useful tool for therapists.

Thorough assessment of the client

It was established in Chapter 7 that occupational therapists and physiotherapists need to undertake a comprehensive assessment of the client's pain. A framework was provided for such assessment, whereby the therapist assesses the description of the pain, the impact of the pain, and the client's response to the pain. The case example in Box 20.6 illustrates a thorough assessment of the pain of a client referred to an occupational therapist for a medicolegal assessment.

Mendelson and Mendelson (1997) have argued the need for a comprehensive assessment of every client with pain problems, irrespective of the presence or absence of compensation or litigation issues.

Establishing effective working relationships with clients

It is important for occupational therapists and physiotherapists to remember that pain is what the client says it is. For this reason, it is crucial for therapists to listen carefully to what their clients may be telling them. It may be that when clients with chronic pain attend your rooms or clinic, they have a history of less-than-satisfactory sequential visits to various health professionals. They may be angry, upset, despairing, questioning, desperate, demanding. Try to be empathetic. Remember the nocebo effect from failed treatments described in Chapter 5, and conversely, the power of human-response analgesia. Put yourselves for a moment in their shoes; how would you be feeling, thinking or acting if this was you or your loved one. Then, empathy can be easier to develop and transmit.

Of course, occupational therapists and physiotherapists must, at all times, be professional and ethical in their dealings with clients. Do not get caught up in taking sides, or denigrating the care or opinion of others. Do be respectful of the client's opinion, and do listen to their story.

People with pain who are clients are often described as 'challenging'. Accept the challenge, and you can learn greatly. If you find that a particular client is very difficult (or that you have difficulties working effectively with that client), speak with your supervisor or consult a colleague. Recognize the boundaries of your own level of competence, and seek additional resources or refer on, when in doubt.

Involve the client as an active agent in their rehabilitation

An important principle in working with clients with chronic pain is to empower the clients to be actively and personally responsible agents in their own rehabilitation process. A shift needs to occur from the acute intervention model of 'passive self-powerful other' to the rehabilitation model of 'active self-partner with other'. This key theme of clients taking charge of their own lives has been endorsed in studies of successful copers (Large & Strong 1997, Strong & Large 1995).

Keep abreast of research findings and evidence-based practice

At this point in time, for some clients with chronic pain, it will not be possible to cure their pain. Given the rate with which our knowledge and understanding of pain science is advancing, we as therapists need to keep informed about new knowledge, new procedures, and new techniques which can help our clients. At the present time, though, we will have clients who will continue to have chronic pain to some degree. We need to work collaboratively with each client to help them improve their functioning and their quality of life.

We need to remember that many of these clients may have been faced with previous disadvantages in life, and may need much support to develop new and more adaptive skills. This issue is discussed more in Chapter 22.

CONCLUSION

In this chapter, an examination has been made of the phenomenon of chronic pain. A distinction was made between the problems faced by someone with persistent pain, which may be successfully managed by a single health professional, and the problems faced by someone with a chronic pain syndrome.

People with a chronic pain syndrome are faced with multiple problems that impact upon their lives in many ways. It was the vision of pioneers such as John Bonica and the other founding members of the International Association for the Study of Pain that management of such patients should be multidisciplinary.

The vexing question as to why some people with persisting pain can manage and some people with pain develop a chronic pain syndrome has yet to be answered. A number of hypotheses have been raised to answer this question, including the use of inappropriate treatment behaviour by health professionals, the presence of pre-existing physical and or sexual abuse, the existence of psychological factors, work-related factors or medicolegal factors. For the moment though, the answers are not clear.

Consideration was given to the question of which clients should be seen in multidisciplinary clinics. Such a decision needs to be predicated on the basis of a careful and comprehensive assessment of each client.

Box 20.6   Case example – Mr SD

Presentation

Mr SD is a 24-year-old man who was referred to an occupational therapist by lawyers for medicolegal assessment. He had sustained a work injury 8 months previously, resulting in alleged injuries to his neck, mid-back and right arm.

History

Mr SD reported that he sustained neck, mid-back and right arm injuries as a result of an accident at work 8 months prior to assessment. He reported that he fell forward, while walking in between carriages, on a train. At the time, he was a Cleaning Supervisor on the train. He recalls that he grabbed onto the side-rails with his right arm, was electrocuted, and could not release the rails for a few moments as a result. He recollects that he stumbled up, when the emergency brakes on the train activated. He recalls smoke in the platform and cabin areas at the time of his accident.

At the time of the accident, Mr SD recalled being disorientated and in shock. He reported that his right arm was 'twitching uncontrollably' and was blackened and chafed. He recalled that he had a headache. An ambulance was called. He stated that there was a delay in the arrival of the ambulance officers, due to authorization problems about entering the railway yard/tracks, due to concerns about electrical exposure. He explained that he must have lost consciousness from the pain as he awoke in a wheelchair at the hospital. He was assessed for a few hours and then driven home by his boss.

Mr SD reported that he then rested for the next 2 weeks. His right arm was painful and continued to 'spasm' and stiffen-up regularly. He consulted his General Practitioner, a Neurologist, an Orthopaedic Specialist and a Psychologist. He explained that he has spent the majority of the time resting since the alleged injury, to allow his right arm to recuperate. Mr SD reported a previous injury to his right arm and neck from a lifting incident at work 2 years prior to the current injury. At that time he was working as a banana picker. He reported that after physiotherapy treatment the problem resolved.

Vocational history

Mr SD completed his secondary education to year eleven. He has worked in a variety of occupations since then, including as a cleaning supervisor, general labourer, banana picker, service station console operator and furniture removalist. His most recent occupation was as a cleaning supervisor.

The physical characteristics of this job were described as prolonged standing, bending, twisting, lifting and carrying to clean the trains. He was required to carry a vacuum pack on his back. There was a small amount of administrative, tendering and delivery work. He attempted to return to work some 2 weeks after the accident but experienced difficulty with his right upper limb and neck. His employer was apparently not able to offer any alternate or suitable duties.

The classifications and the physical strength ratings of the above occupations in the Dictionary of Occupational Titles United States Department of Labor 1991 are as follows:

- Industrial cleaner, classification 381.687.014, strength rating 'heavy'
- General labourer, classification 869.281.014, strength rating 'medium'
- Banana picker, classification 929.687.010, strength rating 'medium'
- Console operator, classification 953.362.010, strength rating 'light'
- Furniture removalist, classification 905.687.014, strength rating 'very heavy'.

Assessment

In order to confirm Mr SD's reports of his functional tolerances, and to better understand how his functional limitations impact upon his ability to work, the Spinal Function Sort (Matheson et al 1993) was administered. His responses to the reliability check items on this instrument indicated that he performed the test reliably. His profile indicated a perception of restriction with any tasks that involved prolonged bending, jarring, and handling over 25 kg. His Rating of Perceived Capacity (RPC) was 128. This RPC also corresponds to the United States Department of Labor (1991) 'light' range of physical capacities.

Mr SD completed the Pain Disability Index (Tait et al 1990). The scores obtained (1 being no disability and 10 total disability) are shown in Table 20.1.

Table 20.1   Mr SD's Pain Disability Index scores

Category	Score	Difficulty(s) experienced
Family and home responsibilities	5/10	Chores around the home and carrying his young son
Recreation	8/10	Sketching, touch football and indoor cricket
Social activity	3/10	Outings with family and friends
Occupation	10/10	Unable to work as industrial cleaner
Sexual behaviour	7/10	Reduced frequency due to distraction of pain
Self-care	2/10	Driving and looking over right shoulder
Life-support activity	4/10	No more than two hours sleep continuously

Box 20.6 (Continued)

Mr SD reported that his neck, mid-back, and right forearm and wrist were constantly sore. Aggravating factors identified were the cold, sleeping on his right arm, sudden forceful movement, squatting, bending his spine and head forward, and heavy impact to his right forearm. He completed the McGill Pain Questionnaire (Melzack 1975), and endorsed the following six adjectives: throbbing, heavy, tight, exhausting, unbearable and nagging.

Mr SD indicated those area(s) where he experiences pain on the pain drawings, shown in Figure 20.2.

Figure 20.2 Mr SD's pain drawings.

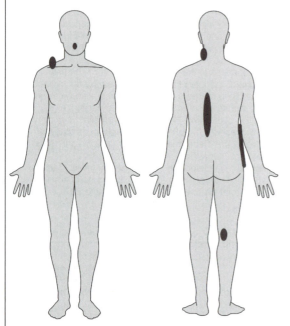

On a Horizontal Visual Analogue Scale (1 being no pain and 10 excruciating pain) Mr SD rated his pain as a constant 3.5 out of 10. It rose to 9 out of 10 when aggravated. He stated that he manages his pain best by having a hot shower, elevating his right arm, stretching his right arm, consuming anti-inflammatory medication and slowing his movements down.

Mr SD had full active range of motion of limbs and trunk. He had mild muscle tightness and weakness over his right wrist and forearm flexors (front of forearm and arm musculature), and right hamstrings (rear thighs). There was generalized reduced sensation over his right upper limb.

Mr SD favoured his right leg during functional transfers and movement. He had demonstrable difficulty squatting through to full range and transferring from a standing to kneeling position. He was able to weight-bear through his right arm in crawling kneeling. He had difficulty manually handling loads over 15 kg. He was limited to handling loads less than 7 kg with his right hand.

Mr SD is right-handed for all tasks. Right grip-strength was considerably reduced when compared to the left using the Jamar Dynamometer.

Social situation and activities of daily living
Mr SD lived with his wife, 15-month-old daughter, and work boss in a four-bedroom home. He experienced difficulties with self-care activities of daily living for a 3-month period after his neck and right-arm injuries. The Modified Barthel Index (MBI) was used as a guide to gauge his level of self-care skills during this time. This yielded a score of 92 out of 100, which represents a level of minimal dependence.

Mr SD described having an active life before the accident, having participated in various physical activities including football and indoor cricket. He reported that he continues to experience difficulty with these activities. Mr SD reported that he had to rely on his wife to assist him with domestic chores for a 3-month period after his accident. He estimated that this equated to some 3 hours per week.

He identified that most physical activity would present some difficulty and increase his pain. He currently favoured his right arm with all activities of daily living. He identified a phobia with most things of stainless steel quality and electrical in nature. He also reported that he has also been easily stressed and bad-tempered towards his wife and family recently.

Comprehensive examination of a patient such as Mr SD would also include detailed evaluation of all joint structures in the upper quadrant, evaluation of muscle function and thorough examination of the upper quadrant using neural-tissue provocation tests.

Study questions/questions for revision

1. Compare and contrast the effect of acute vs chronic pain on the client, and the management approach adopted.
2. Describe the psychosocial complications of chronic pain and how these can influence the presentation and management of the client.
3. Describe the characteristics of a client's presentation that would indicate that a client needed to be referred on to a multidisciplinary pain clinic.
4. What are some of the factors thought to be influential in the development of chronic pain conditions?
5. What are the characteristics of people living successfully in the community with chronic pain problems?

ACKNOWLEDGEMENTS

Sincere thanks are extended to Associate Professor Gwendolen Jull, Helen Rowe, Steve Hoey, Dr Frank New and Dr Bob Large for material used in this chapter.

REFERENCES

Bonica J J 1984 Pain research and therapy: recent advances and future needs. In: Kruger L, Liebeskind J C (eds) Advances in Pain Research and Therapy, Vol 6. Neural Mechanisms of Pain. Raven Press, New York, pp 1–22

Brattberg G, Thorslund M, Wikman A 1989 The prevalence of pain in a general population: the results of a postal survey in a county of Sweden. Pain 37: 215–222

Burns J W, Sherman M L, Devine J, Mahoney N, Pawl R 1995 Association between workers' compensation and outcome following multidisciplinary treatment for chronic pain: roles of mediators and moderators. Clinical Journal of Pain 11: 94–102

Ciccone D S, Bandilla E B, Wu W 1997 Psychological dysfunction in patients with reflex sympathetic dystrophy. Pain 71: 323–333

Craig C D 1994 Emotional aspects of pain. In: Wall P D, Melzack R (eds) Textbook of Pain, 3rd Edn. Churchill Livingstone, Edinburgh, pp 261–274

Croft P, Rigby A S, Boswell R, Schollum J, Silman A 1993 The prevalence of chronic widespread pain in the general population. Journal of Rheumatology 20: 710–713

Crook J, Rideout E, Browne G 1984 The prevalence of pain complaints in a general population. Pain 18: 299–314

Crue B L Jr 1985 Multidisciplinary pain treatment programs: current status. Clinical Journal of Pain 1: 31–38

Cunningham L S, Kelsey J L 1984 Epidemiology of musculoskeletal impairments and associated disability. American Journal of Public Health 74: 574–579

Fishbain D A, Rosomoff H L, Goldberg M, Cutler R, AbdelMoty E, Khalil T M, Rosomoff R S 1993 The prediction of return to the workforce after multidisciplinary pain center treatment. Clinical Journal of Pain 9: 3–15

Goldberg R T, Pachas W N, Keith D 1999 Relationship between traumatic events in childhood and chronic pain. Disability and Rehabilitation 21: 23–30

Hartman L M, Ainsworth K D 1980 Self-regulation of chronic pain. Canadian Journal of Psychiatry 25: 38–43

Jacobsson L, Lindgarde F, Manthorpe R 1989 The commonest rheumatic complaints over six weeks' duration in a twelve-month period in a defined Swedish population. Scandinavian Journal of Rheumatology 18: 353–360

James F R, Large R G, Bushnell J A, Wells J E 1991 Epidemiology of pain in New Zealand. Pain 44: 279–283

Kelly G 1963 A Theory of Personality: the psychology of personal constructs. WW Norton & Co, New York

Kendall N A S, Linton S J, Main C J 1997 Guide to assessing psychosocial yellow flags in acute low back pain: risk factors for long-term disability and work loss. Accident Rehabilitation & Compensation Insurance Corporation of New Zealand and the National Health Committee, Wellington NZ

Kerns R D, Rosenberg R 2000 Predicting responses to self-management treatments for chronic pain: application of the pain stages of change model. Pain 84: 49–55

Kerns R D, Rosenberg R, Jamison R N, Caudill M A, Haythornthwaite J 1997 Readiness to adopt a self-management approach to chronic pain: the Pain Stages of Change Questionnaire (PSOCQ). Pain 72: 227–234

Klapow J C, Slater M A, Patterson T L, Doctor J N, Atkinson J H, Garfin S R 1993 An empirical evaluation of multidimensional clinical outcome in chronic low back pain patients. Pain 55: 107–118

Large R G, Strong J 1997 The personal constructs of coping with chronic low back pain: is coping a necessary evil? Pain 73: 245–252

Loeser J D 1991 Desirable characteristics for pain treatment facilities: report of the IASP taskforce. In: Bond M R, Charlton J E, Woolf C J (eds) Proceedings of the VIth World Congress on Pain. Elsevier, Amsterdam, pp 411–415

Loeser J D 1994 Obituary. Pain 59: 1–3

Loeser J D, Sullivan M 1995 Disability in the chronic low back pain patient may be iatrogenic. Pain Forum 4: 114–121

Main C J, Watson P J 1995 Screening for patients at risk of developing chronic incapacity. Journal of Occupational Rehabilitation 5: 207–217

Melzack R 1975 The McGill Pain Questionnaire: major properties and scoring methods. Pain 1: 277–299

Melzack R, Wall P D 1982 The Challenges of Pain. Penguin Books, Harmondsworth

Merskey H (ed) 1986 Classification of chronic pain. Descriptions of chronic pain syndromes and definitions of pain terms. Pain 24: S1–S211

Mendelson G, Mendelson D 1997 Medicolegal aspects of pain management. Pain Reviews 4: 244–274

Pinsky J J, Griffin S E, Agnew D C, Kamdar M D, Crue B L, Pinsky L H 1979 Aspects of long-term evaluation of pain unit treatment programs for patients with chronic intractable benign pain syndrome: treatment outcome. Bulletin of the Los Angeles Neurological Society 44: 53–69

Pither C E, Nicholas M K 1991 The identification of iatrogenic factors in the development of chronic pain syndromes: abnormal treatment behaviour? In: Bond M R, Charlton J E, Woolf C J (eds) Proceedings of the VIth World Congress on Pain. Elsevier, Amsterdam, pp 429–434

Polatin P B, Mayer T G 1996 Occupational disorders and the management of chronic pain. Orthopedic Clinics of North America 27: 881–890

Rainville J, Bagnall D, Phalen L 1995 Health care providers' attitudes and beliefs about functional impairments and chronic back pain. Clinical Journal of Pain 11: 298–295

Rapkin A J, Kames L D, Darke L L, Stampler F M, Naliboff B D 1990 History of physical and sexual abuse in women with chronic pelvic pain. Obstetrics and Gynecology 76: 92–96

Reitsma B, Meijler W J 1997 Pain and patienthood. Clinical Journal of Pain 13: 9–21

Rey R 1993 History of Pain. Editions la Decouverte, Paris

Roberts M T S 1983 Pain relief clinics. Patient Management 7: 25–32

Roy R 1984 Pain clinics: reassessment of objectives and outcomes. Archives of Physical Medicine and Rehabilitation 65: 448–451

Sanders S H 1994 An image problem for pain centers: relevant factors and possible solutions. American Pain Society Bulletin Jan/Feb: 17–18

Sanders S H, Brena S F 1993 Empirically derived chronic pain patient subgroups: the utility of multidimensional clustering to identify differential treatment effects. Pain 54: 51–56

Schaefer C A 1985 The pain clinic approach. In: Michel T H (ed) The Pain Clinic. Churchill Livingstone, Edinburgh, pp 233–258

Sternbach R A 1974 Pain Patients: traits and treatment. Academic Press, New York

Strong 1989 The occupational therapist's contribution to the management of chronic pain. Patient Management 13: 43–50

Strong J 1992 Chronic low back pain: towards an integrated psychosocial assessment model. Unpublished PhD thesis, Department of Psychology, The University of Queensland

Strong J, Large R G 1995 Coping with chronic low back pain: an idiographic exploration through focus groups. International Journal of Psychiatry in Medicine 25: 361–377

Strong J, Ashton R, Stewart A 1994 Chronic low back pain: an integrated psychosocial assessment model. Journal of Consulting and Clinical Psychology 62: 1058–1063

Sullivan M D, Turner J A, Romano J 1991 Chronic pain in primary care. Journal of Family Practice 32: 193–199

Tait R, Chibnall J, Krause S 1990 The Pain Disability Index: psychometric properties. Pain 40: 171–182

Talo S 1992 Psychological assessment of functioning in chronic low back pain patients. Turku Social Insurance Institution Finland Publications, Turku

Toomey T C, Seville J L, Mann D, Abashian S W, Grant J R 1995 Relationship of sexual and physical abuse to pain description, coping, psychological distress, and health-care utilization in a chronic pain sample. Clinical Journal of Pain 11: 307–315

Turk D C, Melzack R 1992 (eds) Handbook of Pain Assessment. New York, Guilford Press

Turk D C, Rudy T E 1988 Toward an empirically derived taxonomy of chronic pain patients: integration of psychological assessment data. Journal of Consulting and Clinical Psychology 56: 233–238

Turk D C, Rudy T E 1990 The robustness of an empirically derived taxonomy of chronic pain patients. Pain 43: 27–35

United States Department of Labor 1991 Dictionary of Occupational Titles, 4th Edn. United States Department of Labor, Washington

Waddell G, Main C J, Morris E W, DiPaola M, Gray I C M 1984 Chronic low-back pain, psychologic distress, and illness behavior. Spine 9: 209–213

Williams M, Read J, Large R 1999 Child abuse and dissociation in patients with complex regional pain syndrome. Pain Research Management 4: 15–22

Wilson P R 1996 Multidisciplinary . . . transdisciplinary . . . Monodisciplinary . . . where are we going? Clinical Journal of Pain 12: 253–254

Zitman F G, Linssen A C G, Van H R L 1992 Chronic pain beyond patienthood. Journal Nervous Mental Disease 180: 97–1000

21

Cancer pain

Jenny Strong   Sally Bennett

OVERVIEW

Beyond the physical disfigurement and emotional ravages of advanced malignancy, it is the pain of cancer that is most dreaded. (Tigges et al 1984)

Pain is one of the biggest fears of, and a major source of morbidity for, patients with cancer. (Walsh 1991 p 133)

The management of cancer-related pain differs from that of chronic pain of non-cancer origin in many ways. With cancer pain, the intensity or amount is not static. The location and the quality of the pain are more likely to change because of the illness and the treatment. The person with cancer may have multiple pain problems and interrelated symptoms that complicate management.

The meaning of changes in the pain may be more frightening and this fear can exacerbate the experience of pain. Analgesia, surgery and radiotherapy (see Box 21.1) will play a more significant role in the pain-management regime. Therefore, while there are many similarities in management programmes for chronic pain and cancer pain, there are elements that must be considered differently.

Cancer has many personal and/or idiosyncratic emotional and lifestyle ramifications. Working in this area requires therapists to be both sensitive and well prepared in order to work with patients who have cancer pain. To achieve tactful and professional interaction with patients, therapists need to become aware of their own beliefs and values in relation to cancer, to pain, and to death.

Emotional care of the patient is critical in a pain-management programme for patients with cancer. Pain which is not relieved may affect the patient's wellbeing in physical, social, psychological and spiritual ways.

In this chapter, particular pain problems faced by patients with cancer will be outlined, and goals for therapy articulated. The difference in philosophy of pain management for patients with cancer pain

---

Box 21.1 Key terms defined

Adjuvant analgesia – Provided by an agent that is not primarily an analgesic, but has some analgesic properties or enhances the analgesic performance of a primary analgesic.

Palliative care – Any procedure which is performed primarily to provide symptom relief rather than to affect the primary illness. Palliative care is defined by the World Health Organization (WHO) (1990) as 'the active total care of patients whose disease is not responsive to curative treatment'. It includes the physical, psychosocial and spiritual care of patients and support of their families and caregivers (Higginson 1999).

Ventriculostomy – A procedure where a small morphine reservoir is inserted into the lateral cerebral ventricle. This procedure is useful for patients with cancer pain due to head or neck cancer, or those patients with bilateral, midline or diffuse cancer pain (Cramond & Stuart 1993).

Percutaneous cordotomy – A procedure performed to ablate the spinothalamic tract at C1–C2. It is done under local anaesthesia with a thermal coagulation probe. Immediate pain relief is achieved in most

patients, but pain may return in 6 months in half these patients. This procedure can be useful for patients experiencing unilateral cancer pain below the head and neck (Stuart & Cramond 1993).

Radiotherapy – A procedure whereby radiation is used to destroy tumour cells. Radiotherapy may reduce pain by decreasing the tumour's pressure effect on nerves, limiting a tumour's infiltration, and resolving tumour inflammation (Monfardini & Scanni 1987). It is also used to help with well-localized pain due to bony metastases (Janjan 1997).

Chemotherapy – Involves the administration of cytotoxic drugs with the aim of interfering with tumour-cell division. It can relieve pain due to tumour effects such as tissue destruction, enlargement of viscera, and pressure or obstruction. Due to its systemic effects, it is most helpful for relieving pain associated with diffuse metastases in chemo-sensitive tumours (Monfardini & Scanni 1987). Chemotherapy may provide palliation even when there is no survival benefit, in circumstances where the trade-off between symptom reduction and toxicity favours symptom relief (Archer et al 1999).

---

compared to those clients with non-cancer pain will be described. Interventions for both the active treatment and palliation phases will be considered, with an emphasis on palliative-care pain management.

While many different sources of information have been used for this chapter, it is worth noting that a document entitled 'Management of Cancer Pain. Clinical Practice Guideline No. 9', produced by the Agency for Health Care Policy and Research in the USA (Jacox et al 1994), is a useful collation. A more recent report is the 2001 Evidence Report on Management of Cancer Pain.

Learning Objectives

At the completion of this chapter, readers will have an understanding of:

1. The frequency with which pain can occur in people with cancer.
2. The types of pain problems that may occur.
3. The barriers to adequate pain management.
4. The necessity of thorough, frequent but not burdensome pain assessment.
5. The current approaches to pain management.
6. The issues facing practitioners when working with patients with cancer.

INCIDENCE OF PAIN IN PEOPLE WITH CANCER

The fear of pain is a major concern for people being diagnosed with cancer. An examination of the incidence of pain in cancer, and the effectiveness of pain management for people with cancer, suggests that such a fear is not ungrounded.

Moderate to severe pain has been found to occur in 40–50% of patients with early or intermediate stage cancer. For patients with advanced cancer, the incidence of pain is 60–90% (Walsh 1991). Between 25–80% of patients with cancer pain do not receive adequate pain management (Coluzzi 1996, Ferrell et al 1995, Walsh 1991). The World Health Organization (WHO) estimated that around 4 million people were suffering from cancer pain with poor or no relief (Takeda 1991).

As therapists, such knowledge should fuel our resolve to make a contribution to good pain management for patients with cancer. It is not unlikely that many therapists will have had some personal experience of someone dying a painful death with cancer.

DESCRIPTION OF CANCER PAIN

Cancer pain may be long-standing, of more than 3 months' duration, and so has many chronic pain features. It also changes according to tumour-growth damage to tissues, and to the impact of some treatments, and so has acute pain features (Foley 1987). Therefore, cancer pain is in a category of its own when pain syndromes are considered; therapists must be alert to the need to constantly re-evaluate pain status and interventions.

There are three types of pain which may arise for patients with cancer: pain that is secondary to tumour growth and invasion of structures (about 75%); pain that results from treatment of the cancer (about 20%); and pain not associated with the tumour or the treatment (about 5%) (Driscoll 1987).

It is not uncommon for patients with cancer to have a reduced pain threshold with increased sensitivity to other types and sources of pain (Klein 1983). Cancer pain may also be considered as nociceptive or neuropathic (Cherny & Portenoy 1994). Nociceptive pain can be due to somatic or visceral lesions. Somatic pain is usually constant, localized and aching. Visceral pain is also constant and aching, but is poorly localized and may be referred.

Neuropathic pain is due to some abnormal events in the peripheral nervous system or the central nervous system (Cherny & Portenoy 1994). Deafferentation pain may be paroxysmal or burning, and is both difficult to treat and distressing for patients. Some understanding of these different types of pain will help a therapist to be more supportive of, and empathic with, patients. These types of pain are also used as indicators by the physician in identifying the origin of the pain.

Foley (1987) also classified cancer pain by 'patient type'. Her classification can be a useful way to order and conceptualize thoughts about pain. The five types of patients are:

1. Patients with acute pain associated with the cancer or the treatment. Acute pain associated with the cancer heralds the onset or recurrence of the illness, bringing with it associated psychological ramifications. In contrast, acute pain associated with treatment is self-limiting and pain tolerance is often high while the patient is hopeful about outcome, and consequently psychological effects may be limited. In both cases treatment needs to be targeted at the cause of pain.

2. Patients with chronic pain, either from the cancer or the therapy. Chronic pain associated with cancer reflects tumour progression and psychological issues become much more important for these patients. Anxiety and feelings of hopelessness can further exacerbate the pain. Chronic pain may also be due to soft-tissue, nerve or bony injury related to cancer

treatment and be unrelated to the tumour. Identifying this group is important in order to reassure the patient that the pain is not caused by their cancer. Treatment of patients with chronic pain is aimed at the symptom rather than the cause.

3. Patients with chronic pain from another source, generally pre-existing. These patients often already have psychological and functional limitations and require considerable support as the presence of multiple illnesses is very taxing.

4. Patients with pain who are also actively involved with illicit drug use. These patients are very difficult to treat.

5. Patients who are dying and have cancer pain. The focus of treatment is on maximizing comfort and providing psychological care. The family must also be considered in caring for this group.

There are specific pain syndromes which occur in the patient with cancer. These syndromes are related to the type and site of the cancer. Portenoy & Lesage (1999), Foley (1987) and Klein (1983), among others, have provided descriptions of these syndromes, and, as they are outside the scope of this textbook, the reader is referred to these references.

As in all pain situations, it is inappropriate to think of cancer pain as just physical. In addition to physical pain, psychological concerns are probably universal in patients with cancer. Anxiety and depression may be manifest in sleep disturbance, fatigue and worry (Driscoll 1987). Driscoll (1987) also talks of social or environmental pain which may arise if factors in the patient's family and life-situation are such that they become lonely and isolated. Such factors need attention and should be considered in the assessment and management of cancer pain.

Therapists need to take into account the complexity and changing nature of cancer pain. Pain management approaches vary depending on the site of pain, chronicity of pain, characteristics of the individual patient and the stage of disease. Therapists may modify their pain-management approaches according to whether the patient is in active treatment, with the likelihood of recovery, or whether the patient is dying and receiving palliative care. There are different management procedures for treatment and palliation phases. Careful assessment and flexibility in management are vital.

RESPONSES TO CANCER PAIN

Cancer pain customarily leads to some or all of the following effects: decreased quality of life, anger, frustration, decreased food intake (and therefore a poor performance status), and stress on relatives and friends. In turn, these factors can aggravate pain.

Responses to pain associated with having cancer will be modulated by fear, anxiety, depression, and sociocultural factors. Pain associated with malignancy is a constant concern, but patients become more sensitive to it over time. This may be because of associated psychological and emotional influences.

In contemporary management regimes for cancer, many patients are cared for predominantly at home, and their pain management occurs at home. Therefore the patient and/or their family carers are often responsible for medication and other pain-reduction procedures. It has been found that patients are often under-medicated due to beliefs held by themselves and/or their caregivers that they should put up with pain as long as possible, and due to fear of addiction (Ferrell et al 1995, Yeager et al 1997). Responses to cancer pain therefore clearly relate in some part to attitudes and beliefs and knowledge of patients and carers. From reviewing literature, Austin et al (1986) found that if cancer pain was being managed for hospice home-care patients, the parameters of age, social support, living situation, primary cancer site and compliance needed consideration.

Pain from cancer may interfere more with enjoyment of life than pain from other causes (Daut & Cleeland 1982). Cancer pain has the added fear for the person that the disease is getting worse. This is important information for therapists interested in maintaining the highest quality of life possible for their clients. A diagnosis of cancer may lead to a feeling of loss of personal control. The experience of ongoing pain (among other things) may reduce the feeling of control still further. An understanding of this heightened sense of loss of control is important for the therapist to have when working with the person in pain from cancer.

ASSESSMENT AND MEASUREMENT OF CANCER PAIN

Readers are reminded to refer back to Chapter 7 of this book, which covered assessment and measurement issues in more depth. Coluzzi (1996) reported on findings by the American Society of Clinical Oncology that the primary deficiency in cancer pain management was inadequate assessment, which was in turn compounded by patients' reluctance to report pain. It seems that admitting to pain engenders fear about the extent of the illness and the possibility of lack of control. He suggested further that pain assessment should involve:

- A complete history of medical, psychosocial and spiritual aspects
- Pain history (sites, severity, duration, aggravating and relieving factors, mood, previous pain experience)
- Rating scales
- Physical examination
- Diagnostic testing (or review).

Assessment considerations

Assessment of cancer pain should be multi-dimensional and multi-disciplinary. Pain involves a complexity of sensory, cognitive, behavioural, and affective phenomena, requiring a coordinated assessment effort by different disciplines. The source of the pain can be identified by assessing the location, distribution, quality, intensity and duration. Comprehensive assessment of pain should also consider other symptoms that may interact with, and exacerbate pain, such as fatigue (Portenoy & Lesage 1999). Portenoy (1990) suggested that

Just as the impact of pain must be carefully judged in those who are clearly suffering, it is also axiomatic in the clinical management of cancer pain that the degree of suffering, and the factors contributing to it, must be evaluated as a part of comprehensive pain assessment.

It is therefore essential to accurately evaluate the patient's physical, social, and psychological function. This latter type of evaluation is of particular relevance to therapists.

Cleeland (1985) suggested that patients with cancer pain may have 'reporting biases' because cancer is an anxiety-provoking condition. They may fear that a change in pain means more than in other conditions, so there is a need to assess in a way to minimize bias. Clients may under-report their pain, due to a concern about not being a nuisance to ward staff or family members, or due to denial of the increasing seriousness of their condition. A new pain in a patient with cancer should always be investigated thoroughly. It may signal a treatable new problem or the exacerbation of an existing problem that requires re-assessment. A change in the patient's report of pain should be reported immediately to the treating physician, and other members of the team.

Cancer pain needs to be assessed frequently to fully understand changes in the pain and underlying influences, such as proximity to medication, physical activity, anxiety, or time of day (Cherny & Portenoy 1994). Time of day is important, because cancer pain is often worse in early evening, and better in early morning (Klein 1983).

Frequency of assessment will depend to some extent on the setting and type of pain. If the patient's pain is stable and they are being seen as an out-patient, pain can be monitored during appointments, or they can be asked to keep a diary. Patients should be given the opportunity to describe not only their pain at the moment, but also to give an overall picture of the pain at its worst and its best. In this way, the therapist is able to build-up a more complete understanding of the variability in the patient's pain.

The fluctuations in pain relative to various reference points, such as the time of day, medication status, activity level, or anticipation of some event, need to be charted. Patients with uncontrolled pain need frequent assessment. Pain should probably be assessed at least daily, and sometimes more often is necessary (Vallerand 1997).

The implications of this type of assessment regime are that the measurement tools need to be accurate, brief and comprehensive to avoid over-taxing the client. They also need to be appropriate for multiple evaluations and still be reliable, and must be practical for use with severely ill people (Ahles et al 1984).

The guidelines produced by the Agency for Health Care Policy and Research in the USA had as the first recommendation for assessment of cancer pain that 'the patient's self-report should be the primary source of assessment' (Jacox et al 1994). In order for this to be an effective policy to follow, the treatment ethic of the centre must encourage accuracy in patient self-report by acting on information provided by the patient and by providing sufficient education about the aspects of illness and its treatment so that the patient is unafraid to give information about their pain. Simply asking a question such as, 'How is your pain?' does not provide enough opportunity to fully describe it. Various tools which have been shown to be sensitive and reliable should be used (see Chapter 7).

Methods for assessing pain include the Visual Analogue Scale (VAS) and the McGill Pain Questionnaire (MPQ) which were described in Chapter 7. The VAS rates pain intensity and is short and easy to use. Its reliability has been established with patients with cancer. The MPQ is longer, but is multidimensional, and also has good psychometric properties. If the patient is especially ill or fatigued, the short-form MPQ can be used.

Jacox et al (1994) suggested that patients also be asked to describe their pain. The particular descriptive words used can give valuable clues about the cause of the pain. For example, pain described as burning or tingling is likely to involve neural structures.

Assessment of symptoms that may interact with pain may be achieved through symptom-specific measures, or through measures that assess multiple prevalent cancer-related symptoms such as the Memorial Symptom Assessment Scale (Portenoy et al 1994).

There are many approaches to the measurement of function and wider patient concerns. Disease-specific quality of life instruments are one way of ascertaining the interface between cancer pain, other symptoms and functioning. A number of measures of quality of life (QOL) for the patient with cancer have been developed which have acceptable psychometric properties. The Functional Assessment of Cancer Therapy Scale (FACT Scale) is a brief, 33-item, self-report measure of QOL over the past week. It covers physical wellbeing, social/family wellbeing, relationship with doctor, emotional wellbeing, and functional wellbeing (Cella et al 1993).

Another measure is the European Organization for Research and Treatment of Cancer QLQ-C30 (version 2.0) (Aaronson et al 1993, Osoba et al 1997). It consists of 30 items which tap the nine subscales of function (physical, role, cognitive, emotional and social), and associated cancer-related symptoms such as fatigue, pain, nausea and vomiting, and global health, and quality of life.

In general, in assessing a person's pain, a structured or semi-structured questionnaire format is preferable to interview, as it is more objective and reduces the number of details which can be inadvertently forgotten (Cleeland 1985). However, incorporating an interview can be valuable to foster a good working rapport with the patient and their family.

Impact of pain on the occupations of daily life

Pain from cancer can have an impact on an individual's occupations of daily life. Associated fatigue can also impair occupational performance. Patterns of activity, ability to perform functional activities of daily living, ability to meet desired occupational goals, quality of life and coping strategies should be assessed. The impact which the pain and the cancer has had on the person's ability to perform their daily life occupations should be a particular emphasis of the occupational therapist. Again, methods for assessing these features were reviewed in Chapter 7.

Aggravating and alleviating factors of the cancer pain need to be investigated by asking the patient and by observation. A patient's attitudes towards, and beliefs about, pain and taking medication need to be taken into consideration when attempting to gather a true understanding of the patient's level of pain. Therapists should be particularly attuned to the patient's desired occupational goals, and should work to enable patients to attain meaningful occupational goals that are within the capability of the patient.

Family context

The family context is another aspect to be considered. Family members may have many fears and beliefs about cancer, about the 'horribleness' of cancer pain, about the potential for addiction from medication, and about the ways they can best care for their loved one. This requires the careful attention of the treatment team.

For example, the family may be resolute in the need to care for their family member with advanced cancer within the home environment, despite seemingly major obstacles to such management. Both conscious and unconscious interactions between the patient and their family are relevant to the design and implementation of a pain management plan.

In the team, the professional responsibility for gathering information about family relationships and pain may vary. However, it is always necessary for the therapist to be at least aware of the details already gathered in designing their part of the intervention strategies.

INTERVENTION FOR CANCER PAIN

There are number of barriers to providing adequate pain management for patients with cancer. These include:

- The current prevalence of disease/outcome medical models that replaced older system/process models which viewed palliative care more importantly.
- A lack of recognition by health professionals that there are established methods for satisfactory pain management.
- The under-medication of pain.
- The lack of availability of essential drugs in many parts of the world.
- The continuation of the practice of giving analgesia on a prn rather than round-the-clock basis despite the fact that the latter is more effective.
- The lack of systematic training of health professional students in pain management.
- The continued concern of health professionals and patients about side-effects of medication (Coluzzi 1996, WHO 1986).

Fostering multidisciplinary approaches to research, education and training about cancer pain management is seen as central to overcoming some of these barriers (Bonica 1987, Pargeon & Hailey 1999).

Interventions for cancer pain can be broadly classified into five types: medication, non-pharmacological methods, behavioural and counselling approaches, education, and lifestyle adjustments.

In all situations where pain management is required by patients, a collaborative team approach is the preferred method of practice. Beyond this, it has been determined that supporting *active* patient involvement in their therapy is important. That is, patients or clients should be involved in decisions about treatment regimes, and timing of pain interventions around their lifestyle, as much as possible. Such active patient involvement is important, in part, in counteracting the feelings of loss of control.

Medication

While the management of medication regimes is the concern of physicians and nurses, knowledge of the commonly utilized drugs and methods of administration and mechanisms of action is important for therapists to understand. This knowledge can help the therapists to answer questions, to support a patient's understanding of the role of medication, and to structure their therapy around the most optimal times.

A therapist may realize that the patient is not taking the medication appropriately. Fear that addiction might occur or that medication should not be taken until the pain is severe, and other misunderstandings about pain medication may result in the patient receiving poor pain relief.

Therapists should clarify and redirect the patient to their physician if this is required. Therapists may also be more aware of whether the patient has side-effects, or if the medication is improving or hindering the client's occupational performance. Possible side-effects of medications such as opioids may impact upon the patient's safe performance of ADLs such as stairwalking or driving.

The World Health Organization (WHO) three-step analgesic ladder is the recognized standard for drug therapy for cancer pain. It involves the sequential use of non-opioid analgesics plus or minus adjuvant drugs, weak opioids plus or minus non-opiod drugs and adjuvant drugs, and strong opioids plus or minus non-opioid drugs and adjuvant drugs. The reader is referred back to Chapter 16 for a comprehensive consideration of pharmacological methods.

Coluzzi (1996) has provided an excellent review of the most current model of pain management in cancer care and terminal illness. He stresses the need for an 'around-the-clock' dose, and for diligent efforts to be made to select the right dose for each individual. The oral route is the preferred route of administration, and this is obviously best for patients being managed at home. Morphine is the drug of choice (Coluzzi 1996), and the use of slow-release morphine is often recommended for good blood levels and therefore continuous pain cover.

Newer products such as transdermal fentanyl patches, or sublingual products such as buprenorphine, are also available for patients who cannot effectively use the oral route (e.g. patients with colostomies). Alternatively, a continuous subcutaneous infusion of opioids using a portable tranfusion pump may be used.

Patients who are not able to benefit from systemic treatment may find relief from interspinal approaches or ventriculostomy (Portenoy & Lesagel 1999, Cramond & Stuart 1993). Advances in drug therapies are rapid, so therapists are advised to avail themselves of updates through continuing education programmes such as those run by local chapters of professional pain societies.

Non-pharmacological medical methods

Non-pharmacological medical methods may be used for patients in whom adequate relief of pain is not achieved by pharmacological methods. Methods used include radiation therapy, ablative surgery and neurosurgical procedures. An understanding of the reasons for performing these procedures, in the case of each individual patient, is the professional responsibility of the therapist.

Therapists may be involved in the post-procedural rehabilitation of the patient. For example, paraesthesia or dysaesthesia may sometimes occur in patients in whom the pain recurs after a percutaneous cordotomy. Physiotherapists and occupational therapists work with such patients to maximize independence, increase safety in activities of daily living, teach energy-conservation techniques, and work with clients on attaining valued occupational goals (Tigges & Marcil 1988).

Non-pharmacological physical methods

Other non-pharmacological physical methods which are non-invasive, and may be used by a therapist or supported by a therapist as the active choice by the patient, include acupuncture, cutaneous stimulation, cold therapy, heat, exercise, careful positioning, and immobilization. The reader is referred to Chapters 11 and 12 for more detail about these techniques.

Cutaneous stimulation and other types of counter-stimulation may offer relief to a patient at various times through the day, while providing a sense of control over the treatment for the patient. However an increase in the use of such methods initiated by patients should be carefully monitored in case it indicates that inadequate pain control by medication is being provided (Jacox et al 1994). These methods are not intended to replace pharmacological methods.

Cutaneous stimulation includes such methods as massage, pressure, heat, cold and transcutaneous electrical nerve stimulation (TENS). The stimulation may be applied to the painful area if the skin is not compromised. If the skin is not intact, application may be effectively given to the contralateral side of the body.

Psychosocial approaches

These approaches can range from being very sophisticated and requiring special training (such as hypnosis) to being relatively simple, within the expertise of a newly graduated therapist. Some approaches can be taught to the client for self-administration. Distraction, relaxation, guided imagery, music and cutaneous stimulation are some of the recommended methods (Mayer 1985). Relaxation, guided imagery, and systematic desensitization have been shown to reduce nausea and pain (Devine & Westlake 1995). Mindfulness meditation has been shown to be effective in helping to reduce mood disturbance in cancer outpatients (Carlson et al 2000). The reader is referred to Chapters 9 and 15 for earlier coverage of some of these techniques.

A variety of relaxation methods are available, such as progressive muscle relaxation (PMR), yoga and meditation. Guided imagery may be used alone or in conjunction with another relaxation technique. Therapists can train patients in PMR, so that they are able to use the relaxation method at any time needed. Ideally, patients need to be trained in PMR while they are pain-free, or have relatively low pain intensity, but while they are still able to concentrate. Sometimes it will not be possible to teach PMR if patients are concurrently taking analgesic medication. The development of proficiency in muscle relaxation while undistracted by moderate to severe pain will increase the likelihood that the technique will be used with positive result when pain intensity increases.

In similar fashion, the therapist can introduce the patient to guided imagery techniques which patients then have in their repertoire for use as required. Driscoll (1987) has suggested three categories of visual imagery. 'Imaginative transformation of the pain context' is a method where the pain is acknowledged, and then symbolically changed to another object (e.g. a bird) to leave the patient. 'Imaginative inattention' refers to creating a pleasant and relaxing setting in one's mind, with lots of sensory aspects to attend to, but no pain. 'Imaginative transformation' is a method where the patient recodes the pain sensation as something less noxious, such as a tingling or tickling feeling.

A caution must be sounded here. Although patients can become independent in using PMR and guided imagery, it is still valuable for the therapist to monitor use of the techniques, providing re-training and support as required. If such support is not given, the techniques may become ineffective, and the client may feel abandoned and discouraged.

People commonly use distraction in everyday life, often without thinking. It may seem that distraction would not require any particular skill. Any patient may have some methods he or she uses for distraction, which can be supplemented by suggestions from a repertoire of techniques offered by the therapist. Introducing a cognitive component to the use of distraction may be helpful. The patient can be encouraged to develop and elaborate a personal picture of their current use of distraction, and to problem-solve about its effectiveness and methods of possible change. McCaffery (1979) has given an excellent description of distraction as ' . . . a kind of sensory shielding, a protecting of oneself from the sensation by focusing on and increasing the clarity of sensations unrelated to pain'.

Some activities which are useful for distraction include rocking, singing, rhythmic breathing, listening to music, playing games, talking with a specific focus, e.g. to describe a picture (Mayer 1985). Distraction may be most effective when needed for relatively short periods (e.g. until medication works), or with the support of others who understand the real need for distraction.

Psychosocial interventions are a powerful adjunct to physical methods of pain relief. Cognitive–behavioural approaches have been found to be particularly helpful. They have been covered in other parts of the book and will not be re-described here. Group cognitive–behavioural therapy interventions have been used to help the psychological distress associated with cancer, and have been shown to have qualified success (Bottomly 1996). There is value in introducing psychosocial methods early in the course of the illness, while cognitive capacity is still sufficient to understand concepts, or so that the support element of the

intervention is developed early enough to be well established by the time the patient may need supportive psychotherapy.

Peer or self-help groups are a useful resource for patients with cancer. They can provide support, companionship and motivation. They are also invaluable in assisting the education process.

Spiritual intervention from a specialist in this area can reduce the suffering associated with the pain. Supportive counselling is invaluable to help clarify and talk through concerns and plan for the future. Support groups can provide useful companionship, humour, and a forum for canvassing methods used by others to reduce pain and improve quality of life.

Education

Education about pain and pain-management techniques is essential for the person with cancer and the family caregivers (Ferrell et al 1995, Yeager et al 1997). Since much of the care is conducted on an out-patient basis, patients and families will assume considerable responsibility.

Yeager et al (1997) found that outpatients with cancer-related pain have more correct knowledge about pain than those not experiencing pain. From the pattern of responses it was also evident that beliefs and fears about addiction to analgesics existed, which could be corrected with more adequate knowledge. Therefore they suggested that education of patients by a multidisciplinary team is important. The content of education should include:

- Reinforcement of the need to inform staff of pain.
- Education about how keeping a pain diary can help with tailoring an individual regime of analgesics
- Encouragement to talk about all concerns relating to analgesia
- Ongoing education, and re-education, for patients and family.

Coluzzi (1996) suggested that both patients and staff need to be made more aware of the differences between tolerance, dependence and addiction. Readers are referred to Chapter 8 for a detailed discussion of these phenomena. An outline of topics included in one patient education programme is provided in Box 21.2 (Jacox et al 1994).

Lifestyle adjustment

There are several aspects to consider when advising about adjustments to a client's lifestyle in response to

Box 21.2   Education programme for patients with cancer (from Jacox et al 1994, derived from Cancer 72 (II suppl) 1993, 3426–3432. Copyright © 1993 American Cancer Society. Reprinted by permission of Wiley-Liss, Inc., a subsidiary of John Wiley & Sons, Inc.)

Overview
Pain definitions
— pain causes
— pain can be relieved
— how pain is assessed
— telling health professionals about your pain

Drug management
Myths of addiction
Understanding drug tolerance
Understanding respiratory depression
Controlling drug side-effects

Non-drug management
Importance of non-drug treatments
Previous experience with non-drug treatments
Support groups and pastoral care
Demonstration of relaxation, massage, heat/cold modalities, etc

their cancer pain. Some aspects have already been covered in Chapter 15 of this book. Life goals, life roles, and general everyday activities of daily living may all need adjustment. Adjustment may be achieved slowly and thoughtfully in some instances, or may be forced upon an individual quite suddenly by a radical change in health status.

Life goals are often re-determined by the patient, either privately or in discussion with the family, with a counsellor, with a spiritual advisor, and with the oncologist. However, therapists have a responsibility to become aware of the patient's life goals, and to provide the patient with support in achieving them. This may occur through identifying the life roles which are important to the achievement of these goals, and helping achieve maximum efficiency and minimum discomfort from pain in the daily activities associated with these roles.

Methods for adjusting lifestyle so that the pain is least incapacitating include:

- **Setting goals**   Patients can be encouraged to set goals on a daily or weekly basis, and review them frequently, until a manageable number and priority of goals is determined.
- **Adjusting timing or routine**   For example, tasks which require the most energy, or may result in the most pain, might be scheduled for earlier in the day when energy levels are higher, or may closely follow medication so that the pain will be less troublesome. Activities normally completed in one session may be paced to occur over two or more

sessions, and perhaps even over more than one day.
- **Adjusting methods used in task completion**   Adapting the way in which tasks are carried out can can help a patient maintain participation in important life roles essential to maintaining a sense of control. For example, activities normally carried out while standing, such as self-care, can be adapted so they can be completed in a sitting position. Activities may be scheduled to be completed when someone is available to assist.
- **Varying the amount and type of adaptive equipment needed**   If pain is limiting range of motion, for instance, adaptive equipment for dressing may be useful.

Normal principles of activity analysis and task management apply. It is important for therapists to recognize this, and not be distracted from the use of usual therapy techniques by the distress they may feel at the patient's predicament.

DIFFERENT CONTEXTS FOR CANCER PAIN MANAGEMENT

There are many settings in which therapists may encounter patients with cancer, and with cancer pain. If cancer is the primary diagnosis, patients are likely to be either in-patients in hospital, or attending an out-patient service for people with cancer. They may also be in a hospice, or in hospice home-care. In each of these settings the role of the occupational therapist or physiotherapist will vary according to the centre's philosophy and organization. However, the principles of pain management for patients with cancer already outlined will still apply.

Therapists will also encounter patients with cancer in settings where cancer is not the primary diagnosis of all the patients. For instance, a community-based day centre for older people is likely to have clients with a range of diagnoses, and some may have cancer. In such cases, it is important that the therapist does not assume the need to introduce a pain management programme without first checking that this is not already being done by another facility. If there is a pain management program in existence the therapist has a responsibility to follow and support it while the client is in their facility.

PSYCHOLOGICAL FACTORS INFLUENCING MANAGEMENT

When working with patients who have cancer pain, psychological aspects need to be considered. In fact, consideration of psychological aspects are important from both the patient's and the therapist's point-of-view. Therapists working with patients who have cancer should take some time to examine and become comfortable with their own feelings and values about, and understanding of, the issues of potentially terminal illness, dying, pain, and responses to severe pain.

A number of factors can impact upon a therapist and contribute to therapist stress:

1. Their own personal meanings about disease and death, including their personal philosophical or religious beliefs and values
2. Their previous experiences and expectations about the medical system and what can be achieved
3. The complexities, uncertainties, and challenges that arise when caring for patients who are dying.

Macleod (2001) suggested similar issues for doctors entering palliative medicine.

Coping strategies therapists may use include maintaining a personal-support system, examining one's own personal and professional attitudes on death and dying, having realistic expectations about what you can do, using personal stress-management techniques (such as relaxation and exercise), and re-evaluating what the criteria are for successful therapy (Bennett 1991).

Patients who have cancer may exhibit the use of many defence mechanisms, which need to be understood in order to explain their behaviour and to design management and intervention. People develop a personal style of defence mechanisms over their life. For example, one person may use denial or projection more than regression or rationalization. Defence mechanisms are unconscious, and usually operate in a positive way to buffer or protect against stress. However, in some situations use of such defence mechanisms may inhibit communication and decision-making, or may even affect treatment choices.

There are many defence mechanisms, however two of the most commonly seen in major illness are 'projection' and 'denial'. Projection, in essence, involves attributing to others the feeling we are actually experiencing ourselves. For example, if someone is angry that he has cancer, he may see others, usually doctors or nurses or family members, as being angry with him.

Denial means being unable to accept or believe something, despite having been told very clearly, and acting as though it is not true. For example, a patient may insist they have not been told the diagnosis, despite having been told a number of times, or may put-off treatment decisions insisting that there is nothing wrong with their health.

Denial is a common self-protection strategy for easing distress; therapists need to understand its complexity and exercise care when communicating with the patient. Treatment decisions need to be carefully facilitated, while allowing them to face reality at a pace they can cope with.

Due to the presence of defence mechanisms and other types of psychological reaction, it is not uncommon for the patient with cancer, or the family, to react aggressively to various members of the staff with whom they come in contact. It is important that the professional staff member does not take such a reaction personally, but is able to respond to what may be the underlying concern – such as a need for time to talk, need for more information, or a need to express fear and anger.

As well as the operation of defence mechanisms, there are other reasons for patients to be miserable or irritable. There may be events occurring in their private relationships which are stressful, continual coping with pain may become wearisome, or they may be simply 'having a bad day'. All patients have the right to be irritable sometimes, and the therapist has the responsibility to respond maturely, and to be able to provide intervention without always requiring pleasant sociability in return.

CANCER PAIN IN CHILDREN

Children with cancer may experience pain associated with the cancer itself such as bone pain, therapy-related pain such as stomach pain from the side-effects of chemotherapy, and/or procedure-related pain, such as from intramuscular injections (Bryant 1997). The reader is referred to Chapter 6 for a comprehensive coverage of pain in childhood, its assessment, measurement and management.

PALLIATIVE-CARE PAIN MANAGEMENT

Palliative care is defined by the WHO (1990) as:

The active total care of patients whose disease is not responsive to curative treatment. Control of pain, of other symptoms, and of psychological, social, and spiritual problems, is paramount. The goal of palliative care is achievement of the best quality of life for patients and their families.

Palliative care involves working with the patient and their family, usually at home or in a hospice, to minimize suffering, reduce the mechanization of dying, aim for agreement about treatment between the patient, family and health professionals, and to reconcile interpersonal differences.

Box 21.3   Case example – Mr NL

Mr NL was a 61-year-old man diagnosed with prostate cancer. He was married with a 32-year-old daughter and 30-year-old son. He worked full-time as an engineer, consulting on a number of building projects.

During the early stages of his illness he underwent surgery (prostatectomy) and later received a 6-week course of radiotherapy. Mr NL experienced short-lived acute pain related to surgery which resolved within a few weeks.

After 5 years of symptom-free time, Mr NL developed an intense pain in his left hip which significantly affected his mobility. His prostate cancer had recurred with metastatic spread to his left head-of-femur. He was started on hormone treatment (androgen blockade) in an attempt to reduce the effects of the disease.

After a few months he was troubled by increasing pain in his left hip and so received localized palliative radiotherapy which provided temporary relief. Mr NL's pain continued to increase so that he had difficulty with weight-bearing. He started on oral morphine which gave some relief, but this was short-lived. After adjusting dosages of morphine and finding that his sleep was still being interrupted by pain in his left hip, Mr NL was offered a percutaneous cordotomy. This provided instant relief to the pain in his left hip and he was able to mobilize more easily again.

After a few more months Mr NL started developing a central aching pain in his pelvis. On examination, it was clear the primary prostate tumour had significantly enlarged. About this time he became increasingly fatigued. The combination of pain and fatigue severely limited his ability to walk, reduced his endurance for activities of daily living such as showering, and he found it difficult to sit comfortably. He commenced oral morphine again, using a slow-release formula, and eventually needed continuous subcutaneous infusion of morphine using an ambulatory transfusion pump.

It was at this point that he was referred for physiotherapy and occupational therapy.

Physiotherapy input focused on facilitating Mr NL's mobilization throughout this time, advice on positioning to relieve pressure to his groin when sitting, lying and toileting. As his fatigue increased, a walking frame was prescribed which took weight through his arms, decreasing pressure on weight-bearing.

Occupational therapy involvement was initially requested for home-assessment, as Mr NL expressed a desire to stay at home as long as possible. The occupational therapist assessed his occupational status (that is, roles of importance to him, his functional status, and performance components).

Adaptive equipment such as a shower chair and over-toilet seat were prescribed to enable him to perform self-care independently, and ways of conserving his energy conservation were explored. In addition, the therapist worked with Mr NL and his family to find ways of adapting the environment so he could remain involved in family activities. For instance, at times when he was too uncomfortable to mobilize or sit in chairs, a bed was placed in the family room so he could participate in activities when his friends or his children visited. He also found listening to music helped to some extent to distract him from the pain. The therapist discussed other ways of maintaining a sense of control. He used the telephone and Internet for some time to remain in contact with friends and work-mates, following the progress of some of the building projects he had been involved with. Support and education was also provided for his family.

As his disease progressed, he decided to go to a hospice where his pain was closely monitored. Psychosocial and spiritual support became very important to him in the last few weeks of his life.

Mr NL presented as a patient with many common characteristics of cancer pain, that is, varying types and sites of pain as his disease progressed, changing intensities of pain that required constant re-evaluation, and trialing of a number of different methods of pain relief. A multidisciplinary approach with good communication between health carers and family involvement was essential to optimal supportive care as his disease progressed.

Palliative and hospice care are becoming synonymous, as physical surroundings for care are changing – patients are choosing to die at home and hospitals are establishing hospice units. The essential features include recognizing the terminal nature of the illness and the need for the patient to complete unfinished business, offering the patient as much choice as possible, instructing the family in care of their dying loved one, and prevention or maximum alleviation of pain. Pain control should be organized and anticipatory, so that quality of life is enhanced for the patient and the family.

If the patient is at home, or in a situation where his needs and wishes and those of the close relatives and/or friends are paramount, the health professional must often adjust his or her style of practice. One may need to be prepared to follow a more flexible time schedule, to accept that a patient does not wish to be involved in a particular therapy procedure, and to talk more openly about one's own beliefs and feelings than might be typical in some other settings.

Often palliative and hospice care involves a bereavement stage, after the patient has died, for the family and other carers. Therapists may be involved in this stage, following their previous close therapeutic involvement with the patient and the family. See Box 21.3 for a case example illustrating many of these complex issues.

CONCLUSION

In this chapter, it has been established that there are some differences between the management of people with cancer pain and those with non-cancer pain. Cancer pain is not a static phenomenon due to only one cause. Cancer pain is of considerable import to those with cancer. It is important for occupational therapists and physical therapists working with clients with cancer to be well acquainted with the types of cancer pain, and methods for both pain assessment and measurement and management.

While there may be special management strategies to be used with people with cancer pain such as slow-release morphine, radiotherapy and surgical procedures, therapists must remember the value of more-standard therapeutic modalities, such as counterstimulation and energy-conservation techniques.

Particular issues related to working in a palliative care setting may also need to be addressed by therapists.

Study questions/questions for revision

1. What are the different types of cancer pain which patients may present with?
2. Suggest two possible reasons why cancer pain may not be adequately managed in patients.
3. How often should the pain of a person with cancer be assessed?
4. What measurement tools should be routinely used with a patient with cancer pain?
5. Identify five techniques which the physiotherapist might use to help a patient with cancer pain?
6. Identify five techniques which the occupational therapist may use to help a patient with cancer pain?

ACKNOWLEDGEMENT

The authors thank Jennifer Sturgess for her help in the preparation of this chapter.

REFERENCES

Agency for Health Care Research and Quality 2001 Management of Cancer Pain, Evidence Report/Technology Assessment: Number 35, Pub no. a-Eo33. http://www.ahrq.gov/clinic/canpainsum.htm

Ahles T A, Ruckdeschel J C, Blanchard E B 1984 Cancer-related pain–II. Assessment with Visual Analogue Scales. Journal of Psychosomatic Research 28: 121–124

Aaronson N K, Ahmedza S, Bergman B, Bullinger M, Cull A, Duez N J, et al 1993 The European Organization for Research and Treatment of Cancer QLQ-C30: A quality of life instrument for use in international clinical trials in oncology. Journal of the National Cancer Institute 85: 365–376

Archer V R, Billingham L J, Cullen M H 1999 Palliative chemotherapy: no longer a contradiction in terms. Oncologist 4: 470–477

Austin C, Cody C P, Eyers P J, Hefferin E A, Krasnow R W 1986 Hospice home care pain management. Four critical variables. Cancer Nursing 9: 58–65

Bennett S 1991 Issues confronting occupational therapists working with terminally ill patients. British Journal of Occupational Therapy 54: 8–10

Bonica J J 1987 Importance of the problem. In: Swerdlow M, Ventafridda (eds) Cancer Pain. MTP Press Limited, Lancaster, pp 3–7

Bottomly A 1996 Group cognitive behavioural therapy interventions with cancer patients: a review of the literature. European Journal of Cancer Care 5: 143–146

Bryant R 1997 Coping styles and medical play preparation of young children with leukaemia undergoing intramuscular injection. Unpublished Honours Thesis, the University of Queensland Department of Occupational Therapy

Carlson L E, Ursuliak Z, Goodey E, Angen M, Speca M 2001 The effects of a mind fulness meditation-based stress reduction program on mood and symptoms of stress in cancer outpatients: 6-month follow-up. Supportive Care in Cancer 9: 112–123

Cella D F, Tulsky D S, Gray G, Sarafian B, Linn E, Bonomi A, et al 1993. The Functional Assessment of Cancer Therapy Scale: development and validation of the general measure. Journal of Clinical Oncology 3: 570–579

Cherny N I, Portenoy R K 1994 Cancer pain: principles of assessment and syndromes. In: Wall P D, Melzack R (eds) Textbook of Pain, 3rd edn. Churchill Livingstone, Edinburgh

Cleeland C S 1985 Measurement and prevalence of pain in cancer. Seminars in Oncology Nursing 1: 87–92

Coluzzi P H 1996 A model for pain management in terminal illness and cancer care. The Journal of Care Management 2: 45–76

Cramond T, Stuart G 1993 Intraventricular morphine for intractable pain of advanced cancer. Journal of Pain and Symptom Management 8: 465–472

Daut R L, Cleeland C S 1982 The prevalence and severity of pain in cancer. Cancer 50: 1913–1918

Devine E C, Westlake S K 1995 The effects of psychoeducational care provided to adults with cancer: a meta-analysis of 116 studies. Oncology Nursing Forum 22: 1369–1381

Driscoll C E, 1987 Pain management. Primary Care 14: 337–352

Ferrell B R, Grant M, Chan J, Ahn C, Ferrell B A 1995 The impact of cancer pain education on family caregivers of elderly patients. Oncology Nursing 22: 1211–1218

Foley K M 1987 Cancer pain syndromes. Journal of Pain and Symptom Management 2: S13–S17

Higginson I J 1999 Evidence-based palliative care. British Medical Journal 319: 462–463

Jacox A, Carr O B, Payne R, Berde C B, Breitbart W, Cain J H, et al 1994 Management of cancer pain. Clinical practice guidelines. No 9. AHCPR Publication No 94-0592. Agency for Health Care Policy and Research, US Department of Health & Human Services Public Health Service, Rockville M D

Janjan N A 1997 Radiation for bone metastases: conventional techniques and the role of systematic radiopharmaceuticals. Cancer 80: 1628–1645

Klein M E 1983 Pain in the cancer patient. In: Wiernik P H (ed) Supportive Care of the Cancer Patient. Futura Publishing, New York, pp 173–208

Macleod R D 2001 on reflection: doctors learning to care for people who are dying. Social Science and Medicine 52: 1719–1727

Mayer D K 1985 Non-pharmacologic management of pain in the person with cancer. Journal of Advanced Nursing 10: 325–330

Monfardini S, Scanni A 1987 Chemotherapy and radiotherapy for cancer pain. In: Swerdlow M, Ventafridda (eds) Cancer Pain. MTP Press Limited, Lancaster, pp 89–96

Osoba D, Aaronson N, Zee B, Sprangers M, te Velde A 1997 Modification of the EORTC QLQ-C30 (Version 2.0) based on content validity and reliability testing in large samples of patients with cancer. Quality of Life Research 6: 103–108

Pargeon K L, Hailey B J 1999 Barriers to effective cancer pain management: A review of the literature. Journal of Pain and Symptom Management 18: 358–368

Portenoy R K 1990 Pain and quality of life: Clinical issues and implications for research. Oncology 4: 172–178

Portenoy R K, Lesage P 1999 Management of cancer pain. Lancet 15(353): 1695–1700

Portenoy R K, Thaler H T, Korniblith A B, McCarthy Lepore J, Fiedlander-Klar H, Kiyasu E, Sobel K, Coyle N, Kemeny N, Norton L, Scher H 1994 The Memorial Symptom Assessment Scale: an instrument for the evaluation of symptom prevalence, characteristics and distress. European Journal of Cancer Care 30A(9): 1362–1336

Stuart G, Cramond T 1993 Role of percutaneous cervical cordotomy for pain of malignant origin. Medical Journal of Australia 158: 667–670

Takeda F 1991 WHO cancer pain relief programme. In: Bond M R, Charlton J E, Woolf C J (eds) Proceedings of the VIth World Congress on Pain. Elsevier, Amsterdam, pp 467–474

Tigges K N, Marcil W M 1988 Terminal illness and life-threatening illness: an occupational behaviour perspective. Slack, Thoroughfare

Tigges K N, Sherman L M, Sherwin F S 1984 Perspectives on the pain of the hospice patient: the roles of the occupational therapist and physician. Occupational Therapy in Health Care 1: 55–68

Vallerand A H 1997 Measurement issues in the comprehensive assessment of cancer pain. Seminars in Oncology Nursing 13: 16–24

Walsh N E 1991 Cancer pain. Physical Medicine and Rehabilitation: State of the Art Reviews 5: 133–153

World Health Organization 1986 Cancer Pain Relief. WHO, Geneva

World Health Organization 1990 Report of the Expert Committee. Technical Report Series on Cancer Pain Relief and Active Supportive Care. WHO, Geneva

Yeager K A, Miakowski C, Dibble S, Wallhagan M 1997 Differences in pain knowledge in cancer patients with and without pain. Cancer Practice 5: 39–45

22

Chronic pain and psychiatric problems

Robert G. Large   Frank New
Jenny Strong   Anita M. Unruh

OVERVIEW

Patients with chronic pain often face many life difficulties, as was described in Chapter 20. Such patients can benefit not only from conventional medical therapies, but also psychological therapies. An awareness of the particular physical, psychological and social problems that accumulate for people with long-term pain and disability, and an ability to identify and appropriately manage these problems, allows occupational therapists and physiotherapists to obtain more successful outcomes and satisfaction for patients.

In this chapter, the manner in which psychosocial disturbances can develop and present in people with chronic pain will be described. An overview will be given of the association between chronic pain and psychiatric disorders, before a number of specific psychiatric syndromes will be described.

Learning objectives

At the completion of this chapter, readers will have an understanding of:

Box 22.1   Key terms defined

Somatization – The presentation of emotional problems as if symptoms of physical disorders.

Post-traumatic stress disorder – A condition that develops after a person is exposed to a major life-threatening event, whereby the event is frequently re-experienced, with symptoms of persisting arousal.

Dissociation – Where a person reacts to some part of their conscious experience as if detached.

Kinesiophobia – The fear and avoidance of activity.

1. Pain thresholds, pain tolerance and pain behaviours.
2. The influence of psychological and emotional factors on presentations with pain.
3. The relationship between chronic pain and psychiatric disorders.
4. Illness behaviour, normal and abnormal, as it relates to pain.
5. Treatment behaviour, normal and abnormal.

SUBJECTIVITY OF PAIN

Pain is an unpleasant subjective personal experience. We can only understand the pain of another person by listening to his report and understanding it in terms of our own experience. Accordingly, we tend to trust the pain report of someone who can describe their pain in clear, calm terms that fit with our own personal and clinical experience, and academic understanding. When the complaint seems muddled, obscure, and embellished with dramatic statements, gestures and attributions, we feel less sure of our ground. Likewise, we are less sure when the complainant is unusually distressed, or 'odd'. At other times, the intensity of a person's anxiety and depression may subtly pressure us to accept not only her pain, but also her own interpretation and understanding about what the pain represents, whether or not this is correct.

Pain may be a symptom that reflects emotionally difficult aspects of a person's life. When a patient's pain does not seem to fit with an identifiable physical cause, the patient is often told that the pain is 'in their heads', and that it is 'psychogenic'. Such a patient may indeed have symptoms of depression and anxiety, but it does not follow that depression or anxiety *causes* his pain. Pain can be caused solely through psychological mechanisms, as can be demonstrated in hypnosis or in the couvade syndrome, where the husband feels his wife's labour pains. However, these instances are rare. In most clinical presentations psychological and physical processes are simultaneously active.

Pain is a subjective experience. If a person 'feels' it, then, by definition, it is 'real'. Because it is an 'experience', it must involve their mind; it *is* 'in their heads', but not in the sense implied by the rather clumsy reference to the possibility that a person is being foolish or deceptive. This needs to be understood to enable appropriate management. We have a habit of attributing pain to particular parts of the body. However, cases such as referred and phantom pain illustrate that such a conceptualization of pain in a body part can be misleading.

Patients, and not uncommonly doctors, frequently interpret negative investigations as meaning that no pathophysiology was present, rather than the more correct interpretation that these negative tests were unable to identify any pathophysiology being present. This is a significantly different interpretation, which recognizes that our assessments have limitations, and that it is best for us to accept that we cannot remove all doubt. People prefer certainty. Their tolerance of this remaining doubt varies, and is significantly influenced by past and other current experiences.

An appropriate response in this situation is to conduct a careful review to ensure appropriate history, examination and investigations have been conducted. At times, the risk and/or cost is not sufficient to justify the (low) likelihood of benefit of further investigations, leaving a situation in which both the patient, and the therapist, need to acknowledge and to confidently manage the remaining uncertainty. The therapist assists the patient with therapy without a guarantee, developing a judgement of reasonable and unreasonable risks, and an ability to carefully plan and accomplish a range of experiences which would allow redevelopment of confidence and trust.

There are very many **measures** of 'pain', although there are no direct or 'objective' measures of pain. All measure different aspects of the pain experience, and of patients' responses to their pain, with no independent mechanism for absolute verification yet known. All measurement tools have strengths and limitations, and may be misinterpreted. It is the responsibility of therapists to become knowledgeable about assessment issues. Readers are referred back to Chapter 7 for further coverage of assessment issues.

It is important to recognize that it is the **patient's role**, as the only person capable, to define the presence, intensity, type, location, and qualities of the pain.

It is the **therapist's role** to actively listen, and to interpret the significance of the information, in the context of what is known of the patient from other aspects of the history, examination and investigations (Pilowsky 1995). The therapist is not in a position to categorically determine whether a person is experiencing pain or not, even if the pain cannot be understood.

These issues become important in relation to assessing appropriate illness and treatment behaviour, as discussed later.

Pain and the 'pain-prone' patient

In 1959, Engel published his influential paper 'Psychogenic Pain and the Pain Prone Patient' in the American

Journal of Medicine. Engel (1959) argued against the commonly held mechanistic nociceptor stimulation pain pathway view of pain, and suggested that pain is a psychic phenomenon. He proposed that there are some individuals who are prone to developing painful conditions, with psychological factors being very important in their experience of their pain. Such patients typically have repeated painful problems, where the pain is typically chosen symbolically, such as a punishment. For example, it was learned that a man who had unexplained burning pain behind his ear had passively accepted being frequently 'boxed' on his ears by his father and stepmother, as punishment, until he was 21 years-of-age.

Occasionally, in the context of grief, we see people present with pain that seems symbolic of the deceased.

For example, one man developed difficult back pain that appeared to have no physical explanation, after his wife died of cancer. Only when he talked about the harrowing time he had spent nursing her through her last illness did he begin to recover. It transpired that his wife, with secondary involvement of the spine with vertebral collapse, had severe back pain as the dominant feature of her discomfort.

These case examples are illustrative of an important message for the therapist: the therapist cannot fully assess a person's pain without talking with him or her. Although we are bound to accept the person's description of pain (unless we believe he or she is being dishonest), we are not bound to accept his or her explanation of the causes of the pain – that is the professional's task.

In clinical work we must attend to the complaints of our patients. Yet, the complaint of pain is often a problematic communication, particularly when it is chronic in nature.

Pilowsky (1977) has drawn attention to the issue of **altruism** in medicine. He suggested that the pain of another affects the observer, who feels constrained to offer sympathy, support and relief. This response is emotionally demanding, and so we generally want to be sure that our response of care is justified. For these reasons we are very sensitive to any suggestion that the person may be exaggerating, pretending, lying or malingering. Only when we are sure that the complaint is 'genuine' do we respond wholeheartedly.

The degree to which we accept, or are cautious about the complaints of another person, is influenced quite considerably by the nature of our relationship with the person, in turn influencing the degree of confidence about correctly interpreting his or her communications, verbal and non-verbal.

Pain-related concepts

Many clinicians talk of patients having a 'low pain threshold' when they encounter complaints of pain which seem to be exaggerated. Yet this term is derived from laboratory studies, and is of questionable value in clinical work.

In the laboratory, it is possible to apply a noxious stimulus that can be quantified in terms of intensity, and time of exposure. Commonly used stimuli include radiant heat, electric shock, or immersion of an arm in iced water. The point at which the person first reports pain is the **'pain threshold'**. Laboratory experiments suggest that pain threshold is relatively similar for most people with normal central and peripheral nervous systems.

The point at which the person asks for the stimulus to stop is regarded as the **'pain tolerance'**. This varies with mood and motivation, from person to person, and within the same person between different times of testing.

'Pain expression' or **'pain behaviour'** is different again, and refers to the way in which individuals express pain. Again, in a laboratory context, extroverts express their pain more volubly than do introverts, regardless of differences in pain tolerance levels. This means an extrovert may make a terrible fuss over a continuing stimulus, which the introvert quietly asked to be turned off long before!

There is no direct relationship between pain tolerance and pain behaviour. This is an important fact in clinical work. Bond (1971) showed this when postoperative pain relief was administered 'prn'; the extroverts were given more analgesia by their nursing staff than were the introverts. This was in spite of the introverts reporting *higher* levels of pain intensity.

As previously indicated, personal and cultural factors have a strong influence on how people communicate the pain experience, with obvious implications for how we judge the suffering of others. When people are troubled, worried and fearful overall, they more readily notice and attend to bodily sensations. This is consistent with the hyper-vigilance and self-protectiveness of a threatened state, such as when anxious or angry. People often act with a sense of urgency to resolve the problem, which can then influence their judgement. Difficulties can arise if they attribute the cause to the wrong factor, even if it seems to be logical, convenient, and preferable to them at the time.

In this way, people vary considerably, from time to time, and person to person, as to how they respond to what may be very similar, or even identical symptoms. In other words, we will observe differing pain behaviours for the same pain.

The issue of **'salience'** is an important factor in the recognition and reporting of symptoms, for both patients and professionals. Salience refers to a mental behaviour that results in attention being directed to particular aspects, which become very conspicuous in the view of the observer. We are more likely to notice symptoms if we have heard about them recently, through contact with sick people, personal experience, through advertising or education. Hence the well-known hypochondriasis of trainees in the healthcare professions. For patients, noticing 'symptoms', and responding to them, instead of persevering and 'ignoring' them, becomes much more important when their illness has a personal significance for them, particularly if this is threatening, which is very often.

In contrast to the heightened awareness because of salience, **'dissociation'** is a phenomenon that can also dramatically affect the way in which a person responds to his pain, reacting as if it was not present. It occurs when a person reacts to some parts of his conscious experience, but not to other parts, as if these parts were detached.

Dissociation is normal for all people at some time, such as when very tired, when intoxicated or sedated, or when concentrating intensely. Teenagers watching their favourite programme on TV will not hear a request for help in the kitchen, but can hear their friends calling. This phenomenon of dissociation is more likely to occur in states of heightened arousal, such as during a football game, during disasters, or at other times of severe emotional distress.

When distressed, some people may be injured, or may even harm themselves, without experiencing any pain at the time, experiencing a state of **'derealization'**, and **'depersonalization'**. People describe feeling unreal, not connected to the world, as if things were happening in a dream, etc. There may be a sense of numbing in all or part of the body, and a sense of emotional emptiness, as if one has no feelings. Typically there is a time of tension prior to these periods, with the patients reporting relief as if 'real again' when they experience pain. Some people who may be very disturbed actually use self-harm in a very paradoxical manner, as a mechanism to regain this sensation of normality.

Some people are not gifted with an ability to express their emotions, or personal problems. It is then more difficult to solve personal problems, not being able to 'speak the language'. An extreme form of this difficulty is defined as **'alexythimia'**, literally meaning 'no words for emotions'. It has been suggested that such

difficulties may result in patients redirecting painful emotions into physical symptoms (Catchlove et al 1985).

One of the greatest challenges faced by people who become ill is dealing with a loss of **autonomy** and **independence**. The desire to regain independence is usually a strong motivator to return to healthy functioning, and to develop the tolerance of the discomfort involved in this process of recovery. Loss of a sense of hope for recovery, particularly loss of hope for what recovery means to the patients themselves, destroys this motivation and tolerance.

Patients are often in a vulnerable situation, having insufficient knowledge and resources to heal themselves; otherwise they would. They need to allow the involvement of other people, including trained professionals, into their lives, at times very intimately, physically, emotionally and psychologically. Those who have had their trust abused before are likely to have difficulty with this aspect of their care. Others, for various reasons, find life overwhelming, and may become excessively dependent, by relying on others for help with tasks that they could satisfactorily accomplish themselves. A pattern of abnormal illness behaviour may result (Pilowsky 1969, 1976, 1997). **'Illness behaviour'** refers to a pattern of behaviour that is condoned, and expected, of a person deemed to be ill. It is associated with the **'sick role'**, which involves familiar allowances and responsibilities, for the duration of an illness (Parsons 1964, Pilowsky 1995). Illness behaviour and the sick role are most clearly illustrated in short-term physical disorders, and are likely to be much more confused in relation to complex, long-term disorders involving multiple biological, psychological and social contributions, such as with chronic pain.

Consider, for example, the very ordinary situation of a person who becomes ill with pneumonia. It is expected that the person will recognize symptoms of shortness of breath, fever, cough and lassitude as being important, and realize that she will not to recover by her own efforts. As a result she will accept the need to seek skilled help, the responsibility to accurately report all the details of her predicament, and to listen, consider and implement that advice which she regards as being appropriate to return to her usual functioning and wellbeing.

This process might involve giving up some usual activities for the duration of the period of illness, allowing others to help her, and tolerating, to a degree, the discomfort and disadvantages of the situation. In return, those associated with the person are more likely to tolerate her complaints, extend sympathy and support, and to assume her responsibilities, for the (brief) duration.

There is parallel behaviour expected of the therapist, **'treatment behaviour'**. The professional is expected to be available, listen to the patient, recommend examinations and investigations that are necessary, and advise the patient in terms that she can understand. Once an agreement (a **therapeutic alliance**) has been reached, based upon a common understanding of the issues and treatments, then active management can properly commence.

It is quite possible for these roles to become somewhat distorted resulting in abnormal illness behaviour, and/or abnormal treatment behaviour (Pilowsky 1997, Singh et al 1981). There may be insufficient or excessive preoccupation with each of the steps involved, or the patient and/or the therapist might respond to the situation for reasons unrelated to the illness.

Common manifestations include the inappropriate use of medications, aids, relationships and financial support resources, with the common issue that the behaviours in question are not clearly leading to maximizing of the patient's recovery and independence.

THE ASSOCIATION BETWEEN PAIN AND PSYCHIATRIC DISORDERS

Chronic pain occurs in about 10–15% of the general population, with many also having a psychiatric disorder, either pre-existing or consequential (Dworkin & Caligor 1988). Merskey & Spear (1967) reported that pain is as frequent a complaint in the psychiatric clinic as it is in the medical clinics. Spear (1967) found that 45–50% of patients with psychiatric problems attending a psychiatric clinic reported pain problems, with the highest incidence occurring in patients with anxiety states. Large (1986) found that, in a consecutive series of 50 patients presenting for psychosocial evaluation at a pain clinic, 94% had a psychiatric disorder, and 96% had a physical disorder. In other words, most had both psychiatric and physical disorders.

Associations between chronic pain and psychiatric disorders can be:

- Psychiatric disorders coincidental with pain
- Pre-existing factors which predispose to both chronic pain and psychiatric disorders
- Chronic pain causing psychiatric disorders.

Psychiatric disorders coincidental with pain

An illness such as schizophrenia is associated with difficulty defining, understanding and resolving problems. The illness leads patients to have major perceptual, affective and cognitive impairment, which can lead to misinterpretations, at times to a psychotic degree. This distortion might lead to over-reporting or under-reporting of problems. Residents of long-term institutions have been reported as having a higher incidence of 'missed' or 'silent' (painless) heart attacks, appendicitis and brain tumours, which might be attributed in part to these difficulties.

Pain can be a confounding experience for a person with a major psychiatric illness. Occasionally someone with a delusional illness, such as schizophrenia, may develop a delusional misinterpretation of a physical symptom. For example, a patient who had excruciating back pain from degenerative spinal disease 'knew' that this was caused by aliens having implanted electronic stimulators in his spine that they turned on and off at will to break him down.

Less commonly the pain may be a true 'psychogenic' phenomenon, an hallucination, which is associated with a delusional interpretation. However, it has been demonstrated (Whitlock 1967) that when a major psychiatric disorder such as schizophrenia, major depression, or conversion disorder is diagnosed, then it is in fact **more** likely that the person will **also** have an underlying physical illness, rather than the reverse. Increased vigilance in assessing possible physical contributions is indicated, rather than prematurely attributing the patient's complaints to their psychiatric disorder. The case example in Box 22.2 is illustrative of difficulties people with a major mental illness can face when a coincidental pain problem arises.

When depressed, a person's judgement is clouded by a very bleak, pessimistic outlook, a withdrawn, narrow focus, such that the person has difficulty concentrating and conceptualizing, and difficulty shifting focus sufficiently to accurately interpret new information. This point is illustrated by the case example in Box 22.3.

Occasionally, the presentation of depression as pain may have symbolic meaning for the patient. For example, one woman presented with severe burning pain over her entire body, together with profound depression. She eventually revealed some family issues that had caused her great shame and embarrassment, and described that she had been literally 'burning with shame'.

Pre-existing factors predisposing to both chronic pain and psychiatric disorders

People with chronic pain have often experienced more than usual difficulties in life. There is not a direct

---

Box 22.2 Case example – Mrs DB

Mrs DB had been at an international conference in Europe. Post-conference, she sustained a fractured humerus after a bicycle accident. Her arm was set and she returned home. She went to her general medical practitioner for further management. Her regular doctor was unavailable, so she was seen by another doctor.

He couldn't understand why she was in pain. The surgery had a computer system which allowed the doctor to see what medications she was prescribed. He saw that she was taking some psychotropic medication and asked her who her psychiatrist was.

Mrs DB couldn't understand that he needed to speak with the psychiatrist as it was her arm that was broken and not her head. He inferred that the pain she was experiencing was due to her mental illness.

He sent her for an X-ray, commenting that if she insisted on being referred to an orthopaedic surgeon he would do this, but that he was too busy that day to make the referral.

She became angry and decided that she wouldn't push the matter with this doctor.

The pain did not abate and eventually she rang the surgery for a referral to an orthopaedic surgeon after her family and friends insisted that she do this.

Fortunately, she was seen quickly by the orthopaedic surgeon, who expressed surprise at how the bone had been set, and told her that if she had left it much longer she would have had irreversible damage in her left arm. He operated the next day placing two pins in the break.

Mrs DB was impressed at how the orthopaedic surgeon explained the pros and cons of operating prior to the operation and included her in the decision-making process. This involvement allowed her to own the outcome and the rehabilitation process involved.

The surgeon carefully explained to Mrs DB the possible risks involved in surgery and took considerable time in fully explaining these risks. Mrs DB felt like any other person with a broken arm and not a person with a mental illness with a broken arm.

This was in stark contrast to the way Mrs DB felt after her encounter with the GP.

Box 22.3 Case example

A gentleman sat with a handkerchief carefully laid out between the hem of his shorts and his legs, because he found the discomfort of the touch of his shorts against his legs quite intolerable.

He had a recurring unipolar depressive illness, and complained of headache, chest pain and many other physical symptoms with each episode, with relief coinciding with effective treatment of his depression.

It was as if he became exquisitely aware of his body whenever he was depressed.

---

relationship between the severity of a person's illness and either the pain experienced or the response to it. A person's pain and pain behaviour is also reliant on psychosocial factors, many of which are present well before the onset of the pain. This psychosocial contribution to a person's pain is consistent with the IASP definition of pain and with the knowledge of the interaction between physical and psychosocial factors as explained in the Gate Control theory of pain (Melzack & Wall 1965).

Problems such as family dysfunction, substance abuse, emotional abuse, physical abuse and sexual abuse, unemployment, personal and family illness, poverty, isolation and deprivation are all over-represented in the histories of chronic pain patients (Feuerstein et al 1985, Goldberg et al 1999, Katon et al 1985). Such predisposing problems may result in the

patient taking excessive risks, a lack of balance with insufficient attention to personal welfare, and isolation.

A sense of entrapment, and perceived loss of control over one's destiny and wellbeing may lead to defensive reactions, 'fight or flight' responses, including depression and anxiety, dependency or over-activity, instability, and aggression. Patients may have become hurt, cynical, distrustful and reluctant to accept reasonable advice regarding wellbeing, with the pain becoming a symbol of ongoing dissatisfaction and conflict with the world.

People who have been disadvantaged in life are more likely to have occupations and lifestyles with higher rates of injury and illness, and often have fewer personal, financial and social resources to cope with these experiences.

It is worthwhile considering the mechanisms by which these factors can impact upon a person. A person who is stressed, insecure and distracted does not learn well. Unhelpful attitudes and habits may be acquired. This limits the person's ability to develop the academic, vocational, personal and social skills (problem-solving, communication, relationship skills, judgement), resources, choices and supports which would best equip her for life.

Illiteracy, which is often associated with considerable early-life disruption, is an example of a feature which is over-represented among chronic pain patients, but which is not commonly brought to attention without specific enquiry. People who are illiterate have often coped with it as if it had become an ordinary part of life. It is common for people to be so sensitive and embarrassed by their limitation that they conceal it. This results in considerable ongoing difficulty and disadvantage throughout life, with this magnified considerably when needing to participate in any learning process such as is required for rehabilitation and retraining after injury.

The predisposing factors may not have actually caused any problems, distress or dysfunction before the illness or accident, especially as people very often develop coping strategies. However, while able to continue functioning, these factors do make people vulnerable, in the same manner as rust in a car. It may cause no problem to the performance until the extra stress of an accident. At the time of the accident, with the preoccupation of the immediate trauma, the importance of pre-existing factors is often not considered, even though the impact of the trauma is worse because of them.

Accepting a particular behaviour as predisposing to problems can be difficult for a patient, especially if a person previously had a very high level of functioning, such as working 16 hours per day, 6 days per week, sick or not, earning a good reputation and a great income. However this socially encouraged behaviour might conceal significant problems with pacing, time-management, self-care, anxiety, excessive worry about others' approval, or poor management skills.

Many people disregard the effects of earlier life experiences, focusing only on the physical aspects of pain. Others become very sensitive to further disruptions to life, and may find it difficult to muster and maintain the personal strength and courage necessary to confront and deal with further problems, instead becoming avoidant and withdrawn.

In the health system, the dependency of the socially accepted sick role can be a welcome refuge from life's cruelty, especially as the price of remaining ill may remain hidden. Unfortunately the supports offered, particularly financial supports such as compensation payments, can have the unintended effect of reinforcing this state of prolonged illness, a contradiction that continues to trouble society at large.

Therapies aimed at improving function, when accepted and effective, can have a powerful effect in overcoming any sense of threat, and in turn decreasing levels of depression, anxiety and anger in the patient. The benefits of occupational therapy and physiotherapy in relieving the emotional distress experienced by patients should not be underrated.

The case example in Box 22.4 illustrates the unexpected ways in which the crisis of a pain syndrome can uncover premorbid psychopathology, which then requires treatment in its own right. This patient was coping well while her focus was on a successful career in musical performance, and she decompensated in the face of pain and losing her career. Personality issues had not caused her pain, but her pain had severely challenged her habitual ways of coping with the world.

Chronic pain causing psychiatric disorders

Pain is in itself a stressor that may sometimes precipitate the onset of a psychiatric disorder.

Pain is a potent cause of depression in its own right, particularly when combined with a disability which presents to the patient a series of losses – job, lifestyle, friends, interests, income, status, freedom, hopes and dreams, rewards for past effort, etc. Hopelessness and helplessness and fear of the future become a major challenge, along with frustration and irritability, which in turn tend to worsen the situation by discouraging those offering help – it is harder to empathize with someone who is irritable. The insomnia, fatigue, poor appetite and limited activity, as well as many of the medications prescribed, can have a biological 'depressogenic' effect.

At various times, pain has been used to deliberately induce fear and suffering, not only with torture, but with discipline, and even with contact sports. It has a particular cultural symbolism associated with sin, power and control, and has a profound ability to influence people's behaviours. The reference to an association between evil and illness continues despite advances in science, as indicated in the frequent comment by patients, 'what did I do to deserve this?'.

Box 22.4 Case example – AM

AM was a 35-year-old rock musician. Her career was terminated by a debilitating forearm pain and weakness. Occupational overuse syndrome was diagnosed. She faced the grief of losing not only her career, but also the joy of playing the keyboards. She changed to a career of sound engineering, and made some adjustment to her loss, with gradual alleviation of her arm pain.

In the course of treatment, AM revealed intermittent self-mutilation, stormy arguments with her partner and intense mood swings. Psychiatric assessment revealed an atypical dissociative disorder, with significant early childhood sexual abuse.

She engaged in long-term psychotherapy, which helped her gradually integrate her fragmented memories, and she settled into a more stable pattern and relationship with her partner.

In Chapter 20, the chronic pain syndrome and its pervasive and overwhelming nature were described. Very often people remain focused on treatments that may have been unsuccessful, inappropriate or even substandard. People become desperate, and are vulnerable. Judgement may be impaired due to distress and fear, and people may accept approaches offering very dubious promise of return of their health, hopes and wealth.

For example, a lady with 'total body pain' from chronic fatigue syndrome became malnourished and anaemic because she was spending so much of her pension on tests in search of a cure, that she had no money left to buy adequate food. Such situations are often the result of honest, earnest approaches, with good intentions, but with poor judgement.

SPECIFIC PSYCHIATRIC SYNDROMES AND PAIN

Adjustment disorder

Learning to live with pain is a major task. It is remarkable how well most people with chronic pain succeed with this task, and most often without any specific professional help. This reflects a general acceptance of some changes, such as ageing and 'wear and tear' with change being less threatening when not premature, sudden, unexplained or surrounded by conflict, and when occurring in a context of a good life, with good-quality secure supports.

The risk factors for an adjustment disorder are essentially the same as for morbid grief. This is not surprising considering that the function of the grieving process is to accomplish psychological 'healing' after psychological trauma and injury, in a manner analogous to the healing effect of the inflammatory process after physical injury.

Unrelated personal issues, such as family role changes, might inadvertently reinforce an unhelpful pattern of behaviour. Although people may have entitlements to financial support and compensation in some circumstances, there is ongoing concern regarding the effects of compensation and litigation processes on the welfare of the individual involved. Experience suggests that:

- At best, such involvement does not improve the physical and psychological wellbeing of patients
- At worst, such involvement may result in increased pain and disability, and delayed recovery (Greenough & Fraser 1988, Fraser 1996).

The precise situation with regard to financial support and compensation awaits further clarification.

A feature of adjustment disorders is emotional distress, which is more severe and/or prolonged than would usually be expected, especially if the distress becomes worse or interferes with a person's recovery process.

Other manifestations of the disorder can be detected from an understanding of a reasonable and recommended process of adjustment to permanent impairment and suffering. A problem may arise when, while empathizing, we may accept uncritically the patient's own perspective and approach. People with chronic pain are more likely to be too inactive, physically, mentally and socially, or paradoxically too overactive, as if in an attempt to deny and defy their predicament. Both approaches can have attractive short-term gain, but come with too high a risk of complications to be recommended.

Not many people in our community, including health professionals, have the prior training which would equip them to cope with long-term pain, even though models to help us cope with short-term physical disorders have been developed as part of cultural practices in virtually all communities.

This lack of a widely accepted model for appropriate adjustment to chronic pain has led to some criticism of diagnosing an adjustment disorder. It is understandably difficult to cope with chronic pain. Hence, there has been reluctance to consider this as a psychiatric disorder. This is especially so because of the widespread lack of understanding of the important differences between acute, short-term pain and chronic, long-term pain.

Medical practitioners are commonly not aware of, or do not take into account, the important differences between acute and chronic pain. However, it is reasonable to use the diagnosis of adjustment disorder, because it refers to a pattern of behaviour that interferes with the patient's task of re-organizing life to maximize his or her potential for functioning, and which carries considerable risk of future harm.

Treatment involves:

- Identifying the points where a person's progress has departed from that which would be most likely to give the best long-term result
- Identifying the reasons for the departure
- Addressing these.

Lack of appropriate information about pain management is the most common reason for adjustment difficulties. Hence, pain education programmes can be very useful. Associated personal and social problems can be dealt with in the usual way, with the occasional use of psychotropic medication to ease the distress, to allow attention to the process of learning how to develop a new life.

Adjustment disorders can become complicated by the development of other disorders such as depression. Depressive disorders are differentiated from adjustment disorders by being more intense, pervasive and less directly related to the issues of pain and disability.

Adjustment disorders also need to be differentiated from the diagnosis of 'psychological factors causing a physical condition', as pain is not, by definition, a physical condition, but an 'experience' which incorporates both physical and psychosocial elements.

Depression

Patients with chronic pain are often depressed (Brown 1990, Kerns & Haythornthwaite 1998, Rudy et al 1988). The actual incidence of depression among pain patients varies, with reports ranging from 10–100% (Brown 1990, Magni 1987, Rudy et al 1988, Turk et al 1987). Merskey (1999) has suggested that the prevalence of depression in people with pain is approximately 10–30%, while the incidence of depression in the general population ranges from 9–14% (Turk et al 1987). It is likely that the variance observed in surveys reflect different inclusion and exclusion criteria, different definitions of 'depression' and the use of different survey tools.

Some would argue that depression is commonly under-diagnosed in patients with chronic pain, and that treating patients with antidepressants significantly relieves chronic pain. Others point out that antidepressants are also modestly analgesic agents, and that the mild, grumbling depression seen in chronic pain is not the same as the primary depression seen in psychiatric clinics. Very frequently, the presenting picture is a manifestation of grief, demoralization, disillusionment and frustration, rather than a typical melancholic depression. However, these psychological responses can themselves function as strong stressors, leading on to the development of the more typical type of 'biological' depression, especially if a person is also genetically predisposed.

Many different measures have been used to detect depression in the patient with chronic pain. The Beck Depression Inventory (BDI) (Beck 1967, Beck et al 1961) and Zung Self Rating Depression Scale (Zung 1965) are sensitive and specific and correctly classify according to a DSM III (American Psychiatric Association 1980) diagnosis (Turner & Romano 1984). However, the problem with these measures is that they contain somatic items that are also commonly associated with chronic pain and disability, even in the absence of depression, raising the issue of the appro-

priateness of their use with a chronic pain population (Love & Peck 1987, Merskey 1999, Turk et al 1987).

Although there has been much discussion about which comes first, the depression or the chronic pain, recent research supports the view that depression mostly develops after or concurrently with pain, rather than preceding it (Cohen & Marx 1995, Fishbain et al 1997, Merskey 1999). Fishbain et al (1997) have thoroughly reviewed this issue and concluded that the evidence for pain causing depression is quite strong, while the evidence that depression causes pain is relatively weak, although there is some support for the 'scar' hypothesis, that previous depression may predispose patients to recurrence of depression if they develop pain.

The primary focus of intervention may depend upon which problem is more severe and troublesome for the patient; the pain or the depression. However, because the pain itself can have such a profound effect on a person's mood, it is useful to not prescribe antidepressant therapy before there has been an attempt to treat the underlying physical disorder, and the pain. The case example in Box 22.5 illustrates this point.

However, the clinical situation is frequently such that removal of the pain and return to normal ability and lifestyle is not possible. In such situations, treatment of the depression cannot, and should not, be further delayed once initial physical interventions have been adequately trialled.

It is also important to recognize that management of depression encompasses far more than pharmacotherapy. Depression for people with chronic pain is significantly improved by involvement in a comprehensive pain management programme (Maruta et al 1989). Cognitive–behavioural therapy (CBT) is a cor-

---

Box 22.5   Case example

A lady, 67 years-of-age, was experiencing low back pain from osteoporotic crush fractures. She was a widow, lived alone, and was relatively isolated being in a high-set house.

Not surprisingly, she was depressed, though this was severe with imminent suicidal threat, refusal of food and fluids, rejection of visitors and intense pessimism and self-criticism, such that her life was in danger from self-harm and neglect.

Urgent ECT was discussed with the patient and her relatives, with trepidation because of the osteoporosis. During the few days of these discussions, a narcotic infusion was introduced.

Not only did she obtain relief from the pain after being given adequate analgesia, but also there was a return of her usual mood to the extent that even antidepressant medication was no longer required.

ner-stone to most pain management programmes and is efficacious in the treatment of depression (Flor at al 1992). The challenge is to find the right balance of pharmacological and non-pharmacological therapies.

Therapists need to be aware of the possible suicide risk that may be present for patients who have depression in association with chronic pain. Talk about 'the future seeming hopeless' or 'ending all this pain', should never be minimized or disregarded. The message of distress should be recognized, the potential suicide risk should be evaluated, and concerns reported to the patient's doctor.

Therapists need to be aware that *enquiring* about these issues with patients is unlikely to *cause* them to suicide, whereas, *not enquiring* may lead to a serious risk going undetected. The case example in Box 22.6 is illustrative of the importance of secondary depression arising in a patient with chronic pain, and of the danger of suicide.

This case emphasized the importance of secondary depression in chronic pain and the danger of suicide. Depression had intruded upon Mr Brown's functioning, but fortunately he learned how to use the cognitive–behavioural approach, without the need for antidepressant medication. However, the option of pharmacotherapy was still available and could have been combined with the cognitive–behavioural approach.

Anxiety disorders

Anxiety disorders can also be associated with chronic pain, and each can reinforce the other (Gross & Collins 1981). Anxiety makes pain less tolerable, and for many anxious patients, it is the anxiety about the pain itself that becomes the major source of distress, and the main stumbling block to rehabilitation.

This anxiety may present as a heightened state of tension, with persistent worrying without an obvious focus (generalized anxiety disorder), with discrete episodes of overwhelming fear and with profound sympathetic arousal (palpitations, sweating, nausea, vomiting, diarrhoea, hyperventilation – panic disorder) and/or 'kinesiophobia'.

Kinesiophobia refers to the fear of activity, because of the pain it may cause, particularly if the pain is misinterpreted as a signal of more damage. A major thrust of pain management programmes is to help patients overcome their fear of movement and/or re-injury, and to correctly interpret the pains they continue to experience as not necessarily indicating disaster. The problem of fear-avoidance faced by many patients with pain has been discussed earlier in Chapter 9.

Sometimes the withdrawal and loss of confidence associated with pain can lead to the onset of a more generalized social phobia and agoraphobia, and in children to school phobia. Occasionally when the underlying disorder is adequately treated, and when

---

Box 22.6 Case example – Mr Brown

Mr Brown was a 45-year-old farmer, who was married, with three children ranging in age from 5–10 years old. He sustained a lifting injury while baling hay 5 years ago. A disc herniation was shown on imaging and he had back surgery that failed to relieve his pain. He became progressively more disabled with continuing pain and restriction in activities. He sold his farm because he felt incapable of the tough physical work involved.

He continued to search for a surgical solution to his pain, and shied away from offers of non-interventional pain management. When first seen in the pain clinic, he was depressed, with continuous ruminations about his pain, loss of appetite, sleep disturbance and suicidal ideation (but he said he would not act on these ideas because of his commitment to his children).

He was also highly kinesiophobic and had become physically deconditioned.

He declined treatment for depression, because he did not feel he should have to 'accept' his pain. Management consisted of further orthopaedic consultation, where the surgeon fully discussed the surgical facts, and confronted him with the reality that further surgery would not cure his pain.

When reviewed in the pain clinic his depression was worse, he was anhedonic and he showed the slowing of talk and movement seen in severe depression (psychomotor retardation). He had, however, reached the point of accepting that his pain was chronic and expressed a willingness to attend an intensive 4-week programme of pain management involving education, relaxation and activation.

In the initial week of the programme, staff felt that his depression was limiting his ability to participate and benefit from the programme. He was prescribed an antidepressant, but he did not take it. Consistent with his work ethic, and now with improved judgement as the result of the counselling with the surgeon, he elected instead to throw himself more fully into the programme. He also began sharing more of his personal anguish in individual and group sessions.

Within another week his mood started lifting, and he made rapid progress in the gym, with significant gains in activity levels by the end of 4 weeks. At 1-month follow-up, he was smiling, animated, and actively planning his return to work, now managing his back pain much better.

the 'nociception' is reduced or better controlled, the learned phobic behaviours persist. That is, although physical recovery may have occurred, the behavioural response to the pain continues and may still be attributed to pain by the patients, despite their physical improvement. Unless these problems are recognized, therapists may be puzzled as to why the patients remain reluctant to leave their house, or to try suggested therapy activities.

Post-traumatic stress disorders

The events of an accident, illness or treatment can lead to a post-traumatic stress disorder (PTSD), particularly if people regard themselves as having been in a life-threatening situation, with no sense of control, and feeling emotionally overwhelmed.

The experience of ongoing pain, particularly when not well controlled, and interfering with a person's normal functioning, is a major obstacle to a person being able to regain the confidence to recover from the PTSD. In addition, the PTSD makes it more difficult for the patient to become involved in pain management.

Each new advance in a person's therapy involves confronting a reminder of their trauma, with a potential to arouse quite considerable distress, particularly with 'flashbacks' that intrude into the person's consciousness so intensely as to not allow focus and concentration on other more immediate matters. In cases of PTSD, patients may have the experience of 'reliving' the events which caused the pain. They may have panic attacks and nightmares about the event, and they may have a pervasive fear of being hurt.

Up to 10% of patients with chronic pain may have features of PTSD (Muse 1985). Pilowsky (1985) has written about 'crypto trauma', referring to those cases where a significant psychological trauma has gone unrecognized because of the emphasis on the physical presentation. The case example in Box 22.7 illustrates this situation.

The circumstances of injury and its immediate consequences can have long-standing effects on the course of recovery. DeGood and Kiernan (1996) have found that people who attribute the blame to others have a worse prognosis than those who do not. Beliefs and attitudes can be strongly shaped by the behaviour of the employer, the other driver in a motor vehicle accident, accident and emergency department staff, insurance companies, and so on.

Even though at times a person does suffer because of the actions of others, a person needs to accept at

---

> **Box 22.7** Case example
>
> A plumber fell off a roof and injured his back. It was not until the detailed history of the accident was taken, that it was revealed he had clung to the guttering for approximately 1/2 hour, before he lost his grip and fell. He had struggled in this time to regain the roof, all the while only too aware of the height of the drop.
>
> His reluctance to return to roofing was understandable in light of his history, although before more detailed consideration, he had attributed his difficulty returning to work to his pain, despite reasonable functional recovery.
>
> There are many aspects of this man's frightening experience that would have 'hurt' him apart from the impact with the ground.

---

least some degree of responsibility for their own future welfare, no matter what the original cause of their problems. This acceptance is a key for successful rehabilitation. It involves the patient adopting an approach where she:

- Perceives her 'locus of control' as being within her own resources
- Has the confidence that she can actually *do* things
- *Can* make things happen, rather relying on others.

The issue of the appropriate degrees of responsibility, self-control and dependency to adopt can be ambiguous, vexing, and a not-infrequent source of tension. These issues are usually not clearly defined, being unspoken, debatable, and varying with time, context, culture, personal history, and stage of recovery. Agreement about these issues is fundamental to developing good relationships, especially the therapeutic relationship.

The essential element in deciding an appropriate approach is what is in the best long-term interests of the patient, especially in terms of functioning. It may be necessary to use some temporary compromises along the way. For example, a patient may need to accept some dependency temporarily, such as depending initially on adaptive equipment or the advice of professionals. She can then become increasingly independent. If the treatment does not assist progress towards this effect, it needs review.

An occupational therapist and/or physiotherapist can help a person readjust, by helping her to recognize that although there may be activities that she can no longer consider, there are others that remain that do offer self-control. This reflects the choice of deciding 'whether the glass is half empty or half full'.

CHRONIC PAIN, SUBSTANCE ABUSE AND DEPENDENCE

The issue of substance abuse in patients with chronic pain creates many difficulties in management, with prevalence rates for substance abuse in people with chronic pain ranging from 15–40% (Cohen 1995).

There is a range of presentations of patients in this category.

Long-standing prior history of illicit drug abuse

Patients with a long-standing prior history of illicit drug abuse, including opioids, are already familiar with the effects of opioids and may have a high tolerance to these medications. Patients who have been alcohol-dependent also have a high tolerance for opioids because of the induction of liver enzymes for the metabolism of the alcohol.

The consequence of this is that such patients will need higher than usual doses of analgesic medications for acute pain. They are also likely to have a focus on symptom control, with a low tolerance of distress, particularly relying on opioids and benzodiazepines, with all the attendant problems of overuse, abuse and, sometimes, diversion of supplies for trafficking.

The physical focus of such patients is often in the context of very-limited social skills, problem-solving skills and personal skills, frequently with a distorted sense of responsibility and entitlement, and low levels of self-esteem and confidence. People with these problems are usually rather 'damaged' and present extra difficulties in management, with less likelihood of resolving problems by themselves.

Patients who have a history of drug abuse or alcohol addiction prior to the onset of chronic pain have an increased risk of developing addiction when taking opioids for pain. In these cases, analgesic medications need to be offered with extra supervision to reduce the risk of inappropriate use, to ensure **both** appropriate pain management and only appropriate drug use.

When working with patients with chronic pain who have a history of illicit drug abuse, therapists need to be aware of the additional issues of transmissible infectious diseases that need to be considered with physical contact, especially if this involves body fluids such as blood or chest secretions.

Prior history of inappropriate use of prescription drugs

Prescription drugs include analgesic, and hypnotic-sedative medications, most notably the benzodiazepines group.

People misusing these drugs often have similar limitations in the personal skills required to solve their own difficulties, and tend to depend inappropriately on 'external agencies', including medication, rather than developing their own non-pharmaceutical approaches. To encourage use of such approaches requires considerable explanation and encouragement, often because these people lack confidence, experience excessive self-criticism, and have a substantial and unwarranted fear of failure.

Such people usually differ from those abusing illicit drugs in that they have maintained a compliance with community standards, rules and regulations, rather than resorting to covert, illegal or deceitful methods to obtain their supplies. Nonetheless, they require a considerable amount of support to deal with the personal issues contributing to this dependence, before they can make substantial progress. This usually requires a joint approach, which deals with both physical and personal issues simultaneously.

Iatrogenic drug dependence

Patients may have chronic complicated conditions for which their medication has been prescribed, though not always wisely (see Pither & Nicholas 1991). Many people with chronic pain do not use medication appropriately. The ongoing experience of chronic pain can cause patients to feel desperate, and to be vulnerable to well intentioned or sometimes exploitative advice. As a result, patients may take medications that friends, family, or other people have said have helped them.

Recent studies have indicated that herbal remedies are by no means as innocuous as initially considered, and many patients exacerbate their pain due to the interactions of these medications. These drugs might include the use of benzodiazepines for long-term 'muscle relaxation' and for sleep. They may frequently use injections, particularly pethidine, with considerable risk of psychological and physical dependence and complications.

Long-term use of such medications as NSAIDs and steroids, when there is no evidence of inflammation, is also a concern.

Clinicians working in the area of pain need to be as knowledgeable as possible about the effects, short-term and long-term, of analgesic medications. They also need to understand the distinctions between proper use and abuse, drug dependence, addiction and 'pseudo addiction'. Students are referred back to Chapters 8 and 16 where dependence, tolerance, addiction and pharmacological management were discussed.

Some early evaluations of pain management programmes showed that drug withdrawal alone, without any other therapy, resulted in significant improvements in wellbeing and a reduction in the pain experienced. These findings convinced many workers that chronic management called for analgesic withdrawal in most cases.

More recently, this view has been challenged by clinicians experienced in cancer pain management, who have campaigned against the under-usage of opioids (Portenoy & Foley 1986). Their view is that some patients with chronic pain of non-malignant origin may be denied adequate pain control if opioids are withheld.

The few systematic and controlled studies done in this area give only a limited support to the hope that ongoing opioid therapy would be effective for chronic pain of non-malignant origin. Many patients stop the medication because of a lack of effect, or because they dislike the side-effects. The situation is currently unproven. Opioids have not proven to be the long-awaited panaceas (Large & Schug 1995), and the place of opioid medication in the management of people with chronic non-malignant pain remains the subject of debate.

Patients may wait until their pain is severe before taking medication, thinking this to be the right approach, but then use excessively large doses because of the increased pain severity at a time when their ability to tolerate it has been exhausted. This approach is more likely to involve patients in an unstable, fluctuating, 'boom and bust' approach, with a tendency to be excessively preoccupied by their experience, rather than being able to focus their intentions and energies on functioning and the future.

Patients may have been advised by multiple specialists, who may have adopted different approaches and prescribed different medications. Caution is needed at times, as patients with chronic pain who are not using their medication properly may be unfairly regarded as having a problem with addiction, although taking this medication might be at the direction of the prescriber (Fuchs & Gamsa 1997).

A person who is taking medication to relieve pain is not addicted to medication unless there is positive evidence that the patient is engaged in drug-seeking behaviour to obtain opioid medication to achieve a psychological high rather than pain relief. Addiction also involves a person seeking higher and higher doses, with a dramatic preoccupation with medication, which takes over his life.

This process may also involve physical dependence, as indicated by the development of tolerance, with a decreasing effect from the same dose, and a physical withdrawal syndrome if the medication is ceased abruptly.

The patient may, however, be inappropriately psychologically dependent on medication, as may be the prescribing doctor, unless the use is in the context of a well-balanced comprehensive management plan. Any single focus approach, including occupational therapy or physiotherapy alone, has the same risk of inappropriate dependency, by suggesting that there are no other solutions. If the approach does enhance a person's life, the dependency may be appropriate. If, however, it only succeeds in drowsiness and decreased function, such use is debatable.

Inappropriate dependence on treatments can also result from embarking upon prolonged investigations into poorly defined syndromes which have a mainly descriptive basis rather than a well documented pathophysiological basis, such as chronic fatigue syndrome, fibromyalgia, multiple chemical sensitivity, etc. Some have treated these conditions with prolonged use of steroids, resulting in severe and irreversible complications such as proximal myopathy and osteoporosis. Other treatments, such as prescribed rest, activity, manipulation, exercises, aids, splint, braces, wheelchairs, counselling . . . virtually all approaches are capable of being used unwisely without benefit, or worse, resulting in harm if not prescribed and administered wisely. Wise use with respect to chronic pain management requires a focus on functioning, rather than only a short-term relief of symptoms.

Unfortunately, such situations usually reflect good intentions, but a lack of knowledge and appropriate judgement of both the patient and the practitioner with respect to management of chronic pain disorders. Frequently remedies that are appropriate for short-term disorders, when applied to long-term conditions can have unrecognized and unwarranted complications. In short-term situations such complications are inconsequential, easily tolerated, with quick recovery. Over the long term, such complications have a much greater cumulative effect.

Patients dependent on such approaches tend to be very reliant and preoccupied with their physical care, extraordinarily reliant upon obtaining a cure, and very resistant to changes suggested by others. They may have embarked over a long period of time on a very arduous and at times expensive course of action (or inaction!). Particularly when previous therapists had supported their views, sensitive issues of beliefs, trust and confidence can arise for therapists attempting to work within the chronic pain paradigm.

SOMATOFORM DISORDERS

The somatoform disorders are a group of disorders in which the physical complaints are the major presenting focus of the patient, but where the major difficulty is thought to be psychological. The Diagnostic and Statistical Manual (DSM IV) of the American Psychiatric Association (1994) includes pain disorder in this group, but with diagnostic criteria which make it possible to fit most people with chronic pain into this category.

Pain disorder

The DSM IV criteria signify a pain disorder as:

- Pain in one or more site
- Pain causes clinically significant distress, impairment
- Psychological factors play a role
- The symptoms are not intentional
- There is no other psychiatric disorder that better accounts for the pain.

Unfortunately this definition is so broad that it is arguably of little use.

Conversion disorder

Some people present with conversion disorders, which involve a loss of function related to somatic nervous control, such as paralysis, anaesthesia, blindness, deafness, aphonia, etc. Great care is needed when diagnosing these situations. For example, features such as paralysis may be associated with pain secondary to poor posture. The hallmark of conversion disorder is its sudden onset in relation to conflict or emotional trauma, and its symptoms typically resolve a problem for the patient. Box 22.8 outlines an example of this.

It was previously considered that some pain syndromes were manifestations of a conversion disorder. There has, however, been a more recent conceptualization that a patient's pain experience has many different contributions. We recognize that we really do not have the expertise to precisely separate psychological and physical contributions to a person's pain. It is now considered inappropriate to regard pain as a conversion disorder.

Box 22.8 Case example

One patient developed a sudden-onset of paraplegia immediately after her first attempt at Christian Witnessing. She knocked on a door; no one opened it, after which she experienced relief, but then immediate guilt. She felt giddy, and her paraplegia commenced. Her symptoms effectively ended her continuing Witnessing, even though, despite exhaustive investigation, no physical explanation was revealed.

Somatization disorder

A more extreme form of presentation of the somatoform disorders is somatization disorder. Somatization is an important construct. Somatization has been associated with high rates of healthcare utilization (Bacon et al 1994).

This term is used to describe a presentation previously labelled 'Briquette's syndrome', and has been included in the older descriptions of 'hysteria'. Essentially, this is a pattern of presenting with physical complaints involving multiple organ systems, including pain. Repeated examinations and investigations fail to show sufficient organic cause to explain the extent of the symptoms.

Psychosocial evaluation usually reveals a history of interpersonal problems; emotional deprivation in childhood, past abuse, including sexual abuse. This pattern is recognized more often in women. The presentation of physical symptoms is thought to be a manifestation of abnormal illness behaviour, in which the need for care is expressed through illness.

Regular evaluation, at the same time limiting the number of investigations performed to those that have a clear medical indication rather than as a continuing attempt to appease the patient, appears to contain these patients, perhaps preventing iatrogenic harm, but it does little to change the underlying dynamics. These patients have borderline personality traits, and there is a place for intensive psychotherapy where this is available.

Factitious disorders

Uncommonly, there are dramatic presentations of illness in patients who deliberately induce symptoms and who falsify investigations to gain care (Kelly & Loader 1997). Those with factitious disorders have a complex motivation to enter the sick role, and may go to extremes by swallowing sharp objects, taking medications, adding blood to urine, etc, to mimic a clinical syndrome. This is otherwise known as 'Munchausen's syndrome' as described by Asher (1951).

It now seems that a variety of factitious presentations are more frequent than have been previously realized, with both men and woman engaging in this behaviour. Pain may be a part of the presentation but typically there are also more dramatic physical symptoms. Such cases can be perplexing for clinicians in management.

In 'Munchausen's by proxy', a caregiver induces signs and symptoms in a child. This is considered a form of child abuse. Fabricated signs and symptoms may be physical, such as rashes, seizures, facial pain or headaches, but in some cases the fabricated signs and symptoms will be characteristic of psychiatric disease, such as reporting of multiple personalities, delusions and hallucinations (Schreirer 1997, Solomon & Lipton 1999).

Another form of behaviour, **malingering**, has similar manifestations and presentations, with the difference being a demonstration that the deliberate presentation of illness is motivated by material gain, such as obtaining money, or being excused from duty, rather than by more obscure personal motivation.

Diagnosis of factitious disorder and malingering can be difficult, with the definitive diagnoses relying upon the demonstration that the person had organized a deliberate deception, with the intent that observers will believe that she is ill. Suspicion can be aroused by inconsistencies, although it is important not to prematurely come to such a conclusion, as there are many other potential explanations for inconsistencies between expectations and observations.

The presentation with factitious disorder reflects serious psychopathology that needs assessment and intervention. Such people are at considerable risk of iatrogenic complications, and a general principle of chronic pain management is highlighted in their care.

With chronic pain management, a focus on functioning is important, rather than only on symptom-relief. For example, contrary to popular belief, prolonged rest can be very harmful, disabling and potentially fatal. Physical interventions, particularly if there is a likelihood of irreversible consequences, such as with surgery, need to be based upon an identified physical disorder, rather than responding only on the basis of the person's level of distress. The more speculative the understanding of the physical basis, the greater the risk of failure. The more classical the syndrome, the better the result is likely to be.

'DIFFICULT PATIENTS' OR PATIENTS WITH DIFFICULT PROBLEMS?

As in other areas of practice, some patients are difficult to work with. Difficult patient behaviour may be a relationship problem between the professional and the patient, which is exacerbated by the subjectivity of pain, the apparent inconsistencies between the pain complaint and the pain behaviour, poor communications, frustration, resentment, at times because of a difficulty dealing with the sense of failure following the patient's lack of progress (DeGood & Dane 1996).

DeGood & Dane (1996) suggested four principles to guide interaction with patients:

1. Therapists need to recognize that patients may complain about their pain, until they feel that they have been heard and taken seriously. A patient who is certain that his or her account has at least been properly considered will be less concerned with proving the pain to others.
2. Therapists should avoid treating all patients with pain in a stereotypical and automated fashion. Taking the time to understand the patient and his or her context is important to avoid misunderstanding. All communication with patients needs to be comprehensible, in their own 'language' and style. This is best achieved if the therapist has an understanding of their usual lifestyle, preferences, interests, and priorities.
3. Therapists need to avoid personalizing or blaming other health professionals or patients for failures. It is important to decide on first-hand information where possible, rather than other people's recall, perspectives and interpretations of what transpired. Therapists also need to learn to accept their own limitations, and the need for review, revision and/or referral, when progress stops prematurely.
4. Therapists need to remember that changes in behaviour and functioning are likely to be gradual and incremental. Realistic expectations are important for both therapists and patients, to avoid anger and disappointment for both. Therapists need to be mindful of the possibility that their own personal experiences and preferences may influence their reactions to the problems with which the patients present.

Some patients may be more difficult to treat for reasons other than the presence of pain. A person who is usually more difficult to get along with will not be improved by the development of a chronic pain condition. Indeed chronic pain, like other stresses, tends to make it more difficult for a person to manage his or her personal problems. In such cases, involvement of a psychologist, social worker or psychiatrist may be helpful to provide a coordinated approach to managing the difficulties in a person's life.

CONCLUSION

The vast majority of people are honest, well intentioned, and well motivated, but have difficulty managing their pain, particularly because they have not developed the knowledge, skill and judgement required to make the appropriate life-adjustments to their new state. The fact that they have attended is likely to indicate that they are receptive to advice, but it is important not to expect rapid change. This would set them up for yet another failure, disappointment and rejection.

It is often only with the proof that comes from actual performance, especially when carefully guided by an occupational therapist and/or physiotherapist, that such people regain confidence, optimism, and a willingness to take the ordinary risks necessary to emerge from one's 'comfort zone' to again enjoy life.

Guiding people through the 'healing' process of grieving their losses, re-education and retraining to a different but inherently worthwhile lifestyle, can be a challenging but very rewarding task for all involved.

Pain, of all human experiences, is one that strikes at the core of our being. We all fear the possibility of extreme, unending, uncontrollable, unbearable pain. It is the fear of many patients first diagnosed with cancer. Portrayals of inflicted pain, martyrdom and heroism are prominent in the arts, and especially in the movies and television. All cultures strike particular attitudes towards pain, and our understanding of our patient's suffering is filtered through our own cultural heritage. We must try to understand what pain means to us and that it may mean something different to our patients.

To understand the contribution of psychiatry to pain management means understanding the essence of psychiatric methods. This is to listen carefully, setting aside preconceptions, 'bracketing' one's biases, and attempting to stand in the other person's shoes. Only when this has been done are we free to relate the individual's story to the pattern of presentations built by descriptions documented over the past century.

Occupational therapists and physiotherapists need to utilize reflection to ensure that their assessment and management strategies are influenced by patient need, rather than by the bias that all people, including therapists, inevitably have.

The relationship between psychiatric illness and pain is complex. The challenge for clinicians is to deal with the main complaint in the context of the person's understanding and reaction to his predicament, while still taking physical factors into account.

Management of chronic pain is unfortunately often bedeviled by attempts to distinguish between the components of the disorder. Studies demonstrate a very high degree of overlap between the psychiatric and physical diagnosis, which suggests that it is far more practical to consider both psychiatric and physical morbidity concurrently, when assessing patients with pain. Aigner & Bach (1999) found no difference in pain duration, intensity, and type of disability between chronic pain patients whose pain was regarded as associated with a medical condition, and those patients whose pain was regarded as associated with psychological factors.

In other words, in practice pain is pain, and attempting to tease out the causation in a dualistic framework does little to predict appropriate management for the patient. It is more feasible to assess each dimension on its merits, assisted by discussion between those involved, to develop a management approach addressing each of the issues concurrently.

Occupational therapists and physiotherapists need to be aware that acknowledging fears held by patients, offering clear explanations, and acknowledging the limitations of our current knowledge about pain, can often lead to a rebuilding of the trust required before more constructive progress can occur in rehabilitation.

Study questions/questions for revision

1. Describe the mechanisms by which emotional and psychological factors can influence the patient's presentation with pain.
2. In what way can the onset of pain as a result of physical illness contribute to a psychiatric problem?
3. Compare and contrast in acute and chronic pain, the responsibilities and limitations of the role of
   — the therapist
   — the patient
4. Describe the relationship between chronic pain and psychiatric illness.
5. Define illness behaviour, abnormal illness behaviour, treatment behaviour and abnormal treatment behaviour.
6. What should you do if a patient with chronic pain whom you are treating refers to a desire to 'end it all'?
7. You are referred a patient with chronic pain and you are unable to find a demonstrable pathology to explain the pain complaint, despite repeated assessment and treatment sessions. What should you do next?

REFERENCES

Aigner M, Bach M 1999 Clinical utility of DSM IV pain disorder. Comprehensive Psychiatry 40: 353–357

American Psychiatric Association 1980 Diagnostic and Statistical Manual of Mental Disorders, 3rd Edn. American Psychiatric Association, Washington DC

American Psychiatric Association 1994 Diagnostic and Statistical Manual of Mental Disorders, 4th Edn. American Psychiatric Association, Washington DC

Asher R 1951 Munchausen's syndrome. Lancet 1: 339–341

Bacon N M K, Bacon S F, Atkinson J H, et al 1994 Somatization symptoms in chronic low back pain patients. Psychosomatic Medicine 56: 118–127

Beck A T 1967 Depression: Causes and Treatment. University of Pennsylvania Press, Philadelphia

Beck A T, Ward C H, Medelson M, et al 1961 An inventory for measuring depression. Archives of General Psychiatry 4: 561–571

Bond M R 1971 The relation of pain to the Eysenck personality inventory, Cornell medical index and Whiteley index of hypochondriasis. British Journal of Psychiatry 119: 671–678

Brown G K 1990 A causal analysis of chronic pain and depression. Journal of Abnormal Psychology 99: 127–137

Catchlove R F H, Cohen K R, Braha R E D, Demers-Desrosiers L A 1985 Incidence and implications of alexithymia in chronic pain patients. Journal of Nervous and Mental Disease 173: 246–248

Cohen M J 1995 Psychosocial aspects of evaluation and management of chronic low back pain. Physical Medicine and Rehabilitation 9: 725–746

Cohen J M, Marx M C 1993 Pain and depression in the nursing home: corroborating results. Journal of Gerontology 48: 96–97

DeGood D E, Dane J R 1996 The psychologist as a pain consultant in outpatient, inpatient, and workplace settings. In: Gatchel R J, Turk D C (eds) Psychological Approaches to Pain Management – A practitioner's handbook. Guilford Press, London, pp 403–437

DeGood D E, Kiernan B 1996 Perception of fault in patients with chronic pain. Pain 64: 153–159

Dworkin R H, Caligor E 1988 Psychiatric diagnosis and chronic pain: DSM-III-R and beyond. Journal of Pain and Symptom Management 3: 87–98

Engel G 1959 Psychogenic pain and the pain-prone patient. American Journal of Medicine 26: 899–918

Feuerstein M, Sult S, Houle M 1985 Environmental stressors and chronic low back pain: life events, families and work environment. Pain 22: 295–307

Fishbain D A, Cutler R, Rosomoff H L, Rosomoff R S 1997 Chronic pain-associated depression: antecedant or consequence of chronic pain? A review. Clinical Journal of Pain 13: 116–137

Flor H, Fydrich T, Turk D C 1992 Efficacy of multidisciplinary pain treatment centres: a meta-analytic review. Pain 49: 221–230

Fraser R D 1996 Compensation and recovery from injury. Medical Journal of Australia 165: 71–72

Fuchs P N, Gamsa A 1997 Chronic use of opioids for nonmalignant pain: a prospective study. Pain Research and Management 2: 101–107

Goldberg R T, Pachas W N, Keith D 1999 Relationship between traumatic events in childhood and chronic pain. Disability and Rehabilitation 21: 23–30

Greenough C G, Fraser R D 1988 The effects of compensation on recovery of low back injury. Spine 14: 947–955

Gross R T, Collins F L 1981 On the relationship between anxiety and pain: a methodological confounding. Clinical Psychology Review 1: 375–386

Katon W, Egan K, Miller D 1985 Chronic pain: lifetime psychiatric diagnoses and family history. American Journal of Psychiatry 142: 1156–1160

Kelly C, Loader P 1997 Factitious disorder by proxy: the role of the child mental health professionals. Child Psychology and Psychiatry Review 2: 116–124

Kerns R D, Haythornthwaite J A 1988 Depression among chronic pain patients: cognitive–behavioural analysis and effect on rehabilitation outcome. Journal of Consulting and Clinical Psychology 56: 870–876

Large R G 1986 DSM-III Diagnoses in chronic pain: confusion or clarity. Journal of Nervous and Mental Disease 174: 295–303

Large R G & Schug S A 1995 Opioids for chronic pain of non-malignant origin – Caring or crippling. Health Care Analysis 3: 5–11

Love A W, Peck D L 1987 The MMPI and psychological factors in chronic low back pain: a review. Pain 28: 1–12

Magni G 1987 On the relationship between chronic pain and depression when there is no organic lesion. Pain 31: 1–21

Maruta T, Vatterott M K, McHardy M J 1989 Pain management as an antidepressant: long-term resolution of pain-associated depression. Pain 36: 335–337

Melzack R, Wall P D 1965 Pain mechanisms; a new theory. Science 150: 971–976

Merskey H 1999 Pain and psychological medicine. In: Wall P D, Melzack R (eds) Textbook of Pain, 4th Edn. Churchill Livingstone, New York, pp 929–949

Merskey H, Spear F G 1967 Pain: Psychological and Psychiatric Aspects. Baillière, Tindall & Cassell, London

Muse M 1985 Stress-related, posttraumatic chronic pain syndrome: criteria for diagnosis and preliminary report on prevalence. Pain 23: 295–300

Parsons T 1964 Social Structure and Personality. Collier MacMillan, London

Pilowsky I 1969 Abnormal illness behaviour. British Journal of Medical Psychology 42: 347–351

Pilowsky I 1976 A general classification of abnormal illness behaviour. British Journal of Medical Psychology 51: 131–137

Pilowsky I 1977 Altruism and the practice of medicine. British Journal of Medical Psychology 50: 305–311

Pilowsky I 1985 Cryptotrauma and 'accident neurosis'. British Journal of Psychiatry 147: 310–311

Pilowsky I 1995 Pain, disability, and illness. Pain Forum 4: 126–128

Pilowsky I 1997 Abnormal Illness Behaviour. Wiley & Sons, Chichester

Pither C E, Nicholas M K 1991 The identification of iatrogenic factors in the development of chronic pain syndromes: abnormal treatment behaviour? In: Bond M R, Charlton J E, Woolf C J (eds) Proceedings of the VIth World congress on Pain, Elsevier B V, pp 429–434

Portenoy R K, Foley K M 1986 Opioid therapy for chronic nonmalignant pain. Pain Research and Management 1: 17–28

Rudy T E, Kerns R D, Turk D C 1988 Chronic pain and depression: toward a cognitive–behavioural model. Pain 35: 129–140

Schreier H A 1997 Factitious presentation of psychiatric disorder: when is it Munchausen by proxy? Child Psychology and Psychiatry Review 2: 108–115

Singh B, Num K, Martin J, Yates J 1981 Abnormal treatment behaviour. British Journal of Medical Psychology 54: 67–73

Solomon S, Lipton R B 1999 Headaches and face pains as a manifestation of Munchausen syndrome. Headache 39: 45–50

Spear F G 1967 Pain in psychiatric patients. Journal of Psychosomatic Research 11: 187–193

Turk D C, Rudy T E, Steig R L 1987 Chronic pain and depression: I 'Facts'. Pain Management 1: 17–26

Turner J A, Romano J M 1984 Self-report screening measures for depression in chronic pain patients. Journal of Clinical Psychology 40: 909–913

Whitlock F A 1967 The aetiology of hysteria. Acta Psychiatrica Scandinavica 43: 144–162

Zung W W K 1965 A self-rating depression scale. Archives of General Psychiatry 12: 63–70

Index